MRCPCH
MasterCourse
Volume ❷

Commissioning Editors: Ellen Green, Timothy Horne and Pauline Graham
Development Editor: Janice Urquhart
Project Manager: Gail Wright/Emma Riley
Senior Designer: Sarah Russell
Illustration Manager: Merlyn Harvey
Illustrator: Cactus

MRCPCH
MasterCourse
Volume 2

Editor in Chief

Malcolm Levene

MD FRCPCH FRCP FMedSc

Professor of Paediatrics and Child Health,
University of Leeds,
Leeds General Infirmary,
Leeds, UK

Foreword by

Professor Sir David Hall

FRCPCH FRCP FRCP(Edin)

Emeritus Professor of Community Paediatrics,
University of Sheffield;
President of the Royal College of Paediatrics and Child Health
2000–2003

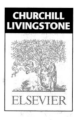

EDINBURGH LONDON NEW YORK OXFORD PHILADELPHIA ST LOUIS SYDNEY TORONTO 2007

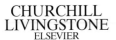

CHURCHILL
LIVINGSTONE
ELSEVIER

An imprint of Elsevier Limited

First published 2007
  Reprinted 2008 (twice)

ISBN: 978-0-443-10190-8

British Library Cataloguing in Publication Data
A catalogue record for this book is available from the British Library

Library of Congress Cataloging in Publication Data
A catalog record for this book is available from the Library of Congress

ELSEVIER your source for books,
journals and multimedia
in the health sciences

www.elsevierhealth.com

Working together to grow
libraries in developing countries

www.elsevier.com | www.bookaid.org | www.sabre.org

ELSEVIER   BOOK AID International   Sabre Foundation

The
publisher's
policy is to use
**paper manufactured
from sustainable forests**

Printed in China

Foreword

Reflecting on their work to establish the structure of DNA, Watson and Crick remarked that 'they knew it would be beautiful'. And so it was — I still remember my biology master reading us their classic letter to *Nature* and explaining the implications of this awe-inspiring discovery, just a few years after it was published. But no-one then could possibly have predicted the progress that would follow in genetics, linking over the next half century with molecular and cell biology and neuroscience, nor the ways in which medicine, and paediatrics in particular, would benefit. Advances in technology have kept pace with biology — ultrasound, CT scanning, magnetic resonance imaging and endoscopic surgery were unheard of when my generation of paediatricians began their training. But some of the most important advances did not need technological genius — just careful listening, acute observation and an open mind. Just a few years after Watson and Crick published their findings, Kempe told a disbelieving medical profession and public that some parents batter their children, sometimes with fatal consequences. We have learned slowly and often reluctantly the full extent of cruelty to children and still find this distressing topic among the hardest aspects of looking after children, whether in general practice or as a paediatrician.

Developments in other areas of the medical sciences have been less dramatic but equally important. Epidemiology and public health have come of age — studies of disease patterns in populations remind us to think of the whole community and to question the way we provide medical care. Continuing advances in the methodology of clinical trials have delivered spectacular improvements in survival for children with conditions like cystic fibrosis and leukaemia. Evidence-based medicine and critical analysis of the literature, backed up by increasingly sophisticated statistics, have revolutionized our attitudes to all aspects of diagnosis and management — the wisdom received from those distinguished older colleagues who taught us when we were junior paediatricians is no longer taken as gospel.

Medical ethics and consumer involvement have had a major influence on the quality and safety of research — in particular, we have learned how to involve children and young people in decisions that affect them or their peers. Issues arising from paediatric and neonatal intensive care, and the nutritional support of profoundly disabled children, present our discipline with sometimes agonizing dilemmas for which we have to seek help from parents, colleagues, and sometimes the Courts.

The picture is less encouraging in the social sciences. We now know far more about the ways in which inadequate nutrition, poverty, bad parenting and soulless communities interact to produce child abuse, educational failure, crime and mental illness. Currently, 10—20% of UK children and young people have mental health problems that are intrusive and cause distress to themselves and their families. These problems are no less common in children who also have organic disease, and unravelling the relative contributions of each to the child's symptomatology is often very difficult. In resource-poor countries around the world, civil unrest, war and extreme poverty combined with the HIV-AIDS epidemic,

TB and malaria have devastating effects on children. Children die from treatable diseases and injuries and often lack even basic symptom relief such as analgesia. Sadly, so far most of these socially determined ills have proved equally resistant to the efforts of professional services and of politicians.

My generation has been privileged to observe and participate in what must be the most exciting period of change in the whole history of medicine. But we also recognize that the explosion of knowledge over the last half century presents enormous challenges to young doctors embarking on a career in paediatrics. The body of scientific knowledge underpinning clinical medicine is now so vast that no-one can hope to acquire a comprehensive knowledge of every topic, yet without some familiarity with the basic biological and social sciences we cannot hope to offer our patients the highest possible standards of care, nor can tomorrow's paediatricians play their full part in the further advances to come.

In many countries, membership by examination of a UK Royal College was, and still is, a highly regarded qualification. Nevertheless, when the British Paediatric Association became a Royal College in 1996, we were aware that the examination system was in urgent need of an overhaul. Candidates needed guidance on how they should apportion their study time between the scientific foundations of paediatrics and the body of clinical knowledge. The exam system encouraged candidates to focus on the complexities of paediatrics and neglect the common problems seen in primary care settings, particularly preventive care, atypical growth and development, and emotional and behavioural problems.

In order to address these problems, the College decided that a new approach to preparation for the Membership examination was needed. After reviewing the experience of other Royal Colleges, we invited Professor Malcolm Levene to lead the development of a project, which we designated 'MasterCourse', that would amalgamate the biological and social sciences with essential clinical practice in a way that would be relevant to any doctor practising paediatrics, whether in primary care or as a hospital general or specialist paediatrician. We wanted something that was not a traditional textbook — there are plenty of those around already, yet they are by their nature out of date almost before they are published, and easy access to the medical and scientific literature over the Internet simplifies searches for the latest information on practically any topic. The aim was rather to create a more interactive product that would make full use of various modes of learning. The result far exceeds my original expectations — Professor Levene and his team in partnership with Elsevier have done a wonderful job, producing a study guide that will smooth the path to Membership and raise the standard of paediatric practice across the country. But those who buy this MasterCourse will need to guard it well, for I have a sneaking suspicion that their seniors will find it a valuable way of keeping up with their trainees!

The project was conceived to meet the needs of UK trainee paediatricians — but my contacts with colleagues in other EU countries and my own experience in Southern Africa have taught me that the fundamentals of our discipline are much the same whether you work in Bristol, Budapest or Blantyre and whether you are working for the UK exams or some other system of assessment. I hope that Professor Levene's work will be of benefit to young doctors studying paediatrics in many parts of the world.

Professor Sir David Hall
Sheffield, 16th January 2007

Preface

MasterCourse is a comprehensive teaching package developed for paediatricians in training to prepare them for admission to the British Royal College of Paediatrics and Child Health by examination. These examinations are taken by young paediatricians after 2–3 years of training at SHO level and are constructed by the College to test aspects of knowledge and skills. The package has also been developed for doctors who do not intend to be full-time paediatricians but whose career aim is in the field of family medicine or with a primary care interest in Child Health. Volume 1 of the package is aimed at primary care paediatrics and Volume 2 at secondary care (hospital-based) paediatrics. Career paediatricians should know the principles in Volume 1 as well as those in Volume 2.

MasterCourse has had a long gestation since the original concept by Professor David Hall, when President of the College, who identified a proportion of paediatric trainees who were presenting to their membership examinations with a poor level of basic science knowledge intended to underpin the practice of Paediatrics and Child Health. It was suggested that a teaching package be developed to incorporate the basic science of Paediatrics together with the clinical science in a single package to help candidates pass their Membership examinations. Hence MasterCourse was conceived. Since then we have seen publication of the College competencies document as well as changes in the structure of the MRCPCH examination. The MasterCourse teaching package has been developed to take account of these changes.

To support the written material an accompanying DVD is provided to give visual and auditory data to supplement the text. This can be played on many desktop or laptop computers or on a stand-alone digital DVD player. A major component of the MasterCourse package is the supporting website, which purchase of the package entitles you to access for 3 years. The website will allow MasterCourse to grow and meet the needs of the trainees between published editions of the books. The website will provide additional data to complement the written material and give links to detailed information as well as useful websites. We will also commission new articles for the website on a regular basis to provide an overview on controversial or rapidly changing areas within our specialty. Finally the website provides extensive self-assessment material to gauge your progress in learning and also to practise for the various parts of the Membership examinations.

In producing the MasterCourse package I am grateful for the great support of three successive Presidents of the College who have seen the project through some rocky times. These include David Hall, Alan Craft and Patricia Hamilton. I am also indebted to Elsevier for their foresight in supporting the project and in particular Martin Delahunty, Ellen Green and Janice Urquhart. Finally a project of this size and complexity would not have been possible without the considerable efforts of the many authors and in particular my co-editors, who have given many hours to help to prepare the finished product. I wish to record my gratitude to the Module editors, Jonathan Darling, Mary Rudolf, Mitch Blair,

Henry Halliday, Martin Ward-Platt and Mike Hall, the DVD editor Andy Spencer and the website editors Ian Spillman and Colin Melville.

Malcolm Levene
Editor in Chief
May 2006

How to use this book

Thank you for purchasing MasterCourse. It has been written to provide you with information and skills that you will require to pass your Membership examination. We hope that as well as passing your examinations, you will adopt a style of working through this package which will stay with you for lifelong learning.

Written material

The written material is contained in two volumes. Volume 1 is directed towards the tool-kit of skills and knowledge that you will require to become proficient in the care of children, both in the community and in hospital. Volume 2 contains material relevant to career paediatricians and those working mainly in a hospital setting. It is essential that aspiring career paediatricians see Volumes 1 and 2 as equally important to pass the College examinations.

Children rarely present with a diagnosis but much more commonly present with a symptom or abnormal sign. The clinical material is initially presented as a 'Problem-orientated topic' abbreviated to 'POT' in both volumes. Each POT contains a short clinical vignette followed by a number of questions. We recommend that you read the POT and think about the answers to each of the questions before reading on. This will allow you to gauge your level of knowledge and understanding at an early stage of your learning. At the end of each POT the answer to each question is provided and the disorders are discussed.

DVD

A numbered DVD icon points to where supporting video clips are provided on the separate DVD to aid learning. These may illustrate a disorder, clinical sign or show a competency that you will be expected to know. These clips can also be used later to prepare for the clinical examination as they may be presented in a similar manner in the MRCPCH examination.

An index of icons describing the contents of each clip is supplied on page xi.

Website

Many paediatricians in training may want more than the core knowledge contained in the text, and the website provides valuable additional pointers as to how to obtain wider information. In many places in the books, a website icon has been placed to signpost towards additional reading. Many of these URLs are linked through the website to the source material. In addition, the website provides further reading at a higher level for those interested in reading around the subject.

The website also contains self-assessment questions similar to those presented in the various parts of the MRCPCH examination and these in turn are designed to cover the range of competencies required to pass the examination. The self-assessment can be accessed on the website by chapter title or can be presented in random format for examination practice. Details on how to access the website are available on the inside front cover. Finally, the website will provide regular updates on topics of current interest to trainee paediatricians, written by experts in the field.

We hope that you enjoy using MasterCourse and, of course, we hope you enjoy working with children in your professional life and that what you learn from the MasterCourse package provides you with life-long skills used for the benefit of children.

Good Luck.

Index of DVD clips

Module editors

Mitch Blair
MBBS BSc MSc FRCP FRCPCH FRIPH MILT
Consultant Reader in Paediatrics and Child Public Health, Imperial College (Northwick Park Campus), London, UK

Jonathan Darling
MB ChB MD FRCPCH
Senior Lecturer in Paediatrics and Child Health, St James's University Hospital, Leeds, UK

Michael A. Hall
MB ChB FRCPCH FRCP DCH
Consultant Neonatologist and Paediatrician, Honorary Senior Clinical Lecturer, University of Southampton Princess Anne Hospital and Southampton General Hospital, Southampton, UK

Henry L. Halliday
MD FRCP FRCPE
Honorary Professor of Child Health and Consultant Neonatologist, Regional Neonatal Unit, Royal Maternity Hospital, Belfast, UK

Malcolm Levene
MD FRCPCH FRCP FMedSc
Professor of Paediatrics and Child Health, University of Leeds, Leeds General Infirmary, Leeds, UK

Mary Rudolf
MB BS BSc DCH FRCPCH FAAP
Professor of Child Health and Consultant Paediatrician, University of Leeds, Leeds, UK

Martin Ward-Platt
MB ChB MD FRCP FRCPCH
Consultant Paediatrician, Newcastle upon Tyne Hospitals NHS Foundation Trust; Reader in Neonatal and Paediatric Medicine, Newcastle University, Newcastle upon Tyne, UK

DVD Editor

S. Andrew Spencer
BM BS BMedSci MRCP DM FRCPCH
Consultant Paediatrician, University Hospital North Staffordshire; Honorary Reader in
Neonatal Medicine, Keele University, North Staffordshire, UK

Website Editors

Ian Spillman
FRCPCH DA DCH DTM&H
Consultant Paediatrician, Macclesfield District General Hospital, UK

Colin Melville
MB ChB MMedEd FRCPCH
Senior Lecturer in Paediatrics and Consultant Paediatrician, Keele University, UK

Contributors

Noura Faital Al-Aufi
MB ChB DCH Dip Arab Board Peds
Consultant Paediatrician, Maternity and Children's Hospital, Jeddah,
Saudi Arabia

Huda Al-Hussamy
MB BS DCH Dip Arab Board Peds
Consultant Paediatrician, Maternity and Children's Hosptial, Jeddah,
Saudi Arabia

Sabah Alvi
MB ChB MD MRCP MRCPCH
Consultant in Paediatric and Adolescent Endocrinology, Department of Paediatric and
Adolescent Endocrinology, Leeds Teaching Hospitals NHS Trust, Leeds, UK

Paul Arundel
MB BS MRCPCH DCH
Specialist Registrar in Paediatric Diabetes and Endocrinology, Leeds Teaching Hospitals
NHS Trust, Leeds, UK

Dr Jason Barling
MBBS BSc MRCPCH
Paediatric A&E Consultant, Epsom & St Helier's NHS Trust, Surrey, UK

Ravindra Bhat
MB BS MD MRCPCH
Specialist Registrar, Neonatal Unit, St George's Hospital NHS Trust, London, UK

Susan Bunn
MB ChB MRCPCH MD
Consultant Paediatric Gastroenterologist, Newcastle upon Tyne Hospitals NHS
Foundation Trust, Newcastle upon Tyne, UK

David M. Burge
FRCS FRCPCH
Consultant Paediatric Surgeon, Southampton General Hospital, Southampton, UK

Frank Casey
MD FRCP MRCPCH BSc
Consultant Paediatric Cardiologist, Royal Belfast Hospital for Sick Children, Belfast;
Honorary Senior Lecturer, Department of Child Health, Queen's University, Belfast, UK

Julia Clark
BMedSci BM BS DCH FRCPCH
Consultant in Paediatric Immunology and Infectious Diseases, Newcastle upon Tyne
Hospitals NHS Foundation Trust, Newcastle upon Tyne, UK

Anthony Costello
MA FRCP FRCPCH
Professor of International Child Health; Director of International Perinatal Care Unit,
Institute of Child Health, London, UK

Melanie Drewett
RCN RSCN MSc
Clinical Nurse Specialist, Neonatal Surgery, Neonatal Surgical Service, Department of
Neonatal Medicine and Surgery, Princess Anne Hospital, Coxford Road, Southampton

Susan M. Gentle
FRCPCH
Consultant Paediatrician, Ryegate Children's Centre, Sheffield Children's NHS Trust,
Sheffield, UK

Brian Grant
MD MRCPCH
Specialist Registrar in Paediatric Cardiology, Department of Paediatric Cardiology,
Royal Belfast Hospital for Children, Belfast, UK

Anne Greenough
MD FRCP FRCPCH DCH
Professor of Neonatology and Clinical Respiratory Physiology, Guy's,
King's and St Thomas School of Medicine, King's College, London, UK

Valerie A. Harpin
FRCP FRCPCH MD
Consultant Paediatrician (Neurodisability), Ryegate Children's Centre,
Sheffield Children's NHS Trust, Sheffield, UK

Carl J. Harvey
BMedSc MBChB MRCPCH
Specialist Registrar, Birmingham Heartlands Hospital, Birmingham, UK

Breda Hayes
MB BCh NUI MRCPCH
Neonatology Registrar, Rotunda Hospital, Dublin, Eire

Chris J. Hendriksz
MB ChB MSc MRCPCH
Consultant in Clinical Inherited Metabolic Disorders, Birmingham Children's Hospital,
Birmingham, UK

Therese Hesketh
MRCPCH MFPHM MPH PhD
Senior Lecturer in International Child Health, Institute of Child Health,
University College London, London, UK

Stephen Hodges
MB ChB FRCP FRCPCH DCH
Consultant Paediatric Gastroenterologist, Newcastle upon Tyne Hospitals NHS
Foundation Trust, Newcastle upon Tyne, UK

Neil Kennedy
BSc MB ChB MRCPCH MRCP DTMH
Senior Lecturer in Child Health, Queen's University, Belfast; Consultant Paediatrician, Royal Belfast Hospital for Sick Children, Belfast, UK

Heather Lambert
PhD FRCP FRCPCH
Consultant Paediatric Nephrologist, Newcastle upon Tyne Hospitals NHS Foundation Trust, Newcastle upon Tyne, UK

Malcolm Levene
MD FRCPCH FRCP FMedSc
Professor of Paediatrics and Child Health, University of Leeds, Leeds General Infirmary, Leeds, UK

Vernon Long
FRCOphth
Consultant Ophthalmologist, St James' University Hospital, Leeds, UK

Niamh Lynch
MB BCh BAO MRCPI(Paeds)
Specialist Registrar in Paediatrics, Our Lady's Hospital, Dublin, Ireland

Florence McDonagh
MB BCh BAO LRCPSI(Irel)DipCommunityPaed MSc FRCPCH
Consultant Community Paediatrician Audiology, St Mary's Hospital, Leeds, UK

Sachin Mannikar
MB BS MD MRCPCH
Specialist Registrar in Paediatrics, Queen Elizabeth Hospital, Gateshead, Tyne and Wear, UK

Michael J. Marsh
MB BS MRCP FRCPCH
Director of Paediatric Intensive Care Unit, Southampton General Hospital, Southampton, UK

Thomas G. Matthews
MD FRCPI FAAP DCH
Professor, Children's University Hospital, Dublin, Eire

Neena Modi
MB ChB MD FRCP FRCPCH
Professor of Neonatal Medicine, Faculty of Medicine, Imperial College, London; Honorary Consultant in Neonatal Paediatrics, Chelsea and Westminster Hospital, Hammersmith and Queen Charlotte Hospitals, London, UK

Matthew Murray
MA MB BChir MRCPCH DCH
Clinical Research Fellow in Paediatric Oncology, Addenbrooke's Hospital, Cambridge, UK

James C. Nicholson
DM MA MB BChir MRCP FRCPCH
Consultant Paediatric Oncologist, Addenbrooke's Hospital, Cambridge, UK

B. S. O'Connor
MB MRCPCH
Senior Paediatric Registrar and Research Fellow, Royal Belfast Hospital for Sick Children, Belfast, UK

Mary O'Sullivan
MB BCh BAO MSc DCH FRCPCH
Consultant Community Paediatrician, Audiology, St Mary's Hospital, Leeds, UK

David Osrin
MRCPCH
Clinical Research Fellow, International Perinatal Care Unit, Institute of Child Health,
University College London, London, UK

Janet M. Rennie
MD FRCP FRCPCH DCH
Consultant and Senior Lecturer in Neonatal Medicine, Elizabeth Garrett Anderson
Obstetric Hospitals, University College London Hospitals, London, UK

Edward Michael Richards
MA BM BCh DM MRCP FRCPath
Consultant Paediatric Haematologist and Honorary Senior Lecturer,
Leeds Teaching Hospitals Trust, Leeds, UK

Martin Samuels
MB BS BSc MD FRCP FRCPCH
Consultant Paediatrician, University Hospital of North Staffordshire;
Senior Lecturer in Paediatrics, Keele University, UK

Saikat Santra
MB BChir BA MRCPCH
Specialist Registrar, Worcester Royal Hospital, Worcester, UK

Neela Shabde
FRCP FRCPCH DCH DCCH
Consultant Paediatrician/Clinical Director of Children's Services,
Northumbria Healthcare Trust, UK

Michael D. Shields
MF FRCP FRCPCH
Senior Lecturer in Child Health, Queen's University of Belfast and Royal Belfast Hospital
for Sick Children, Belfast, UK

Andrew Tomkins
MB BS FRCP FRCPCH FFPHM FMedSci
Head, Centre for International Child Health, Institute of Child Health,
University College, London, UK

Sabita Uthaya
MBBS MD MRCP FRCPCH
Consultant and Honorary Senior Lecturer in Neonatal Medicine,
Chelsea and Westminster Hospital, Imperial College, London, UK

Julian L. Verbov
MD FRCP FRCPCH FIBiol FLS
Honorary Professor and Consultant Paediatric Dermatologist, Royal Liverpool Children's
Hospital, Liverpool, UK

Richard B. Warren
BSc MB ChB MRCP
Specialist Registrar in Dermatology, Royal Liverpool and Broadgreen University Hospitals
NHS Trust, Dermatology Unit, Broadgreen Hospital, Liverpool, UK

David W. Webb
MB BCh BAO MD MRCP(Edin)(Lon) FRCPI FRCPCH
Consultant Paediatric Neurologist, Our Lady's Hospital for Sick Children, Dublin, Eire

List of abbreviations

AABR	(automated) auditory brainstem responses
AAP	American Academy of Paediatrics
ABC	airway, breathing, circulation
ABPA	allergic bronchopulmonary aspergillosis
AC	air conduction
ACE	angiotensin-converting enzyme
ACPC	Area Child Protection Committee
ACTH	adrenocorticotrophic hormone
AD	autosomal dominant
ADEM	acute disseminating encephalomyelitis
ADH	antidiuretic hormone
ADHD	attention deficit/hyperactivity disorder
ADPKD	autosomal dominant polycystic kidney disease
AFP	alpha-fetoprotein
AGA	antigliadin antibody
AIDS	acquired immune deficiency syndrome
ALCL	anaplastic large cell lymphoma
ALI	acute lung injury
ALL	acute lymphoblastic leukaemia
ALP	alkaline phosphate
ALSG	Advanced Life Support Group
ALT	alanine aminotransferase
ALTE	apparent life-threatening event
ANA	antinuclear antibodies
ANCA	antineutrophil cytoplasmic antibody
ANF	antinuclear factor
ANP	atrial natriuretic peptide
AOM	acute otitis media
AP	antero-posterior
APC	antigen-presenting cell
APLS	advanced paediatric life support
APTT	activated partial thromboplastin time
AR	autosomal recessive
ARDS	acute respiratory distress syndrome
ARF	acute renal failure
ARI	acute respiratory infection
ARPKD	autosomal recessive polycystic kidney disease
ASD	atrial septal defect
ASOT	antistreptolysin O titre
AST	aspartate aminotransferase

ATN	acute tubular necrosis
ATP	adenosine triphosphate
AVP	arginine vasopressin
AV(SD)	atrioventricular (septal defect)
AXR	abdominal X-ray
BAL	bronchoalveolar lavage
BBB	blood–brain barrier
BC	bone conduction
BCG	bacille Calmette–Guérin
BDR	bronchodilator responsiveness
BG	blood glucose
BHR	bronchial hyper-reactivity
BMI	body mass index
BMT	bone marrow transplant
BNF	*British National Formulary*
BP	blood pressure
BPD	bronchpulmonary dysplasia
BSER	brainstem evoked response
BSPED	British Society for Paediatric Endocrinology and Diabetes
BTS	British Thoracic Society
CAH	congenital adrenal hyperplasia
CAMHS	Child and Adolescent Mental Health Services
CBD	common bile duct
CBF	cerebral blood flow
CBT	cognitive behavioural therapy
CCAM	congenital cystic adenomatoid malformation
CD	conduct disorder
CDC	children in difficult circumstances; Centers for Disease Control
CDD	Control of Diarrhoeal Disease
CDH	congenital diaphragmatic hernia
CEDC	children in especially difficult circumstances
CF	cystic fibrosis
CFAM	cerebral function activity monitor
CFS	chronic fatigue syndrome
CFTR	cystic fibrosis transmembrane regulator
CGD	chronic granulomatous disorder
cGMP	cyclic guanosine monophosphate
CHD	congenital heart disease
CHT	congenital hypothyroidism
CJD	Creutzfeldt–Jakob disease
CK	creatine kinase
CLO	*Campylobacter*-like organism
CML	chronic myeloid leukaemia
CMV	cytomegalovirus
CNS	central nervous system
CNSP	children in need of special protection
CO	cardiac output
CONS	coagulase-negative streptococci
CP	cerebral palsy
CPAP	continuous positive airway pressure
CPP	cerebral perfusion pressure
CPR	cardiopulmonary resuscitation
CRF	chronic renal failure
CRH	corticotrophin-releasing hormone
CRP	C-reactive protein

CRT	capillary refill time
CSC	children in special circumstances
CSF	cerebrospinal fluid
CT	computed tomography
CTG	cardiotocograph
CTZ	chemoreceptor trigger zone
CVA	cough variant asthma
CVC	central venous catheter
CVID	common variable immune deficiency
CVL	central venous line
CXR	chest X-ray
CYP	cytochrome P450
DCD	developmental coordination disorder
DEXA	dual-energy X-ray absorptiometry
DHEAS	dihydroepiandrosterone
DHS	Demographic and Health Survey
DI	diabetes insipidus
DIC	disseminated intravascular coagulation
DIDMOAD	diabetes insipidus, diabetes mellitus, optic atrophy, deafness
DJ	duodenojejunal
DKA	diabetic ketoacidosis
DMSA	demercaptosuccinic acid
DOT(S)	directly observed therapy
DPPC	dipalmitoyl phosphatidylcholine
DSM	Diagnostic and Statistical Manual of Mental Disorders
DTaP/IPV/Hib	diphtheria, tetanus, acellular pertussis, polio and Hib
DU	duodenal ulcer
DVLA	Driver and Vehicle Licensing Authority
EB	epidermolysis bullosa
EBV	Epstein–Barr virus
ECF	extracellular fluid
ECG	electrocardiography
ECMO	extra-corporeal membranous oxygenation
EEG	electroencephalography
EHEC	enterohaemorrhagic *E. coli*
ELISA	enzyme-linked immunosorbence assay
EMA	endomysial antibody
EN	erythema nodosum
ENMR	early neonatal mortality rate
ENT	ear, nose and throat
EPI	Expanded Programme on Immunization
ESR	erythrocyte sedimentation rate
EVD	extraventricular drain
FBC	full blood count
FDG	flurodeoxyglucose
FEV$_1$	forced expiratory volume in 1 second
FRC	forced residual capacity
FSGS	focal and segmental glomerulosclerosis
FSH	follicle-stimulating hormone
FTT	failure to thrive
FVC	forced vital capacity
G6PD	glucose-6-phosphate dehydrogenase
GABA	gamma-aminobutyric acid
GABHS	group A β-haemolytic streptococci
GAD	glutamic acid decarboxylase

GALT	gut-associated lymphoid tissue
GAS	group A streptococci
GBM	glomerular basement membrane
GBS	group B streptococci
GCS	Glasgow Coma Scale/Score
GCS-F	granulocyte colony stimulating factor
GET	graded exercise therapy
GFAP	glial fibrillary acidic protein
GFR	glomerular filtration rate
GGT	gamma-glutamyl transferase
GH(D)	growth hormone (deficiency)
GHIS	growth hormone insensitivity syndrome
GHRH	growth hormone-releasing hormone
GMC	General Medical Council
GMH	germinal matrix haemorrhage
GnRH	gonadotrophin-releasing hormone
GOR(D)	gastro-oesophageal reflux (disease)
GP	general practitioner
GTP	guanine triphosphate
GTT	glucose tolerance test
GU	gastric ulcer
GvHD	graft versus host disease
HAART	highly active antiretroviral therapy
HAV	hepatitis A virus
HBCO	carboxyhaemoglobin
HBV	hepatitis B virus
hCG	human chorionic gonadotrophin
HCOM	hypertrophic obstructive cardiomyopathy
HCV	hepatitis C virus
HD	Hirschsprung's disease; high-dose
HDN	haemolytic disease of the newborn
HELPP	haemolysis, elevated liver enzymes and low platelets
HFJV	high-frequency jet ventilation
HFOV	high-frequency oscillatory ventilation
HHV	human herpes virus
HiB	*Haemophilus influenzae* type B
HIE	hypoxic–ischaemic encephalopathy
HIV	human immunodeficiency virus
HLA	human leucocyte antigen
HMA	homovanillic acid
HMSN	hereditary motor sensory neurophathies
HPI	haemorrhagic periventricular infarction
HSP	Henoch–Schönlein purpura
HSV	herpes simplex virus
HUS	haemolytic uraemic syndrome
ICAM	intercellular adhesion molecule
ICD-10	International Statistical Classification of Diseases—10th revision
ICF	International Classification of Functioning and Disability; intracellular fluid
ICH	intracranial haemorrhage
ICP	intracranial pressure
ICU	intensive care unit
IEM	inborn error of metabolism
IFN	interferon
IL	interleukin

ILO	International Labour Organization
i.m.	intramuscular
IMCI	Integrated Management of Childhood Illness
IMR	infant mortality rate
INR	international normalized ratio
INSI	International Life Sciences Institute
IPEC	International Programme for the Elimination of Child Labour
IPL	intraparenchymal lesion
IPPV	intermittent positive pressure ventilation
IRT	immunoreactive trypsinogen
ISKDC	International Study of Kidney Disease in Children
i.t.	intrathecal
ITP	idiopathic thrombocytopenic purpura
IUGR	intrauterine growth retardation
i.v.	intravenous
IVH	intraventricular haemorrhage
JIA	juvenile idiopathic arthritis
JVP	jugular venous pressure
KSADS	Kiddie Schedule for Affective Disorders and Schizophrenia
LA	left atrium
LGA	large for gestational age
LH(RH)	luteinizing hormone (releasing hormone)
LIP	lymphocytic interstitial pneumonitis
LKM	liver, kidney, microsomal (antibodies)
LNMR	late neonatal mortality rate
LOC	loss of consciousness
LOS	lower oesophageal sphincter
LP	lumbar puncture
LPD	lymphoproliferative disease
LPS	lipopolysaccharide
LRTI	lower respiratory tract infection
LSCB	Local Safeguarding Children Board
LV	left ventricle
LVH	left ventricular hypertrophy
MAG3	mercaptoacetyltriglycine
MAP	mean arterial pressure
MAS	meconium aspiration syndrome
MCAD(D)	medium chain acyl CoA dehydrogenase (deficiency)
MCH	mean cell haemoglobin
MCUG	micturating cystourethrogram
MCV	mean cell/corpuscular volume
MD	muscular dystrophy
MDI	multiple daily injections
MDR-TB	multidrug-resistant tuberculosis
MEE	middle ear effusions
MHC	major histocompatibility complex
mIBG	meta-iodobenzylguanidine imaging
MIF	migratory inhibition factor
MIP	macrophage inflammatory protein
MMR	measles/mumps/rubella vaccination
MODY	maturity-onset diabetes of the young
MPGN	membranoproliferative glomerulonephritis
MRA	magnetic resonance angiography
MRCPCH	Membership of the Royal College of Paediatrics and Child Health
MRD	minimal residual disease

MRI	magnetic resonance imaging
MRV	magnetic resonance venography
MSU	midstream urine
MTB	*Mycobacterium tuberculosis*
MTCT	mother-to-child transmission
MTX	methotrexate
NAHI	non-accidental head injury
NAI	non-accidental injury
NAITP	neonatal alloimmune thrombocytopenia
NDI	nephrogenic diabetes insipidus
NEC	necrotizing enterocolitis
NF	neurofibromatosis
NGT	nasogastric tube
NHL	non-Hodgkin's lymphoma
NHSP	newborn hearing screening programme
NIBP	non-invasive blood pressure
NICE	National Institute for Clinical Excellence
NICU	neonatal intensive care unit
NIH	National Institutes of Health
NK	natural killer
NMR	neonatal mortality rate
NNT_B	number needed to treat for benefit
NO	nitric oxide
NPV	negative predictive value
NSAID	non-steroidal anti-inflammatory drug
NSE	non-specific enolase
NSPCC	National Society for Prevention of Cruelty to Children
NTD	neural tube defect
OA	oesophageal atresia
OAE	oto-acoustic emissions
OCD	obsessive–compulsive disorder
ODD	oppositional/defiant disorder
OGTT	oral glucose tolerance test
OHC	outer hair cell
OM(E)	otitis media (with effusion)
OMIM	Online Mendelian Inheritance in Man
OPV	oral polio vaccine
ORS/T	oral rehydration solution/therapy
OSAS	obstructive sleep apnoea syndrome
OT	occupational therapy
OVC	orphans and vulnerable children (made vulnerable through HIV)
PA	pulmonary artery; postero-anterior
PAF	platelet-activating factor
PALS	paediatric advanced life support
PAN	polyarteritis nodosa
PBSCT	peripheral blood stem cell transplants
PC	phosphatidylcholine
PCA	post-conceptual age
PCP	*Pneumocystis carinii (jirovecii)* pneumonia
PCR	polymerase chain reaction
PCV	packed cell volume
PCWP	pulmonary capillary wedge pressure
PDA	patent ductus arteriosus
PEEP	positive end-expiratory pressure
PEFR	peak expiratory flow rate

PET	positron emission tomography
PFT	pulmonary function testing
PG	prostaglandin; phosphatidylglycerol
PICU	paediatric intensive care unit
PIE	pulmonary interstitial emphysema
PIP	peak inspiratory pressure
PIVKA	proteins produced in vitamin K absence
PKU	phenylketonuria
PMA	post-menstrual age
PML	polymorphonuclear leucocyte
PMR	perinatal mortality rate
PMTCT	perinatal mother-to-child transmission
PN	parenteral nutrition
PNET	primitive neuroectodermal tumour
PNMR	post-neonatal mortality rate
PPH	primary pulmonary hypertension
PPHN	persistent pulmonary hypertension of the newborn
PPI	proton pump inhibitor
PPV	positive predictive value; patent processus vaginalis
PRL	prolactin
PSGN	post-streptococcal glomerulonephritis
PT	prothrombin time
PTH	parathyroid hormone
PTU	propylthiouracil
PTV	patient-triggered ventilation
PUO	pyrexia of unknown origin
PVL	periventricular leukomalacia
PVR	pulmonary vascular resistance
PVS	pulmonary valve stenosis
QS	quiet sleep
RA	right atrium
RAAS	renin–angiotensin–aldosterone system
RAST	radioallergosorbence testing
RCP	Royal College of Physicians
RCPCH	Royal College of Paediatrics and Child Health
RDS	respiratory distress syndrome
REM	rapid eye movement
RF	rheumatoid factor
RMS	rhabdomyosarcoma
ROP	retinopathy of prematurity
RP	retinitis pigmentosa
RRT	renal replacement therapy
RSV	respiratory syncytial virus
RTA	road traffic accident
RV	right ventricle; residual volume
RVOT	right ventricular outflow tract
SALT	speech and language therapy
SBR	stillbirth rate
SCBU	special baby care unit
SCID	severe combined immunodeficiency disease
SD	standard deviation
SGA	small for gestational age
SIDS	sudden infant death syndrome
SIGN	Scottish Intercollegiate Guideline Network
SIMV	synchronous intermittent mandatory ventilation

SIOP	International Society of Paediatric Oncology
SIP	spontaneous isolated intestinal perforation
SIRS	systemic inflammatory response syndrome
SLE	systemic lupus erythematosus
SLT	speech and language therapist
SM	severe malnutrition
SNHL	sensorineural hearing loss
SNP	single nucleotide polymorphism
SP	surfactant protein
SPA	suprapubic aspiration
SPF	sun protection factor
SRSV	small round structured virus
SSNS	steroid-sensitive nephrotic syndrome
SSPE	subacute sclerosing panencephalitis
SSRI	selective serotonin reuptake inhibitor
STBI	severe traumatic brain injury
STD/I	sexually transmitted disease/infection
SUDI	sudden unexplained death in infancy
SVC	superior vena cava
SVT	supraventricular tachycardia
T_3	tri-iodothyronine
T_4	thyroxine
TB	tuberculosis
TBG	thyroid-binding globulin
TBI	total body irradiation
TCA	tricyclic antidepressant
TCR	T-cell receptor
TGF	transforming growth factor
Ti	inspiratory time
TLC	total lung capacity
TNF-α	tumour necrosis factor-alpha
TOF	tracheo-oesophageal fistula; tetralogy of Fallot
TORCH	toxoplasmosis, rubella, cytomegalovirus, herpes simplex
TPN	total parenteral nutrition
TRALI	transfusion-associated lung injury
TRH	thyrotrophin-releasing hormone
TS	tuberous sclerosis
TSH	thyroid-stimulating hormone
TSS	toxic shock syndrome
tTG	tissue transglutaminase
TTN	transient tachypnoea of the newborn
TTP	thrombotic thrombocytopenic purpura
TTTS	twin-to-twin transfusion syndrome
U5MR	under-5 mortality rate
UDPGT	uridine diphosphate glucuronyl transferase
U&Es	urea and electrolytes
UKCCSG	UK Children's Cancer Study Group
UNAIDS	Joint United Nations Programme on HIV/AIDS
UNCRC	United Nations Convention on the Rights of the Child
UNHS	universal newborn hearing screening
UNICEF	United Nations Children's Fund
URTI	upper respiratory tract infection
US	ultrasonography
UTI	urinary tract infection
vCJD	variant Creutzfeld–Jakob disease

VCT	voluntary counselling and testing
VKDB	vitamin K deficiency bleeding
VLCFA	very long chain fatty acids
VMA	vanillylmandelic acid
VSD	ventricular septal defect
VT	ventricular tachycardia
VUR	vesico-ureteric reflux
vWF	von Willeband factor
VZV	varicella zoster virus
WBC/WCC	white blood/cell count
WHO	World Health Organization
XLA	X-linked agammaglobulinaemia

Contents

Contents

Edited by Henry L. Halliday

Childhood Disorders I

MODULE SIX

David W. Webb   Niamh Lynch

Central nervous system

LEARNING OUTCOMES

By the end of this chapter you should:

- Have an understanding of central nervous system embryology and brain development
- Be familiar with the principal disorders of brain development
- Be able to identify common episodic events in childhood
- Be familiar with the common epilepsy syndromes in children
- Be familiar with the common electroencephalogram patterns of childhood epilepsy
- Be aware of the common causes of epilepsy
- Know how to manage a child with status epilepticus
- Know how to assess and manage a child with hemiplegia
- Be familiar with the common childhood brain tumours and their presentation
- Know the causes of acute and chronic ataxia in childhood
- Be familiar with the common muscle diseases of childhood
- Know how to assess a child with neurodevelopmental regression
- Know how to evaluate a child with macrocephaly
- Have an understanding of neural tube defects and their management.

MODULE SIX

Basic science of brain development

Embryology of the central nervous system (Table 28.1)

In the third and fourth weeks of gestation the nervous system begins on the dorsal aspect of the embryo as a plate of tissue differentiating in the middle of the ectoderm. This differentiation results in formation of the neural plate and is induced by the underlying mesoderm at about 18 days of gestation. The lateral margins of this plate invaginate to form the neural tube, which in turn gives rise to the central nervous system (CNS); the cavity of this tube becomes the ventricular system. Neuralation, or fusion of the neural folds, begins at 22 days and is complete by 28 days. Neural tube defects arise as a result of the failure of the neural plate to form the neural tube during the first 28 days of gestation; they can vary in severity and occur at any level between the rostral and caudal ends.

Development of the prosencephalon (future brain) and its cleavage into two hemispheres (prosencephalic cleavage) occur in the second and third months and are induced by factors that influence development of the face; thus severe disorders of brain development at this time may result in facial anomalies.

The ventricular zone is the site of proliferation of neurons and glial cells, which occurs between 3 and 4 months. Neuronal cells migrate outwards from the area of the primitive ventricles and are guided as they travel by a network of glial fibres. This process ultimately results in the formation of the six-layered cerebral cortex. Subplate neurons are the first to migrate and act as the trigger for neuronal organization, which begins from the fifth month of gestation and continues into early childhood. During this phase there is glial differentiation and an orientation of neurons and their dendritic synaptic contacts, including a process of selective cell death and pruning. Myelination in the human nervous system begins in the peripheral nerves, where motor roots myelinate before sensory roots. Central brain myelination begins to appear prior to birth and is most prominent in the major sensory systems of vision and hearing and in the major motor systems of the brainstem. Higher-level myelination progresses over decades.

Disorders of brain development and their consequences are listed in Table 28.2.

Table 28.1 Major events in human brain development and their timing

Event	Timing
Primary neuralation	Weeks 3–4
Prosencephalic development	Months 2–3
Neuronal proliferation	Months 3–4
Neuronal migration	Months 3–5
Neuronal organization	Month 5–years postnatal
Myelination	Birth–years postnatal

Source: Volpe 2001.

Table 28.2 Disorders of brain development and their consequences

Disorder	Consequence
Neuralation	Neural tube defects (spina bifida)
Prosencephalic development	Holoprosencephaly
	Agenesis of the corpus callosum
	Agenesis of the septum pellucidum
	Septo-optic dysplasia
	Fetal hydrocephalus (some cases)
Neuronal proliferation	Microencephaly
	Macroencephaly/cerebral gigantism
	Hemi-megaloencephaly
Neuronal migration	Schizencephaly
	Lissencephaly
	Polymicrogyria
	Heterotopias
	Focal cortical dysplasia
	± Agenesis of the corpus callosum
Neuronal organization	Learning disability, autism and epilepsy

Neurons and synapses

Nervous tissue contains two distinct classes of cell: the neuron cell and the glial cell, both of which arise from the ectoderm. Neurons consist of a cell body, axon and dendrites that transmit impulses. Neurons are classified functionally as afferent (sensory), efferent (motor) and interneurons. The excitable nature of their resting membrane potential allows them to act as signalling units for behavioural responses.

The synapse is the point where neurons transmit signals between each other and consists of a presynaptic and post-synaptic membrane. Electrical synapses are extremely rapid and are facilitated by gap junction channels in the neuron membrane. Chemical synapse transmission is mediated by neurotransmitters that are stored in vesicles in the axon terminal. The main excitatory neurotransmitter in the brain and spinal cord is glutamate, while the major inhibitory neurotransmitters are gamma-aminobutyric acid (GABA) and glycine. To transmit impulses, neurotransmitters must attach to receptors, and it is the receptor and not the transmitter that decides whether the synaptic response is excitatory or inhibitory. Receptors are either ligand-gated ion channels or are coupled to an intracellular guanosine triphosphate (GTP) binding protein.

Neural pathways

The major functional systems in the human nervous system are the motor and sensory systems. The corticospinal (pyramidal) tract and corticonuclear fibres are the pathways of voluntary movement. These tracts arise in the primary and premotor cortex of the frontal lobe, travel down the posterior limb of the internal capsule, and then tightly bundle as they exit the cerebral hemispheres to form the cerebral peduncles. As they pass through the pons, the tracts rotate so that the corticonuclear fibres lie dorsally. In the medulla the corticonuclear fibres terminate on the cranial nerve nuclei, and the corticospinal fibres come together to form the pyramids. At the caudal end of the medulla 70–90% of the fibres decussate to form the lateral corticospinal tract, while the uncrossed fibres form the anterior corticospinal tract. Once in the ventral (or anterior) horn, fibres synapse with interneurons (most common) or directly with the α-motor neuron.

The two main sensory pathways in the spinal cord are the dorsal columns that carry the sensations of vibration, fine touch and proprioception, and the lateral spinal thalamic tracts that carry the more vaguely interpreted signals of pain, crude touch and temperature. The dorsal column fibres are well myelinated to transmit fast and accurate impulses. They travel up the cord without crossing until the medulla, and continue to the thalamus via the medial lemniscus and on to the post-central gyrus via the posterior limb of the internal capsule. The lateral spinal thalamic tracts cross over immediately on entering the cord and then follow a similar pathway.

Episodic events

Problem-orientated topic:

the child presenting with funny turns

(See also Chapter 24 for a more detailed description.)

Emma is a 3-year-old girl who is brought to the accident and emergency department after a fall from her bike. After the fall she became extremely pale and floppy, then stiffened, extended her neck and jerked her arms and legs. She was incontinent. The episode lasted less than a minute and she was upset afterwards. She is otherwise a normal child.

Q1. Has this girl had an epileptic seizure?

Q2. What investigations are needed?

BOX 28.1 History-taking in the assessment of clinical events: the 'five Ss'

Scene	What was the setting in which the event happened?
Start	How did it begin?
Sequence	What actually happened and in what order?
Stop	How did it stop?
Sequelae	Were there any after-effects?

Q1. Has this girl had an epileptic seizure?

This event involved truncal stiffening, limb jerking and incontinence, and on the surface might appear to be an epileptic seizure. However, there are several features that should raise suspicion of an alternative mechanism and the case highlights the importance of taking the whole event in context. The 'five Ss' will help with this (Box 28.1).

Q2. What investigations are needed?

This girl's episode occurred in the context of a minor injury, began with pallor and hypotonia and was brief. The history would be compatible with a reflex anoxic syncopal event (Ch. 24) and this should be considered. It would also be important to exclude a prolonged QT interval and electrocardiography (ECG) should be undertaken; electroencephalography (EEG) in this situation may be misleading.

Other paroxysmal events seen in childhood

There are a number of non-epileptic paroxysmal conditions that occur in childhood. Those associated with anoxia/hypoxia and syncope are most likely to be confused with epilepsy (Box 28.2).

Epileptic seizures, epilepsy and status epilepticus

Problem-orientated topic:

the child with an epileptic seizure

John is a 2-year-old boy who is admitted following an episode of loss of consciousness associated with stiffening of his trunk, cyanosis, salivation, eye rolling and limb jerking for 4 minutes. He is febrile on admission. He is otherwise a normal child.

Q1. What is this clinical event?

BOX 28.2 Non-epileptic paroxysmal events

Anoxic syncope (Ch. 24)
- Blue breath-holding
- Pallid syncope (reflex anoxic syncope)
- Vasovagal syncope
- Cardiogenic syncope (prolonged QT interval)
- Obstructive syncope (Sandifer's syndrome, suffocation)

Involuntary movements
- Rigors, jitteriness, shuddering
- Paroxysmal dyskinesias
- Alternating hemiplegia of infancy

Migraine equivalents (Ch. 24)
- Benign paroxysmal vertigo
- Cyclical vomiting
- Paroxysmal torticollis

Behaviour
- Day-dreaming
- Hyperventilation
- Pseudoseizures
- Gratification phenomena

Sleep disorders (Ch. 24)
- Night terrors
- Sleep myoclonus
- Narcolepsy/cataplexy

Q1.   What is this clinical event?

This boy has had a symptomatic epileptic seizure. The most common cause of this in his age group would be a 'febrile seizure'. Hypoglycaemia, electrolyte disturbances and intracranial infection or trauma may also cause symptomatic seizures and should be considered.

Precipitating factors to be considered
- Fever
- Meningo-encephalitis
- Head injury
- Hypoxic–ischaemic injury
- Toxin (endogenous/exogenous)
- Metabolic and electrolyte disturbance.

Febrile convulsions are considered in detail in Chapter 24.

Problem-orientated topic:

the child with epilepsy

Colin is seen in clinic with a history of events occurring in sleep. These began at the age of 7 years and cluster in the early morning. He comes to his parents' room and is upset. His face is twitching and he is salivating and cannot talk. He appears to remain awake throughout these events, which last 3–4 minutes.

Q1.   Does this boy have epilepsy?
Q2.   What type of epileptic seizure is he having?
Q3.   What is the management?
Q4.   What causes epilepsy?

Q1. Does this boy have epilepsy?

Epilepsy is the tendency to have recurrent unprovoked epileptic seizures. These are clinical events that arise from abnormal cerebral electrical activity. They are paroxysmal, stereotypical and unpredictable, and are characterized by their clinical manifestations and their effect on consciousness. Other non-epileptic causes of 'funny turns' must be considered (Ch. 24).

Q2. What type of epileptic seizure is Colin having?

See Box 28.3.

BOX 28.3 Classification of seizures

- Partial:
  - Simple
  - Complex partial
  - Secondary generalized
- Generalized:
  - Tonic–clonic, tonic, clonic
  - Absence
  - Atonic
  - Myoclonic
  - Infantile spasms
- Unclassifiable

Simple and complex partial seizures

 Partial seizures have a focal onset. In a simple partial seizure the child remains fully aware and, if old enough, will recall the event in detail. In a complex partial seizure the child has altered consciousness with minimal recollection of the event. Both simple and complex partial seizures may progress to loss of consciousness. The typical simple partial seizure might involve a localized sensation, with associated motor or autonomic activity that the child is aware of and cannot suppress. The typical complex partial seizure might involve staring, confusion and automatic behaviours such as fumbling. Complex partial seizures of temporal lobe origin are often preceded by an aura of fear or an epigastric discomfort. Gustatory, visual or auditory hallucinations may occur.

Generalized seizures

Seizures without focal onset and with loss of consciousness from the onset are called primary generalized seizures:

- *Generalized tonic–clonic seizures.* The generalized tonic–clonic seizure is characterized by a sudden loss of consciousness, associated with stiffening of the trunk and limbs (tonic phase) that lasts about 10 seconds and is followed by rhythmic jerking of the limbs that is usually symmetrical (clonic phase). The patient may bite the tongue or be incontinent of urine and faeces. This phase usually lasts 2–5 minutes, and is followed by a post-ictal period of unconsciousness and confusion that can last up to 1 hour. The patient usually has no recollection of the seizure or the post-ictal period.
- *Absence seizures.* Absence seizures involve an abrupt brief cessation of activity, followed by a vacant stare and unresponsiveness. The child has no recollection of the event and will resume activity as if nothing has happened. There are no major motor phenomena, but the eyes may roll upwards and there may be automatisms such as lip smacking or picking at clothes. The events can be induced by hyperventilation and this can be a useful observation in the clinic.
- *Atonic, myoclonic and infantile spasms.* The atonic seizure involves an abrupt loss of tone usually associated with a head nod and/or fall. Myoclonic seizures involve single brief jerks. Infantile spasms, also known as 'salaam attacks', are brief forceful episodes of truncal flexion or extension, associated with elevations of the arms and legs. They typically occur in clusters on waking from sleep and appear to upset the child. Their usual age of onset is 3–12 months. Infantile spasms can be associated with prior brain injury, infection or cerebral malformation, but remain unexplained in about 25% of cases. Idiopathic cases and those with previously normal development have a better prognosis.

Epilepsy syndromes

The combination of seizure type, age, developmental profile, family history and EEG features is used to identify epilepsy syndromes (Box 28.4).

- *Childhood absence epilepsy.* Onset is between 3 and 12 years and is characterized by frequent brief absence seizures lasting 5–20 seconds. The

---

BOX 28.4 Epilepsy syndromes

Idiopathic
- Benign neonatal convulsions
- Benign infantile myoclonic epilepsy
- Childhood absence epilepsy
- Benign Rolandic epilepsy
- Juvenile myoclonic epilepsy

Cryptogenic/symptomatic
- West's syndrome
- Lennox–Gastaut syndrome

Source: Roger et al 2005.

BOX 28.5 EEG findings in benign Rolandic epilepsy

- High-voltage diphasic centro-temporal spikes
- Unilateral or bilateral
- Activated by drowsiness and sleep
- Do not relate to seizure frequency or duration
- May be found in unaffected siblings

BOX 28.6 EEG findings in juvenile myoclonic epilepsy

- Polyspike and wave complexes
- Generalized discharges at > 3 Hz
- Photosensitivity is common

---

child is developmentally normal and there is a strong genetic predisposition. Seizures tend to remit in adolescence. EEG findings are bilateral, synchronous and symmetrical spike/wave discharges, at a frequency of 3 Hz.

- *Benign Rolandic epilepsy* (Box 28.5). Onset is at 3–13 years with a peak at 9 years and intelligence is normal. Seizures are typically nocturnal and begin with unilateral paraesthesia of the face, lips and tongue, associated with an ipsilateral motor seizure of the face. Awareness is maintained but the child is unable to speak and may salivate. Seizures last 1–2 minutes and nocturnal episodes may become generalized. Daytime seizures are rare and do not tend to result in loss of consciousness. Most children do not require treatment and the seizures typically resolve spontaneously during puberty.
- *Juvenile myoclonic epilepsy* (Box 28.6). Onset is between 8 and 26 years of age and intelligence is normal. Generalized tonic–clonic seizures provoked by sleep deprivation and brief absence seizures bring the child to medical attention. A specific enquiry about early morning brief extensor upper limb myoclonic jerks confirms the diagnosis.

- High-voltage disorganized and chaotic background
- High-voltage asynchronous spike/polyspike wave discharges
- A decremental (drop in voltage) seizure pattern

- *West's syndrome* (Box 28.7). A triad of infantile spasms, developmental regression and a specific EEG pattern is the hallmark of this syndrome. The prognosis is poor. There is an associated mortality of 5%, with half of the survivors having severe developmental delay and half suffering from persistent seizures.

Q3. What is the management?

See Table 28.3.

http://www.nice.org.uk/CG020

NICE guidelines for epilepsy

Q4. What causes epilepsy?

See Box 28.8.

Neurofibromatosis

Neurofibromatosis type 1 (NF-1) has an incidence of 1/3000 to 1/4000, with 50% of cases representing new mutations. It is linked to a gene on chromosome 17q11.2 that encodes a protein thought to act as a tumour suppressor gene.

Clinical features

The earliest features are multiple café au lait macules over the trunk and limbs, and freckling in the axilla (Fig. 28.1) and perineum. Pigmented nodules in the iris (Lisch nodules) may be visible with the assistance of a slit lamp and these increase in frequency through

Table 28.3 Treatment of childhood seizures

Seizure type	First-line drug
Generalized tonic–clonic	Carbamazepine, sodium valproate, lamotrigine
Absence	Ethosuxamide, lamotrigine, sodium valproate
Myoclonic	Sodium valproate
Tonic	Lamotrigine, sodium valproate
Atonic	Lamotrigine, sodium valproate
Partial	Carbamazepine, lamotrigine
Infantile spasms	Steroids, vigabatrin

Idiopathic (genetic)	80%
Symptomatic	20%

- Acquired:
  - Post-infectious
  - Post-traumatic
  - Post-ischaemic
- Developmental:
  - Cerebral dysgenesis
  - Chromosomal
  - Neurocutaneous syndromes

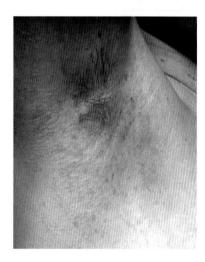

Fig. 28.1 Axillary freckling in neurofibromatosis type 1 (NF-1)

childhood. Neurofibromas are benign subcutaneous nodular tumours located along peripheral nerves. These increase with age and are rarely seen in childhood. Plexiform neurofibromas represent a rare but serious and disfiguring complication of NF-1, particularly when they involve the head and neck. Bone involvement can lead to pseudoarthrosis and bowing of the long bones, and there is also an increased risk of scoliosis.

Complications

These include optic gliomas, which may be bilateral. These lesions tend to behave benignly, particularly when located anterior to the optic chiasm. Other intracranial or intraspinal tumours are uncommon in NF-1 but there is an increased risk of malignancies in general. There is also a higher risk of mild learning difficulties and of hydrocephalus (as a consequence of aqueduct stenosis). There is an association with renal artery stenosis and systemic hypertension, and a higher rate of vascular accidents.

Diagnosis

The diagnosis is clinical and based on the finding of two or more of the following:

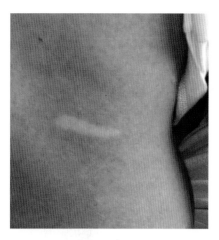

Fig. 28.2 **Depigmented ash-leaf macule in tuberous sclerosis**

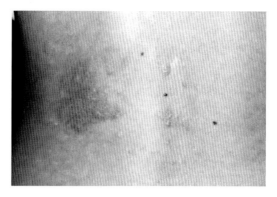

Fig. 28.3 **Shagreen patch**

- Six or more café au lait macules > 5 mm in diameter in prepubertal children or > 15 mm in diameter in post-pubertal children
- One plexiform neurofibroma or two or more neurofibromas of any type
- Axillary or inguinal freckling
- Optic gliomas
- Two or more Lisch nodules
- Distinctive osseous lesion
- First-degree relative with NF-1.

Management
This includes genetic counselling and annual surveillance for complications. Some children with NF-1 will require neuroimaging with input from paediatric neurosurgery, orthopaedic surgery, plastic surgery and/or ophthalmology.

Tuberous sclerosis

Tuberous sclerosis (TS) is a dominantly inherited neurocutaneous syndrome with a high spontaneous mutation rate (70%). Affected parents may not be aware that they have the condition and require careful examination and brain imaging before the risk of recurrence in future pregnancies can be given. The incidence is about 1/20 000. Gene loci have been identified on chromosomes 9q and 16p, and are believed to represent 'tumour suppressor genes'. The condition is named after the cerebral 'potato-like' hamartomas (tubers) in the brain that become calcified (sclerosis).

Clinical features
The earliest cutaneous features of the condition are ash-leaf-shaped depigmented macules (Fig. 28.2), seen best with the aid of a Wood's lamp in a darkened room. These may be followed by the development of a shagreen patch (a roughened area of skin over the lumbar spine, Fig. 28.3), facial angiofibromas (over the nasolabial folds, cheeks and chin) and periungual fibromas. The latter only become evident in late childhood and early puberty.

The majority of affected individuals (80%) develop epilepsy and onset is most commonly before the age of 5 years. Cognitive difficulties are seen in 50% and are associated with infantile spasms, early onset of intractable seizures and multiple cerebral tubers. The condition is also associated with cardiac rhabdomyomas (fetal hydrops, neonatal heart failure), polycystic kidneys, renal and hepatic angiomyolipomas and retinal astrocytomas.

Diagnosis
Diagnosis is made on the presence of two or more of the following features:
- Facial angiofibromas or forehead plaque
- Non-traumatic ungual or periungual fibromas
- Hypomelanotic macules (≥ 3)
- Shagreen patch (connective tissue naevus)
- Retinal astrocytomas
- Cortical tuber
- Subependymal nodule
- Subependymal giant cell astrocytoma
- Cardiac rhabdomyoma, single or multiple
- Lymphangiomyomatosis
- Renal angiomyolipoma.

Management
This requires a multidisciplinary approach. The major issues are control of seizures, surveillance for cognitive deficits and management of behavioural difficulties. There is a higher incidence of autistic behaviour. Vigabatrin for infantile spasms in children with TS has improved seizure control significantly, although this has to be weighed against the risk of potentially irreversible peripheral visual field defects with this drug. Facial angiofibromas may be disfiguring and may benefit from laser therapy.

Sturge–Weber syndrome

Sturge–Weber syndrome is the association between a facial angiomatous naevus (port-wine stain) and a venous angioma of the leptomeninges or glaucoma of the eye. Only 8% of all children with facial port-wine stains have the syndrome, but this increases to 25% of those with a port-wine stain in the ophthalmic division of the trigeminal nerve and 33% of children with bilateral facial angiomas. The disorder is sporadic.

Clinical features

The facial lesion is variable in size and does not correlate with the size of the intracranial angioma. Among children with Sturge–Weber syndrome 75% will develop seizures. The onset of epilepsy is usually in the first year of life and seizures are frequently resistant to anticonvulsant therapy. Cognitive difficulties occur in 80% and 30% have profound learning disability. The risk of cognitive difficulties is associated with early onset of polymorphous and resistant seizures and the presence of bilateral cerebral lesions. A hemiplegia develops in 50% of children on the contralateral side to the angioma. It is often first noticed after a seizure and may progress in severity with subsequent seizure events.

Diagnosis

Children who present with focal seizures should have the eyelids and skin above the eye carefully examined for evidence of haemangiomas. Computed tomography (CT) of the brain may reveal 'railroad track' calcification of the cerebral cortex. Contrast-enhanced magnetic resonance imaging (MRI) will demonstrate the pial angioma and local cerebral atrophy.

Management

Among those with intractable epilepsy who fail to respond to standard anticonvulsant medication, a functional hemispherectomy should be considered. Laser therapy for the facial lesion may be of cosmetic benefit. Regular ophthalmology review for glaucoma is also important.

Problem-orientated topic:

status epilepticus

Anna is a 9-year-old girl with a previous history of epilepsy and mild learning difficulties. She presents to accident and emergency in a generalized tonic–clonic seizure that has lasted at least 35 minutes. You are called to the accident and emergency department to help control her seizures.

Q1. What is the emergency management of this clinical scenario?

Q2. What are the potential causes of this medical emergency?

Q3. What investigations should be undertaken?

Q4. What anticonvulsant drugs should be used?

Q5. What are the potential complications of status epilepticus?

Q1. What is the emergency management of this clinical scenario?

This girl is in status epilepticus. This is defined as a prolonged seizure lasting over 30 minutes or repeated seizures without inter-ictal recovery. Generalized tonic–clonic status is a medical emergency that requires immediate action.

Management goals are:
- Maintain vital functions.
- Terminate the seizure.
- Identify and treat causal or precipitating factors.

Management protocol is:
- Place the child in lateral prone position.
- Secure airway with soft mouthpiece.
- Administer 100% oxygen.
- Obtain intravenous access.
- Administer emergency anticonvulsant therapy.
- Obtain urgent blood investigations.

Status epilepticus can occur as a consequence of an acute cerebral insult or may be provoked in a child with an underlying seizure tendency by factors such as intercurrent illness, sleep deprivation or anticonvulsant withdrawal.

Q2. What are the potential causes of this medical emergency?

See Box 28.9.

Q3. What investigations should be undertaken?

See Box 28.10.

Q4. What anticonvulsant drugs should be used?

See Table 28.4.

Q5. What are the potential complications of status epilepticus?

See Box 28.11.

BOX 28.9 Aetiology of status epilepticus

Idiopathic (50%)
- 25% febrile seizures
- 25% epilepsy

Acute symptomatic (25%)
- Infection
- Trauma
- Anoxia
- Metabolic or electrolyte disturbances
- Drug toxicity

Chronic symptomatic (25%)
- Previous cerebral injury
- Cerebral malformation
- Progressive encephalopathy

BOX 28.10 Investigations in status epilepticus

Mandatory
- Blood glucose
- Blood gas
- Serum electrolytes, calcium, magnesium
- Full blood count
- Blood culture (if febrile)

Others to be considered
- Liver function tests
- Anticonvulsant drug levels if on treatment
- Urine toxicology and organic acids
- Serum ammonia, lactate and amino acids

Status epilepticus is a life-threatening event, with a mortality of 3–6% and a morbidity of 20%, depending on the aetiology of the seizures. Outcome is affected by duration of the seizure, age (worse under 3 years) and the cause of the status epilepticus.

BOX 28.11 Complications of status epilepticus

- Cerebral:
  - Hypoxic–ischaemic injury
  - Cerebral oedema and raised intracranial pressure
  - Hippocampal sclerosis
- Cardiorespiratory:
  - Central respiratory failure
  - Aspiration, pneumonia, pulmonary oedema
  - Cardiac failure, arrhythmias
  - Hypertension/hypotension
- Metabolic:
  - Dehydration
  - Electrolyte imbalance: hyponatraemia, hyperkalaemia
  - Hypoglycaemia
- Multi-organ failure
- Disseminated intravascular coagulation

Hemiplegia

Problem-orientated topic:

acute onset hemiplegia

Peter is 7 years old and presents with a 6-hour history of right-sided weakness that seems to be getting worse. He can no longer stand unsupported and has stopped using his right hand.

Q1. What are the possible causes of this boy's acute hemiplegia?

Q2. What investigations will you order?

Table 28.4 Drug management in status epilepticus

	Intravenous access	No intravenous access
Immediate	Lorazepam 0.1 mg/kg i.v. (give over 30–60 sec)	Diazepam 0.5 mg/kg PR
Seizure continuing at 10 minutes	Lorazepam 0.1 mg/kg i.v. (give over 30–60 sec)	Paraldehyde 0.4 ml/kg PR in same volume of olive oil
Seizure continuing at 20 minutes	*Call for senior help* Phenytoin 18 mg/kg i.v. (give over 20 min) OR (if already on phenytoin) Phenobarbital 20 mg/kg i.v. (give over 10 min) AND (if under 3 years with unexplained afebrile status) Pyridoxine 100 mg i.v.	*Call for senior help* Use intra-osseous route
Seizure continuing at 40 minutes	*Contact anaesthetist and paediatric ICU* Consider thiopental 4 mg/kg i.v.	*Contact anaesthetist and paediatric ICU*

PR = per rectum

- Epilepsy: Todd's paresis
- Migraine: hemiplegic variant
- Stroke: ischaemic, haemorrhagic
- Tumour: brainstem in particular
- Trauma: extradural or subdural haematoma
- Infection: focal encephalitis, abscess
- Demyelination: acute disseminated encephalomyelitis, multiple sclerosis
- Diabetes: acute hypoglycaemia
- Metabolic: mitochondrial disorders

Q1. What are the possible causes of this boy's acute hemiplegia?
(Box 28.12)

There is a broad differential diagnosis here and a child presenting with acute hemiplegia requires a careful history and examination. In the absence of a history of head trauma, headache, seizure activity or infection the most likely explanation is an acute ischaemic stroke.

Q2. What investigations will you order?

Ultimately the findings on brain imaging will guide further management. CT brain scan is usually the first form of brain imaging; an ischaemic lesion is seen as an area of low density that may not be visible in the first 24 hours post-insult but may with time enhance with intravenous contrast. The infarction is usually in the distribution of a single artery. MRI is preferred for imaging in childhood stroke; with an ischaemic lesion it will reveal an area of low density on T1-weighted images and high signal on T2-weighted images. Brain haemorrhage is seen as an area of increased density on a non-contrast CT scan and may be associated with significant oedema and midline shift.

Stroke

Childhood stroke is rare, with an incidence of 2.6 and 3.1 per 100 000 white and black children per year, respectively. Ischaemic stroke usually presents as a sudden-onset hemiparesis or focal neurological disturbance in a previously well child. Additional clinical features vary and are related to the age of the child and location of the stroke. They may include hemisensory loss, hemianopia, dysphasia and ataxia. With involvement of the vertebrobasilar vessels, features may also include quadriplegia, vomiting, tremor, vertigo, dysarthria, oculomotor palsies and lower cranial nerve involvement. Haemorrhagic stroke is most commonly seen with structural anomalies of the cerebral vasculature and disorders of coagulation. While hemiparesis is also common with haemorrhagic stroke, the dominant symptoms are often headache, vomiting and seizures. There may also be features of raised intracranial pressure.

Risk factors for childhood stroke
Risk factors for stroke in children are very different from those in adults (Table 28.5). With thorough evaluation, one or more risk factors can be identified in about 75% of children with ischaemic infarction and an even higher number of those with haemorrhagic stroke. Sickle cell disease is one of the most common causes world-wide and varicella infection is increasingly recognized as a risk factor.

Investigations in a child with ischaemic stroke
- ECG, echocardiography (cardiac consultation)
- MR angiography
- Carotid Doppler studies
- Thrombophilia screen (haematology consultation)
- Sickle screen
- Varicella serology
- Homocysteine levels
- ± Cerebrospinal fluid (CSF) lactate.

Table 28.5 **Conditions predisposing to stroke in children**

Condition	Examples
Ischaemic stroke	
Congenital heart disease	Aortic lesions, complex congenital heart defect
Acquired heart disease	Endocarditis, cardiomyopathy
Vasculitis	Meningitis, varicella, HIV, Kawasaki disease
Vasculopathy	Moyamoya, fibromuscular dysplasia, Sturge–Weber syndrome
Vasospasm	Migraine
Haematological	Sickle cell anaemia, disseminated intravascular coagulation (DIC), thrombotic tendency
Metabolic	Homocystinuria, mitochondrial disorders
Trauma	Arterial dissection, child abuse
Haemorrhagic stroke	
Vascular lesions	Arteriovenous malformations, fistulas, aneurysm
Haematological	Haemophilia, thrombocytopenia, sickle cell anaemia
Lesional	Brain tumour, haemorrhagic infarction

BOX 28.13 Management of childhood stroke

- Ischaemic stroke: consider low-dose aspirin prophylaxis
- Ischaemic stroke in a hospital setting: consider tissue plasminogen activator
- Sickle cell disease: exchange transfusion
- Haemorrhagic stroke: immediate referral to unit with neurosurgical facilities

Source: Kirkham 1999.

Management and prognosis (Box 28.13)

Treatment depends on the cause of the stroke and the underlying condition in the period immediately after the stroke. If the child is left with a persisting neurological deficit, multidisciplinary input is required, including physiotherapy, occupational therapy, speech therapy and psychological support. Adverse outcomes after childhood stroke include death in 10%, recurrence in 20%, and neurological deficits in two-thirds of survivors.

Headaches

Problem-orientated topic:

the child with headaches

(See also Ch. 24.)

Harry is 8 years old. For the past 2 months he has been complaining of headaches, which are particularly severe in the mornings. He was initially thought to have school refusal but recently has started to vomit. His examination appears normal.

Q1. What is the likely cause of this boy's headache?
Q2. What is the most appropriate investigation?

Q1. What is the likely cause of this boy's headache? (Box 28.14)

This is a sinister history and suggests raised intracranial pressure. The headache associated with raised intracranial pressure is worse when lying down, typically peaks in the early morning and may be associated with neck stiffness, vomiting and/or irritability. Harry should be specifically questioned on the presence of diplopia and carefully examined for evidence of papilloedema.

BOX 28.14 Causes of raised intracranial pressure in childhood

- Cerebral tumour
- Hydrocephalus
- Cerebral oedema
- Cerebral abscess
- Idiopathic intracranial hypertension (pseudotumour)
- Cerebral venous obstruction (venous thrombosis)
- Intracranial haemorrhage
- Hypercarbia

BOX 28.15 Brain tumours in children

- Astrocytomas (40%):
  - Juvenile cystic astrocytoma (Fig. 28.4) — cerebellar, slow-growing, good prognosis with surgery
  - Non-juvenile — often cerebral hemispheres, prognosis variable
- Embryonal tumours (25%):
  - Medulloblastoma — cerebellar, can have spinal metastases, prognosis poor
  - Primitive neuroectodermal tumour (PNET)
  - Atypical teratoid/rhabdoid
- Ependymoma (8%)
- Others:
  - Oligodendrogliomas
  - Glioneural/neuronal tumours
  - Choroid plexus tumours
  - Pineal tumours
  - Craniopharyngioma

Q2. What is the most appropriate investigation?

The absence of neurological findings is not reassuring and you need to image this boy immediately to rule out a space-occupying lesion or hydrocephalus. A posterior fossa tumour would be the most common cause of acquired hydrocephalus with raised intracranial pressure. CT scan with contrast will establish whether a lesion is present or not. If an abnormality is identified, one would proceed to further imaging with MRI. Space-occupying lesions within the cerebral hemispheres in children will usually present with focal neurological deficits, seizures or signs and symptoms of raised intracranial pressure.

Brain tumours (Box 28.15) (see also p. 413)

Brain and spinal tumours are the most frequent solid tumour in children under 15 years of age. They are almost always primary as opposed to metastatic and

MODULE SIX

13

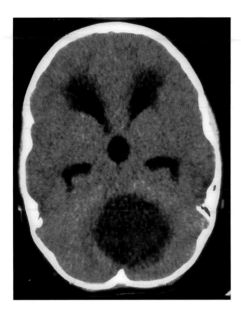

Fig. 28.4 **Cystic astrocytoma in posterior fossa**

the majority are infratentorial. The prognosis for brain tumours depends on the location and histology. Brainstem gliomas have a particularly poor prognosis.

Ataxia

Problem-orientated topic:

the child who goes off his feet

Jack, who is 18 months old and has been walking since the age of 1 year, is referred to the emergency department by his GP because his mother reports that he is unable to stand up. She noticed some unsteadiness a week ago but he has deteriorated and now can no longer walk. He had an MMR vaccination 2 weeks previously but has been well since and there is no history of trauma.

He is irritable but afebrile. His balance is poor, even when sitting. When his mother hands him his pacifier (dummy), he has difficulty placing it in his mouth. He cannot stand or walk, but appears to have normal power in his limbs. Reflexes are normal. It looks as if he has nystagmus.

Q1. Why is Jack ataxic?
Q2. What investigations would you perform?

Q1. Why is Jack ataxic?

The term ataxia is used to imply a disturbance in gait. In its strictest sense, ataxia is caused by a dysfunction in the cerebellum or its major input systems from the frontal lobes or posterior columns of the spinal cord. The ataxic child will be unable to stand with two feet together and will have a broad-based and staggering gait. There may be associated limb ataxia with intention tremor and past pointing, bobbing of the head (titubation), dysarthria and nystagmus.

It is important to remember that an unsteady child may have pathology outside of the cerebellum, including:

- Non-convulsive status epilepticus
- Bifrontal white matter disease
- Vestibular dysfunction
- Peripheral weakness.

It can be difficult to distinguish between cerebellar, sensory, vestibular and other causes of acute ataxia, and other signs of CNS dysfunction need to be carefully sought.

The most common causes of acute ataxia in childhood are post-infection and drug ingestion. The differential diagnosis is outlined in Box 28.16. Brain tumours usually cause a slowly progressive ataxia but many slowly progressive ataxias may be noticed acutely to begin with (Box 28.17).

This boy could have post-infectious/vaccine-related ataxia but there are unusual features, including the subacute onset, marked irritability, nystagmus and upper limb signs. On closer inspection the boy's abnormal eye movements are not nystagmus but rather the jerky and chaotic movements of opsoclonus–myoclonus syndrome. This is associated with a significant risk of occult neuroblastoma and further investigation is needed, including urinary catecholamines and MRI of the thorax and abdomen. If these investigations are negative, an isotope MIBG scan should be considered.

Q2. What investigations would you perform?

See Box 28.18.

Friedreich's ataxia

Friedreich's ataxia is an autosomal recessive disease with a prevalence of about 1/50 000 and accounts for half of all cases of hereditary ataxia. It affects the central sensory pathways in the posterior columns and spinocerebellar tracts of the spinal cord and the efferent cerebellar and corticospinal tracts. Large myelinated peripheral sensory nerves are also affected.

after onset of symptoms. Cognitive function usually remains intact.

Diagnosis

MRI reveals atrophy of the spinal cord but cerebral imaging is usually normal until disease is advanced. Sensory nerve action potentials are severely reduced or absent, while sensory and motor nerve conduction velocities are normal. Most patients are homozygous for the expansion of a GAA triplet repeat sequence in the *Frataxin* gene on chromosome 9.

Management

There is no specific therapy. Multidisciplinary supportive care is helpful and surveillance for cardiac involvement, diabetes and scoliosis is important.

Ataxia telangiectasia

This is an autosomal recessive, progressive neurodegenerative disorder associated with significant immunodeficiency in most patients and a risk of malignancy. It is the most common recessive ataxic disorder in children under 5 years of age. The gene has been mapped to chromosome 11q22–23 and produces a protein, ATM, which has a role in DNA repair.

Clinical features

Onset of symptoms is typically around puberty but early- and late-onset cases exist. Ataxia with a broad-based gait and clumsiness are among the first manifestations. Scoliosis and hypertrophic cardiomyopathy may precede neurological symptoms. Limb dysmetria, action tremor and dysarthria develop with time. Absent deep tendon reflexes and diminished joint position and vibration sensation, with extensor plantar responses and pes cavus, are typical findings. The eyes show abnormalities in smooth pursuit and saccadic movement. The majority of patients develop a cardiomyopathy, and other complications include optic atrophy, deafness and diabetes. The disease progresses throughout childhood and the patient is usually wheelchair-bound an average of 10–15 years

---

BOX 28.19 Conditions associated with cerebellar hypoplasia

- Dandy–Walker malformation: agenesis of the cerebellar vermis, 4th ventricular cyst and hydrocephalus
- Joubert's syndrome: vermis agenesis, neonatal breathing disturbance, abnormal eye movements
- Smith–Lemli–Opitz syndrome: dysmorphic syndrome, learning disability and low plasma cholesterol
- Fetal alcohol syndrome
- Trisomies 13 and 18, fragile X syndrome

Clinical features

Truncal ataxia is usually evident before the age of 3 years, and choreoathetosis and oculomotor apraxia (limitation of ocular movement to command) are other prominent early neurological features. Telangiectasia usually develops after the onset of neurological symptoms and can be seen on the bulbar conjunctivae, neck and ears. Intelligence is usually normal but motor disability is progressive, with the typical child requiring a wheelchair by the age of 10 years. The leading causes of death are infection, malignancy and non-specific pulmonary failure.

Diagnosis

In infancy ataxia telangiectasia can be confused with mild cerebral palsy, acute infectious or episodic ataxia, ataxia with oculomotor apraxia or other rare genetic and mitochondrial disorders. By the age of 10 years a clinical diagnosis is usually readily apparent. Cerebellar atrophy is usually not seen on MRI in young patients. Three routine tests support a diagnosis: serum alpha-fetoprotein levels, karyotyping with special attention to translocations involving chromosomes 7 and 14, and B- and T-cell immune studies. Deficiencies in IgE, IgA and IgG2 may also be found.

Management

This is focused on neuro-rehabilitation and medical management of immunodeficiency and malignancy. It is important to limit exposure to radiation and provide genetic counselling to the family.

Cerebellar hypoplasia (Box 28.19)

The cerebellar hypoplasias are a group of developmental disorders of the cerebellum arising during fetal life and diagnosed on brain MRI. They should be distinguished from acquired and especially progressive cerebellar atrophies (Box 28.20). The cerebellar hypoplasias may be isolated or seen in association with a more

---

BOX 28.20 Conditions associated with progressive cerebellar atrophy

- Pontocerebellar atrophy
- Carbohydrate-deficient glycoprotein syndrome
- Spinocerebellar degenerative conditions
- Tay–Sachs disease
- Menkes' disease
- Rett's syndrome
- Phenylketonuria

---

widespread CNS malformation, structural congenital myopathies or congenital muscular dystrophies. They present with gross motor developmental delay and truncal hypotonia that is usually moderate or severe. Titubation of the head usually predicts future ataxia when the child eventually walks at 18 months to 2 years. More widespread CNS involvement is common and additional features may include epilepsy, language delay, learning disability, autism and other psychiatric disorders.

The weak child

Problem-orientated topic:

the weak child

Emily is 9 years old and has been referred with a 4-month history of generalized weakness and malaise. She had not been well since a bad cold last winter. Her teacher noticed that Emily has stopped running with her friends at break time and seems to have difficulty with physical activity. Emily's mother tells you that she is often too weak to climb the stairs at home and her father has to carry her to bed.

Emily is a polite, anxious little girl. She has subtle periorbital oedema and an erythematous rash on extensor surfaces of both elbows. There is proximal muscle weakness and she has difficulty in moving from lying prone to standing. There is some wasting of the shoulder girdle muscles. Reflexes, coordination and sensation are normal.

Q1. What are the causes of weakness in childhood?

Q2. How would you investigate this child?

BOX 28.21 Investigations in a weak child

Serum creatine kinase (CK)

- Markedly elevated CK can be seen with muscular dystrophy, inflammatory muscle disease, hypothyroidism and defects of carnitine metabolism

C-reactive protein (CRP) and erythrocyte sedimentation rate (ESR)

- Elevated CRP and ESR would support an inflammatory process

Myositis-specific antibodies

- Antinuclear antibody (ANA), anti-Mi-2 antibodies and anti-Jo-1 antibodies may be elevated in inflammatory muscle disease but results will take some time to obtain

Nerve conduction studies

- Demyelination is associated with conduction block and slow nerve conduction velocities; in axonal neuropathy conduction is normal but amplitudes are reduced

Electromyography

- Low-amplitude short-duration muscle unit potentials support muscle pathology

Muscle biopsy

- In Emily's case, this showed perivascular and interfascicular inflammatory infiltrates with groups of muscle fibre degeneration and regeneration, confirming dermatomyositis

Q1. What are the causes of weakness in childhood?

- *Limb girdle muscular dystrophies*. Emily could have an inherited muscular dystrophy, although the subacute onset of symptoms and absence of a family history make this unlikely.
- *Inflammatory muscle disease*. Dermatomyositis occurs in children and is associated with irritability and a rash.
- *Myasthenia gravis*. Fatiguable ptosis is the most common presentation but more generalized weakness can occur.
- *Peripheral neuropathy*. Normal reflexes and the presence of proximal weakness make this less likely.
- *Non-organic cause*. The presence of muscle wasting and definite weakness makes this untenable.

Q2. How would you investigate this child?

See Box 28.21.

Muscular dystrophies

These are a group of hereditary myopathies caused by defects in muscle structural proteins. The limb girdle muscular dystrophies (MDs) have onset after birth and present with progressive weakness of predominantly proximal distribution. They are now known to be associated with defects in dystrophin, dystrophin-associated glycoproteins and other sarcolemmal proteins along the muscle membrane. There have been recent advances in understanding the basic biology and genetics of this group of disorders, which are now classified into defects of either sarcolemmal or nuclear envelope proteins.

Basic science

The sarcolemma is the microscopic sheath covering muscle fibres and is composed of the plasma membrane, basement membrane and the adjacent reticular lamina that also contains fibrillar collagens.

Duchenne and Becker muscular dystrophy

Duchenne and Becker are the commonest limb girdle MDs and are X-linked recessive disorders resulting from a defect in the *dystrophin* gene at Xp21. This gene codes for dystrophin, a muscle membrane protein thought to strengthen muscle cells by anchoring elements of the internal cytoskeleton to the surface membrane. Dystrophin deficiency weakens the integrity of the muscle cell wall, leading to irreversible destruction of muscle cells. Duchenne MD is the more severe phenotype, with less than 3% of the normal dystrophin content present.

Clinical features

Duchenne MD affects 1 in 4000 boys and usually presents with delayed walking. There is hip girdle weakness leading to an inability to run, jump or climb stairs. The gait is characteristically 'waddling' due to hip muscle weakness and there is an associated lumbar lordosis and a tendency to toe-walk. With progressive weakness the child will have difficulty standing from the lying position and to do this will first turn prone, then raise the buttocks and, using the arms, climb up along the thighs until upright (Gower's sign). In the calves, deltoids and buttocks, muscle fibres are replaced by fat and connective tissue, leading to pseudohypertrophy.

Boys with Duchenne MD may also present with speech delay or early learning difficulties, and as a cohort have a lower than average IQ.

Diagnosis

Serum creatine kinase is markedly elevated before the age of 5 years. Following this, there is a decline in the level, due to loss of muscle. Genetic diagnosis is

MODULE SIX

17

based on mutation analysis, and carrier detection and antenatal diagnosis is possible.

Clinical course

The ability to walk is usually lost between the ages of 9 and 12 years, with progressive weakness and limb contractures. Patients usually die in their late teens or early twenties due to progressive respiratory failure or associated cardiomyopathy. Boys with Becker MD have a later onset of symptoms, follow a more slowly progressive course and remain ambulant into their late teens. They survive into adult life.

Management

There is no cure for MD. The use of oral steroids has been shown to delay functional deterioration in muscle strength and may prolong the ambulatory period. A multidisciplinary approach to management is needed.

Other limb girdle muscular dystrophies

The identification of the dystrophin-associated glycoproteins and other sarcolemmal proteins that are relevant to the functional integrity of the muscle membrane led to recognition of an increasing number of new genetic limb girdle MDs. These are predominantly autosomal dominant and recessive, and have varying ages of onset and rates of progression. There is considerable overlap in the clinical presentation of this group of disorders and specific diagnosis often requires histopathological and molecular analysis in a tertiary neuromuscular centre.

Myotonic dystrophy

This is an autosomal dominant disorder resulting from an unstable trinucleotide repeat expansion on chromosome 19. Myotonia refers to the failure of the muscle to relax after sustained contraction and can be demonstrated: for example, following a handshake. A severe neonatal presentation is recognized, with weakness, hypotonia, bulbar paresis and respiratory failure requiring ventilatory support and tube feeding. The mother is always affected.

Adolescents presenting with the condition may have a characteristic pattern of weakness involving the face and peripheries (hands and feet). There is typically ptosis and drooping of the corners of the mouth. Other features include premature frontal baldness, cataracts, cardiomyopathy, multiple endocrinopathies and, for some, significant learning difficulties. Weakness is progressive and disabling, with more than half of those developing symptoms in adolescence dying before the age of 50 years.

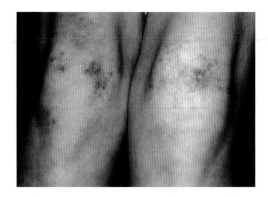

Fig. 28.5 Skin lesions of dermatomyositis over knees

Dermatomyositis (see also p. 89)

Dermatomyositis is a symmetrical, rapidly progressive inflammatory disease of muscle with associated skin inflammation. Onset of symptoms may be insidious or fulminant, and typically there is a proximal weakness associated with marked pain, stiffness and irritability. A heliotrope facial rash may be seen and in children is commonly associated with periorbital oedema. It may also affect the extensor surface of joints (Fig. 28.5), with the skin then becoming scaly and atrophic. Contractures and calcinosis of the skin can occur. Corticosteroids are the first line of treatment for this condition.

Myasthenic syndromes

Myasthenia gravis is an acquired autoimmune disease that results in the destruction of acetylcholine receptors on the post-synaptic membrane, leading to fatiguability with repeated muscle contractions. It is associated with abnormalities of the thymus but the exact nature of the autoimmune process remains unclear. Maternal transmission of acetylcholine receptor antibodies can result in a transient but severe neonatal myasthenia.

The child with prepubertal onset of myasthenia gravis is usually male and seronegative for acetylcholine receptor antibodies. Presentation is with ptosis and/or diplopia that affects both eyes, although not always equally. Ocular myasthenia can follow a relapsing and remitting course, with 20% having a complete remission. Post-pubertal onset of myasthenia is more common in girls and is associated with seropositivity and generalized myasthenia. This may also begin with ocular involvement but generalized weakness usually becomes apparent within a year of ocular symptoms. There may be bulbar involvement, with dysarthria, dysphagia and difficulty chewing. Limb fatiguability becomes evident with time and there is a risk of respiratory insufficiency and myasthenic crisis if not treated.

The edrophonium chloride (Tensilon) test is used as a standard of diagnosis for both ocular and generalized myasthenia gravis. This is an inhibitor of acetylcholinesterase. An endpoint for the study should be determined before it begins; the best endpoints are those that can be measured objectively, such as resolution of ptosis or restoration of ocular motility. Some children are hypersensitive to edrophonium chloride, and a test dose should be given and administered with the use of an oxygen saturation monitor. Atropine and ventilatory support should be to hand. Ocular myasthenia may resolve spontaneously. If it does not, anticholinesterases (neostigmine) or corticosteroids may be helpful. Thymectomy should be considered in generalized myasthenia with acetylcholine receptor antibodies.

Peripheral neuropathies

Most neuropathies have a gradual onset and are slowly progressive, with symmetrical predominantly distal mixed sensory and motor manifestations. An acute onset of neuropathy is seen in a small number of conditions and in children is most commonly due to vincristine toxicity during chemotherapy, Guillain–Barré syndrome or a critical illness polyneuropathy.

Guillain–Barré syndrome

This is an acute inflammatory demyelinating polyneuropathy of autoimmune origin. The majority of cases present 2–3 weeks after an upper respiratory tract or gastrointestinal infection, with an ascending weakness of the lower limbs associated with absent reflexes and sometimes paraesthesia of the hands and feet. The weakness should have reached its peak within 4 weeks of onset. Progression to respiratory failure is associated with cranial nerve involvement and a short incubation period, and mechanical ventilation is required in 7–15% of cases.

CSF examination typically reveals a markedly elevated protein with normal white cell count, although protein elevation may not be apparent until week 2 of the illness. Nerve conduction studies show slowed conduction secondary to demyelination.

Treatment is supportive, with careful vigilance of respiratory function. Steroids have not been shown to be beneficial. Intravenous immunoglobulins may be used in severe, rapidly progressive disease. Virtually complete recovery is seen in two-thirds of patients and begins after a plateau of weakness.

Hereditary motor sensory neuropathies (HMSN)

 This group of disorders leads to a slowly progressive muscular wasting that is distal and symmetrical.

Inheritance can be autosomal dominant, recessive or X-linked. The most important assessment is to examine the child's siblings and parents. The most common condition in this group is HMSN type 1 (Charcot–Marie–Tooth disease). This is an autosomal dominant condition with a gene locus on chromosome 17p11.2; it initially presents with delay in motor milestones, toe-walking, frequent falling or foot deformity (pes cavus). There is progressive atrophy of the muscles supplied by the peroneal nerve, with weakness of ankle dorsiflexion resulting in foot drop and a high-stepping gait. Thigh muscles are spared in comparison with the wasted calf muscles, giving rise to an 'inverted champagne bottle' appearance. Deep tendon reflexes are present initially but disappear later. As the disease progresses, the distal muscles of the hands may become involved. Nerve conduction studies reveal a demyelinating neuropathy with a decrease in nerve conduction velocities.

Spinal muscular atrophy

See page 318.

Neurodevelopmental regression

Problem-orientated topic:

the child with neurological regression

Priya is a previously healthy 10-year-old girl who has undergone a change in behaviour and deterioration in school work in the past 4 months. Her parents have also noted jerking movements of the arms. She was adopted from Nepal at the age of 3 years and did not have vaccinations prior to adoption.

She is a quiet, small child with little spontaneous speech. She follows simple instructions but struggles with more complex commands and has difficulty reading. She has some cogwheel rigidity in her upper limbs and myoclonic jerks are noted. These do not appear to be associated with altered awareness.

Q1. What are the causes of regression in childhood?

Q2. What investigations would you undertake in a child who is regressing?

BOX 28.22 Causes of childhood regression

Epilepsy	Non-convulsive status, Landau–Kleffner syndrome, epileptic encephalopathy
Increased intracranial pressure	Hydrocephalus, brain tumour
Endocrine	Hypothyroidism
Inflammatory	HIV, subacute sclerosing panencephalitis (SSPE), acute disseminating encephalomyelitis (ADEM), Creutzfeldt–Jakob disease (CJD)
Vascular	Moyamoya syndrome
Toxic	Lead poisoning, drug ingestion
Nutritional	Thiamine deficiency, B_{12} deficiency, pellagra
Psychiatric (Ch. 30)	
Inherited metabolic disorders (see Ch. 34)	

Q1. What are the causes of regression in childhood? (Box 28.22)

The two essential features in considering a child who has regressed are the observance of a 'free interval' or period where the child is not affected, followed by demonstration of a 'progressive loss of skills'. While we immediately associate childhood regression with inherited metabolic neurodegenerative disorders, there are a number of 'non-metabolic' causes of regression in childhood that should always be considered, as some of them are treatable.

Priya was born in Nepal and did not have measles immunization. Asia has a higher incidence of subacute sclerosing panencephalitis (SSPE) than Europe. She may also have been exposed to HIV infection. Chronic lead ingestion through the chewing of leaded paint is a cause of toxic encephalopathy in childhood, but presents subacutely with vomiting, irritability and ataxia, usually in the under 3-year age group. Priya may not have had screening for hypothyroidism and this should be excluded. Wilson's disease is an autosomal recessive condition that can present with hepatic, neurological or haematological signs and is treatable. In the neurological form there is mental deterioration, and dystonic movements are common. Myoclonus is frequently observed. This child has SSPE.

Q2. What investigations would you undertake in a child who is regressing?

Precise investigations should be tailored to the individual case. Below is an outline in this child:

- Full blood count:
  - Lead poisoning can give rise to anaemia
  - Wilson's disease can cause haemolytic anaemia
  - HIV infection is associated with a low CD4 count
- Toxicology:
  - Serum lead levels and urine toxicology
- Serum ceruloplasmin:
  - Serum ceruloplasmin levels will be low in Wilson's disease
- Metabolic screen:
  - Serum amino acids, blood gas, lactate, ammonia and urinary organic acids
  - Metabolic consultation may also be needed
- Virology screening:
  - Measles antibody titres
- Ophthalmology review:
  - Wilson's disease — Kaiser–Fleischer rings or metabolic retinopathy
- EEG:
  - SSPE — periodic bursts of spike/wave complexes with the myoclonic jerks
- MRI scan:
  - SSPE — can be normal or reveal patchy focal abnormalities
  - Wilson's — symmetrical hypodensity in the thalami and basal ganglia
- CSF analysis:
  - Measles antibody titres and/or polymerase chain reaction (PCR).

Subacute sclerosing panencephalitis (SSPE)

This is due to chronic persistent measles infection of the CNS following exposure to the measles virus, typically in the first 2 years of life. It has become very rare in the developed world due to vaccination, although this may change with falling vaccination rates. Symptoms usually occur within 6 years of the initial infection and involve subtle personality change, intellectual decline and behaviour change. There is a progressive decline in cognitive function, and within months of onset of symptoms the patient develops myoclonic jerks followed by dementia and spasticity. The majority of those affected die within 3 years of the onset of symptoms. CSF contains anti-measles antibodies. There is no cure as yet.

Acquired immune deficiency syndrome (AIDS) encephalopathy

AIDS-related encephalopathy is now the most common cause of neurodegenerative disease in childhood world-wide. Maternal intravenous drug abuse and prostitution are risk factors in the Western world. Antiretroviral drugs have greatly reduced the risk of an infant contracting HIV due to transplacental or perinatal transmission but are not readily available world-wide. Children with untreated HIV are likely to show evidence of infection within the first year of life. Neurological disease can arise from opportunistic infections in the brain or HIV encephalitis that causes a progressive loss of developmental milestones, microcephaly, dementia and spasticity, and is associated with an elevated CSF protein (0.5 to 1 g/l) and slightly reduced CSF glucose. Neuroimaging may reveal calcification of the basal ganglia. HIV encephalopathy carries a very poor prognosis.

Inherited metabolic neurodegenerative disorders
(See also Ch. 34.)

The inherited metabolic conditions associated with childhood regression are largely autosomal recessive, so that familial incidence or consanguinity may be important clinical clues. The clinical syndromes associated with these disorders presenting in the first few years are relatively non-specific, so that different diseases present in very similar ways. To complicate the situation further, the same disease can manifest differently at different ages. The most helpful approach is to classify the conditions clinically on the basis of age at onset of symptoms: during the neonatal period, during the first 2 years of life, or in the older child.

Presentation in the neonatal period is usually with reduced alertness, coma, seizures, hypotonia and feeding difficulties (Box 28.23).

In the infant and young child with neurological regression it is possible to distinguish disorders with predominant involvement of specific areas of the CNS (Boxes 28.24 and 28.25). Cerebral MRI, EEG, evoked potentials and peripheral nerve conduction studies can be helpful in localizing nervous system involvement. It is also helpful to establish whether there are features to suggest multi-organ involvement (organomegaly, skeletal and/or connective tissue involvement). The mucopolysaccharidoses are unique in having a characteristic phenotype that can be readily recognized. This includes coarse facial features, viscero-megaly, hernias and joint contractures.

BOX 28.23 The most common neonatal inherited metabolic disorders

- Amino acid disorders: galactosaemia, maple syrup urine disease
- Urea cycle disorders
- Peroxisomal disorders (p. 96): Zellweger's syndrome, neonatal adrenoleucodystrophy
- Mitochondrial disorders (p. 96): Leigh's disease
- Ketotic and non-ketotic hyperglycinaemia (p. 94)
- Sulphite oxidase deficiency

BOX 28.24 Inherited metabolic disorders with onset under 2 years (see also Ch. 34)

- Amino acid disorders: phenylketonuria (p. 97), homocystinuria
- Lysosomal disorders:
  - Sphingolipidoses (p. 96): GM1/GM2 gangliosidoses; Gaucher's (type II), Niemann–Pick (type A); metachromatic leucodystrophy, Krabbe's
  - Mucopolysaccharidoses (p. 96)
  - Mucolipidoses
  - Glycoproteinoses
- Neuronal ceroid lipofuscinoses
- Mitochondrial disorders (p. 22): Leigh's, Alpers', Menkes'
- Neuroaxonal dystrophy
- Lesch–Nyhan syndrome
- Rett's syndrome
- Alexander's disease (p. 23), Canavan's disease
- Pelizaeus–Merzbacher disease

BOX 28.25 Clinical patterns in childhood neurodegenerative conditions

White matter disease
- Spastic paralysis ± ataxia
- Loss of tendon reflexes
- Blindness + optic atrophy (normal retina)

Grey matter disease
- Seizures, myoclonus
- Dementia
- Blindness with retinal changes

Basic science

Lysosomes are cytoplasmic vesicles that contain enzymes responsible for degrading the products of cellular cata-bolism. When these enzymes are deficient, abnormal storage of material occurs. Each condition is associated with an enzyme deficiency (Table 28.6).

Table 28.6 Enzyme deficiencies associated with specific lysosomal disorders

Disorder	Enzyme
GM1	Beta-galactosidase
GM2	Hexosaminidase
Gaucher's	Glucocerebrosidase
Niemann–Pick	Sphingomyelinase
Metachromatic leucodystrophy	Arylsulphatase
Krabbe's leucodystrophy	Galactosylceramidase
Mucopolysaccharidoses	Multiple enzymes
Mucolipidoses	Multiple enzymes
Glycoproteinoses	Multiple enzymes

The neuronal ceroid lipofuscinoses are a group of genetically determined neurodegenerative disorders associated with the accumulation of autofluorescent lipopigment inclusions. Seizures, dementia and visual impairment are the prominent clinical features (Boxes 28.26 and 28.27).

The mitochondrial encephalomyopathies

These are a diverse group of disorders associated with defects in the oxidative metabolism of pyruvate or in the five respiratory chain complexes.

Leigh's disease

This is characterized clinically by the combination of hypotonia and regression, with nystagmus or ophthalmoplegia and abnormal breathing. There may be evidence of a raised CSF lactate concentration and abnormalities on MRI in the deep grey nuclei and brainstem.

Menkes' syndrome

This is an X-linked disorder of copper transport and metabolism, associated with early intractable seizures, dementia and abnormalities of scalp hair (sparse, poorly pigmented and wiry hair). Plasma copper concentrations and ceruloplasmin levels are decreased.

Lesch–Nyhan syndrome

This is an X-linked disorder caused by a deficiency of the enzyme hypoxanthine guanine phosphoribosyltransferase. It presents with motor delay followed by progressive limb rigidity, spasticity and chorea. Self-mutilation is a prominent feature and high uric acid levels are a marker.

Rett's syndrome

Rett's syndrome (see also p. 32) is an important cause of neurological regression in girls, with loss of language, gait ataxia and autistic features to begin with, followed by the loss of purposeful hand function associated with stereotypical hand movements (wringing and clasping). Breath-holding and hyperventilation may

BOX 28.26 Clinical syndromes associated with inherited metabolic disorders with onset before 2 years

Myoclonus and/or intractable seizures
- GM2 (Tay–Sachs)
- Neuronal ceroid lipofuscinoses (Batten's)
- Alpers'
- Menkes'

Macrocephaly spasticity
- Alexander's
- Canavan's
- GM2 late

Motor syndrome (can mimic cerebral palsy)
- Metachromatic leucodystrophy
- Krabbe's
- Pelizaeus–Merzbacher
- Leigh's
- Lesch–Nyhan
- Neuroaxonal dystrophy

Hurler's phenotype
- Mucopolysaccharidoses
- Mucolipidoses
- Glycoproteinoses

Isolated cognitive regression
- Phenylketonuria
- Homocystinuria
- Maple syrup urine disease
- Rett's syndrome (girls)

Visceromegaly
- GM1/GM2
- Gaucher's
- Niemann–Pick

BOX 28.27 Inherited metabolic disorders with onset after 2 years

- Lysosomal enzyme disorders:
  - Mucopolysaccharidoses
  - Glycoproteinoses
  - Sphingolipidoses:
      GM2 gangliosidoses (juvenile Tay–Sachs)
      Gaucher's (type III)
      Niemann–Pick (type C)
      Metachromatic leucodystrophy (late onset)
      Krabbe's (late onset)
  - Neuronal ceroid lipofuscinoses (late infantile, juvenile)
- Huntington's disease
- Adrenoleucodystrophy
- Alexander's disease
- Mitochondrial

be prominent features and there is a fall-off in head growth with microcephaly. Diagnosis is confirmed by evidence of a mutation on the *MECP2* gene on the X-chromosome present in 70–80% of cases. The late stages are characterized by spasticity, dystonia and scoliosis. Cognitive function is severely diminished. Treatment is supportive.

Alexander's disease

This is caused by a mutation in the gene for glial fibrillary acidic protein (GFAP), a component of the astrocyte intermediate filament structure, and is associated with the presence of Rosenthal fibres. Canavan's disease is caused by a deficiency of the enzyme aspartoacylase, leading to tissue accumulation of N-acetylaspartic acid. Measurement of this metabolite in urine is a good marker of the condition. Both conditions present clinically with hypotonia and megalencephaly, with evidence of a leucodystrophy on MRI.

Pelizaeus–Merzbacher syndrome

This is an X-linked dysmyelinating encephalopathy caused by a defect in a structural protein of the myelin sheath. It is associated with mutations in the *PLP1* gene. The clinical features include early hypotonia, evolving spasticity, intermittent head-bobbing, nystagmus and stridor.

Huntington's disease

This is an autosomal dominant disorder caused by an expanded trinucleotide repeat on chromosome 4. Symptoms begin before the age of 20 years in 10% and usually involve behavioural disturbance, cognitive decline, rigidity, lack of facial expression, and abnormal eye movements (oculomotor apraxia). Death usually occurs within 8 years of onset of symptoms.

Adrenoleucodystrophy

This is an X-linked recessive condition resulting in the accumulation of saturated very long chain fatty acids (VLCFAs) in all tissues of the body. The cerebral form of the disease usually has its onset between the ages of 5 and 10 years, with deterioration in behaviour and school work, followed by a disturbance of coordination and gait and a decline into a persistent vegetative state within 3 years of the onset of symptoms. CSF protein is increased and MRI reveals high-signal intensity in the periventricular white matter. Analysis of VLCFAs provides the definitive diagnosis. Bone marrow transplant has been shown to be beneficial in some isolated presymptomatic cases.

Macrocephaly

Basic science

Cerebrospinal fluid (CSF) is produced in the choroid plexus of the lateral, third and fourth ventricles. From the lateral ventricles it flows through the foramen of Munro to the third ventricle, and into the fourth ventricle via the aqueduct of Sylvius. From there it flows through the foramina of Luschka and Magendie into the basal cisterns, out over the surface of the brain and down the spinal cord. It is reabsorbed into the blood stream in the superior sagittal sinus through the arachnoid villi. This circulation occurs 6–7 times per day.

Problem-orientated topic:

the child with a large head

Matthew is referred by his GP at the age of 8 months because of concerns about the size of his head. Having started on the 50th centile, his occipito-frontal head circumference is now above the 98th centile. His anterior fontanelle is large and pulsatile but not bulging. He is well and appears to be developing normally. His height and weight are on the 50th centile.

Q1. What is the likely cause of this boy's macrocephaly?

Q2. What investigations would you undertake?

Q1. What is the likely cause of this boy's macrocephaly? (Box 28.28)

This is a common clinical scenario. The child is well and does not have symptoms or signs of raised intracranial pressure. The most helpful assessment is measurement of the parents' head circumferences, as the likely aetiology is benign familial macrocephaly. This is commonly associated with a benign enlargement of the subarachnoid spaces (communicating hydrocephalus) in the first 2 years of life.

BOX 28.28 Causes of macrocephaly in childhood

- Large baby
- Benign familial macrocephaly
- Hydrocephalus
- Subdural effusions
- Megaloencephaly:
  - Anatomical — Soto's, Weaver's, neurocutaneous syndromes
  - Metabolic — Alexander's, Canavan's, glutaric aciduria type 1, storage disorders, leucodystrophies
- Skull vault disorders

BOX 28.29 Causes of hydrocephalus

Communicating hydrocephalus

- Benign enlargement of subarachnoid spaces (Fig. 28.6)
- Post-haemorrhagic
- Post-meningitic
- Achondroplasia
- Sagittal sinus thrombosis
- Venous obstruction

Non-communicating hydrocephalus

- Aqueduct stenosis: genetic/acquired
- Dandy–Walker malformation
- Arnold–Chiari malformation
- Mass lesions: tumour, haematoma, abscess, vein of Galen malformation

BOX 28.30 Clinical features of hydrocephalus with raised intracranial pressure

Infant

- Increase in the rate of head growth
- Macrocephaly
- Splaying of the sutures
- Tense anterior fontanelle
- Dilated scalp veins
- Vertical gaze paresis (sun-setting eyes)

Older child

- More typical features of raised intracranial pressure
- Headache, vomiting, irritability
- Papilloedema and bilateral abducens paresis
- Lower limb spasticity and ataxia

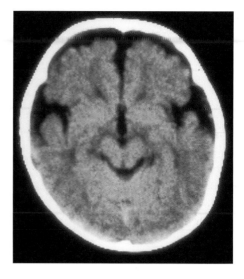

Fig. 28.6 CT scan showing benign external hydrocephalus

neonates, repeated aspiration of CSF may be helpful as a temporary measure.

Craniosynostosis

Craniosynostosis (Table 28.7) is a skull vault abnormality associated with premature closure of one or more cranial sutures. If multiple sutures are involved, raised intracranial pressure is a complication. Skull X-ray reveals increased density along the prematurely fused suture. Referral should be made to a craniofacial surgeon.

Spina bifida

Q2. What investigations would you undertake?

Hydrocephalus (Boxes 28.29 and 28.30)
Obstruction of CSF flow or failure of CSF reabsorption gives rise to hydrocephalus (an excess of CSF in the ventricular system). Non-communicating hydrocephalus results from obstruction in the ventricular system at a point at or above the level of the fourth ventricular outflow. Communicating hydrocephalus occurs as a result of failure to reabsorb CSF.

Treatment of hydrocephalus associated with raised intracranial pressure requires placement of a shunt from one of the ventricles to the peritoneum (ventriculoperitoneal shunt). The catheter in the peritoneum is coiled to allow for growth. Shunt drainage can become ineffective because of infection (typically *Staphylococcus aureus*), obstruction or breakage. In cases where surgery is not possible or must be delayed, e.g. in premature

Problem-orientated topic:

the child with spina bifida

You are asked to see a term infant in the neonatal unit who has just been born. She has a congenital anomaly of her back with a large defect in the spinal column and is not moving her legs. She has evidence on examination of a myelomeningocele at L3 and has a flaccid paraparesis. Her parents have a number of questions.

Q1. How common is this and what are the risk factors?

Q2. What other associated problems should be investigated?

Q3. What is the likelihood of future disability?

Q4. What are the important points of management?

Table 28.7 **Head shapes associated with suture synostosis**

Head shape	Suture involved
Scaphocephaly	Sagittal suture
Brachycephaly	Both coronal sutures
Plagiocephaly	One coronal or lambdoid suture
Trigonocephaly	Metopic suture
Oxencephaly	All sutures

BOX 28.31 Risk factors for neural tube defects

- Maternal diabetes
- Sodium valproate in pregnancy
- Previously affected child (recurrence risk = 5%)

BOX 28.32 Types of neural tube defect

- Anencephaly
- Encephalocele
- Meningocele
- Myelomeningocele

Q1. How common is this and what are the risk factors? (Boxes 28.31 and 28.32)

The incidence of neural tube defects (NTDs) varies widely; in continental Europe it is about 1/1000 live births, compared with 0.5/1000 in the USA. The causes of NTDs are multifactorial, with both genetic and environmental factors being important. The use of preconceptual supplementary folic acid (0.4 mg/day) reduces the risk by 70%.

An encephalocele is a sac-like protrusion of brain and meninges through a midline skull defect anywhere from between the nose and forehead to the back of the skull, and is often associated with other cerebral malformations or craniofacial abnormalities. Posterior defects are more common. Small frontal encephaloceles in the nasal or forehead regions can go unnoticed and may present with rhinorrhoea and/or intracranial infection. Treatment of the defect is surgical.

A meningocele is the protrusion of meninges and CSF through a vertebral defect without neural tissue. It is covered by skin and usually has a good prognosis following surgery. A myelomeningocele is a complex NTD with involvement of the spinal cord, meninges, nerve roots, vertebral bodies and overlying skin. Neural tissue develops abnormally (myelodysplasia) and results in neurological deficits that correspond to the level of the lesion. There may be additional developmental anomalies in the brain and there is a strong association with the Arnold–Chiari type II malformation, characterized by cerebellar hypoplasia and associated displacement of the hindbrain through the foramen magnum. The result is an obstruction of CSF flow causing hydrocephalus in 90% of children with a myelomeningocele.

Q2. What other associated problems should be investigated?

See Box 28.33.

Q3. What is the likelihood of future disability? (Table 28.8)

Most infants will have surgery to repair the skin defect soon after birth. The majority will have a neuropathic bladder and are usually incontinent, with impaired emptying and high voiding pressures. Recurrent urinary tract infections, impaired renal function and hypertension are potential complications. Neuropathic bowel with

---

BOX 28.33 Anomalies associated with neural tube defects

- Cerebral malformations
- Brainstem dysfunction
- Hydrocephalus
- Neurological deficits
- Cardiac malformations
- Genitourinary tract malformations
- Orthopaedic deformities

Table 28.8 Neurological outcomes of myelomeningocele

Type	Level	Effect
Non-ambulant	Low thoracic/high lumbar	Flaccid complete lower limb paresis
		Absent reflexes and sensation
		Retained upper limb movement
		Normal head/neck movement
		Varying truncal control
	High lumbar (L1–L3)	Hip flexion/adduction preserved
		Hip extension/abduction absent
		No knee or ankle movements
Usually ambulant	Low lumbar (L3 or lower)	Hip/knee movements present but variable strength
		Ankle movement variable

constipation and faecal impaction may also be a problem. Cognitive problems occur in 25% of children with myelomeningocele, and up to 15% of children with ventriculoperitoneal shunts for hydrocephalus develop epilepsy.

The spinal cord lesion leads to paraplegia, the severity of which is dependent on the level of the lesion (Table 28.8). Children with thoracic or high lumbar lesions will be confined to a wheelchair, with no lower limb function. Children with low lumbar or sacral lesions may walk with the assistance of devices such as splints and walking aids. Many children develop joint contractures and scoliosis.

Q4. What are the important points of management?

- A multidisciplinary team approach
- Closure of skin defect
- Shunt insertion for associated hydrocephalus
- Surveillance for brainstem dysfunction
- Orthopaedic intervention
- Management of neuropathic bladder/bowel.

References

Kirkham FJ 1999 Stroke in childhood. Archives of Disease in Childhood 81:85–89

Roger J, Bureau M, Dravet C et al 2005 Epileptic syndromes in infancy, childhood and adolescence, 4th edn. John Libbey Eurotext

Volpe JJ 2001 Neurology of the newborn. W.B. Saunders, Philadelphia

Valerie A. Harpin   Susan M. Gentle

Neurodevelopmental disability

29

LEARNING OUTCOMES

By the end of this chapter you should:

- Understand the causes of learning disability, attention deficit/hyperactivity disorder (ADHD), cerebral palsy and communication disorders
- Understand the principles of management of learning disability, ADHD, cerebral palsy and the different types of language impairment and communication disorder
- Understand the concept of the autistic spectrum and what it includes.

You should also take the opportunity to ensure that:

- You can make an initial assessment of a child with learning difficulties, ADHD, delayed walking and cerebral palsy, and delayed language development
- You are aware of the different ways of assessing of language impairment and communication disorder
- You are aware of appropriate management.

MODULE SIX

Introduction

The prevalence of physical and multiple disabilities in children is estimated to be approximately 10–20 per 1000. Chapter 18 describes the concepts and causes of disability, and emphasizes that its management requires a multidisciplinary approach, often focused on a Child Development Centre. This chapter concentrates on the causes, investigation and management of common specific neurodisabilities of childhood. Although each disability is considered separately, multiple disabilities in the same child are common.

Learning disability

Problem-orientated topic:

the slow learning child

Thomas is a 3-year-old boy who is referred because of suspected developmental delay. His vision and hearing are normal. There is no family history of learning disability, fits or serious illness. His parents are not

Continued overleaf

related. Thomas was born at term weighing 3.5 kg, following a normal pregnancy. He had no neonatal problems. There is no relevant past medical history and no evidence of fits. He smiled at 8 weeks, sat by 8 months and walked at 15 months. He has had no feeding difficulties. His early social interaction was normal. On examination he is not dysmorphic. His head circumference is on the 70% centile. He has no neurocutaneous lesions; his gait, fundi and deep-tendon reflexes are normal, and his plantar reflexes are down-going. Arm and leg tone is normal and symmetrical. He shows good eye contact, early turn-taking and uses his index finger to point for a drink or food. The only word he uses is 'Mum', with some other early babble.

Q1. What is the definition of learning disability?

Q2. How do you make the diagnosis of learning disability?

Q3. What are the pros and cons of investigating a child with a learning disability?

Q4. What investigations would you perform, if any?

Q5. How would you manage this child and family?

Q1. What is the definition of learning disability?

A child or young person has a learning disability if he or she has 'a difficulty in learning than the majority of children of the same age' (Box 29.1).

The International Statistical Classification of Diseases–10th revision (ICD-10) defines it as 'a condition of arrested or incomplete development of the mind which is especially characterized by impairment of skills manifested during the developmental period contributing to the overall level of intelligence, i.e. cognitive, motor and social abilities'. This is not a helpful definition for parents.

For research and study it is sometimes necessary to have a definition that can be measured. Average intelligence quotient (IQ) is 100, with a standard deviation (SD) of 15. Learning disability may then be defined as > 2 SD below the mean or the ICD-10 definitions:

- Mild   IQ 50–69
- Moderate   IQ 35–49
- Severe   IQ 20–34
- Profound   IQ < 20.

In practice, people in the UK often use the definitions shown in Table 29.1.

BOX 29.1 Definitions in learning disability

In the UK, the term 'learning disability' is currently used in preference to 'mental subnormality' or 'mental retardation', whereas in the USA the term 'learning disability' means 'specific learning disability' and 'mental retardation' is still the term used to denote 'general learning difficulties'.

Table 29.1 UK definitions and incidence

Definition	IQ	Incidence (per 1000)	Cause identified*
Mild/moderate	50–70	5	68%
Severe	< 50	3.8	96%
Severe (developing countries)		9.3	

* This is higher, however, than in routine clinical practice (Whiting K 2001 Investigating the child with learning difficulty. Current Paediatrics 11:240–247).

We will use the abbreviations 'SLD' for severe learning disability and 'MLD' for mild/moderate learning disability.

Some psychometric tests

The following two tests are commonly used by paediatricians. Both require training and special equipment:

- *Griffiths*. This has been standardized on 0–8-year-old British children but relies on parental reporting; many items are timed. It has recently been updated.
- *Bayley II*. This scale (age range 0–42 months) is used to assess developmental age and has been standardized on American children.

Q2. How do you make the diagnosis of learning disability? (Box 29.2)

Mild/moderate learning disability

While children with SLD often have associated problems such as cerebral palsy, those with MLD often have no other problems. Many will be the tail-end of the normal distribution; others will have learning difficulties as a result of environmental factors (lack of early opportunities or iron deficiency) and be functioning below their genetic potential; some will have an identifiable remediable cause such as vision or hearing problems; some will have an intrinsic problem such as neurofibromatosis or a chromosome abnormality.

BOX 29.2 A point to remember

History and examination are the main ways in which a diagnosis is made. Investigations are most useful in confirming or clarifying a diagnosis.

All children with significant learning difficulties should have at least some paediatric assessment to contribute to identification of special educational needs.

When seeing a child referred from school with MLD enquire about:

- History
- Birth
- Progress from birth
- Family
- Other concerns
- Hearing and vision
- Behaviour
- Poor general health
- Time off school, leading to under-achievement
- Whether children are working at their best in school
- Epilepsy (absences, minor status).

Look for dysmorphism or other clues to aetiology.

Severe learning disability

It is important to ask or examine for:

- Genetic abnormalities:
  – Dysmorphism
  – Malformations
- Metabolic defects:
  – Failure to thrive
  – Hypotonia
  – Consanguinity
  – Recurrent unexplained illness (especially anorexia and vomiting)
  – Loss of skills
  – Coarse facies
  – Ocular abnormalities
  – Macro- or microcephaly
  – Family history of unexplained illness or death
- Brain malformation:
  – Abnormal skull
  – Focal deficit
  – Loss of skills
  – Micro- or macrocephaly
  – Seizures
  – Visual abnormality.

Syndromes

These are more likely in children with SLD but should be considered in all children with learning difficulties. In children with SLD, about one-quarter have a chromosomal disorder; 80–90% of these have Down's syndrome. The next most common disorder is fragile X syndrome (p. 32).

There are now over 2000 syndromes and the number continues to increase. From a practical day-to-day perspective they fall into two broad groups: the more common or easily recognized syndromes, such as Down's, Edwards' and Sturge–Weber; and others with a number of abnormal features not immediately recognizable as a syndrome but in whom it is possible to make a diagnosis.

 http://www.ncbi.nlm.nih.gov/Omim/

OMIM (Online Mendelian Inheritance in Man) dysmorphology database

Developmental regression

If there is progressive loss of skills (Ch. 28) it is important to consider:

- Hydrocephalus
- Poorly controlled epilepsy
- Metabolic disorder/neurodegenerative disorder
- Rett's disease
- Infection, particularly in an immunocompromised host (e.g. AIDS)
- Vascular problem, e.g. repeated minor strokes from moyamoya or sickle cell disease; malformations causing vascular 'steal'.

True regression can be hard to ascertain because development is taking place at the same time. All children, and particularly those with a learning disability, will sometimes learn something new and then appear to forget it for a while.

Reasons to ask for further assessment

- To obtain an objective assessment of abilities
- To identify strengths and weaknesses that may help with management
- To assess progress
- For the court, such as in cases of neglect
- For research.

Q3. What are the pros and cons of investigating a child with a learning disability?

Pros

- Treatable cause, e.g. hypothyroidism
- Genetic counselling may be useful
- For prognosis
- The parents may be helped by knowing the cause.

Cons

- False positives and false negatives
- Pain and complications of investigations (especially anaesthesia)
- Financial cost.

Q4. What investigations would you perform, if any? (Box 29.3)

Investigations should be performed on the basis of clues from the history and examination. The following investigations may be indicated, particularly in children with SLD:

- Chromosome analysis
- Brain imaging
- Metabolic investigations.

Q5. How would you manage this child and family?

The neurodevelopmental paediatrician's role is:

- *Establishing whether there is a learning disability* (usually done with a multidisciplinary team). In younger children it is the health services that are primarily involved in this. In older children it is primarily school-based.
- *Identifying the cause*. This may be from the history and examination or may include investigation.
- *Referral to other professionals as appropriate*. These may include:
  - Speech and language therapy (SLT), occupational therapy (OT), physiotherapy
  - Psychology
  - Other medical specialties
  - Education
  - Social services.
- *Looking for and managing associated difficulties*. There may be problems with hearing, vision, motor function, behaviour or epilepsy. Some are specific, e.g. hypothyroidism in Down's syndrome.
- *Counselling parents*. The neurodevelopmental paediatrician may be the initial person to do this, although others may take up the role later.
- *Liaison with education*.
- *Explanation to child and parents of the likely effects of the disabilities*.
- *Responding to concerns*.

In metabolic disorders some pharmacological treatments may have an effect on progress. This is a very specialized area and one that is constantly changing, but it is a good reason for trying to make a specific diagnosis.

Down's syndrome (Tables 29.2 and 29.3)

Incidence is approximately 1 in 1000 live births. The risk of having a child with Down's syndrome increases with maternal age, so that for a mother in her twenties the risk is less than 1 in 1000, but greater than 1 in 100 in mothers over 40. However, most babies are born to mothers in their twenties and thirties.

Almost everyone can recognize a child or adult with Down's syndrome. One of the problems with a well-recognized syndrome is that people can have preconceived ideas about what a child with Down's syndrome is like. Children with Down's syndrome can be as different from each other as any other group of children in the population. Some children are able to follow a mainstream curriculum and achieve GCSE passes. Others may never develop language. Some have very limited exercise tolerance, while others achieve sporting excellence.

Genetic types (see also Ch. 9)

Most are caused by non-disjunction in meiosis, resulting in an additional chromosome 21 (47 XY with additional chromosome 21). In 20–25% the extra chromosome is paternal. When Down's syndrome is caused by trisomy 21, the recurrence risk is about double that of a woman of the same age without a previous history.

Three to four percent result from translocation of material from chromosome 21 on to another chromosome. A parent may often have a balanced translocation (one of their chromosome 21s is attached to another chromosome), but this causes no problem because they have a normal total amount of chromosome material. However, this tagged-on chromosome may be present in a gamete in addition to a normal chromosome 21, giving rise to extra chromosome material in the offspring. There is a greatly increased risk of a couple having a second affected child.

Mosaicism accounts for 2–6% and such individuals are usually affected to a lesser degree.

Diagnosis

If the diagnosis is not made on antenatal screening, it is usually made early in the neonatal period by recognition of the typical features of Down's syndrome. It may be a midwife, a paediatrician or the parents who first recognize that there is a problem with the baby. There is strong evidence from parents to suggest that disclosure should be made as soon as the diagnosis is suspected, preferably with both parents present. The diagnosis is confirmed by chromosome analysis.

Management

Down's syndrome has possible effects on all body systems. Management of children therefore needs

Table 29.2 Down's syndrome

Feature	Comments

Facial features
    Prominent epicanthic folds
    Flat nasal bridge
    Small nose
    Protrusion of tongue
	
	This is not a large tongue but poor tone

Brachycephaly	
Wide hands, short fingers Distal tri-radius, clinodactyly Single palmar crease Wide gap between first and second toes	 Simian crease may be present in normal individuals
Brushfield spots	Spots on iris
Fine soft hair Dry, hyperkeratotic skin Other skin problems	Can have alopecia Helped by simple emulsifying cream and appropriate bath oil Such as vitiligo, papular erythema, mottled skin (cutis marmorata)
Hypotonia	Prominent in the neonatal period. Influences motor development. May result in joint dislocation
Orthopaedic problems	Atlanto-axial instability (see below) Hip dysplasia/dislocation Dislocation/displacement of other joints
Cardiac problems	See below
Bowel problems	Duodenal atresia presents neonatally Also look out for constipation (Hirschsprung's disease, hypothyroidism) and malabsorption
Infections	More prone to infections, e.g. bacterial pneumonia, otitis media
Hypothyroidism	Higher incidence of autoimmune hypothyroidism; important to screen for this
Leukaemia	About a 10–20-fold increase. Children may cope badly with intensive treatment
Low fertility	Females are fertile Males often have undescended testes and hypogonadism
Behaviour difficulties	Management should be appropriate to developmental age
Poor growth and weight problems	Frequently poor feeders in infancy. Later a tendency to become overweight and attention to diet and activity levels is needed N.B. Use growth charts for children with Down's syndrome
Presenile dementia	Important for long-term support, as carers may be elderly with an affected young adult

Table 29.3 Average milestones for children with Down's syndrome

Milestone	Mean age	Range
Sitting	13 months	6–30 months
Standing	22 months	9–48 months
Walking	30 months	12–60 months
Single words	34 months	12–72 months

40% of children with Down's syndrome are able to learn to read

a multidisciplinary approach. Of the many other potential problems in a child with Down's syndrome, there are two that deserve particular mention:

- *Congenital heart disease*. This occurs in 40–50% of babies with Down's syndrome. All newborn babies should be evaluated, with observation (of feeding etc.), physical examination, electrocardiogram (ECG), chest X-ray (CXR) and echocardiogram.

Atrioventricular (AV) canal defects (endocardial cushion defects) occur very specifically in children with Down's syndrome (p. 215). Any newborn found to have an AV canal defect should have chromosomal analysis.

Patent ductus arteriosus (PDA), ventricular septal defect (VSD) and atrial septal defect (ASD) are also more common in children with Down's syndrome.

Damage to pulmonary vasculature with irreversible pulmonary hypertension can occur much earlier in children with Down's syndrome than expected from the size of the shunt alone. PDA, ASD, VSD and AV canal defects should be considered for early surgical intervention.

- *Atlanto-axial instability*. Routine cervical spine X-ray used to be recommended but review of X-rays of the same child taken minutes apart could give rise to completely different advice. Spinal cord damage in Down's syndrome is rare and usually insidious rather than acute. It is important not to frighten parents and cause children to be wrapped in cotton wool and prevented from joining in appropriate activities; however, parents do need relevant information to enable them to recognize symptoms that should be reported. The three most common symptoms are:

- Deterioration/change in gait or manipulation skills
- Neck pain/stiffness
- Difficulties with sphincter control.

Children with any of these should be investigated urgently.

Advice should be given to other regular carers of children with Down's syndrome and included in medical advice for assessment of special educational needs.

 http://www.dsmig.org.uk

Guidelines on surveillance for people with Down's syndrome

Fragile X syndrome

This is probably the second most common known syndromic cause of global learning disability (about 1 in 1360 males and 1 in 2000 females; a further 1 in 1000 females are asymptomatic carriers). The degree varies from mild to severe in boys, and mild to moderate in girls. The defect in fragile X is now known to be an expansion in a specific DNA triplet repeat (CGG) on the X chromosome.

Physical features include:

- Long face and slightly increased head circumference
- Macrognathia
- Large protuberant ears
- Flattened nasal bridge
- Abnormal dermatoglyphics
- Macro-orchidism
- Infantile hypotonia
- Connective tissue dysplasia (joint laxity and soft velvety skin)
- Aortic dilatation and mitral valve prolapse
- Recurrent otitis media
- Failure to thrive in infancy
- Tonic–clonic or partial epilepsy, temporal spikes on electroencephalogram (EEG)
- MRI scan abnormalities (especially cerebellum).

Psychological features include:

- Variable intellectual impairment
- Language delay
- Social impairments, such as those seen in autism
- Attention and concentration difficulties.

Features are very variable and some are only evident in adolescent or adult life. Clinical diagnosis in a young child is difficult.

Families need careful genetic advice.

Other sex chromosome abnormalities in which learning disability may occur are discussed in Chapter 9.

Neurocutaneous syndromes

These may also cause learning disability (pp. 8–10).

Rett's syndrome

This presents as a neurodegenerative disorder but is probably a neurodevelopmental disorder. It is sometimes classified with the pervasive development disorders such as autism. Genetic advances in Rett's have been rapid in recent years. Milder cases and cases in boys are being described. It constitutes about 10% of SLD in girls.

Specific learning difficulties

The Education Code of Practice defines children as having specific learning difficulties when they have 'significantly' more difficulty in a specific area than most children of the same age that is not due to general learning disabilities.

ICD and DSM (*Diagnostic and Statistical Manual of Mental Disorders*) definitions depend on the child having a normal IQ and no other problems, but there is no reason why a child with generalized learning difficulties cannot have specific difficulties in one particular area, over and above their general level of difficulty.

Specific reading disorder

The term 'dyslexia' is used, but very loosely, for a wide variety of difficulties at school.

Writing disorder

There is a lot of overlap between reading and writing problems (dysgraphia).

Mathematics disorder (dyscalculia)

Incidence is probably similar to dyslexia and dysgraphia but there are interesting differences:

- Dyscalculia is seen equally in boys and girls (though recent work suggests that dyslexia may also be equally represented).

- It is seen more in fragile X carriers, Turner's syndrome, phenylketonuria (PKU) and ADHD.
- It is the most common learning difficulty in epilepsy.

Developmental coordination disorder (DCD)

Currently, this is the term used most commonly for children with motor coordination problems. A number of conditions can present with clumsiness other than DCD and these need to be excluded because management is different. Evidence of deterioration should be sought at presentation and at reviews.

Differential diagnosis
- Muscular dystrophies
- Cerebral palsies
- Brain tumours
- Brain injury
- Hydrocephalus
- Ataxias, such as Friedreich's ataxia (p. 14)
- Metabolic disorders
- Polyneuropathies
- Seizure disorder (p. 5)
- Vestibular disease
- Tremors and other involuntary movements.

History, examination and, if appropriate, investigation should exclude these diagnoses.

Presentation
This is variable and depends on the age of the child, though most patients do not present until school age. There is a mixture of gross and fine motor problems.

Gross motor problems include:
- Awkward gait, ungainly running
- Falling a lot
- Bumping into things
- Poor balance
- Poor balancing on one leg, inability to hop
- Slow (or failure of) learning to ride a bike
- Difficulty learning to swim
- Poor at catching, throwing, batting a ball.

Fine motor problems include:
- Difficulty dressing (clothes on the wrong way round or in the wrong order, difficulty with buttons and zips)
- Feeding messy; difficulty using a knife and fork
- Poor at building with bricks, jigsaws, drawing
- Poor pencil control for writing
- Difficulty using scissors and rulers.

Secondary problems include:
- Behaviour problems
- Poor self-esteem
- School failure.

When a child first presents at the clinic, a general paediatric and neurological assessment is needed, particularly to exclude other causes. There are no specific signs on neurological examination. Assessments specifically for DCD are best carried out by an occupational therapist, but the paediatrician should perform some initial screening.

Management
The mainstay of treatment is occupational therapy and physiotherapy. Management can be considered under the following headings:
- Explanation to child, parent and teacher
- Specific advice to parents and teachers to help in specific areas such as handwriting and dressing
- Improving self-esteem
- Specific therapy.

Problem-orientated topic:

disruptive behaviour (ADHD)

Connor is 7 years old. His mother, a single parent to Connor and his 4-year-old sister, has always struggled with his behaviour. Now things are going very badly at school. Connor has barely started to acquire literacy skills, although he seems a bright child. His disruptive behaviour in class is now such a problem that he is frequently sent home. His class teacher has advised his mother to seek a medical appointment. He was initially slow to acquire language but other milestones were normal. Last week he set fire to his bedroom carpet.

Q1. What is attention deficit/hyperactivity disorder?

Q2. How would you assess Connor for this condition?

Q3. How should you manage Connor and his family?

Q4. What is Connor's prognosis?

Q1. What is attention deficit/hyperactivity disorder?

This is not a new disorder explained by environmental pollutants or 'made up' to explain away naughty children. Frederick Still described children in 1902 with a 'defect in moral control', which almost certainly was ADHD.

Individuals with ADHD have:

- Inattention
- Hyperactivity
- Impulsivity: excessive in the context of age, sex and cognitive ability.

For a diagnosis to be made these symptoms should be:

- Present in more than one situation
- Present before the age of 6/7 years
- Impairing the child's educational or social functioning.

Inattention

There is poor regulation of attention and this is manifest particularly in difficult, imposed tasks that are not immediately rewarding. A child may attend to a video game or watch a TV programme with sustained attention but be unable to concentrate in school.

Hyperactivity

This is manifest differently at different ages:

- The preschool child will rush around, jumping and climbing noisily and being unable to settle in play.
- The school-age child may be fidgety, squirming and having difficulty remaining seated.
- The adolescent is restless, with foot-tapping and twiddling, and is unable to sit quietly.

Impulsivity

Impulsivity means not thinking before acting; it often results in getting into trouble for being cheeky or reckless. The child may have frequent accidents.

Secondary problems

Most children have secondary problems, including:

- Poor self-esteem
- Poor peer relationships
- Poor relationship with parents
- Sleep/wake problems
- Dietary problems (will not settle to eat).

Epidemiology (Table 29.4)

ADHD is almost certainly still under-diagnosed in parts of the UK, depending on where the child lives. All studies show a predominance of boys, but this may be over-estimated because boys show more obvious aggressive behaviour and girls have more inattention.

The underlying problem

This appears to be an executive function deficit. Executive functions include:

- Self-regulation
- Sequencing of behaviour
- Flexibility in response
- Response inhibition
- Planning
- Organization.

Pathology

Development of the frontal lobes is relatively late and myelination is not complete until adolescence. Neuroimaging studies have been inconsistent but the frontal cortex and its connections, as well as intracerebral connections via the corpus callosum, have abnormal activity. There may be differences in brain volume and size of the cerebellum. Functional magnetic resonance imaging (MRI) shows diffuse and decreased activity when individuals with ADHD undertake tasks requiring concentration. There is abnormal handling of noradrenaline (norepinephrine) and dopamine in the brain. This theory is supported by response to treatment with drugs affecting these neurotransmitters.

Aetiology

- *Genetics.* Genetics is the major factor governing whether or not a child has ADHD. It has been estimated that there is between 54% and 98% heritability.
- *Environment.* This also plays a part, particularly maternal depression and social disadvantage. It is likely that there is an interplay of genetics and environment, with environmental factors maintaining or exacerbating ADHD rather than causing it.
- *Central nervous system damage.* ADHD is also more frequent following:
  - Perinatal problems and prematurity
  - Antenatal insults, such as fetal alcohol syndrome or maternal smoking
  - Head injury, especially frontal lobe damage
  - Encephalitis and meningitis
  - Hypoxic episodes, such as drowning and strangling
  - Cerebrovascular accidents
  - Chronic neurological illness, such as epilepsy, metabolic problems (e.g. PKU)
  - Medical treatments, such as cerebral irradiation, anticonvulsants
  - Certain conditions such as Williams' syndrome, hypothyroidism, tuberous sclerosis, XYY, XXY and fragile X syndrome.

Table 29.4 **Epidemiology of ADHD**

Population	Incidence
UK (inner city)	1.5% of 7-year-olds
UK (general)	0.5–1% (hyperkinetic) 3–7% ADHD

Q2. How would you assess Connor for this condition?

Diagnosis is made by assessing information from a variety of sources. This is time-consuming and more than one clinic visit is usually needed.

History

- Current concerns, with specific examples, onset of problems and situation
- Antenatal and perinatal history for possible risk factors
- Early development: babies may be hyperactive with sleep problems, feeding difficulties, colic, waking early
- Medical problems for risk factors and differential diagnosis
- Educational problems for difficulties in different environments
- Relationships with parents and peers
- Family history
- Social situation, looking for other causes of difficulties
- Possible comorbidities (see below).

Examination

- Physical and neurological examination for associated problems (e.g. clumsiness), other problems (e.g. hearing, vision) and other diagnoses putting the child at risk (e.g. dysmorphism, tuberous sclerosis)
- Mental state looking for poor self-esteem, depression, anxiety
- Developmental assessment: behaviour inappropriate for developmental age.

    Observation in different settings is vital:
- During the initial assessment
- In school/playground/nursery/playgroup
- At home (parental report may be adequate).

    Structured questionnaires, e.g. Conner's Scales, play an important role in the screening and diagnosis of ADHD.
    Psychometric testing is helpful in identifying those children whose primary problem is a learning difficulty and comorbid specific learning difficulties.

Differential diagnosis

- Physical illness
- Drugs (either prescribed or of abuse)
- Attachment difficulties
- Social issues (e.g. family break-up)
- Child abuse (especially if change in behaviour)
- Depression/anxiety
- Hearing problems

- Unrealistic expectations on the part of parents or teachers
- Poor parenting
- Bullying
- Bored bright child
- Learning difficulties
- Sleep problems
- Conduct disorder.

Investigations

These are rarely indicated but you may need to exclude other causes of hyperactivity or inattention, such as hearing loss, epilepsy, thyroid disorders, side-effects of drugs:

- Test chromosomes if the child is unusually tall (XYY) or has learning difficulties (fragile X) or dysmorphism.
- Order an EEG if there is suspicion of subclinical epilepsy or absence epilepsy (poor concentration rarely is absence epilepsy).

Comorbidities

Comorbidity appears to be the rule rather than the exception in ADHD. The common additional problems are:

- Reduced cognitive ability (IQ on average is 5–15 points lower)
- Specific learning difficulties (particularly in reading)
- Delayed language development and poor language skills
- Developmental coordination difficulties (DCD)
- Oppositional/defiant disorder and conduct disorder (ODD/CD)
- Mood disorders (anxiety, depression)
- Obsessive–compulsive disorders (OCD)
- Tourette's syndrome
- Autistic spectrum disorders.

    It is important to identify these to optimize treatment.

Q3. How should you manage Connor and his family?

Information is an important aspect of management. Making the diagnosis and making this known to all involved may, in itself, help the child, parent and teachers to cope with the ADHD:

- Oral and written information should be made available.
- The child should be informed as well as the parents.
- Teachers should be informed about the diagnosis and, if necessary, about what it means.

Support groups

These can be very helpful to parents and child.

Educational measures

Simple suggestions can be very helpful such as:
- Having the child sit near the teacher
- Removing distractions where possible
- Clear, frequent and small rewards and discipline
- Working alone or in small groups
- Addressing any learning difficulties.

Behaviour modification

Positive reinforcement is very important. Children with ADHD often have low self-esteem. Children respond best to a well-structured, predictable environment where expectations and rules are clear and consistent, and consequences are set down ahead of time and delivered immediately.

Medication

Medication is the single most effective approach in severe ADHD.

Stimulant medications (methylphenidate, dexamphetamine) affect the dopamine pathways in the brain but the exact mechanism of action is unclear. They may stimulate areas of the brain that are not functioning properly. They do not affect the underlying pathology but control some symptoms, so that behavioural management can be more effective, school work can progress and social relationships can develop better. They work best in controlling hyperactivity and impulsivity but are less effective in controlling inattention. Methylphenidate, the most frequently used medication, is usually started at a dose of 2.5–5 mg twice or three times a day, increasing by 2.5–5 mg weekly until the desired effect is achieved. A maximum of 20 mg per dose, or 45–60 mg per day, should be used. If there is no effect after 3 weeks at maximum dose, it should be stopped.

Sustained-release products are now available. These have a lower incidence of side-effects and, as they are long-acting, do not need to be given in school.

Between 60 and 80% of children are helped by stimulant medication. Side-effects occur but are not usually severe and include:
- Stomach ache and headache
- Decreased appetite
- Sleep disturbance
- Cardiovascular effects (blood pressure should be checked before starting treatment and at follow-up)
- Unhappiness/withdrawal
- Growth suppression (0.5–1.0 cm if treatment is continued throughout puberty)

- Rebound behaviour difficulties
- Tics, although it is not certain that these are a true side-effect or constitute a coexistent tic disorder
- Marrow aplasia (very rare).

Atomoxetine is a non-stimulant selective noradrenergic reuptake inhibitor, which was licensed for use in ADHD in the UK in 2004. Research suggests that it has a significant effect in around 70% of individuals with ADHD. It is used as a once- or twice-daily medication (and therefore does not need to be given in school). Side-effects may include somnolence, gastrointestinal effects and rarely liver problems.

 http://www.nice.org.uk//page.aspx?o=TA098guidance

Diet

Diet has long been suggested as an important cause of behaviour problems. Additives in the diet worsen hyperactivity but do not cause ADHD. It is worth checking whether the parents have noticed any foods that cause deterioration in behaviour and removing them from the diet.

Sleep

Many children and young people with ADHD have poor sleep patterns and cannot usually stop themselves waking others when they are awake. It is seldom safe to leave such a child unattended for long and families are often very sleep-deprived. This may greatly limit their capacity to cope with their constantly active offspring in the daytime! Although stimulants may cause insomnia in some children, a teatime dose may actually help a child to get off to sleep by calming a racing mind. In other children, the use of melatonin to regulate sleep patterns and quality is very useful.

4. What is Connor's prognosis?

Some children continue to have difficulties in adult life. Various groups have reported similar findings, with approximately 30% within the normal range as adults, 50–60% continuing to have problems with concentration, impulsivity and social interaction, and 10–15% having significant psychiatric or antisocial problems (depressed, suicidal, drug and alcohol abuse, convictions for assault, armed robbery etc.).

The prognosis is best for those children with 'pure' ADHD and worse for those with severe symptoms, comorbidities, and poor family and educational support.

The cerebral palsies

Cerebral palsy (CP) is defined by the Oxford Register of Early Childhood Impairments as:

BOX 29.4 Exercise: terminology in cerebral palsy

Have a go at defining these commonly used terms:
- Tone
- Spasticity
- Ataxia
- Athetosis
- Chorea
- Dystonia

BOX 29.5 Feedback on terminology

- *Tone* is the resistance of a muscle to passive stretch (hypertonia — increased resistance, hypotonia — reduced resistance)
- *Spasticity* is a velocity-dependent increase in resistance to passive stretch. Spastic muscles are not necessarily hypertonic. The key is the velocity dependency; spasticity is an abnormal response to rapid stretch. Usual associated features are clonus, increased deep tendon reflexes and extensor plantar responses
- *Ataxia* is an abnormality in the smooth approach to an object, with wide-amplitude corrections during the movement. In relation to gait, ataxic means broad-based, poorly coordinated
- *Athetosis* is the characteristic of slow writhing movement, usually seen in the distal part of the limb during voluntary activity
- *Chorea* is rapid, high-amplitude, sudden involuntary movement
- *Dystonia* is abnormal tone, either high or low. It usually refers to abnormal sustained contractions of agonists and antagonists resulting in an unusual and abnormal posture, e.g. inversion of foot, retraction of shoulders etc.

A permanent impairment of voluntary movement or posture presumed to be due to permanent damage to the immature brain. Children with progressive disorders and those with profound hypotonia and no other neurological signs (often associated with severe intellectual delay) are excluded. It is an umbrella term which includes a heterogeneous group of conditions and can arise at any point during brain development.

There are three main types:
- *Spastic* CP, which can be divided into diplegia, hemiplegia and quadriplegia depending on areas affected
- *Ataxic* CP
- *Dyskinetic* CP.

Terminology

See Boxes 29.4 and 29.5.

Classification

CP refers to a group of disorders. Classification is based upon clinical descriptions of neurological signs. It is commonplace to find mixed patterns with one predominant aspect, e.g. hemiplegia with some involvement of the good side, diplegia with asymmetry in the upper limbs etc.:

- *Spastic diplegia.* Recent magnetic resonance studies show that the underlying lesion in most cases of spastic diplegia is periventricular leucomalacia (p. 367).
- *Spastic hemiplegia.* Spastic hemiplegia constitutes about 25% of all cases of CP. The cause is usually an infarction within the distribution of the middle cerebral artery (p. 367).
- *Total body involvement CP.* In these cases the brain pathology most commonly originates in the prenatal period and may be due to a variety of abnormalities such as primary cerebral dysgenesis (lissencephaly/pachygyria), early pregnancy infections (e.g. cytomegalovirus (CMV), toxoplasmosis), or vascular malformations and vascular accidents (e.g. hydranencephaly). *Spastic tetraplegia* with bilateral cerebral hemisphere infarction, sometimes with extensive cyst formation (multicystic encephalomalacia) and

severe learning difficulties, may occur as a result of brain injury in late third trimester. Prolonged partial asphyxia in a term infant may be the cause (p. 365). Acute profound asphyxia may develop in the third trimester as a consequence of antepartum haemorrhage, cord prolapse or uterine rupture and may lead to damage in the basal ganglia and thalami which may be confirmed on MR scanning. The clinical correlate is the later development of dyskinetic cerebral palsy, often with relatively preserved cognitive function. The contribution of perinatal asphyxia to the overall prevalence of CP is debatable, but most agree an estimate of about 10% of all cases.

Dyskinetic CP may also arise due to bilirubin encephalopathy in the neonatal period. These cases were more common in the past, but prevention and improved management of rhesus iso-immunization have resulted in a dramatic fall in the number of cases.

Ataxic CP (about 5% of CP) is mainly of prenatal origin. There may be strong familial patterns, with autosomal dominant, X-linked and autosomal recessive modes of inheritance. Sporadic cases are also seen. Children show ataxia, intention tremor and dyskinesia, usually before 2 years of age. Some may achieve independent walking by 4–6 years, although in these cases handwriting remains problematic and, in more severe cases, learning difficulties and seizures may complicate the presentation. About 30% show normal or borderline intellectual function. A magnetic resonance study of ataxic CP showed that over 50% were unclassifiable, 23% were genetic, and only 4% (3 cases) may have had a perinatal cause.

Epidemiology

Prevalence of the cerebral palsies is about 1.7–3 cases/1000 live births. There may have been a trend of increase in the overall prevalence of CP in children born in the 1970s and 1980s. The main area of increase has been in the most immature babies weighing under 1 kg. The reasons for this increase are unclear but probably relate to dramatic changes in survival of very immature infants.

Another important aspect of epidemiology is survival. Most children with CP now survive to adult life, even when disease is severe. This is having an impact on services for adults as well as children.

Problem-orientated topic:

delay in walking

Matthew is 18 months old and his mother is concerned that he is not yet walking. He is a bright, sociable child, who has several single words. He was born at 27 weeks' gestation and had a difficult neonatal course.

Q1. What questions would you ask to elucidate a cause?

Q2. What are the possible diagnoses?

Q3. What are the principles of management?

Q1. What questions would you ask to elucidate a cause?

An underlying cause may not be apparent, but the following should be considered in history-taking:

- Prenatal:
  - Genetic
  - Infection (e.g. CMV, rubella, chorioamnionitis)
  - Toxins (e.g. drugs)
  - Trauma
  - Nutritional ('placental insufficiency')
- Perinatal:
  - Prematurity (intraventricular haemorrhage/ periventricular haemorrhage/periventricular leucomalacia)

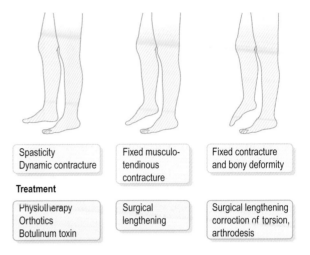

| Spasticity Dynamic contracture | Fixed musculo-tendinous contracture | Fixed contracture and bony deformity |

Treatment

| Physiotherapy Orthotics Botulinum toxin | Surgical lengthening | Surgical lengthening correction of torsion, arthrodesis |

Fig. 29.1 **Spasticity: management**

- Infection (e.g. meningitis)
- Toxins (e.g. hyperbilirubinaemia)
- Perinatal asphyxia
- Postnatal:
  - Infection
  - Vascular accidents
  - Head injury (accidental or non-accidental)
  - Encephalopathy
  - Anoxic event.

Q2. What are the possible diagnoses?

One likely cause for this history is CP and this is confirmed by abnormal physical signs. A familial delay should also be considered, as well as rarer causes such as Duchenne muscular dystrophy (p. 17) in boys.

It is important to remember that everything that looks like CP may not be. Many infants with complex congenital abnormalities (dysmorphic syndromes) will display central motor impairment. These children will require similar services.

Q3. What are the principles of management?

This depends upon the stage of the disorder (Fig. 29.1).

Different approaches to treatment have, from time to time, attracted considerable interest and enthusiasm, as well as opposition. Only recently have attempts been made to study the relative merits of each in objective ways. No single approach will suit all children with a particular form of CP. In most centres in the UK staff follow an eclectic approach, deriving therapeutic ideas from a variety of 'methods'. No study has convincingly shown benefits of one approach over another.

Management involves regular assessment of the child (with parent/carer involvement) and close multi-disciplinary working.

Key professionals

- *The physiotherapist* is responsible for development of motor skills, and assessment for lower limb orthoses and specialized supportive equipment, such as standers and mobility aids. In the early stages physiotherapy is aimed at interrupting the circle of malachievement caused by abnormal muscle tone. The child's carers are shown methods of handling and carrying out everyday tasks that help this.
- *The speech and language therapist* plays these key roles in CP:
  - Most importantly, helping with feeding early in life
  - Helping early communication development
  - Help with speech, which may be severely impaired
  - Management of dribbling
  - Provision of communication aids.
- *The occupational therapist* will assess the need for equipment to facilitate aspects of daily living, e.g. bathing, toileting, static seating, feeding etc., and fine motor skill function, perceptual skills and the use of upper limb orthoses. Adaptations may also be required in the home.

Specialized equipment

- *Orthoses.* The purpose of an orthosis is to restore the normal distribution of forces acting through the limb, thereby normalizing musculoskeletal relationships and establishing a normal pattern of motion and/or prevention of progressive deformity. Hence children with a persistently equinus foot may wear an ankle orthosis. Other orthoses facilitate hand function. Some children experience upper limb spasticity at night; a night resting splint will hold the hand in a neutral position in children, thus optimizing functional use during the day.
- *Special seating, standing and lying frames.* These are used to try to maintain good posture and to give the child optimal positioning and support for feeding and play.
- *Supportive bracing.* This may be needed in some quadriplegic patients to prevent progression of spinal deformity.

Specific drug treatment

Drugs are now being used more widely in CP:

- *Botulinum toxin A (BT A).* This works by chemically denervating the muscle, allowing it to relax, which may enable improved gait or easier care, for example. Relaxation of the muscle may also enable it to grow better by allowing stretching and thereby reducing contractures. The duration of effect is usually 10–14 weeks, and measurable effects may persist for up to 26 weeks.
- *Baclofen.* This analogue of gamma-aminobutyric acid (GABA) impedes excitatory neurotransmission at a spinal level. Oral baclofen is rapidly absorbed, but is protein-bound and has poor penetration into CSF because of poor lipid solubility. The half-life is 3–4 hours, requiring regular dosing (3 times daily). Response to oral baclofen is unpredictable; a number of children will show a satisfactory response, with reduction in muscle tone, but others will develop unacceptable side-effects, including somnolence, confusion, difficulties with oral control, ataxia and increased frequency of micturition. Recently, baclofen by continuous infusion has been given by an intrathecal catheter and pump delivery system to achieve higher and continuous CSF baclofen levels. Baclofen is perhaps most useful when there is generalized increase in tone, which would require multiple injections of botulinum toxin, e.g. in the child with severe spastic tetraplegia.

Surgery

The orthopaedic surgeon has a major role to play in management of CP. Orthopaedic surgery may be indicated to improve function, to prevent deterioration, to relieve pain and to facilitate care.

There are two surgical aspects to the management of CP:

- *Selective posterior rhizotomy.* Two groups of patients are most suitable: children who are of good intelligence, well motivated and sufficiently strong to achieve walking after spasticity is reduced, and severely affected, non-ambulant patients in whom painful spasm can be reduced.
- *Single event multilevel surgery with associated gait analysis.* When fixed contracture of muscles occurs, surgical release has been required to correct the deformity. The traditional approach has been to undertake soft tissue surgery in a 'phased' manner, dealing with one area at a time. Recently it has become clear that this approach of repeated operations, often on a yearly basis, frequently does not improve long-term function. As a result, techniques of thorough pre- and post-operative assessment have been developed, in particular gait analysis. The latter has led to a better understanding of normal gait in children and hence the abnormal gait of the child with CP. Detailed surgical planning is based upon objective rather than subjective information. Gait analysis also allows proper objective review after surgery.

Associated problems

Difficulty may arise from motor problems:

- *Feeding difficulties.* Feeding may be a considerable problem, leading to inadequate quantity and quality of intake. Children with spastic quadriplegia or athetoid CP may have such severe feeding difficulties that they fail to thrive. Recurrent aspiration during feeding may lead to serious chest complications, and children with severe CP commonly suffer from significant gastro-oesophageal reflux (up to 70% having oesophagitis). It is important to address positioning and consistency of food, and to consider the need for gastrostomy feeding. A multidisciplinary approach is essential for significant feeding problems and many places will have a 'feeding clinic'.

- *Drooling.* This is associated with speech and feeding problems and can be a significant cosmetic handicap, as well as being very messy and affecting the skin around the mouth and neck. It is usually due to a problem with swallowing saliva rather than excessive production. Techniques used to help it are:
  - Prompting and rewards for swallowing
  - Positioning and exercises to improve oro-motor function and sensory awareness, now sometimes aided by intra-oral training appliances
  - Medication with anticholinergics to reduce secretions
  - Surgery to direct the ducts further towards the back of the mouth
  - Occasionally, removal of salivary glands
  - Intraglandular botulinum toxin injections.

- *Dislocated hips.* These are an important complication in CP and routine screening by X-ray is needed. Good postural management will help to prevent dislocation.

- *Bowel and bladder problems.* Incontinence may result from learning difficulties, but may be a problem of not being able to get to the toilet in time or undress quickly enough. Constipation is common, particularly in the immobile child and those with restricted diets. It may also be associated with abnormal gut sensitivity and motility. It is important to try to prevent problems by explaining to the parents and child about normal bowel function and giving dietary advice. If constipation occurs, the earlier it is treated, the better.

- *Osteopenia.* The increased risk of bone fractures in children with motor disabilities is linked to reduced bone density. Measures such as weight-bearing, particularly ambulation, good nutrition (especially calcium, vitamin D and magnesium) and sunlight will help.

Other associated problems include:

- *Vision problems.* These are common (50%), particularly myopia, cortical visual impairment and squint.

- *Hearing problems.* These occur in 20–30%, particularly sensorineural deafness. It is also important to look for conductive problems.

- *Learning disabilities.* These are found in all types of CP. Generalized learning difficulties tend to be related to severity of physical problems; however, not all children with severe motor problems have learning difficulties and children with relatively mild motor problems may have significant learning difficulties.

- *Specific learning difficulties.* These are also seen more frequently in CP and can easily be overlooked. Assessment can be very difficult if there are severe motor problems.

- *Epilepsy.* Around 21% of children with CP develop epilepsy, which may be difficult to control.

- *Psychological problems.* These may be due to physical difficulties, or children may have problems directly related to the underlying brain disorder.

- *Educational issues.* Most children will go to mainstream school and need a minimum of help. Some adaptations may be necessary, e.g. ramps, handrails, lifts, special toilet facilities and adapted working surfaces in the classroom.

Communication and its disorders

Basic science

When thinking about speech and language development, you must address the different skills necessary for communication. These include the following.

Attention control

The child must have adequate listening skills and attention.

Symbolic understanding

Words are symbols, so unless children can understand the concept of symbols, they will not understand speech.

Comprehension

Does the child understand spoken language?

Expressive speech

This is the area of communication most easily identified by both parents and professionals, and so tends to be what people concentrate on in the early stages.

Phonology

The development of sounds proceeds largely in the same order in all children, the easier sounds being acquired earlier.

Oromotor skills

These depend on normal orofacial development and functioning bulbar innervation.

Grammar/syntax

The rules of language (e.g. plurals, tenses, word order) need to be acquired.

Semantics

Semantics is about the meaning of words. Children can just learn words by rote and not be able to use them appropriately in context.

Pragmatics

Pragmatics is the way in which language is used in the social context. It includes turn-taking, keeping to the subject, selection, context, verbal jokes and negotiation. This is an area that children with developmental language difficulties, and in particular autism, find hard to learn.

Non-verbal communication

A lot of non-verbal communication occurs without thought, but in children with autism it has to be taught. It includes:

- Tone of voice, pauses etc.
- Facial expression, including eye contact
- Body posture
- Gesture and signing
- Physical contact.

These become more important in children with speech problems and may be the predominant form of communication in some, such as those with profound deafness.

Problem-orientated topic:

delay in speaking

Alex is 2¹/₂ years old. His parents are concerned that he is still only using a few single words. He has achieved his motor milestones within the average range and has no significant previous medical history.

Q1. How would you assess this child?
Q2. What other information would you seek?

Q3. What investigations would you perform?
Q4. How would you manage this child?

Q1. How would you assess this child?

History

Ask in particular about:

- *Pregnancy and birth history.*
- *Family history of language problems or learning difficulties.* There is certainly a strong genetic component in language disorder and possibly in the normal range of language acquisition.
- *Early input.* Carer/child interaction is clearly vital.
- *Bilingualism.* This was thought to be a problem for children first learning language but there is no evidence for this.
- *General development.* Language delay is often a marker for general delay.
- *Any worry about hearing?* Has the hearing been checked? Is there intermittent hearing loss or high-frequency loss? Profoundly deaf children will not learn spoken language without considerable help. Some children with mild hearing losses are delayed in their language development.
- *Any feeding problems in early life?*
- *Any problems now with chewing or dribbling?*
- *Any difficulties with social relationships?*

Observation

- Is there any clumsiness?
- Observe the child's attention span.
- Watch children in a free play situation. Do they make good eye contact with their parent and with other people in the room? Do they turn to share enjoyment of a toy with their parent? How does the parent respond? Is there imaginative play?
- What spontaneous sounds, words or phrases do they use?
- Is there good non-verbal communication?

Examination

- Do the ears look normal? Undertake a full ear, nose and throat examination (Ch. 5).
- Are there local problems in the mouth? Submucous cleft or problems with tongue movements?
- Assess hearing in your clinic (Ch. 5).
- Associated disorder. Any evidence of a movement disorder, e.g. CP?
- Try to engage the child in some one-to-one activities. Some children may appear to have poor auditory attention. Does this improve when you work one-to-one with the child (as in a child

with an attention disorder) or is the child unable to tolerate this one-to-one direction (raises the possibility of autistic spectrum disorder)?

These factors may interplay.

Q2. What other information would you seek?

There are a number of aspects of language that need to be addressed separately.

Listening and attention
Can the child attend to language?

Verbal comprehension
What level of verbal comprehension has the child developed?
- From the history, get particular examples and make sure that they show verbal rather than non-verbal comprehension. Beware the child understanding from context alone. Can the child identify single objects (from objects or pictures)?
- Can the child understand prepositions (in/on/under/behind) and concepts (big/little)?
- How many key words can the child follow? For example:
  - 'Put the *big* pencil in the box' — 1 key word. There are only pencils and a box and it is automatic to put things in boxes.
  - 'Put the *cat under* the *chair*' — 3 key words.

Non-verbal strategies
What non-verbal strategies does the child use to communicate, both for comprehension and expression?
- Pointing and facial expression plus non-speech sound to indicate needs?
- Common gestures, such as pointing, arms up for wanting to be lifted up and waving bye-bye?
- More complex gestures as a means of self-expression?

Verbal expression (Box 29.6)
- Pre-speech babbling or only open vowel sounds?
- Some symbolic noise or word approximations: e.g. 'hiya' (for 'here you are') or 'brrmm brrmm' (for car play)?
- How many single words is the child using that Mother understands (not necessarily other people)?
- Are there some learned phrases that are two- or three-word combinations learned together, e.g. 'all gone', or has the child started flexible word joining, e.g. 'teddy gone' or 'daddy car'?
- Are longer structures used, e.g. 'my teddy gone' or 'my teddy's called Joe and he's going to bed now'?
- Does the child ask questions?

BOX 29.6 Pitfalls in assessing verbal competence

Beware of the echolalic child or the child using chunks of 'late echoing', which will give the impression of a verbally competent child. This may indicate delayed verbal comprehension or semantic–pragmatic problems.

Beware of children who initially appear to have good expressive language using appropriate social phrases but who demonstrate a lack of variety or range in their speech. These may be children with general delay or with very little language stimulation.

- Can the child tell you what he or she has been doing?
- Does he or she tend to copy what you say?

Phonology
This is an area that parents often get worried about, but which has the best prognosis:
- Is it dysarthria (due to abnormal neurology, e.g. CP)?
- Is it dysphonia (e.g. hoarseness due to disorder of the voice box)?
- Is it delay (the way a younger child would talk) or deviance?

Semantics and pragmatics (Box 29.7)
This is an area of difficulty that may only become evident as the child develops more language. It is rare for children to have semantic or pragmatic disorders with completely normal early language development:
- Does the child have difficulties following instructions, particularly complicated ones?
- Does the child understand tenses?
- Are conversational skills age-appropriate? Can the child turn-take? Is the content of speech pertinent?

BOX 29.7 Pitfalls in parental descriptions

Parents often *underestimate* their child's expressive language and *overestimate* their comprehension.

Standardized assessments of language

Numerous standardized tools for language assessments exist and these are described on the MasterCourse website.

Q3. What investigations would you perform?

- Hearing should be tested in all children.
- Test chromosomes only if there are other indications.

- Order an EEG if there is loss of language or some other reason to suspect epilepsy.

Any child with severe language impairment or complex problems should be seen by a paediatrician.

Q4. How would you manage this child?

The role of the doctor in the management of language difficulties is:
- To identify and address any possible causes (e.g. hearing loss, submucous cleft)
- To identify and address associated difficulties (e.g. epilepsy).

Management of language impairments lies predominantly with the speech and language therapist (SLT), whose role is:
- To advise parents on how they can help the child
- To monitor young children or those with mild delay
- To work with nursery or school, advising how to help language development
- To work with groups of children who have similar problems, to encourage language development
- To work with individual children, usually for short intensive bursts of speech therapy
- To advise on and implement alternative communication systems.

 Details of these alternative communication systems are given on the MasterCourse website.

Education

Fortunately, most language difficulties have resolved by school age or soon after. Some children will go on to have reading difficulties.

A small number of children need specialist educational input, which may be available locally at nursery or primary school, but by secondary school age the numbers are so small that the child may need to travel some distance and occasionally even board at a special school to obtain this level of specialist education.

English as a second language

Special problems may arise for children whose first language is not English. These include:
- *Late recognition.* People assume that there are no problems, or that any difficulties in English result from it being the child's second language.
- *Assessment.* Is there a problem in the first language or is the problem only in English? Trying to assess this means having an interpreter.
- *Treatment.* Should this be in the first language? Can this be achieved?

Children with profound and multiple learning difficulties

The SLT will be part of a team caring for these children. He or she may be involved initially with feeding difficulties and can anticipate language problems.

Key elements for aiding communication in children with profound and multiple difficulties are:
- Using all senses to give messages about the child's world: hearing, vision, touch, taste, smell
- Helping the child to learn to control the environment at a basic level: making simple choices, turn-taking
- Helping the child to develop relationships: limiting numbers of professionals involved directly with the child and working through other people
- Using augmentative communication systems.

Language disorders

Definitions

The terms 'communication' and 'language' are sometimes used interchangeably. Communication problems encompass a wider range of disorders, including difficulties in non-verbal communication and ability to use language (as in autism). We will discuss language problems other than autism here, although this is not always a simple distinction:
- *Delay* implies that language is slow to develop; it is progressing in a normal pattern but is like that of a younger child.
- *Disorder* implies that language contains elements that are not part of normal development.
- *Impairment* is the term that is currently preferred and encompasses both delay and deviance. Specific language impairment is used for children who have isolated language impairment with non-verbal learning skills at a higher level. However, studies show that children with 'specific' language impairment have a high incidence of other neurodevelopmental disorders.

Prevalence

Studies on prevalence vary, depending on definition and whether children with intellectual difficulties are included. About 5–7% of children have significant language difficulties without other learning difficulties. Around 1% have severe persisting difficulties.

There is a wide variation in normal development of language. This can make it hard to decide when there is an abnormality, particularly when there is delay rather than deviance and it affects verbal expression and phonology. Many (though not all) of these children will have corrected themselves by school age or soon after.

Classification

There are problems with classification of communication disorders; children often overlap categories or change from one to another. There is also difficulty because of the wide spectrum of normal development.

A practical classification can be used to assist assessment and investigation:

- Disorders affecting speech production:
  - Neurological problems, e.g. CP
  - Structural problems, e.g. cleft lip and palate ('tongue-tie' rarely, if ever, causes speech problems)
  - Dysphonia, e.g. abnormalities of the vocal cords
  - Dysfluency (stammering), a frequently normal stage of development between 2 and 4 years
  - Elective (or selective) mutism
- Specific language impairments:
  - Expressive language delay
  - Articulatory dyspraxia, possibly associated with feeding difficulties
  - Difficulties in producing sounds accurately, in comprehension or in finding a word
  - Semantic–pragmatic difficulties. These children may have had normal early development of language but often have had delay or deviance that resolved. Difficulties become apparent later with inability to maintain a conversation, 'getting the wrong end of the stick', going off at a tangent, misunderstanding rules of conversation, or difficulty with puns and jokes. There are often problems with social interaction, which may overlap with the autistic spectrum.
- Children who stop talking:
  - Usually associated with loss of other skills, e.g. neurodegenerative disorders
- Impaired language and social interaction:
  - These are considered in the section on autistic spectrum disorders.

 http://www.afasic.org.uk

The Afasic website has information sheets on different types of disorder

Aetiology

Most children with language difficulties not linked with other major disabilities have no identifiable cause for their problems.

Children with language disorders are known to have an increased family history of language disorders and twin studies suggest strong heritability.

Associated problems

- *Epilepsy* has a higher incidence in children with language disorders. This supports the idea that language disorders are due to problems with brain development.
- *Left-handedness* (especially in girls) is often noted but not always confirmed. The significance is unclear; it may sometimes be a pathological left-handedness.
- *Clumsiness* is found in 90% of children with severe language disorder. Studies and clinical observation confirm this link.
- *Educational difficulties* are complicated and depend on the type of language impairment.

Autistic spectrum disorders

Problem-orientated topic:

the isolated child

Robbie is 3 years of age and has been referred by his GP because he has recently started nursery school and his teacher has expressed concern that he may be autistic. Robbie is his mother's third child and he has always acted differently to the other two. Since the age of 6 months he stopped making eye contact and is now a very solitary child, preferring his own company to that of his family. He spends hours spinning a toy top and becomes inconsolable if interrupted. His speech development is immature and he tends to echo phrases made by his brothers.

Q1. What are the three core impairments seen in autistic spectrum disorders?

Q2. How would you assess this child?

Q3. What alternative conditions do you need to consider?

Q4. What investigations should be considered?

Q5. What are the advantages/disadvantages of finding a diagnostic label for Robbie and his family?

Q6. What are your management options?

Q7. What is the prognosis for this condition?

Q1. What are the three core impairments seen in autistic spectrum disorders?

Autism is a specific type of communication disorder, which has some overlap with semantic–pragmatic disorders of language (p. 41) and also with other types of neurodevelopmental disorder. The present concept is of an 'autistic spectrum', in which the three core features are:

- Impairment of social interaction
- Impairment of communication
- Rigidity of thought.

It can be useful within this spectrum to define the type (classic autism, high-functioning autism, Asperger's syndrome) while accepting that some children do not fit any one of these labels but still show significant features within the spectrum.

Impaired social interaction

Eye contact may be present but is abnormal in its nature (fixed and staring, held too long). However, there may be good reasons for a child to have poor eye contact in the clinic, such as shyness, embarrassment, wilfulness.

Lack of cuddliness is another popular concept, but autistic children may be willing to be cuddled and even give cuddles back, especially with their parents, though the parents may describe it as 'on the child's terms' or 'too intense'.

Key indicators of impaired social interaction are:

- Lack of sharing and directing attention
- Poor recognition of others' affect
- Poor understanding of social situations.

Impaired communication

In classic autism there will be delayed development of communication, though many autistic children develop some language. About 33% of children with autism develop some early words and then lose them. It is often apparent that they had social interactional problems from the outset and/or never used their words really communicatively. Only 7–8% of autistic children have a setback in language development following completely normal development in the first couple of years with acquisition of two-word phrases. Children with Asperger's syndrome may have normal language development, but content and use of language may be unusual.

Rigidity/stereotyped thought and behaviour

These include the hand flapping and turning in circles seen in classic autism and the intense narrow interests of children with Asperger's syndrome. Some children have no imaginative play; others will have restricted imaginative play, such as going through the same routine, probably copied from a video.

Q2. How would you assess this child?

With practice it becomes relatively easy to identify most children within the spectrum in the informal clinic situation and many parents have already suspected the diagnosis. In some children it is less easy, and it is important to have reliable methods of assessment so that the diagnosis can be made or excluded with confidence and backed up with evidence.

History

Diagnosis depends greatly on history, so it is important to have a framework that will cover the triad of impairments. In addition a standard medical, developmental and family history may indicate a different diagnosis, associated problems or a possible cause for the autism.

There are formal scored interviews for the autistic spectrum, which have diagnostic cutoff points and may also give an indication of where in the spectrum the child lies.

Examination

This may identify possible causes, including:

- Dysmorphism
- Neurological abnormality, including head size
- Skin markers (should include examination under Wood's light for depigmented patches, p. 9).

Informal observation in the clinic setting will often give clues as to diagnosis, but children may act fairly normally in this structured one-to-one situation, so it is helpful to observe them in different settings and over time.

Assessing where on the spectrum a child lies

The formal scored tools will help with this. Beware of being too precise early on because this may change as time goes by and as you obtain more information about the child.

Assessing the child's strengths and weaknesses

Each aspect of the child's difficulties is assessed:

- Its nature
- Its degree
- Whether it is primary or secondary
- Whether it is changing over time.

Other aspects can be assessed, such as:

- Rigidity/routines
- Motor abilities
- 'Dangers' of special interests
- Motivation/reliability
- Obsessional–compulsive behaviours
- Insight
- Depression/anxiety
- Temperament
- Support systems.

Children are presenting younger with possible autistic spectrum disorder and this may present difficulties around stability of the diagnostic label over time.

Q3. What alternative conditions do you need to consider?

Social impairment may be secondary to other disorders:

- Learning difficulties, leading to social immaturity
- Dyspraxia, leading to invasion of other people's social space
- Psychopathy (p. 52)
- Shyness, leading to social awkwardness
- Conduct disorder, bullying, abuse, depression, which may all lead to abnormal social relationships
- Semantic–pragmatic disorders (p. 41), leading to abnormalities in social relationships; there is overlap between these and autism
- Secondary social impairment, which may occur as a result of ADHD (p. 33), depression, bullying or abuse
- Rett's syndrome (p. 22), but the relationship to autism is debatable; certainly, these children develop features of severe autism but also tend to lose them as the condition progresses.

Comorbidity

Children with an autistic spectrum disorder have a greater incidence of other developmental and psychiatric disorders and these should be sought:

- Learning difficulty is the most common associated problem in classic autism (70–75%). Also, children with learning disorders may show features of autism and it is important to ascertain whether this is sufficient to give an additional diagnosis of autism.
- ADHD.
- Depression.
- Affective disorder.
- Anxiety disorder.

Q4. What investigations should be considered?

Children with autism find investigations very difficult to cope with; therefore consider the reasons for ordering them. These reasons are:

- To identify a treatable cause
- To identify genetic implications
- Parental 'need to know'
- Research.

Investigations are most likely to be positive in children with a severe cognitive impairment.

Cytogenetics

Around 3% of children with autism have an abnormal karyotype. This figure is higher in children with dysmorphisms, severe learning difficulties and identifiable syndromes.

Imaging

Most common abnormalities are of the cerebellum but the significance of this is unknown. Cortical migration anomalies may sometimes be seen, but they are non-specific and will not help in diagnosis of autism or discovery of the cause. Features of tuberous sclerosis and neurofibromatosis may be recognized. Routine imaging is not recommended.

EEG

Between 21 and 43% of children with autism have an abnormal EEG. The longer the EEG, the more likely it is to reveal abnormalities, but these do not necessarily have implications for clinical care.

Q5. What are the advantages/disadvantages of finding a diagnostic label for Robbie and his family?

Advantages

- Changes attitudes towards the child positively (more understanding and appropriate responses)
- Mobilizes resources
- Indicates type of management for specific problems
- Gives an explanation to the child and parents
- Gives access to support networks.

Disadvantages

- Changes attitudes towards the child negatively (inappropriate lowering of expectations, assumptions about what diagnosis means)
- A label for life
- The label may need to change with passage of time.

Q6. What are your management options?

These include:

- Management of the child:
  - Medical and psychological
  - Social skills (group work)
  - Educational
- Management of the family:
  - Parent courses
  - Parent support
- Information/education about the condition:
  - For the parent
  - For the child.

Goals for management include:
- Fostering of development
- Promotion of learning
- Reduction of stereotypy
- Elimination of maladaptive behaviours
- Alleviation of family distress.

There are different approaches to management, which will be used in conjunction with each other.

Pharmacotherapy
In the US 30% of children with autism and 55% of children with high-functioning autism and Asperger's are on medication. The corresponding figures in the UK are only 5% and 10%.

Drugs will not generally affect the core symptoms of autism (and there is no evidence at present of long-term benefits) but they can ameliorate symptoms. It is important when considering medication that you are clear about the specific symptoms you are targeting and that ongoing behavioural and educational management is continued. Ensuring safe and consistent administration and monitoring for side-effects is essential. You also need to consider who you are treating (child, parent, doctor, teacher) and make sure you have informed consent as far as you are able. Substances suggested as a general treatment for autism are:
- *Secretin.* There is no evidence from randomized controlled trials of any benefit.
- *Vitamins, minerals, essential fatty acids and metals.* No studies have shown any effect.
- *Gluten- and casein-free diets.* These have their supporters but robust evidence is not yet available. Some children with autism have distressing bowel problems and a gluten- or casein-free diet may decrease bowel symptoms and greatly improve general wellbeing.

Family support
This is important from the start. Some support will come from the medical and educational teams but families should also be made aware of local and national parent groups. There are practical issues that can be addressed and which will make life easier.

Behaviour management
Difficult behaviours can be analysed as follows:
- Instrumental: in order to get something
- Social: in order to get attention
- Self-stimulatory.

The first two types of behaviour are most amenable to behaviour therapy and the last type to drug treatment.

Educational management
Many educational intervention programmes are advocated in autism; some claim to provide a 'cure' but most claim only improvement. Most approaches have in common a high degree of one-to-one intervention, often with highly structured activities. Some focus on parent intervention and some use professionals or trained workers.

Multidisciplinary teams
Many children will benefit from going through a formal multidisciplinary assessment and management. This may be at the local Child Development Centre or may be within the community.

 http://www.cafamily.org.uk/NAPFront.PDF

National Initiative for Autism: Screening and Assessment

 http://www.nelh.nhs.uk

National Service Framework for Children. Autism is one of the topics picked out as an exemplar condition

Q7. What is the prognosis for this condition?

The degree of independence reached by a child within the autistic spectrum depends to a major extent not only on the degree of intellectual impairment, but also on severity of the autism. Parents have a real anxiety that some children with high-functioning autism and Asperger's syndrome will find it hard to manage on their own. Undoubtedly some people with autism do very well, and there are a number of accounts written by autistic people about their experiences that give an insight into what autism is like from the inside.

Classic autism

Classic autism has a prevalence of about 0.5/1000. This rate has remained fairly steady over the years. The corresponding figure for Asperger's syndrome is around 0.25/1000.

Autistic spectrum disorder prevalence is between 3 and 6/1000, rising to nearly 1 in 100 in studies seeking out the whole range of disorders. It appears to be rising but this is likely to be because the diagnosis is being more readily recognized.

Aetiology of autism
A long list of associated conditions have been found in studies of children with autistic spectrum disorder:
- Fragile X syndrome (p. 32; either some autistic impairments or full autism)
- Tuberous sclerosis (p. 9; 43–60% of children with tuberous sclerosis will have autism or pervasive developmental disorder)

- Phenylketonuria (p. 97)
- Neurofibromatosis (p. 9)
- Down's syndrome (p. 30)
- Williams' syndrome
- Duchenne muscular dystrophy (p. 17)
- Non-specific dysmorphisms and other chromosomal abnormalities
- West's syndrome (p. 8)
- Hydrocephalus (p. 24; 23% have autism)
- Severe sensory deficits
- Congenital infections
- Encephalitis (p. 292)
- Hypothyroidism (p. 108)
- Fetal alcohol syndrome
- Neurometabolic disorders (p. 93).

Autism is probably under-diagnosed in many of these conditions because, once a child has a label, there may be reluctance to pursue an additional label.

A variety of possible aetiological agents have been proposed, but convincing evidence for any of these is not available. There is no evidence linking measles/mumps/rubella (MMR) vaccination to autism.

High-functioning autism and Asperger's syndrome

These are not 'mild' autism! The distress caused to the child can be greater than with 'classic' autism because of the awareness the child has of the difficulties without the ability to understand them.

What worries me is that when Jonathan leaves school he'll have 6 or 7 GCSEs but he won't be able to go out and buy himself a shirt. (Parent of a boy aged 15 years)

David knows that when he walks into the tennis club he 'gets it wrong', whilst his younger brother Peter is fine. He doesn't understand why this is and he gets very depressed. (Parent of a boy aged 11 years)

The characteristics are as follows:

- Presentation is usually after 3 years of age but, with hindsight, indicators can be identified in the first 3 years of life.
- Language may be normal, at least superficially.
- Presentation is often via the school with behavioural difficulties, school failure and 'oddness'. The difficulties become apparent with the pressures for social conformity at school.

The terms high-functioning autism and Asperger's syndrome are sometimes used interchangeably but there are differences.

Asperger's syndrome is characterized by:

- Highly developed special interests
- Verbal IQ being greater than performance IQ
- Frequent clumsiness
- More social interest than in high-functioning autism
- Socially approaching (but may be unusual or inappropriate)
- More insight into own thoughts and feelings
- Greater desire to fit in
- Cognitive (but not empathic) understanding of social rules.

These difficulties can give rise to:

- High levels of anxiety
- Psychiatric morbidity
- Socially manipulative behaviour, such as school exclusion
- Problems gaining independence
- Vulnerability, both socially and practically.

Acknowledgement

We would like to thank the Sheffield Distance Learning Programme for Paediatric Neurodisability and in particular Dr Hilary Cass, Professor David Hall, Dr Mike Smith, Dr Connie Pullon, Dr Peter Baxter, Sian Bell and Dr Karen Whiting for their kind permission to use materials they have written.

CHAPTER

30

Child mental health

LEARNING OUTCOMES

By the end of this chapter you should:

- Know the diagnostic criteria of chronic fatigue syndrome (CFS)
- Know the basic investigations that are necessary in cases of possible CFS
- Know the principles of management of CFS
- Be able to recognize children at risk of suicide
- Know the principles of management of self-harm
- Know how to assess suicide intent in adolescents
- Know the differential diagnosis of acute psychosis in children.

Introduction

Children with symptoms of a severe emotional or apparent psychiatric nature are commonly referred to paediatricians, who must decide whether the child can be managed in a paediatric clinic or should be referred to the Child and Adolescent Mental Health services (CAMHS). In fact, most of the children with emotional-based problems are seen and managed by paediatricians and are discussed in Chapter 20. Sometimes children with more serious psychiatric problems are referred directly to the paediatrician, often through the accident and emergency department when an acute crisis develops, and it is important that paediatric trainees develop a knowledge of these disorders in order to decide when referral to the CAMHS is appropriate.

Chronic fatigue syndrome

Problem-orientated topic:

a child with chronic fatigue

Naomi is a 13-year-old girl who is referred to your outpatient clinic because of a 2-month history of tiredness, which began after an episode of 'possible glandular fever'. She is 'exhausted all the time' but finds sleep at night difficult. She regularly complains of limb pain, headache and poor concentration. She has missed 4 weeks of school. Prior to this episode she was well, lively and active. On examination you find some small cervical lymph nodes but otherwise no abnormality.

Continued overleaf

Q1. Could this child be suffering from chronic fatigue syndrome?

Q2. What is the differential diagnosis and what investigations should be done?

Q3. What are the principles of management?

Q1. Could this child be suffering from chronic fatigue syndrome?

Epidemiology
- Prevalence is estimated at 0.5–1% in 12–16-year-olds.
- It is perhaps the most common cause of long-term school absence through illness in UK adolescents.
- Female:male ratio in some studies is 3:1.
- Mean duration of symptoms is 3–4 years.

Pathophysiology
- This is unknown but many theories exist.
- Slightly higher rates are reported in monozygotic than in dizygotic twins.
- Inconsistent findings of immune system abnormalities have been reported. Subtle defects in the hypothalamic–pituitary axis and muscle pathology are detected in some studies.
- Recent viral infection is common, particularly with Epstein–Barr virus (EBV), but the significance of this is uncertain given the ubiquitous nature of this infection in this age group.

Diagnosis
The first step is a careful history and thorough examination. Pay particular attention to the fundi, muscle bulk, lymph nodes, presence of hepatosplenomegaly, and lying and standing blood pressure.

There is no single diagnostic feature in this condition. The Royal College of Paediatrics and Child Health (RCPCH) has published diagnostic criteria (Box 30.1).

http://www.rcpch.ac.uk/publications/clinical_docs/cfs.pdf

Q2. What is the differential diagnosis and what investigations should be done?
(Table 30.1)

Secondary investigations may be required if symptoms or signs suggest an alternative diagnosis.

Q3. What are the principles of management?

The key components of management are likely to include:

BOX 30.1 RCPCH diagnostic criteria for chronic fatigue syndrome
- Persisting debilitating generalized fatigue, for which no other cause can be found
- (RCPCH criteria do not prescribe a minimum duration of fatigue prior to diagnosis in children; adult criteria require fatigue > 6 months)
- Fatigue exacerbated by effort

Common associated symptoms
- Headache/myalgia
- Sleep disturbance
- Memory impairment/concentration difficulties
- Sore throat/tender lymph nodes
- Depressed mood
- Nausea/abdominal pain

Rarer associated symptoms
- Dizziness
- Hyperacusis/sensitivity to light
- Weight loss/gain
- Diarrhoea

- *A multidisciplinary approach.* Involve the child and parents at every stage.
- *Graded exercise therapy (GET).* Using a detailed diary, establish a baseline of activity. Gradually increase activity levels in partnership with the patient.
- *Sleep hygiene.* (Advice on establishing a helpful sleep pattern).
- *Cognitive behavioural therapy (CBT).*
- *Pain management.* Simple analgesics for most cases. Amitriptyline may be necessary.
- *Treat accompanying mood disorders.* Referral to the CAMHS team may be necessary if there is significant evidence of low mood.
- *Liaison with education services.* For home tuition and gradual reintegration into school.

Attempted suicide

Problem-orientated topic:

a child who has attempted suicide

Holly is 13 years old and presents to the accident and emergency department with her older sister (aged 18). She reports that she took six paracetamol tablets 2 hours ago 'because I was so fed up I wanted to kill myself'. She has never attempted suicide in

Table 30.1 Differential diagnosis and *minimum* investigation required in chronic fatigue syndrome

Test	Aims to exclude
Full blood count (FBC)/film	Anaemia, iron deficiency, leukaemia
Erythrocyte sedimentation rate (ESR)/C-reactive protein (CRP)	Autoimmune disorder, chronic infection
Urea and electrolytes (U&Es), glucose	Renal impairment, Addison's disease, diabetes
Thyroid function	Hypothyroidism (increasingly common in this age group)
Liver function	Hepatitis
Viral serology (EBV, IgM, IgG)	Recent viral illness
Urinalysis (glucose, white blood cells (WBC), protein)	Urinary tract infection (UTI), renal disease, diabetes

the past. You note (a) several old transverse scars and (b) a 3 cm long superficial abrasion on the anterior aspect of her left forearm. Her paracetamol levels 2 hours later are below the treatment threshold for N-acetylcysteine.

Q1. How do you assess suicidal intent in children such as Holly?

Q2. What are the principles of management of self-harm in children?

Q1. How do you assess suicidal intent in children such as Holly?

- Actual suicide is rare in children < 12 years old.
- Age-specific mortality from suicide rises from 1.6/100 000 per year in 10–14-year-olds to 9.5/100 000 in 15–19-year-olds in the USA.
- It is more common in males and there is no trend in social class.
- Methods of suicide in males differ from those in females (for example, violent methods such as hanging in males, self-poisoning in females).
- There is evidence for a pre-existing mental illness in ~90% (mood disorder (depression) or anxiety disorder). A previous suicide attempt is common.
- Suicide is precipitated by common, 'minor' stressful events: e.g. trouble at school, argument with parents/friends/boyfriend or girlfriend.

 http://www.surgeongeneral.gov/library/ mentalhealth/chapter3/sec5.html

More information on suicide

Attempted suicide is common (4/1000 per year in 15–19-year-olds), and more common in females and lower socioeconomic groups. Mental illness is found in ~50% (depression), and alcohol and drug misuse are common.

Q2. What are the principles of management of self-harm in children?

Medical/surgical management (see also Ch. 50)
- Consider activated charcoal if the patient presents within 2 hours of ingestion of a poison, is conscious and is able to maintain an airway (see also p. 397).
- Obtain samples for toxicology (blood, urine, vomitus). Measure paracetamol levels in all children with suspected overdose or self-harm.
- Do *not* use cathartics (ipecac) or laxatives, unless directed by TOXBASE.
- Consult TOXBASE and manage accordingly.
- Treat superficial wounds with tissue adhesive or skin closure strips.

Further management of acute episode
- Admit overnight under care of a named paediatrician to allow full assessment the next day.
- Obtain consent from the parents (or other legally responsible adult) for mental health team assessment.
- Arrange a multidisciplinary CAMHS assessment of needs and risks.
- Check to see if there are child protection issues.

Assessing suicidal intent in adolescents

Circumstances of the attempt

- Precipitating factors
- Did you actually want to die?
- Detailed history of the attempt: where, when, how, who else was around?
- Was there any planning?
- Was anyone else told?
- Was help sought, and if so, when?

Current mental state

- Evidence of depression/anxiety
- Do you still want to die?

Attitude towards the future

- Has the attempt changed your attitude to the future or the attitude of your carers?
- How do you feel about the future? Do you feel hopeless?

 http://www.rcpch.ac.uk/publications/clinical_docs/self_harm.pdf

RCPCH appraisal of NICE guidelines

 http://www.rcpsych.ac.uk/mentalhealthinformation/mentalhealthandgrowingup.aspx

Royal College of Psychiatrists: Mental Health and Growing Up. Sheet 26 Suicide and attempted suicide; sheet 26 Deliberate self-harm in young people

Acute psychosis

Problem-orientated topic:

a child with acute psychosis

Gary is urgently referred to you by his GP. He is 12 years old and has mild learning difficulties. He attended speech therapy until he was 7 years old. He goes to a mainstream school. He has always been a quiet boy with few friends, but over the last 3 months his mother has noticed him becoming increasingly withdrawn. She wonders if he is depressed because he 'doesn't seem to react to anything'. Two days ago she found a collection of canned food and biscuits in Gary's bedroom. When questioned, he told her he was keeping them because a ghost had been telling him to.

Q1. How do you clinically assess Gary?
Q2. What investigations should be ordered?

Q1. How do you clinically assess Gary?

- Obtain a detailed history, paying particular attention to behaviour, emotions, relationships, family history, developmental progress and recent loss of skills.
- Perform a detailed neurological examination.

- Perform a mental state examination. You may consider using a standardized instrument such as the 'Kiddie Schedule for Affective Disorders and Schizophrenia' (KSADS, see below).
- Request an urgent psychiatric opinion.
- Consider and test for differential diagnoses (Table 30.2 below).

 http://www.wpic.pitt.edu/ksads/ksads-pl.pdf

KSADS

Q2. What investigations should be ordered?

See Table 30.2.

Schizophrenia in childhood/adolescence (Box 30.2)

- This is a rare disorder affecting 3/10 000 adolescents; it is much rarer before puberty.
- There is a large genetic component in the aetiology; 20% have a first-degree affected relative.
- One-third have a long-standing history of difficulty in making and keeping friends.
- Mean IQ of patients at initial presentation is 80–85.
- Insidious onset is common, with gradual social withdrawal.

> **BOX 30.2 Symptoms of childhood/adolescent schizophrenia**
>
> **Positive ('florid')**
> - Delusions
> - Hallucinations (auditory > visual)
> - Distortions of thinking (thought insertion)
>
> **Negative**
> - Social withdrawal
> - Lack of motivation
> - Poverty of speech
> - Slowness of thought

Management

Treatment is generally with newer antipsychotic drugs (risperidone, olanzapine), as these have fewer side-effects (extrapyramidal effects and drowsiness) than traditional antipsychotics.

Prognosis is probably worse than in those who present as adults. Poor premorbid functioning, predominance of negative symptoms and a long period of untreated illness are associated with a poor prognosis.

Table 30.2 Differential diagnosis and investigation of psychotic symptoms in children

Diagnosis	Test
Schizophrenia	Clinical diagnosis
Psychosis associated with bipolar/mood disorder	Clinical diagnosis
Drug misuse (especially hallucinogens)	Toxicology
Brain tumour (p. 413)	MRI brain scan
Late-onset neurodegenerative disorder (e.g. metachromatic leucodystrophy)	MRI brain scan
Wilson's disease (p. 188)	Copper/ceruloplasmin
Porphyria	Urinary porphobilinogen
Subacute sclerosing panencephalitis (p. 20)	EEG/CSF measles titres

Further reading

Crawley E, Chambers T 2005 It's not all in ME mind, doc.
Archives of Disease in Childhood, Education and Practice
Edition 90: ep92–ep97

MODULE SIX

The eye and vision

LEARNING OUTCOMES

By the end of this chapter you should:
- Be able to undertake a fundoscopic examination
- Be able to assess a child for a squint
- Know the common causes of a red eye
- Understand the causes of visual impairment
- Know how to examine for a cataract and its common causes.

MODULE SIX

Basic science

The eye is the organ of vision and is highly specialized in its structure and function. Many disorders of vision can be explained by understanding the embryology of the eye and visual development.

Normal visual development depends on normal structure of the eyes and an intact visual system to the striate cortex in the occipital lobe. Also, the midbrain and cerebellum play an important role in eye movements.

The eye is the sensory organ that focuses light on the retina and works much like a camera focusing light on to photosensitive film. For an image to be in focus on the retina, the cornea and lens bend the light, a process called refraction; the refractive power of the lens is measured in dioptres. The refractive power of the lens is altered by changes in its shape effected by the ciliary muscles. This process of the lens changing shape to focus light on the retina is described as accommodation.

Visual disturbance as a result of ocular problems can be described as:
- *Myopia* (near-sightedness), in which images are focused in front of the retina because the eye is too long for the refractive process
- *Hypermetropia* (long-sightedness), in which images are focused behind the retina because the eye is relatively short

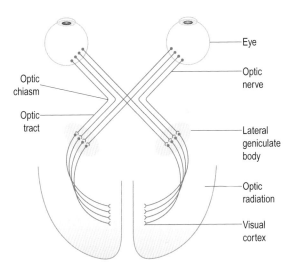

Optic chiasm

Optic tract

Eye

Optic nerve

Lateral geniculate body

Optic radiation

Visual cortex

Fig. 31.1 **Visual pathways**

- *Astigmatism*, in which there is asymmetrical focusing due to distortion of refraction.

The retina is the most metabolically active tissue in the body for its size and depends on many biochemical reactions for its normal function. It contains different photoreceptor cells called rods and cones. Both types of cell contain a photosensitive pigment called rhodopsin, which is dependent on normal levels of vitamin A. The rods are particularly sensitive to light (photons) and the cones provide the ability to discriminate colours. Colour blindness, a genetic disorder, results from the loss of one or more of the cone cell types.

The optic nerves take visual impulses from the retina to the central visual projections in the brain (Fig. 31.1). The optic nerves decussate at the optic chiasm into optic tracts, which then synapse at the lateral geniculate body and project to the visual cortex via the optic radiation. The lateral geniculate body acts as a filter for visual information before it is conducted to the visual cortex in the occipital lobes of the brain.

Interruption to the visual pathway at different points will result in different types of visual field defect. A lesion affecting the optic chiasm causes loss of vision in both temporal fields and is referred to as bitemporal hemianopia. Damage to an optic tract causes loss of vision in the contralateral half of the visual field of each eye, a condition referred to as homonymous hemianopia.

The processing of visual information in the cortex of the occipital lobe is a complicated process that needs to be learned by light stimulation. Amblyopia (see below) occurs as a result of failure to stimulate the occipital cortex at a critical phase of development in early postnatal life.

Strabismus

Problem-orientated topic:

a child with a squint

David, a 4-year-old boy, has been identified by the school nurse as having a possible squint. His vision appears to be normal on gross testing in the GP surgery, and the GP is not certain whether David has a squint or not. He refers the child to the paediatric department for advice.

Q1. How would you assess whether David has a squint?

Q2. How would you classify squints?

Q3. What is the management of a definite squint?

Q1. How would you assess whether David has a squint?

Assessment includes all of the following:
- Corneal light reflex
- Ocular movements (is there an increasing angle of squint with different eye movements?)
- Visual acuity (each eye separately)
- The cover test (Box 31.1)
- Fundoscopy (Box 31.2).

Q2. How would you classify squints?

Strabismus (squint) is defined as a misalignment of one eye in relation to the other. It may have its onset in

BOX 31.1 Skill: cover test

 See also Chapter 5

BOX 31.2 Skill: fundoscopy

Take an ophthalmoscope and set the lens dial to zero. From an arm's distance, look through the eyehole towards the patient's pupils. Note the presence and relative brightness of the red reflex (reflection). Use your right eye and right hand to look at the subject's right eye. Change your hand and eye to view the subject's other eye. Looking through the eyepiece, move towards the red reflex of the right eye. Move the lens dial to focus on a blood vessel. Follow the blood vessel to find the optic disc.

infancy or in later childhood. It is a common disorder in childhood.

Some young children with a prominent nasal bridge give the appearance of a squint. On testing, the child does not have strabismus and the term used to describe this condition is therefore 'pseudosquint'.

Most true strabismus in childhood is inturning (esotropia). Exotropia is less common in childhood, although children with neurological problems may have a tendency to develop it. The strabismus may be present some of the time (latent) or all of the time (constant). A latent squint is the most likely cause in David's case.

The most common childhood strabismus is an accommodative esotropia. This is usually seen in hypermetropia (all images focused behind the retina). Without glasses, the child can still see by using a lot of accommodative effort to focus distant or near images. This excess accommodative effort causes the eyes to converge and gives an esotropia. Continuous wearing of the correct glasses can improve the angle of strabismus, and in some cases can cause the eyes to straighten completely.

Sudden onset of strabismus in childhood should be referred to the eye department. If the findings are consistent with an accommodative esotropia, then corrective glasses may be given and no other investigations may be required. Sudden onset of esotropia can sometimes be a manifestation of a sixth nerve palsy (e.g. raised intracranial pressure) and this needs urgent investigation.

Q3. What is the management of a definite squint?

Binocular vision cannot develop while the visual axes are not aligned.

Management of a squint is as follows:

- Testing for amblyopia and patching of the good eye to stimulate visual input into the affected eye
- Assessment for hypermetropia, as glasses may be required
- Strabismus surgery, often carried out early to help in the development of binocular vision by aligning the eyes.

Ptosis

This is the term given to the lowering of the upper eyelid.

The upper lid is normally elevated by the levator muscle that is innervated by the third cranial nerve, which also innervates most of the ocular movements and constricts the pupil. It also receives a contribution from the sympathetic system, which dilates the pupil.

Ptosis may be caused by the following problems: lesions in the central nervous system, sympathetic chain (e.g. neuroblastoma), structural (congenital disinsertion of levator into eyelid) or muscular (myasthenia gravis).

Horner's syndrome

Horner's syndrome is the term given to ptosis caused by a lesion of the sympathetic system. The main signs are ptosis (about 2 mm) and a constricted pupil. The lesion may be anywhere along the sympathetic system, e.g. along the carotid artery or in the lung apex.

Proptosis

This term refers to forward displacement of the eye due to the presence of a mass behind the eye. The most common primary malignant tumour that can cause this is a rhabdomyosarcoma. The most common secondary tumour is a neuroblastoma. Other conditions that can give rise to proptosis in childhood include capillary haemangioma, lymphangioma, orbital pseudotumour (idiopathic orbital inflammation) and, rarely, thyroid eye disease.

Orbital imaging is required and prompt biopsy may be indicated if rhabdomyosarcoma is suspected.

Amblyopia

Amblyopia (lazy eye) is caused by a lack of visual experience on the part of one or both eyes during the developmental stages of vision. Visual experience of visual cortex cells is required for them to perceive light normally. It is the most common cause of visual loss in childhood and in young adults.

The amount of amblyopia a child experiences depends on its time of onset, duration and severity of the amblyopic stimulus. Different types of amblyopic stimuli include refractive (light not focused on the retina), strabismic (eyes misaligned; see below) and sensory deprivation (light blocked from entering the eye, e.g. cataracts or ptosis). So a cataract that affects a child at 7 years of age is less likely to be as amblyogenic as a congenital one. This is why all babies have their red reflex tested as part of their first-day check.

Amblyopia is treatable by clearing the visual axis, prescribing glasses if required and encouraging the child to use the amblyopic eye. Patching or atropine drops to the fellow eye will achieve this in selected cases.

Children affected by amblyogenic stimuli early in their development should be urgently referred to the ophthalmology department for optimization of their vision. This may require early cataract surgery, with visual rehabilitation and close follow-up throughout childhood.

Nystagmus

This is a rhythmic to-and-fro movement of the eyes, a disorder of fixation of vision. There is usually slow movement, as fixation is lost with a rapid refixation movement. It is rarely seen from birth but becomes more apparent after about 2 months of age.

Nystagmus may be caused by a problem in the anterior visual system affecting vision or by a central motor problem causing fixation to be lost (e.g. in the midbrain or cerebellum). Nystagmus may result from poor vision, and may be the reason for presentation. Ocular albinism is a common cause of nystagmus. If the eye examination is otherwise normal, a retinal dystrophy should be considered.

In many cases, there is no obvious cause and this may be congenital idiopathic motor nystagmus. New onset of nystagmus may sometimes herald an optic nerve glioma; intracranial imaging should be considered, along with early referral to ophthalmology.

Infantile glaucoma

Glaucoma is a condition that results in optic nerve damage from increased intra-ocular pressure. It can rarely present in the first years of life. It is a serious problem because, without treatment, severe irreversible visual loss would be expected.

The most common symptoms are an aversion to lights (photophobia) and watering eyes (epiphora).

Because the intra-ocular pressure is raised during a period in which the eye would be enlarging, the most noticeable sign of infantile glaucoma is enlarged corneal diameter. The cornea is noted to be cloudy, which may give a reduction in the red reflex.

The most common cause of infantile glaucoma is a congenital abnormality in the formation of the anterior chamber angle that normally removes aqueous fluid from the eye. This results in an increase in intra-ocular pressure. Generally speaking, an operation is required to overcome this drainage problem.

Cataract

Problem-orientated topic:

a child with cataract

Hannah, a 2-year-old child, is referred because she is thought by her parents to have impaired vision in her left eye. On examination she has an obvious opacity in her left eye, which you think might be a cataract.

Q1. Why is evaluation urgently required?

Q2. What are the important causes to consider?

Q3. What would you look for in your clinical examination?

Q4. What investigations are required?

Q5. What is the management of cataract?

Q1. Why is evaluation urgently required?

Cataracts that cause reduced vision in childhood can result in permanent blindness due to amblyopia if not removed promptly. Adult-onset cataracts can be removed years after their onset with a complete return of vision. This is because normal visual development will have occurred during childhood. Normal development requires the exposure of neurons in the visual system to stimulation from visual experience during the development of the visual system.

Childhood cataracts (Fig. 31.2) are a very potent amblyopic stimulus. They should be operated on appropriately and early. Significant cataracts at birth are generally operated on in the first few weeks of life to allow visual development to occur.

Q2. What are the important causes to consider?

The causes of cataracts in childhood are many. Some may be related to systemic conditions (Box 31.3).

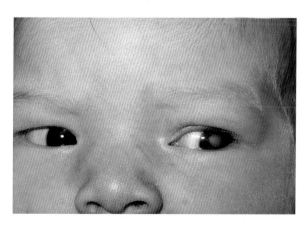

Fig. 31.2 Cataract of left lens in a 3-month-old baby

- Autosomal dominant/recessive isolated cataract
- Rubella
- Galactosaemia (p. 374)
- Total body irradiation
- Steroids
- Iritis
- Metabolic, e.g. Lowe's syndrome

baby definitely fixes on a face intermittently. Examination of the eyes is unremarkable. There is no history of any other medical problems.

Q1. What is the likely cause of reduced vision?
Q2. What should be noted on clinical examination?
Q3. What investigations should be considered?

Q3. What would you look for in your clinical examination?

Most congenital cataracts will be picked up on the first-day examination by the paediatrician checking the red reflex. Developmental cataracts that are not present at birth will be picked up later due to reduced vision. Very advanced cataracts may present when the parent notices a white pupil (leucocoria). This is also a presentation of retinoblastoma and should always be promptly referred to the ophthalmology service.

Q4. What investigations are required?

A complete physical examination is recommended but further investigations are usually not required unless some other abnormality is detected. Often, examination of the parents and the history will reveal an autosomal dominant isolated cataract that requires no further investigation. Investigations that are worth considering include urine for reducing substances, amino acids and organic acids. Rubella, calcium and glucose may also be considered.

Q5. What is the management of cataract?

Cataract surgery involves removing the cataract and either placing an intra-ocular lens or fitting the child with contact lenses if a lens cannot be placed inside the eye. Frequent follow-up in the eye clinic is needed, as visual development must be carefully monitored.

Reduced vision

Problem-orientated topic:

the child who appears not to see

Amy, a 4-month-old baby, was noticed not to be making eye contact from birth. The parents say that her vision has improved in the past week. Vision testing shows that the

Q1. What is the likely cause of reduced vision?

In this case of reduced vision from birth in the absence of any other medical problems, delayed visual maturation is most likely.

Conditions affecting the apparently blind child with a normal eye examination can generally be divided into those affecting the anterior visual pathway and those affecting the posterior visual pathway (see below).

Q2. What should be noted on clinical examination?

Each child with visual loss should have a careful examination to detect any other physical signs that may be associated with the condition.

Q3. What investigations should be considered?

Any eye abnormality should initially be ruled out. Presence or absence of nystagmus and pupil reactions to light are important to note.

In Amy's case, where the vision is improving, no further testing is required. Tests that would otherwise be considered include visual electrophysiology and brain imaging.

Anterior visual pathway problems

These can be located anywhere from the eye to behind the optic chiasm. While other causes of reduced vision, like corneal opacities and cataracts, are also anterior visual pathway problems, they are not included in this section because they are easily detected on clinical examination. This section will deal with the child who has reduced vision due to an anterior visual pathway problem with an apparently normal eye examination.

Anterior visual pathway disorders in infancy are associated with nystagmus (see above), whereas posterior visual pathway disorders are not.

Table 31.1 Examples of systemic conditions associated with retinal dystrophies

Condition	Other systems/organs affected
Isolated retinal dystrophy	None
Leber's congenital amaurosis	None
Senior–Loken syndrome	Renal
Usher's syndrome	Hearing and balance
Kearns–Sayre syndrome	Cardiac, liver and central nervous system (CNS)
Batten's disease	CNS
Alstrom's syndrome	Cardiac, endocrine

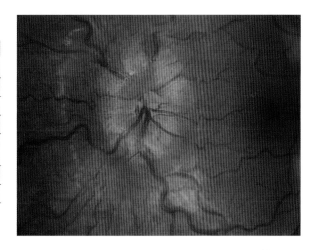

Fig. 31.3 **Papilloedema**

Retinal dystrophies (Table 31.1)

Retinal dystrophies involve a progressive inherited reduction in retinal function. This usually results from reduced cone and/or rod retinal function. With a cone dystrophy, the person will prefer dark conditions to optimize rod function; with a rod dystrophy, the converse is true. In some retinal dystrophies, and especially in childhood, the retina may have a relatively normal appearance. Electrophysiology may be useful in identifying retinal dysfunction.

Retinitis pigmentosa (RP) is a form of retinal dystrophy that may present in childhood. There are various forms of RP, which affects the rods more than the cones. Visual function is affected in dark conditions more than in light conditions. RP is usually associated with relatively good central vision. While progression may occur, it is unlikely that all vision would be lost.

Retinal dystrophies have a typical appearance of pigmentary changes in the retina, narrowing of the retinal vessels and a pale optic disc. They may be inherited as an isolated disease or may be associated with other systemic conditions.

Optic nerve

Optic nerve disorders can also cause reduced vision. Some examples of causes are:

- Congenital
- Inherited
- Neoplastic
- Toxic
- Metabolic
- Traumatic.

Raised intracranial pressure from any cause, e.g. hydrocephalus or idiopathic intracranial hypertension, may result in reduced optic nerve function. Treatment is to normalize the raised intracranial pressure. Optic nerve function in these cases should be followed by assessing visual acuity and visual fields and monitoring the optic disc appearance. Papilloedema is shown in Figure 31.3.

Posterior visual pathway problems

Children who do not appear to see due to a posterior visual pathway problem may have cortical visual impairment or delayed visual maturation.

Cortical visual impairment

Cortical visual impairment is reduced vision from a posterior visual pathway problem that results from a neurological cause. Causes of this condition may include:

- Seizures
- Metabolic
- Ischaemic
- Neuronal migration disorders.

Generally speaking, some improvement in visual performance occurs as the child gets older. The amount of improvement can range from a small change to full development of normal visual function. The timing of return of vision can be only a few days or it may take several weeks or months, depending on the cause and severity of injury. Treatment of the underlying cause is paramount to helping visual outcome to improve. Visual electrophysiology is useful in these cases. An electroretinogram measures function of the retinal layers and should be normal in this condition. A visual evoked potential will usually be reduced and delayed. Improvement in the visual evoked potential may precede clinical visual improvement.

Delayed visual maturation

Delayed visual maturation is usually a retrospective diagnosis. It is a congenital condition whereby the timing of myelination of the posterior visual pathway neurons is delayed but will develop fully with time. This may take 3–6 months to occur. Full visual function is expected with this condition. A comprehensive ophthalmology clinical examination is mandatory to rule out treatable and amblyogenic ocular causes of reduced vision.

Retinopathy of prematurity

Some premature infants are vulnerable to the development of retinopathy of prematurity (ROP). The normal retina begins vascularization from the optic disc towards the periphery after the ninth week post-conception. The entire surface area of the retina should be vascularized by term. Premature birth exposes the infant to higher oxygen tensions than would have been experienced in utero. This creates a relative ischaemia between the better-oxygenated, vascularized retina and its less oxygenated, non-vascularized periphery. This results in the non-vascularized retina releasing various angiogenic factors that cause the changes seen in ROP. ROP can cause retinal detachment and severe visual loss in its severest form.

Factors that seem to predispose infants to ROP include prematurity, low birth weight, chronic lung disease, intraventricular haemorrhage and necrotizing enterocolitis. It is important that all infants who are at risk of developing ROP are screened by an ophthalmologist. Children born at less than 32 weeks' gestation or weighing less than 1.5 kg at birth are usually screened. Screening usually commences 4–6 weeks after birth.

 http://www.site4sight.org.uk/Quality/RGov/ Guidelines/Retinop.htm

Treatment of infants who are deemed to have sufficient ROP (stage 3 plus) are treated by laser. The aim of treatment is to destroy the ischaemic retina in an attempt to stop the liberation of further ischaemic products. This usually results in resolution of the condition.

The red eye

Problem-orientated topic:

a child with a red eye

Ewan, a 3-week-old term baby, presents with a 1-week history of bilateral red sticky eyes. On examination, there is a conjunctivitis. The child is otherwise clinically well.

Q1. What is the likely diagnosis?
Q2. What investigations would you perform?
Q3. Is treatment required, and if so, when?
Q4. What follow-up may be required?

Q1. What is the likely diagnosis?

The most likely diagnosis in this case is neonatal conjunctivitis (ophthalmia neonatorum). This may be caused by various organisms and may have been picked up during delivery. Organisms that may be implicated include *Chlamydia trachomatis*, *Neisseria gonorrhoeae* and herpes simplex.

Infection of a blocked nasolacrimal duct may present in a similar manner. Corneal ulcers (caused, for example, by *Pseudomonas aeruginosa*) may present in the neonatal period.

Silver nitrate drops are sometimes routinely instilled in the eyes of newborns at birth to reduce the risk of infectious conjunctivitis. The silver nitrate itself can sometimes cause conjunctival irritation and redness.

Q2. What investigations would you perform?

Conjunctival swabs or scrapes should be taken for Gram stain, *Chlamydia* polymerase chain reaction (PCR) and culture.

Q3. Is treatment required, and if so, when?

Immediate treatment of suspected neonatal conjunctivitis is indicated because there is a risk to vision and to the child. Systemic therapy is usually required because neonatal conjunctivitis is considered to be a systemic condition.

Q4. What follow-up may be required?

Follow-up is needed to check for resolution of the signs in the baby. The results of laboratory investigations should be checked. The parents should be informed of the results, as sometimes they may also require treatment.

Uveitis

The most common uveitis in childhood is iritis due to juvenile idiopathic arthritis (JIA). A characteristic feature of the ocular inflammation is that there are no symptoms. Also, the eye may remain white. Similar iritis in an adult would be expected to cause photophobia and a red eye. For this reason, the eyes of children with JIA should be checked for the presence of iritis (p. 83).

Visual loss may occur due to glaucoma, cataract or swelling of the central vision part of the retina.

Treatment involves frequent steroid eye drops. If this is insufficient, then commencement or alteration of systemic immunosuppressive medications should be considered to control the iritis.

Mary O'Sullivan   Florence McDonagh   Neil Kennedy

Disorders of hearing, the ear and throat

LEARNING OUTCOMES

By the end of this chapter you should:

- Know when to be concerned about a child's hearing and refer appropriately
- Understand the implications of a report on a hearing assessment
- Know the causes of children's hearing difficulties
- Know what difficulties a deaf child may encounter
- Understand the implications of communication difficulties
- Understand the importance of working closely with other agencies
- Understand screening of children's hearing and its limitations
- Understand the natural history of adenotonsillar enlargement
- Know the indications for adenoidectomy and tonsillectomy
- Know when to use antibiotics for tonsillar exudate and sinusitis.

MODULE SIX

Basic science

A basic knowledge of the embryology of the ear is helpful in understanding how and why children have hearing problems as a result of trauma or teratogenic agents at specific stages in embryonic development. The severity of deafness depends on the site of involvement and hence the degree of difficulty with, for example, speech acquisition.

Embryology

Inner ear

Early in week 4 of embryonic development, a thickening (the otic placode) forms on each side of the head. The gross structures of the inner ear develop from the otic placode at between 5 and 8 weeks of embryonic life and continue to mature until between 25 weeks and term.

Middle ear

Around 32 days the middle ear begins to develop from the first pharyngeal pouch, which expands to form the middle ear cavity. Medially it forms the Eustachian (auditory) tube. Later the middle ear cavity expands by programmed cell death (apoptosis) and the ossicles become suspended in the cavity.

External ear

The external ear develops from the first pharyngeal groove, from three pairs of auricular hillocks that fuse to form the pinna. The cartilage of the otic capsule begins to ossify in the sixth month.

Physics of sound

Sound is the pattern of changes in pressure caused by movement or vibration of an object. From a central source it travels outwards in all directions in waves like ripples on a pond. The pitch or frequency of a sound is the number of waves that pass in 1 second (known as cycles). The more cycles per second, the higher the pitch. Cycles per second are called Hertz (Hz). Most sounds, including speech, are a mixture of frequencies. A drum makes a low-frequency sound and a whistle is a high-frequency sound. A sound of a single frequency is called a pure tone.

In general, the closer one is to a sound source, the louder the sound. Loudness (or intensity) is measured in decibels (dB). Figure 32.1 shows examples of everyday sounds, with their frequency and intensity plotted on an audiogram. An audiogram is a chart used to plot the quietest sound (threshold) that can be heard at given frequencies. If levels are obtained in the sound field (i.e. without the use of headphones or insert earphones), the loudness is usually described in 'dBA', but units are related to how the equipment is calibrated. If headphones are used, the levels are described in 'dBHL'. Thresholds of <20 dBHL are considered normal in the UK.

How does the ear work? (Fig. 32.2)

The ear is the organ of hearing and balance. It receives sound, amplifies it and converts it into neural impulses. The pinna funnels sound waves into the ear canal. These sound waves cause the tympanic membrane to vibrate. The middle ear improves sound transmission because of the difference in size of the tympanic membrane relative to the oval window, and by the lever action of the ossicles (malleus, incus and stapes). The ossicles

transmit this vibration through the footplate of the stapes to the inner ear, where it creates an action potential in an afferent neuron that is transmitted via the eighth nerve to the brain.

Hearing loss can be:
- *Conductive*, i.e. there is a problem in the external or middle ear
- *Sensorineural*, i.e. there is a problem with the cochlea or eighth nerve
- *Mixed*, i.e. both types occur concurrently.

Clinical assessment of hearing

The purpose of audiological assessment is to establish hearing thresholds, and if a hearing loss is present, to establish its type, configuration and severity.

Observation of the child's play (which can be done while listening to the history) will indicate how to pitch the testing so it is appropriate to the child's developmental age.

Routine hearing assessment is usually accompanied by:
- *Otoscopy* (Box 32.1): aids clinical decision-making (see above)
- *Tympanometry* (Box 32.2, Fig. 32.3): gives an indication of middle ear function.

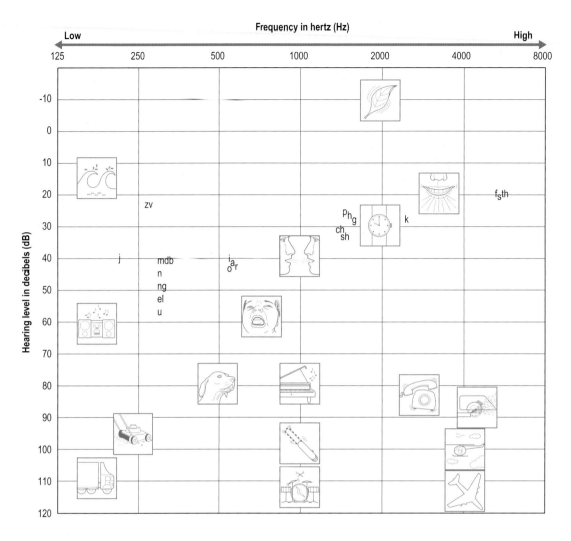

Fig. 32.1 Frequency and loudness of some everyday sounds
(Source: Deafness. HMSO. This figure is reproduced under the terms of the click-use licence.)

A full assessment by an audiologist may include:
- *Oto-acoustic emissions (OAEs)*, which can be used throughout childhood to assess cochlear function when middle ear function is normal.
- *Electric or brainstem evoked response (BSER) audiometry*, which can be used from birth if indicated.
- *Distraction testing*, which can be used when a child can sit unaided and turn to locate a sound until awareness of object permanence makes it unreliable. This is being phased out as a screening tool.
- *Visual reinforcement audiometry*, which can be used from 5 months of age once a child can locate a sound.
- *Performance testing*, which can usually be used by 2¹/₂ years if a child can wait for a sound stimulus

and perform an action reliably in response to it.
- *Pure-tone audiometry*, which can be used once a child will perform an action in response to hearing a sound and will accept headphones or insert earphones (Fig. 32.4).

Hearing assessments should be carried out in a child- and family-friendly environment. Parents can be included in 'playing the games' in clinic, and can observe when the child responds to a sound. The hearing thresholds at each frequency are discussed and related to the loudness of certain sounds in running speech. Some parents will welcome confirmation of a hearing loss they have suspected, while others will be shocked to find their child is deaf. For some parents there is only one interpretation of the word 'deaf', so it

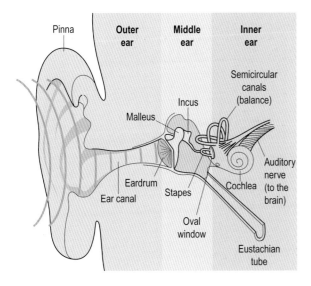

Fig. 32.2 **Diagram of the ear**
(Source: Deafness. HMSO. This figure is reproduced under the terms of the click-use licence.)

BOX 32.2 Skill: tympanometry

Middle ear problems are very common in childhood and tympanometry is a quick and reliable indicator of middle ear function. The assessment of middle ear function is an essential part of the test battery so that hearing thresholds are correctly interpreted. Before commencing, the audiologist will check for contraindications such as tenderness or the presence of discharge. After the procedure is explained to the parent, the child should be seated sideways on the parent's knee; the pinna is pulled gently backwards and an appropriately sized probe tip is placed at the entrance to the child's ear canal. Movement and excess noise can give spurious or inconclusive results. If abnormal shapes are obtained, the test should be repeated.

Figure 32.3 shows the most common types of tympanogram in paediatric practice.

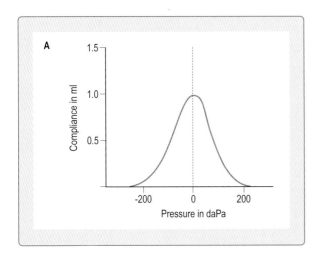

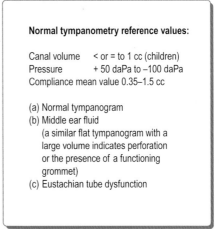

Normal tympanometry reference values:

Canal volume   < or = to 1 cc (children)
Pressure   + 50 daPa to –100 daPa
Compliance mean value 0.35–1.5 cc

(a) Normal tympanogram
(b) Middle ear fluid
     (a similar flat tympanogram with a large volume indicates perforation or the presence of a functioning grommet)
(c) Eustachian tube dysfunction

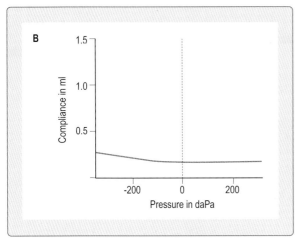

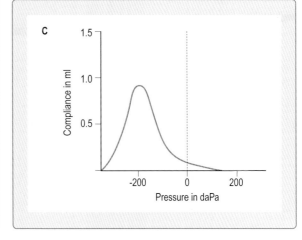

Fig. 32.3 **Tympanometry**

Disorders of hearing, the ear and throat

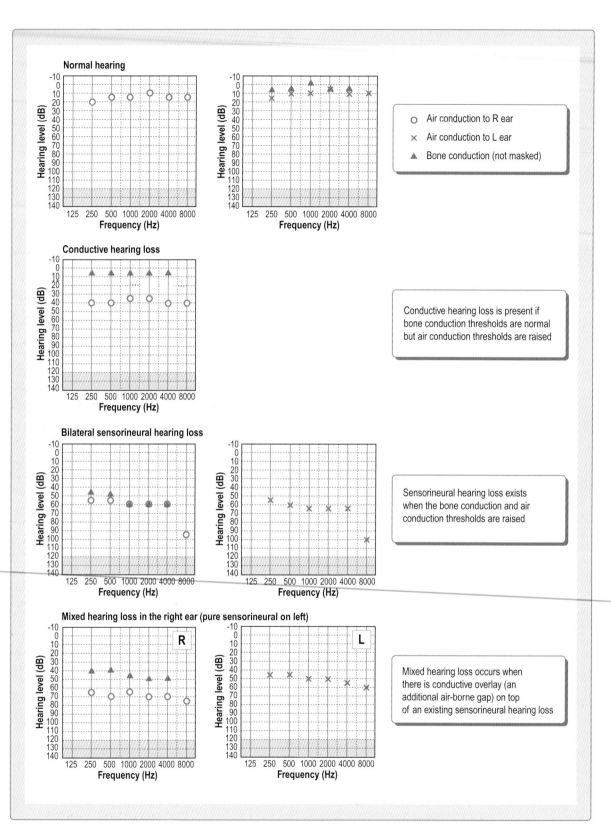

Fig. 32.4 **Pure tone audiometry**

is important to explain carefully the degree of hearing loss and the implications in relation to specific speech sounds.

Screening for hearing impairment

Deafness affects the linguistic, social, emotional and educational development of a child. The incidence of significant permanent congenital hearing impairment (> 40 dB across speech frequencies in the better ear) is about 1 per 1000. Deafness is the most common birth defect, having a greater incidence than cystic fibrosis and hypothyroidism. Approximately 840 children are born in the UK each year with a moderate to profound degree of deafness. Acquired and late-onset cases add to this number. Over 50% of these children will have a moderate deafness, with approximately equal numbers of children having severe and profound deafness. Almost 30% of deaf children have no known history of risk factors for hearing impairment.

Neonatal screening

A universal newborn hearing screening programme (NHSP) will pick up children with hearing problems and adequately fulfils the criteria for a screening programme. All districts in the UK were to have a universal newborn hearing screen in place by 2006. The health visitor distraction test, which was previously carried out on all babies between 7 and 9 months, was to run in parallel with this screen for the first year and was then to be discontinued. Although neonatal screening will detect children who are deaf at birth, professionals need to continue to be vigilant regarding the possibility of acquired, progressive and late-onset deafness.

The aim of a universal newborn hearing screen is the early identification of children who have a significant permanent hearing impairment in the neonatal period. Early detection of hearing impairment and early intervention lessen the impact of deafness on the child, the child's family and society. Studies have highlighted the importance of diagnosis and introduction of early support programmes before 6 months of age for the future speech and language abilities of the child.

Two non-invasive, quick and reliable screening tests are available for screening for hearing impairment in the newborn period. Descriptions are available on the NHSP website. All newborn babies will have an oto-acoustic emission (OAE) test and some will go on to have an automated auditory brainstem response (AABR) test.

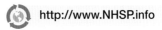 http://www.NHSP.info

Oto-acoustic emissions

OAEs are tiny sounds that can be measured in the ear canal in 98% of normally hearing people by placing a small probe in the ear. They originate in the inner ear and are thought to be produced as a by-product of the amplification action of the outer hair cells (OHCs). They are only present in ears with normal OHCs and correlate highly with normal hearing. Since the vast majority of hearing impairment is due to OHC damage, recording an OAE provides a sensitive and accurate means of identification of cochlear hearing impairment. Since the test is robust and easy to perform, it is an excellent screening test. OAEs are not normally present when the hearing loss is greater than 30 dB. The presence of a clear response on OAE testing suggests normal cochlear function in an ear. An automated OAE system has been designed for screening and indicates the presence or absence of a clear response.

Auditory brainstem response test

ABR records the electrical activity in the auditory nerve and in the brainstem when sounds are presented in the ear. An automated ABR system has been designed for screening. A click stimulus at 35 dBnHL (n = normal) is presented into the ear via a probe or ear cuffs, and the machine automatically registers the presence or absence of a clear response. Some infants are at greater risk of damage to the auditory pathway. ABR is the test of choice for these infants, as it tests the integrity of the auditory pathway as well as the cochlea. For this reason babies admitted to neonatal units will have an OAE test and an AABR test as routine, as these infants are at greater risk of developing retrocochlear hearing problems. Some babies who are at risk of developing late-onset or progressive hearing problems will be identified at birth and will require a targeted infant distraction test when they are 7–9 months old.

Children whose newborn screen indicates bilateral clear responses should have follow-up if they meet one or more of the criteria specified in Box 32.3.

Later screening

Intermediate screening between the newborn screen and school entry is no longer recommended, but it is important to ask parents about hearing concerns at routine health checks. The school entry sweep test of hearing, which checks hearing using a pure-tone audiometric screen, continues to be recommended. The sweep screen is undergoing review in 2007. This

- Parental or professional concern
- Meningitis, chronic middle ear effusion and craniofacial abnormalities
- Family history of sensorineural hearing loss (SNHL) in parents or siblings
- Special care baby unit (SCBU)/neonatal intensive care unit (NICU) child with no clear responses on OAEs despite clear responses on ABR
- SCBU/NICU child who had intermittent positive pressure ventilation (IPPV) for more than 5 days
- Jaundice, where bilirubin levels indicate a need for exchange transfusion
- Congenital TORCH (*toxoplasmosis, rubella, cytomegalovirus, herpes simplex*) infection
- Neurodegenerative or neurodevelopmental disorders
- Confirmed syndromes related to hearing loss, e.g. Down's syndrome (see Box 32.4)

BOX 32.4 Hearing surveillance for children with Down's syndrome

Over 50% of people with Down's syndrome have deafness of a mild/moderate/profound degree.

- Newborn hearing screen
- Full audiological assessment between 6 and 10 months
- Review audiological assessment at 18 months
- Yearly audiological assessment until 5 years old
- Thereafter, 2-yearly review for life
- Assessment should include 8 kHz in view of early onset of presbycousis

screen should pick up late and acquired losses not present at the time of the targeted distraction test.

Babies who are found to have permanent congenital deafness as a result of neonatal screening and subsequent evaluation require early intervention. Developments that may improve speech and language and communication are shown in Box 32.5.

BOX 32.5 Developments in the management of permanent congenital deafness

- Newborn hearing screening and targeted follow-up
- Early cochlear implantation
- Guidelines on support in the early years
- Digital signal processing hearing aids

Hearing loss

Problem-orientated topic:

poor speech development

Jamie, aged 18 months, has been referred by his health visitor because he is not making progress with his speech. The referral indicates that he had started to babble but this has ceased. His mum gives a history of bilateral ear infection with discharge at age 1 year.

Hearing assessment with visual reinforcement audiometry indicates a flat loss across the thresholds of 50–60 dBHL at 500–4000 Hz. Otoscopy and tympanometry indicate middle ear effusions (MEE) bilaterally.

Q1. What are the possible causes of Jamie's hearing loss?

Q2. How would you manage this condition?

Q3. What factors in Jamie's history would contraindicate the normal practice of watching and waiting for improvement?

Q1. What are the possible causes of Jamie's hearing loss?

Conductive deafness occurs when sound transmission through the outer or middle ear is not efficient. The causes of conductive loss include:

- Blockage of the ear canal (atresia, wax, foreign body)
- Perforation of the tympanic membrane
- Otitis media with effusion (OME), also called middle ear effusion (MEE) or 'glue ear' (by far the most common cause in children)
- Ossicular problems: e.g. disarticulation or necrosis
- Otosclerosis: i.e. bridge formation from footplate to oval window (unlikely in young children).

Jamie has MEE.

Q2. How would you manage this condition?

Initial management, in the absence of significantly raised hearing thresholds or indicators of persistence or other causes for concern, will be watching and waiting for spontaneous resolution. Arrangements should be made to reassess the hearing in 3 months. Meanwhile, advice with regard to risk factors is given to parents/carers and information can be gathered about school progress and speech and language development, which will be useful for the review appointment. If there is a significant hearing loss, advice to school is useful, once parental consent is obtained. Balance may be affected temporarily.

Early referral to an ear, nose and throat (ENT) surgeon is prompted by:
- The possibility of a mixed hearing loss
- Significantly raised hearing thresholds
- Speech and language difficulties
- Educational difficulties
- Recurrent ear infections
- Persistent snoring or sleep apnoea syndrome
- Behavioural difficulties linked to hearing.

Q3. What factors in Jamie's history would contraindicate the normal practice of watching and waiting for improvement?

Concerns in Jamie's case include:
- Lack of progress with speech
- Likely duration of condition (6 months)
- Significantly raised hearing thresholds.

The latter raises the possibility of a mixed hearing loss.

With children like Jamie, it is important to assess their hearing after intervention or resolution of glue ear (MEE, OME) in order to rule out a sensorineural hearing loss. Children who have a first episode of glue ear in their first 18 months are more prone to recurrence.

Otitis media with effusion (OME)

OME is an accumulation of fluid behind an intact tympanic membrane in the absence of acute infection. It is the most common cause of hearing difficulty in childhood, with peak prevalence at around 1 year of age, rising again around the age of 3–5 years. Spontaneous resolution occurs in most cases in about 3 months. Persistence is more likely in children who first present early in life. Most children with conductive hearing loss have a mild loss (< 45 dBHL). Even mild losses, however, can have an effect on speech discrimination and hence on language acquisition. The duration of the loss is important, as is adequate exposure to language. There is an increasing body of evidence to suggest that OME puts children at risk with regard to language acquisition and subsequent schooling.

Risk factors for OME include:
- Age
- Season (more likely in winter)
- Sibling history
- Group childcare (possibly due to cross-infection)
- Environmental smoke exposure
- Bottle feeding (breastfeeding is protective in the first year)
- Race
- Anatomical predisposition (including cleft palate, craniofacial abnormalities).

The infant's Eustachian tube is more horizontal than that of the adult. Eustachian tube dysfunction is causally linked to OME. Microorganisms have been cultured in the effusion in a significant proportion of cases. OME is associated with adenoidal hypertrophy (p. 74) and adenoidectomy is a treatment option. When OME is suspected, it is obviously important to assess the child's hearing. If there are no signs of acute infection (pain or signs of inflammation, red and bulging tympanic membrane), antibiotics are not indicated.

Management decisions then depend on:
- Hearing levels
- Whether there are indicators of persistence
- Whether there is parental, carer or professional concern
- Presence of other symptoms and signs, e.g. recurrent ear infections, snoring
- Presence of other issues, e.g. learning difficulties.

The hearing levels in OME are prone to fluctuate. This has been linked to the poor listening skills that are evident in some of these children. It is also helpful to consider whether hearing difficulties are having an adverse effect on the parent–child relationship. If hearing difficulties persist after a period of watching and waiting, treatment options such as grommet insertion or trial of hearing aids need to be considered and this usually necessitates a referral to ENT. Close liaison with ENT is helpful, especially for children with particularly poor speech or where there are learning difficulties and complex needs that are associated with more adverse outcomes.

It is helpful for children who have been adversely affected by OME to be followed up, and this can sometimes be usefully done by the family doctor, who can monitor for recurrence, persistent perforation, significant tympanic membrane retraction and cholesteatoma. Certain groups are at particular risk, e.g. children with Down's syndrome or cleft palate (see also Boxes 32.3 and 32.4). Thus there is a need for vigilance and routine review in these groups. Surveillance guidelines are helpful. Parents are often unaware of children's hearing difficulties and notice a difference only after intervention.

Evidence suggests that persistence is more likely if children are first seen at ENT between July and December, if the hearing level is ≤ 30 dBHL and the route of referral includes prior audiometry.

Acute otitis media (OM)

Acute OM is a common infection in childhood and usually presents with pain in the ear, fever and sometimes deafness. The diagnosis is made by otoscopy, when a red, bulging tympanic membrane is seen. An effusion may be evident behind the membrane.

Bacteria cause the majority of cases of acute OM and the most common are:

- *Streptococcus pneumoniae*
- *Haemophilus influenzae*
- *Moraxella catarrhalis*
- Group A streptococcus
- *Staphylococcus aureus.*

Viruses cause a minority of infections in the middle ear.

Antibiotic management remains controversial. Spontaneous recovery occurs in 80% of cases, whether treated or not, and in only 13% has 'primary control' with antibiotics been noted, with shortening of the duration of symptoms. Nevertheless, in view of the small risk of serious complications (mastoiditis, meningitis), most doctors treat symptomatic children with amoxicillin to shorten the duration of symptoms.

 http://www.cps.ca/english/statements/ID/id97-03.htm

Problem-orientated topic:

failed hearing screening test at 8 months

Alice, aged 10 months, has been referred by her health visitor because she did not pass her hearing screen at 8 months of age. On testing, Alice responds at 75 dB throughout the frequencies tested. On examination she has middle ear effusions bilaterally. She is referred immediately to a joint clinic with an ENT surgeon, who agrees to see her urgently in view of the severity of her hearing loss. He confirms middle ear effusions and Alice is listed for grommet insertion within the week. On retesting afterwards she has a 60 dB loss.

Q1. What type of hearing loss does Alice have?

Q2. What are the most likely causes of Alice's sensorineural hearing loss?

Q3. How should a deaf child be managed?

Q4. What is Alice's prognosis?

Q1. What type of hearing loss does Alice have?

Alice has mixed hearing loss and has been urgently referred to ENT services because of the severity of her hearing loss. Although her long-term prognosis is expected to be reasonably good, she requires to be carefully followed up to manage her sensorineural hearing loss (SNHL) and to detect any recurrence of middle ear effusion.

Mixed hearing loss occurs when a conductive loss is superimposed on a sensorineural loss. Hearing assessment shows air conduction (AC) thresholds to be poorer than the (abnormal) bone conduction (BC) thresholds (Fig. 32.4). When the conductive element is treated or disappears, AC thresholds revert to BC levels.

SNHL is caused by abnormality of the cochlea or ascending neural pathways. Most often it is due to hair cell damage in the cochlea. SNHL is less common than conductive loss, with a prevalence of about 1.2 per 1000 live births for moderate loss and above. Most SNHL is congenital and is usually permanent. The prevalence of SNHL increases with increasing age due to acquired and progressive losses. When a hearing loss is purely sensorineural, AC and BC thresholds are the same, i.e. there is no air–bone gap (p. 66). Hearing loss is described as unilateral or bilateral and also by the degree of the impairment, as follows:

- Mild hearing loss: < 40 dBHL
- Moderate: 41–70 dBHL
- Severe: 71–95 dBHL
- Profound: > 95 dBHL.

When children are able to cooperate with pure-tone audiometry, the presence of the mixed loss is shown by a gap between the AC threshold and the BC threshold (Fig. 32.4). If the conductive element is due to OME, it is important to remedy this as soon as possible with a referral to an ENT specialist. It has been shown, however, that the necessity for an ENT operation can significantly delay the age of identification and hearing aid fitting in children with severe hearing loss. Thus there is a need for clear communication and urgency in liaison between professionals and departments. Not all conductive components are due to effusions, however. Permanent conductive losses occur infrequently but are more likely in certain syndromes, e.g. Treacher Collins syndrome.

Q2. What are the most likely causes of Alice's sensorineural hearing loss?

Investigation of the cause of SNHL is important because:
- Parents want to know why their child is deaf.
- They may want to know about the risk of deafness in further siblings.
- Deafness may be associated with medical problems that need to be identified.
- The cause of deafness may influence management.

The relative prevalence of the causes of hearing loss has changed with time because of immunization programmes (e.g. rubella), improvements in neonatal intensive care and improvements in genetics. The most common causes of isolated hearing loss are:
- Neonatal problems (asphyxia, prematurity)
- Toxicity (aminoglycosides, Ch. 10; hyperbilirubinaemia, p. 323)
- Genetic (see below)
- Craniofacial abnormality
- Infection (post-meningitis, p. 287)
- Trauma.

Post-meningitis (bacterial) deafness

This remains an important cause of severe deafness. The important points are as follows:
- Deafness of any degree follows bacterial meningitis in 10% of children.
- The onset of deafness may occur late after the infection has been treated.
- Optimum time for assessment of hearing is 4–6 weeks post-infection.
- 1–4% have bilateral profound deafness.
- The deafness may be progressive.
- There is a risk of cochlear ossification.

With the advent of universal neonatal screening, which has led to earlier identification of childhood hearing impairment, it is likely that more precise diagnosis will be achieved; for example, congenital infection may be identified with greater certainty.

 http://www.nhsp.info
Medical Management of Infants with Significant Congenital Hearing Loss Identified

Vestibular investigations should be performed on all children.

Progressive hearing loss can be familial but can also be due to viral infections (e.g. rubella, cytomegalovirus), metabolic causes or bacterial meningitis.

Genetic considerations

Following aetiological assessment of deafness, referral to a geneticist is indicated if:

- There is a positive family history
- There are complex needs, learning difficulties or other medical problems
- There are dysmorphic features
- The family request it.

It is estimated that the cause of permanent congenital deafness in at least 50% of cases is genetic. Most of these are likely to be recessive, some dominant. About 30% of genetic deafness is syndromal; less frequent are X-linked and mitochondrial inheritance. A common mutation in the *connexin 26* gene, referred to as 30delG (sometimes called 35delG), is frequently implicated in non-syndromal deafness. When this is homozygous, it is likely to be the cause of deafness in a particular child. When the child is heterozygous, it is useful to seek a genetic opinion, as another mutation may need to be excluded. Mitochondrial inheritance is implicated in deafness due to the A1555G mutation. Deafness may occur regardless of exposure to aminoglycosides, although this was how the gene was first discovered. The prevalence of deafness increases with increasing age when this mutation is present.

Q3. How should a deaf child be managed?

Professionals involved in the management of deaf children want the best outcome for the child and family, i.e. a well-rounded individual who communicates well, is healthy and happy, is learning appropriately in school, and has good relationships with peer groups and family alike. Specific goals include:
- Early identification of deafness
- Optimal habilitation, i.e. appropriate aiding and family support
- Appropriate communication strategies and support.

The multidisciplinary team managing a deaf child includes:
- Audiologist: hearing assessment, hearing aid work
- Parent
- Doctor: examines, treats, investigates, refers, advocacy work
- Teacher: with a special qualification for teaching the deaf
- Speech and language therapist
- Nurse (health visitor, school nurse)
- Social worker (may be a 'specialist' working with deaf children only).

How confirmation of deafness is imparted to the family, the language used by professionals, good listening skills and treating parents as partners all play an important part in managing the stress and anxiety for the family around the time of identification of deafness. Confident parental involvement will facilitate successful hearing aid use, encourage successful communication and enable the child to reach his or her potential.

Once the degree and nature of the hearing loss is apparent, the team, together with the parents, can meet and plan intervention. Initial work will include:

- Fitting of appropriate hearing aids
- Supply of information about voluntary organizations
- Ongoing recursive assessment (to verify hearing aid fitting)
- Involvement of the early intervention team
- ENT and paediatric assessment
- Aetiological assessment and investigation
- Communication assessment and input as needed
- Referral for ophthalmological assessment.

The degree and configuration of the loss will determine hearing aid fit. It is important that parents understand the potential effect of the hearing loss on the child's ability to communicate and thus accept the need to wear hearing aids. If the child shows no benefit after 3 months of hearing aid wear, consideration should be given to referral with a view to cochlear implantation if appropriate.

As the child approaches 2 years of age, there needs to be consideration of schooling options in consultation with parents. When a deaf child is born to hearing parents, there is a sense of loss and grief. This may show as anger against professionals and parents may seek alternative opinions. While parents are working through these emotions, they will not be able to take in all the information given to them by professionals. Thus they need time and space to talk about their feelings and a sympathetic and supportive attitude from the multidisciplinary support team. Some parents may need psychological counselling or intervention. Meanwhile, they need to be encouraged to work with their child to improve communication and may themselves need to consider alternative strategies, e.g. learning sign language so they can begin to communicate appropriately with their child.

There is a higher prevalence of child abuse in deaf children, and it is more difficult for the deaf child to disclose abuse. Mental health problems are more prevalent in deaf children, and mental health services with appropriate communication and professional skills should be available as necessary.

Q4. What is Alice's prognosis?

When children are learning to talk they need to be able to hear all of the individual sounds of speech in order to reproduce them properly. Some speech sounds are significantly quieter than others: for example, 's', 'f'

and 'th' (Fig. 32.1). Therefore even mild hearing losses make it difficult for children to hear plurals, tenses and voiceless consonants. Children with moderate losses cannot hear most of conversational speech sounds. Children with SNHL need to be monitored in case the loss progresses, i.e. hearing gets worse.

Children with SNHL are more dependent on their vision to access the environment and education. They are more likely to have visual problems. Aetiological clues may sometimes be evident to the ophthalmologist. Thus ophthalmological assessment and oversight is essential for deaf children.

Deaf awareness

Deaf children need to understand and communicate as hearing children do. Going to the doctor or into hospital can be a frightening experience. Paediatricians need to understand the implications of a child's deafness for communication (see p. 70 for definitions):

- A child with mild deafness may find it difficult to understand quiet speech, particularly in background noise, and the use of a sound field system in the classroom may need to be considered.
- A child with moderate deafness will find it difficult to follow conversational speech without the use of a hearing aid.
- A child with severe deafness will not be able to follow conversational speech without the use of a hearing aid.
- A child who is profoundly deaf will be unable to hear speech, and will only hear loud environmental sounds without amplification.

Professionals need to be aware of and sensitive to the child's preferred communication mode, and to make sure children understand planned investigations and treatment. An interpreter should be available for the child who signs. Communication should be effective, i.e. the speaker should avoid jargon, explain clearly, write things down as necessary, and be aware that deaf children's literacy skills may be limited if English is their second language.

Minimizing the effects of permanent hearing impairment in children

As already stated, about 840 children are born in the UK each year with significant permanent hearing loss. Until the introduction of the NHSP, identification of these children was significantly delayed. They were deprived of much auditory experience during the first year(s) of life at a stage when environmental stimulation is necessary for the development of neuronal connections in the auditory nervous system. Even though it may not be obvious to the casual observer, receptive language is developing in the first year of life, leading to understanding and production of first words at around 1 year of age.

It is anticipated that early identification through NHSP and early intervention, including the Early Support Programme, will facilitate language acquisition in this group and improve outcomes, i.e. will reduce the linguistic, social, educational and cognitive sequelae as well as the mental health implications of deafness for this group.

It has been shown that approximately 40% of deaf children have another disability in addition to their deafness and over 60% of these will have more than one additional disability. Visual problems are four times as common in deaf children, who depend largely on their vision to access the environment.

Children with complex needs are more likely to have hearing difficulties. They are also more likely to be adversely affected by hearing difficulties, either permanent or temporary. Children with unilateral hearing loss have problems with learning and with discriminating speech in noisy environments.

Even children with mild hearing loss that may not be considered to be 'significant' in terms of need for support by Educational Hearing Impairment services or who would not be fitted with hearing aids may be at risk of 'academic failure'. There are links between minor hearing difficulties and self-esteem and peer status, and thus it becomes clear that the management of the child with even minor hearing difficulties needs to involve many disciplines working together.

Cochlear implantation

Cochlear implantation aims to provide hearing sensation for children who are severely and profoundly deaf and derive no useful benefit from conventional hearing aids. A cochlear implant has the potential to deliver hearing sensation at levels of 30–45 dB across speech frequencies that will enable children to 'hear' speech in a way that is not possible with conventional aids. Each Cochlear Implant Centre has its own referral guidelines and needs to work closely with local services with regard to individual children. If implantation goes ahead, the implanted electrodes, which are surgically placed in the cochlea, stimulate afferent cochlear neurons directly; the resultant impulse travels along the auditory pathway to the cortex, where it is interpreted as sound. Selection of children for implantation follows a detailed assessment.

Pre-lingually and post-lingually deaf children will derive benefit from a cochlear implant. Children with profound deafness who receive a cochlear implant early

on derive most benefit from it. Cochlear implantation is also an option for children who have progressive deafness or who suddenly become deaf, e.g. post-meningitis. Post-meningitis patients need to be fast-tracked. Around 40% of deaf children have additional complex needs and cochlear implantation will offer an important management adjunct for some of these children. Cochlear implantation is usually carried out on one side only.

Every child's experience with a cochlear implant is unique. Cochlear implantation does not restore hearing but it does provide an auditory sensation that has been described by some people who were hearing previously as mechanical or synthetic. The first experience of audition comes about 1 month after implantation, when the speech processor and coil are fitted and switched on. With support over time, children will hear and understand everyday environmental and speech sounds through their cochlear implant, which means they may develop speech themselves. Some users may advance to understand speech without the help of lip reading and go on to use the telephone.

 http://www.bcig.org

Criteria for referral for cochlear implantation

- Bilateral severe/profound sensorineural hearing impairment (≥ 90 dBHL at 2 kHz and 4 kHz in the better ear)
- Clinical ABR thresholds ≥ 90 dBHL
- No minimum age for referral
- Children with additional needs should be referred
- Post-meningitis patients need to be fast-tracked
- Children of any age who fulfil the audiological criteria should be discussed with the cochlear implant team.

Factors that influence outcome of cochlear implantation

- Age of the child and duration of deafness at time of implantation
- Aetiology of deafness
- Type of device implanted
- Auditory environment post-implantation, i.e. rich in spoken language
- Degree of engagement in the habilitative process
- Consistent use of the cochlear implant over time.

Balance disorders

Balance problems and hearing problems often coexist. Delay in establishing head control, sitting and walking can indicate vestibular dysfunction. A history of ototoxic medication or meningitis (or both) may be significant aetiological factors in the genesis of vestibular dysfunction. Children with vestibular areflexia do not suffer from motion sickness. Walking is delayed until after 18 months of age in children with bilateral vestibular areflexia.

Children may not complain of vertigo; therefore it is important to elicit from parents whether the child has signs or symptoms suggestive of vestibular dysfunction. These may include sudden onset of nystagmus, vomiting, pallor and falling without loss of consciousness, or the older child may complain that the environment is moving.

Afferent information from the vestibular system, visual information and proprioceptive information are integrated in the brainstem, pons and cerebellum. This generates efferent signals that facilitate coordinated movement. Vestibular assessment aims to isolate these components. Teamwork by paediatricians, neurologists, audiological physicians and others may be needed in individual cases.

The presence or absence of vestibular dysfunction can be helpful in separating genetic syndromes. Rehabilitation (which may simply include playing and sport) facilitates central compensation.

Tonsillar and adenoidal hypertrophy

Problem-orientated topic:

tonsillar and adenoidal hypertrophy

Najimee, a 4-year-old, is brought to her GP by her mother. She is having frequent episodes of tonsillitis, which cause her to miss school. She is chronically tired, sleeps poorly and snores loudly. On examination she is thriving. She is a persistent mouth breather. Her tonsils are non-inflamed but large enough to obstruct over 60% of her airway.

Q1. What features in the history suggest that she should be referred to an ENT surgeon?

Q2. What are the indications for adenoidectomy/tonsillectomy?

Q1. What features in the history suggest that she should be referred to an ENT surgeon?

The tonsils and adenoids begin to develop in the third month of gestation. Their maximal period of enlargement is in the first and second years of life. They continue to grow until, at around 8 or 9 years, they begin a slow process of involution. Only a remnant remains by early adulthood. Some genetic disorders predispose to adenoidal airway obstruction, e.g. trisomy 21.

Historically, many children underwent adenotonsillectomy for recurrent tonsillitis or adenoiditis. UK tonsillectomy rates have fallen from 120 per 10 000 children (age ≤ 14 years) in 1967 to 65 per 10 000 in 1998. Obstructive sleep apnoea syndrome is an increasingly common indication for surgery.

Adenoidal obstruction of the nasopharynx (Fig. 32.5) can present as:

- Prolonged (3–4 weeks) upper respiratory tract infections, with purulent rhinorrhoea
- Persistent mouth breathing with hyponasal ('adenoidal') speech
- Recurrent otitis media/otitis media with effusion
- Obstructive sleep apnoea syndrome.

Obstructive sleep apnoea syndrome (OSAS)

Symptoms of OSAS include noisy breathing at night and/or loud snoring accompanied by nocturnal apnoeic pauses, poor sleep quality and daytime somnolence. In contrast to adults, episodes of airway obstruction in children usually occur in rapid eye movement (REM) sleep. A reduction of time in REM sleep can lead to cognitive or behavioural disorders. Untreated, OSAS is associated with chronic hypoxia, secondary pulmonary hypertension, cor pulmonale and failure to thrive.

OSAS can be confirmed by a 'sleep study'. The gold standard is polysomnography: continuous concurrent recording of oxygen saturation, heart rate, end-tidal CO_2, abdominal and thoracic breathing movements, nasal airflow, oculograms and electroencephalogram (EEG). This is rarely available in practice and overnight oxygen saturation monitoring is substituted. Compared with polysomnography, oximetry has a positive predictive value (PPV) of 97% and a negative predictive value (NPV) of 47%, i.e. it has a high false negative rate. The American Academy of Pediatrics has published evidence-based guidelines for the diagnosis and management of OSAS.

 http://aappolicy.aappublications.org/cgi/content/full/pediatrics;109/4/704

Q2. What are the indications for adenoidectomy/tonsillectomy? (Box 32.6)

Reasonable evidence exists for adenoidectomy/tonsillectomy in the treatment of OSAS. There is some evidence for adenoidectomy as a treatment for OME. A large multicentre trial is ongoing.

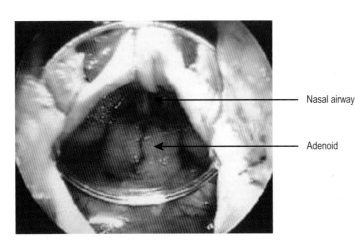

Fig. 32.5 **Adenoidal obstruction of the nasopharynx**

Nasal airway

Adenoid

BOX 32.6 Relative indications for adenoidectomy

- Obstructive sleep apnoea syndrome (often with tonsillectomy)
- Recurrent acute otitis media
- Otitis media with effusion and hearing loss
- Severe persistent nasal obstruction

BOX 32.7 Referral criteria for recurrent tonsillitis in children

All the following criteria should be met:

- Five or more definite episodes of tonsillitis per year
- Symptoms for at least 1 year
- Episodes of tonsillitis that are disabling and prevent normal functioning, e.g. school attendance

Enlargement of the tonsils alone is not an indication for surgery. Clear criteria exist for referral to ENT services for recurrent tonsillitis (Box 32.7).

 http://www.rcpch.ac.uk/publications/clinical_docs/GGPsorethroat.pdf

Following referral, a 6-month period of 'watchful waiting' is recommended to establish the symptom pattern and to allow time to consider the implications of surgery (Box 32.8).

Complications of adenotonsillectomy

Post-operative bleeding occurs in 0.5–1.5%. Treatment of primary post-operative haemorrhage (within the first 24 hours) consists of local pressure, fluid or blood replacement, and return to theatre for diathermy/ligature of the bleeding vessel. Secondary haemorrhage (usually day 6–10) is associated with wound infection.

Rare complications include damage to the soft palate or Eustachian tube.

BOX 32.8 Indications for tonsillectomy

- Recurrent tonsillitis (see above)
- One or two episodes of quinsy
- Obstructive sleep apnoea syndrome
- Suspicion of other pathology, e.g. lymphoma

The effects of adenotonsillectomy on the immune system have been debated. Most studies do not show any significant alteration in immune function following surgery.

Tonsillar exudates

Problem-orientated topic:

the child with tonsillar exudate

Martin, a 5-year-old, is brought to the accident and emergency department by his mother, who is concerned about his high temperature. On examination, temperature is 38.9°C. He has bilateral red swollen tonsils with exudate. His superior cervical lymph nodes are swollen and tender. He has no rash and appears systemically 'well'.

Q1. What are the causes of tonsillitis with exudate?
Q2. What investigations (if any) should be done?
Q3. Should Martin be treated with antibiotics?

Q1. What are the causes of tonsillitis with exudate?

The palatine tonsils and adenoids are part of a protective ring of lymphoid tissue in the oropharynx and nasopharynx. A surface lining of stratified squamous epithelium is invaginated by 15–20 deep grooves or crypts. Deeper lie multiple lymphatic nodules, several of which coalesce and contain germinal centres. The crypts frequently contain 'cheesy' debris consisting of food particles, mucus, neutrophils and lymphocytes. A dense connective tissue capsule separates the tonsil bed from the pharyngeal wall. Efferent lymphatics drain to the jugulodigastric (behind the angle of the mandible) and upper cervical lymph nodes. Sensation is supplied by the glossopharyngeal and vagus nerves.

Functionally, both tonsils and adenoids serve to detect and defend against oral or inhaled pathogens. Antigens presented to T-helper cells are in turn presented to B cells within the germinal matrix of a lymphoid nodule. IgA is secreted as a result.

In cases of tonsillitis with exudates consider:
- Bacterial infection
- Epstein–Barr virus infection (glandular fever)
- Diphtheria.

Q2. What investigations (if any) should be done?

Organisms cultured from the tonsils are listed in Box 32.9. Most episodes of tonsillitis are caused by viral infection. Group A β-haemolytic streptococci (GABHS) are isolated in approximately 30% of people with a sore throat. However, GABHS is also isolated in 5–40% of asymptomatic carriers.

BOX 32.9 Organisms cultured from the tonsils

Viruses
- Epstein–Barr (EBV)
- Adenovirus
- Respiratory syncytial virus (RSV)
- Influenza A and B
- Parainfluenza
- Herpes simplex
- Coxsackie A

Bacteria
- Group A β-haemolytic streptococci
- Other β-haemolytic streptococci
- *Streptococcus pneumoniae*
- *Haemophilus influenzae*
- *Moraxella catarrhalis*
- *Staphylococcus aureus*
- Anaerobes (*Bacteroides* spp, peptostreptococci etc.)
- Occasionally, *Mycobacteria* spp, *Neisseria* spp, *Corynebacterium diphtheriae*

BOX 32.10 Differential diagnosis of tonsillitis: non-specific features suggesting viral infection

- Age < 3 years (GABHS unusual in this age group)
- Extrapharyngeal signs and symptoms (rhinorrhoea, cough, hoarseness)
- Conjunctivitis (exudative tonsillitis and conjunctivitis suggest adenovirus)
- Fatigue, generalized lymphadenopathy, splenomegaly (suggest EBV)
- Vesicular/ulcerative lesions (suggest Coxsackie A: herpangina or herpes simplex)

It is not possible to distinguish bacterial from viral infection reliably by clinical examination. Tonsil exudate is not specific for bacterial infection. Other non-specific features suggesting a viral origin are listed in Box 32.10.

Throat swab culture cannot reliably distinguish streptococcal disease from carriage. Furthermore, swabs have low sensitivity and take 48 hours to be reported. Rapid antigen tests also have poor sensitivity.

Current UK evidence-based guidelines suggest that throat swabs or rapid tests should not be carried out routinely in children with tonsillitis. Further research into the role of rapid tests is required.

http://www.rcpch.ac.uk/publications/clinical_docs/GGPsorethroat.pdf
http://www.sign.ac.uk/pdf/qrg34.pdf

Group A β-haemolytic streptococcal (GABHS) throat infection

GABHS species, which include *Streptococcus pyogenes*, can cause disease by direct invasion or toxin production. Several strains produce an erythrogenic toxin responsible for the rash of scarlet fever. Complications are listed in Box 32.11.

GABHS infection is the most common bacterial cause of tonsillitis in the UK. It is usually a self-limiting illness, resolving in 90% of patients within 1 week regardless of whether or not antibiotics are used.

BOX 32.11 Complications of streptococcal tonsillitis

- Otitis media
- Sinusitis
- Cervical adenitis
- Peritonsillitis or abscess (quinsy)
- Scarlet fever
- Streptococcal toxic shock syndrome
- Rheumatic fever (p. 88)
- Post-streptococcal glomerulonephritis (PSGN, p. 201)

> **BOX 32.12 Specific indications for antibiotics in children with tonsillitis**
>
> - Marked systemic upset with sore throat: scarlet fever, streptococcal toxic shock syndrome
> - Peritonsillitis or abscess (quinsy)
> - History of rheumatic fever
> - Increased risk from acute infection: e.g. child with diabetes, immunodeficiency, congenital heart disease

Q3. Should Martin be treated with antibiotics?

A Cochrane review concluded that antibiotics confer only modest benefit, reducing symptom duration by an average of only 16 hours. Over-prescribing risks the harms of antibiotic resistance, diarrhoea and rash. Current UK guidelines therefore do not recommend 'routine' antibiotic treatment. This raises several questions:

- *Should antibiotics be prescribed to prevent complications?* Not in countries with a low incidence of complications. Although the complication rate is reduced by antibiotics, the absolute risk of secondary otitis media, quinsy, sinusitis, rheumatic fever or glomerulonephritis is low in the UK. For instance, the number needed to treat for benefit (NNT_B) to prevent one case of otitis media is approximately 200. However, in developing countries, where complication rates are significantly higher, antibiotics may be indicated.
- *Should antibiotics be prescribed to prevent cross-infection?* Yes, if the index case is returning to a closed institution, e.g. boarding school. No, for children from the general community.
- *Should antibiotics ever be prescribed?* Yes, in the specific situations listed in Box 32.12. Antibiotics should not be withheld if the clinical condition of the patient is causing concern.

 http://www.cochrane.org/reviews/en/ ab000023.html
http://www.sign.ac.uk/pdf/qrg34.pdf

Choice of antibiotic
Penicillin for 10 days is still the drug of choice (erythromycin if allergic to penicillin).

Scarlet fever

See page 292.

Quinsy

This is uncommon in children. Infection spreads into the surrounding pharynx and soft palate (peritonsillitis).

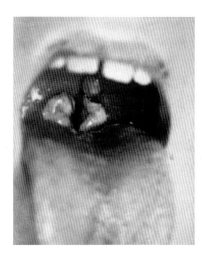

Fig. 32.6 Diphtheria pseudomembrane
(Courtesy of Centers for Disease Control, Atlanta)

Untreated, an abscess may form (quinsy). The child with quinsy usually presents with unilateral marked pain and swelling, dysphagia and otalgia. Trismus may make examination difficult. The affected tonsil is inflamed and displaced medially by a swelling in the lateral pharyngeal wall, which can occasionally cause airway obstruction. Treatment is by surgical drainage and antibiotics.

Diphtheria

Corynebacterium diphtheriae (a Gram-positive bacillus) infection is rare in the UK but should be considered in the differential diagnosis of children recently in Eastern Europe, Russia or South-East Asia. After 1–2 days of malaise, fever and sore throat, a 'pseudomembrane' (Fig. 32.6) forms over the tonsils, palate or larynx. The grey–green membrane adheres firmly to underlying tissues. Significant soft tissue swelling and cervical lymphadenopathy ('bull neck') occur. Mortality without treatment (diphtheria antitoxin and penicillin) is high.

Sinusitis

> **Problem-orientated topic:**
>
> **sinusitis**
>
> Ben is 5 years old. Last week he developed a 'viral upper respiratory tract infection', which has not resolved. Yesterday he developed poorly localized facial pain and fever. His father has brought him to the accident and emergency department of his local hospital because his right eye seems swollen. On
>
> *Continued overleaf*

examination, temperature is 39.4°C. There is a non-tender boggy swelling around his right eye. The periorbital skin is not inflamed. On rhinoscopy he has a thick purulent nasal discharge, with inflamed nasal mucosa. He is alert, without any meningism.

Q1. What is the differential/most likely diagnosis?
Q2. What are the factors predisposing to sinusitis?
Q3. What investigations and treatment are required?
Q4. What are the major complications of sinusitis?

Q1. What is the differential/most likely diagnosis?

The four paranasal sinuses (ethmoid, mastoid, frontal and sphenoid) are air spaces within the anterior skull, draining via narrow openings (ostia) into the middle or superior meatus of the nasal cavity (Fig. 32.7). They are lined by pseudostratified ciliated columnar epithelium. Mucus produced within the sinuses is continually moved towards the ostia by ciliary action.

The maxillary and ethmoid sinuses are present at birth, and are the main site of sinusitis in young children over 3 years old. The frontal sinuses develop from the anterior ethmoid sinus in mid-childhood. Although difficult to see on X-ray before the age of 12 years, the frontal sinuses can cause symptoms after the age of 10 years.

Symptoms
- Prolonged upper respiratory tract infection associated with fever and purulent nasal discharge

Table 32.1 Differential diagnosis of sinusitis

Condition	Distinguishing features from sinusitis
URTI	Discharge less purulent, less systemic upset
Allergic rhinitis	Watery discharge, repeated episodes, seasonal variation
Periorbital cellulitis	Tenderness, fewer nasal symptoms

- Cough
- Malodorous breath
- Less commonly:
  - Facial pain/headache
  - Painless periorbital swelling due to ethmoid sinusitis.

Signs
- Thick mucopurulent nasal discharge
- Inflamed nasal mucosa
- Pyrexia
- Occasionally:
  - Non-tender periorbital swelling (particularly young child with ethmoid sinusitis)
- Rarely:
  - Tenderness on palpation or percussion of sinuses.

Differential diagnosis
See Table 32.1.

Q2. What are the factors predisposing to sinusitis?

Sinusitis is a result of ostial obstruction, defective ciliary function or abnormal mucus production (Box 32.13), leading to poor drainage and subsequent infection. Typical organisms recovered include *Haemophilus influenzae*, *Streptococcus pneumoniae* and *Moraxella catarrhalis*.

> **BOX 32.13 Pathophysiology of sinusitis in children**
>
> **Ostial obstruction**
> - Viral URTI*
> - Allergic rhinitis*
> - Nasal polyps
> - Foreign body
> - Trauma
> - Unilateral choanal atresia
>
> **Defective cilia**
> - Ciliary dyskinesia (e.g. Kartagener's syndrome)
>
> **Abnormal mucus**
> - Cystic fibrosis
>
> * Common cause.

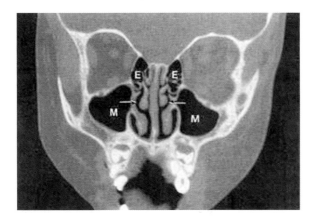

Fig. 32.7 Coronal CT of normal sinuses (maxillary ostia arrowed)
(M = maxillary; E = ethmoid)
(© Texas Tech University)

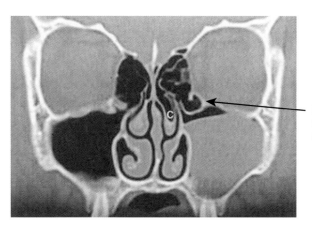

Fig. 32.8 Maxillary sinusitis with visible air/fluid level on coronal CT

Maxillary sinusitis with visible air/fluid level on coronal CT

Q3. What investigations and treatment are required?

Investigations include:
- Culture of nasopharyngeal secretions
- X-rays ('sinus views' must be requested); false negatives are common
- CT scan (Fig. 32.8): the gold standard, particularly if orbital involvement is suspected.

Treatment is:
- Antibiotic for 10–14 days: oral amoxicillin or erythromycin if mild disease; cefuroxime or co-amoxiclav i.v. if more severe
- Topical ephedrine (to reduce mucosal oedema blocking ostia)
- Surgery if local abscess formation.

Q4. What are the major complications of sinusitis?

Important complications include:
- Orbital:
  - Periorbital oedema
  - Orbital abscess, subperiosteal abscess: may cause proptosis
  - Periorbital cellulitis
- Intracranial:
  - Cavernous sinus thrombosis
  - Meningitis
  - Intracranial abscess.

Mastoiditis

Problem-orientated topic:

mastoiditis

A 21-month-old girl, Janie, is referred by her GP. She developed otitis media 1 week ago. Her fever has persisted despite 5 days of amoxicillin. She has developed a tender swelling behind her left ear. On examination, she has a swelling, as shown in Figure 32.9. Her temperature is 39.4°C. The left tympanic membrane is inflamed and bulging.

Q1. What is the most likely diagnosis?
Q2. What else could it be and how will you confirm the diagnosis?
Q3. How should Janie be treated?
Q4. What complications should you look out for?

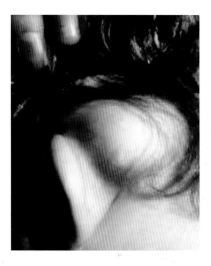

Fig. 32.9 Mastoiditis

Q1. What is the most likely diagnosis?

Mastoid pneumatization occurs shortly after birth and is complete by age of 10 years. The mastoid air-cell system communicates with the posterior aspect of the middle ear through the narrow aditus ad antrum.

Acute mastoiditis is a result of infection spreading from the middle ear. The antrum is blocked by inflamed mucosa, inhibiting drainage and triggering mastoid empyema. Bacteria causing otitis media are usually responsible: *Streptococcus pneumoniae, Haemophilus influenzae*, group A streptococci (rarely *Moraxella catarrhalis, Mycoplasma, Pseudomonas* or anaerobes).

Mastoiditis is usually a disease of young children. It is uncommon. Symptoms include:

- Recent otitis media
- Fever despite adequate antibiotic treatment
- Pain located in or behind the ear
- Less commonly: purulent otorrhoea, hearing loss.

On examination there is:

- Pyrexia
- Otitis media with or without tympanic perforation
- Tender swelling behind the ear, which displaces the auricle laterally and obliterates the post-auricular skin crease (Fig. 32.9).

Q2. What else could it be and how will you confirm the diagnosis?

The differential diagnosis includes:

- *Otitis externa*: less systemic upset, no post-auricular swelling
- *Post-auricular lymph node abscess*: post-auricular skin crease is preserved.

Investigations are directed towards identifying the responsible organism, monitoring the response to treatment and detecting spread outside the mastoid. Therefore:

- Culture any discharge (some surgeons suggest myringotomy to obtain a sample).
- Order blood culture, full blood count, erythrocyte sedimentation rate/C-reactive protein.
- Organize a CT scan if there is evidence of complications, i.e:
  - Facial palsy
  - Persistent fever despite parenteral antibiotics
  - Reduced level of consciousness
  - Recurrent vomiting with headache
  - Signs of meningism.

BOX 32.14 Complications of mastoiditis

- Subperiosteal abscess
- Meningitis
- Facial (seventh nerve) palsy
- Cavernous/sigmoid sinus thrombosis
- Osteomyelitis of the petrous temporal bone
- Intracranial abscess
- Labyrinthitis

Q3. How should Janie be treated?

- *Antibiotics*. Prescribe a parenteral third-generation cephalosporin. Consider adding vancomycin or clindamycin and/or anaerobic cover. Oral antibiotics may be substituted after 18–72 hours if the temperature settles. Give 14 days of antibiotics.
- *Obtain an ENT opinion*. Surgery (myringotomy and/or mastoidectomy) was necessary in approximately 25% of children in a UK series. Indications for surgery include failure to respond to medical treatment or complications.

Q4. What complications should you look out for?

Complications (Box 32.14) arise when infection spreads beyond the mastoid into local structures.

Further reading

Bamiou DE, Macardle B, Bitner-Glindzicz M et al 2000 Aetiological investigations of hearing loss in childhood: a review. Clinical Otolaryngology 25:98–106

Fortnum HM 1992 Hearing impairment after bacterial meningitis: a review. Archives of Disease in Childhood 67:1128–1133

Hall DMB, Elliman D 2003 Health for all children, 4th edn. Oxford University Press, Oxford

Medical Research Council Multi-centre Otitis Study Group 2001 Risk factors for persistence of bilateral otitis media with effusion. Clinical Otolaryngology 26:147–156

Neil Kennedy   Malcolm Levene

Disorders of bones and joints

LEARNING OUTCOMES

By the end of this chapter you should:
- Be able to screen a child for joint disorders
- Be able to undertake an examination of the major joints
- Be able to undertake a screening test for neonatal development dysplasia of the hip
- Know the common causes of limp
- Know the presentation and management of bone and joint infection
- Know the common causes of joint swelling
- Know the presentation, classification and management of juvenile idiopathic arthritis.

MODULE SIX

Clinical assessment

Examination of the joints is often only a cursory part of a routine clinical examination (Ch. 5). If a child presents with joint or bone pain, then more careful history and examination are required.

History

Important questions in the history include:
- *What is the nature of the pain (arthralgia)?* Ask about location, exacerbating and relieving factors, radiation and timing of onset of the pain (whether it is related to times of the day). Pain or immobility (stiffness) first thing in the morning is suggestive

of an inflammatory cause. Pain exacerbated by exercise suggests a mechanical cause and usually resolves with a period of rest.
- *Are there constitutional symptoms?* These include fever, fatigue, anorexia, weight loss and rashes.
- *Are there emotional, family or school-related problems?* Non-organic causes of limb pain are common and are discussed in Chapter 24.

Examination

- *Gait.* With an antalgic (painful) gait the child spends as little time as possible during the walking cycle on the painful leg. Important points include the ability to weight-bear on a joint.

1. Walk on tip-toe and on heels.
2. Sit cross-legged on floor and then jump up.
3. Extend arms straight out in front and make a fist.
4. Place palms and fingers flat together with wrists extended to 90° in a 'saying prayers' position.
5. Raise arms straight above head.
6. Turn head to look over each shoulder.

- *Rash.* Look carefully for rashes (in particular on the face, eyelids, flexor surfaces of joints and knuckles).
- *Muscle tenderness or wasting.* Assess muscle strength.
- *Joint examination.* Look for:
  - Evidence of wasting or limb length differences
  - Redness of the joint
  - Swelling
  - Range of movements (are there joint contractures?).

It may be useful to perform a screening musculoskeletal examination if in doubt as to whether the child has an organic cause for the joint pain (Box 33.1). A child who can perform all these functions without difficulty is unlikely to have a significant musculoskeletal problem.

Developmental dysplasia of the hip

This refers to a disorder of hip development that may predispose to dislocation either at birth or later. Hip instability is present in 1:60 neonates and, before the introduction of widespread clinical neonatal hip screening, late dislocation occurred in 1–2 per 1000 live births. This incidence has fallen with routine screening but the condition still occurs in 0.8 per 1000 live births.

Risk factors for developmental dysplasia include:
- Gender: it is six times more common in girls than boys
- First-born children
- Breech position in utero
- Maternal oligohydramnios.

Screening

All newborn infants should be routinely examined for hip dysplasia. Repeat screening is recommended at 6 weeks and 6 months of age by the GP or health visitor.

Newborn screening involves the following elements.

Is the hip in joint?

Inspect gluteal folds. Are they symmetrical? Are the legs of equal length? If either of these is abnormal, it suggests the hip may be dislocated.

Test hip abduction. If the hip abducts fully, it is not dislocated.

Is the hip stable?

If the hip is not dislocated, then its stability should be tested by Barlow's test. The essence of this test is to exert downward pressure through the femur to see whether the hip can be dislocated backwards. If the hip is unstable, a 'clunk' is felt as the head of the femur is pushed over the lip of the acetabulum.

Can a dislocated hip be relocated?

If the hip cannot be fully abducted and dislocation is suspected, then the Ortolani test is used to attempt to relocate the hip into joint. Upward traction on the femur is used to relocate the hip in the acetabulum. Relocation is accompanied by a 'clunk' sensation. Once the hip is relocated, then the hip can be gently abducted.

Ultrasound assessment

Ultrasound examination of the hips is a very useful way of determining hip architecture and is widely used to assess the child who is at high risk of hip dysplasia or where there is an equivocal screening test.

Management

The dislocated or dislocatable hip should be reduced into the acetabulum and maintained in the position of flexion and abduction until it becomes stable. A variety of harnesses are used to maintain stability, including the Pavlick harness, the most widely used. The hips are located into the harness under the supervision of an orthopaedic surgeon and the harness is worn continuously for 12–16 weeks. Regular adjustments to ensure appropriate fitting of the harness are required.

Dislocation diagnosed after 4 months of age will require specialist orthopaedic attention. Initially a 2-week period of traction is initiated, followed by surgical intervention to ensure the hip is relocated and remains stable.

Complications

Avascular necrosis of the femoral head is the most important serious complication. This may arise as the result of forceful reduction or immobilizing the hip too fully in an abduction harness or splint.

Arthritis

Problem-orientated topic:

the child with a limp (see also Ch. 24)

Conor is 4. He is brought to the accident and emergency department having developed a right-sided limp a day ago. He has had a recent 'cold'. His mother tells you that he fell off his scooter 4 days ago, but other than cutting his knee, he had no major injury. On examination, he is pyrexial (38.3°C) and appears mildly unwell. He has a healing abrasion on the right knee, which does not appear to be infected. When asked to stand, he will weight-bear only on his left leg and holds his right leg flexed at the hip. When lying down, he will allow you to flex, extend, adduct and abduct his hips. However, passive internal flexion of the right hip causes him pain.

Q1. What is the differential diagnosis of a child with a limp?

Q2. How can you differentiate septic arthritis from 'irritable hip'?

Q3. What are the causative organisms of septic arthritis?

Q1. What is the differential diagnosis of a child with a limp?

These are listed in Box 33.2.

Q2. How can you differentiate septic arthritis from 'irritable hip'?

'Irritable hip' occurs in up to 3% of children between 3 and 8 years, more commonly in boys. Typically a child will develop a limp a few days after an upper respiratory tract infection. The child remains systemically well. On examination, internal rotation of the hip may be limited. The child rests with the hip held in flexion and external rotation. Ultrasound will often show an effusion of the hip. The syndrome is probably caused by a transient reactive hip synovitis. Most cases settle in 5–10 days, with symptomatic treatment only. The

BOX 33.2 Causes of acute limp in children

- Transient synovitis (sometimes known as 'irritable hip')*
- Septic arthritis/osteomyelitis of hip, femur or knee*
- Trauma*
- Perthes' disease
- Slipped capital femoral epiphysis
- Juvenile idiopathic arthritis
- Idiopathic chondrolysis
- Neoplastic: osteosarcoma/bony infiltrate of other malignancy

* Common cause.

Table 33.1 Features differentiating septic arthritis from irritable hip

Feature	Irritable hip	Septic arthritis
Fever	Mild	High
Systemic upset?	None/mild	Moderate/severe
White cell count (WCC)	Mild ↑	↑↑↑
Erythrocyte sedimentation rate (ESR)	Mild ↑	↑↑
Ultrasound	Effusion	Effusion
Improves with rest?	Yes	No

important differential diagnosis is septic arthritis and the main distinguishing features are shown in Table 33.1.

Conor probably has 'irritable hip'.

Q3. What are the causative organisms of septic arthritis?

- *Staphylococcus aureus* (75% of cases)
- Group A β-haemolytic streptococcus (*Strep. pyogenes*)
- *Strep. pneumoniae*
- Group B β-haemolytic streptococcus (neonates only).

Osteomyelitis and septic arthritis

In this condition there is infection in the bone. It most commonly arises as the result of haematogenous spread and rarely following trauma. Septic arthritis may develop as a result of direct spread from adjacent osteomyelitis, especially in younger children and neonates. The most common site of involvement is the metaphysis of long bones or vertebral bodies.

Osteomyelitis may be acute, subacute or chronic. Subacute is usually the result of less virulent organisms and chronic usually arises as a result of inadequately treated infection.

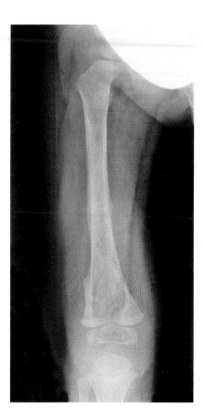

Presentation

Pain and loss of function are the most common presenting features. The pain can usually be localized by the child, and if a lower limb is involved, limp or refusal to walk is common. Hip infection results in the child lying with the hip flexed and in internal rotation, with the knee in flexion. Localizing signs are less obvious when the primary infection arises in pelvis or spine.

Neonates present with non-specific signs, including unstable temperature, poor feeding, pallor, recurrent apnoea and pseudoparalysis (maintaining the limb completely immobile). The affected limb may be swollen and tender to touch. Diagnosis requires awareness of osteomyelitis as a cause of severe infection in a non-specifically unwell baby.

Infecting organisms

In Europe *Staph. aureus* causes 75% of osteomyelitis infection. Other infecting organisms include group A β-haemolytic streptococcus (*Strep. pyogenes*) and *Strep. pneumoniae*. In the neonate, group B β-haemolytic streptococcus is relatively common. *Haemophilus influenzae* type b (Hib) is now very rare due to widespread immunization. Other organisms to be considered include tuberculosis (usually insidious in onset), brucellosis and *Mycoplasma pneumoniae* (these latter two may both cause low-grade septic arthritis).

Investigations

Full blood count, ESR and C-reactive protein (CRP) usually suggest infection. Blood cultures should be taken prior to starting antibiotics. Culture from bone or a joint effusion may identify the organism, together with a marked pleocytosis in the synovial fluid.

The first X-ray change is periosteal reaction (Fig. 33.1) and is seen within a few days of infection with bone changes later. Radionuclide bone scanning may reveal areas of multiple infection. In septic arthritis the early radiological features are osteopenia of the epiphysis, increased joint space and soft tissue swelling. Ultrasound imaging may reveal fluid in the joint.

Management

Early administration of antistaphylococcal antibiotics (flucloxacillin and cefotaxime in a neonate or child below 2 years; flucloxacillin and ampicillin in an older child) in appropriate dosage is essential. A broader-spectrum choice is recommended in immunosuppressed children until the organism has been identified. It is recommended that intravenous antibiotics are used for at least 3 days, followed by an oral course for 3–4 weeks if the fever has settled. Neonates require a longer intravenous course.

The role of bone drilling in the management of this condition is controversial. Biopsy for microbiological diagnosis may be useful.

Fig. 33.1 X-ray of femur showing periosteal reaction in acute osteomyelitis

Aspiration of a septic joint is always recommended for diagnostic purposes. Surgical drainage is necessary for septic arthritis of the hip to minimize risk of avascular necrosis of the femoral head.

An ill child will require supportive care, often on an intensive care unit.

Complications

Outcome is usually good with early treatment. Disturbance of bone growth may occur following septic arthritis or if osteomyelitis involves the epiphysis. Chronic osteomyelitis may lead to bone necrosis and sequestration.

Reactive arthritis

Arthralgia and joint swelling may occur directly or indirectly as a result of a number of infections. Viruses such as rubella, parvovirus (erythrovirus) and varicella commonly cause a short period of arthralgia.

True 'reactive' arthritis occurs after enteric infection with *Salmonella*, *Shigella*, *Yersinia* and *Campylobacter* and is often associated with the child expressing the HLA B27 antigen. Joint(s) of the lower limb are usually involved in an asymmetrical manner. Dactylitis (swelling and pain of interphalangeal joints) may also occur. Non-steroidal anti-inflammatory drugs (NSAIDs) are indicated until pain and swelling regress.

Swollen joints

Problem-orientated topic:

swollen joints

Stacey (3 years old) presents in the outpatient department. She has been complaining of pain in her knee on and off for several weeks. The pain is mainly in the morning, and gets better over the day. In the last 10 days, her left knee has swollen. She is otherwise well. On examination she has an effusion of the left knee. There is mild pain when you passively flex the knee by more than 60°.

Q1. What is the differential diagnosis for inflammatory arthritis in children?

Q2. What is the classification of juvenile idiopathic arthritis (JIA)?

Q3. What type of JIA does Stacey have?

Q4. What are the principles of treatment of JIA?

Q1. What is the differential diagnosis for inflammatory arthritis in children?

The differential diagnosis is listed in Box 33.3.

Q2. What is the classification of juvenile idiopathic arthritis (JIA)?

The most recent classification proposes the following subtypes of JIA:
1. Systemic arthritis
2. Oligoarticular arthritis
   (a) Persistent
   (b) Extended
3. Polyarthritis: rheumatoid factor (RF) negative
4. Polyarthritis: RF positive
5. Enthesitis-related arthritis (inflammation at insertion of tendons into bones)
6. Psoriatic arthritis
7. Other arthritis.

 http://www.medscape.com/viewprogram/5690

Juvenile Idiopathic Arthritis: Insights into Classification, Outcomes and Treatment

Q3. What type of JIA does Stacey have?

Stacey probably has the oligoarthritis form of JIA (see below for a description of this condition).

BOX 33.3 Differential diagnosis of a child with limp and joint effusion

- Infection
  - Viral arthritis
  - Septic arthritis
  - Reactive arthritis
- Juvenile idiopathic arthritis (JIA)
- Vasculitis
  - Henoch–Schönlein purpura (HSP)
  - Kawasaki disease (p. 286)
  - Polyarteritis nodosa
- Trauma
- Autoimmune disorders
  - Systemic lupus erythematosus
  - Juvenile dermatomyositis
- Malignancy
  - Leukaemia (p. 418)
  - Neuroblastoma (p. 421)
- Blood disorders
  - Sickle cell disease (p. 263)
  - Haemophilia (p. 268)
- Drug reactions

Q4. What are the principles of treatment of JIA?

These are summarized as follows:
- An NSAID is the first-line drug.
- Intra-articular corticosteroids are very effective at relieving pain.
- Methotrexate is indicated for persistent synovitis.
- There is only a very limited role for systemic corticosteroids.
- Management must be within a multidisciplinary team under the supervision of a paediatric rheumatologist.

More details of management are discussed below in the section on JIA.

Juvenile idiopathic arthritis (JIA)

This represents a spectrum of disorders most recently classified as JIA. It is a disease of children with onset below 16 years of age and presents as synovitis (joint swelling, limitation of movement, or pain) persisting for at least 6 weeks. In addition, varieties of JIA include different distributions of synovitis and sometimes other clinical involvement such as skin, eyes and heart.

The incidence of JIA is 10–20 per 100 000 children in Europe and the USA. Twice the number of girls as boys are affected. There are two peak ages of onset: early and late. In the early group presentation is at 1–3 years and is mainly of the oligoarthritis form, affecting girls. The second age peak is at 9 years, and boys and girls are equally affected.

Basic science

There is a strong genetic basis to JIA based on single nucleotide polymorphisms (SNPs, Ch. 9) of the major histocompatibility complex (MHC) on chromosome 6. The human leucocyte antigen (HLA) genes comprise an important part of the MHC and susceptibility to JIA is particularly associated with HLA A2, DR5, DR8 and DPB1*0201. In older boys, oligoarthritis is associated with HLA B27. Genetic susceptibility may require a second environmental trigger to induce disease. Triggers such as infective agents may account for seasonal variations in the onset of this disease.

Inflammation is mediated through expression of cytokines, a family of soluble proteins that exert either pro-inflammatory or anti-inflammatory activity. In JIA certain pro-inflammatory cytokines, such as tumour necrosis factor-alpha (TNF-α), induce release of tissue-destroying metalloproteinases and stimulate release of other members of the pro-inflammatory cytokine cascade. TNF-α is produced by activated macrophages, T-lymphocytes and synovial cells, and contributes to joint destruction.

Clinical features

The classical presentation of JIA is joint swelling, redness, pain or tenderness in the affected joint, and limitation of joint movement. Morning stiffness is a common complaint in children. The presentation may be dramatic or protean, and systemic features are seen in systemic arthritis.

The form of JIA can be defined on the basis of joint involvement as well as involvement of other organs.

Oligoarthritis

Oligoarthritis refers to disease affecting 1–4 joints during the first 6 months of the illness. It is the most common form of JIA and accounts for 50% of affected children: mainly girls, with peak age of onset at 1–3 years. It most commonly presents insidiously with isolated joint involvement, particularly of knee or ankle, or more rarely an upper limb joint. Eye involvement (uveitis) may occur and all affected children should be regularly screened by an ophthalmologist.

The child may present with a limp but rarely complains of severe pain. On examination the joint is hot and swollen and an effusion may be present. Clinical signs include reduction in passive movement, which may result in contractures in long-standing disease.

Affected children usually have positive antinuclear antibodies (ANA).

Polyarthritis

This refers to disease affecting five or more joints during the first 6 months of illness, and occurs in about 25% of children with JIA. It usually involves joints symmetrically. The polyarthritis can be further subdivided into seropositive and seronegative forms, based on whether or not IgM rheumatoid factor is present. Seronegative disease is much more common than seropositive disease in children.

Seronegative polyarthritis has a peak incidence at 6–7 years and may be insidious or more aggressive in some children. Seropositive disease starts later in late childhood or adolescence and affects smaller joints of hands and feet.

Systemic arthritis

In this form, joint involvement is accompanied by fever and other systemic features. It accounts for about 10% of cases of JIA and occurs at a peak age of 5 years. The fever usually follows a characteristic pattern, being present for at least 2 weeks, and spiking once or twice a day, usually in the evening, and returning to normal between spikes (Fig. 33.2). A pale pink macular rash and malaise are particularly common when the child is pyrexial. Lymphadenopathy, hepatomegaly or splenomegaly is also commonly present. Because of the similarity to malignancy in the way this disease presents, other conditions must be carefully excluded (Ch. 51).

Joint manifestation is variable but is most commonly of the polyarthritis form. Some children have a very aggressive form, with joint destruction within 2 years.

Investigations

The presence of antinuclear antibody factor (ANF) and rheumatoid factor (RF) is important in classifying the disease. A positive ANF in oligoarthritis is a risk factor for uveitis.

Ultrasound is a sensitive investigation for joint effusions and may help guide needle aspiration of fluid.

Radiology may show the following features:
- *Early signs*: periarticular osteopenia (Fig. 33.3)
- *Intermediate signs*: cortical erosions (Fig. 33.4), joint space narrowing and subchondral cysts
- *Late signs*: destructive changes with ankylosis and growth anomalies.

Management

The management of children with chronic disorders must be within a multidisciplinary team (Ch. 18) and under the supervision of a paediatric rheumatologist.

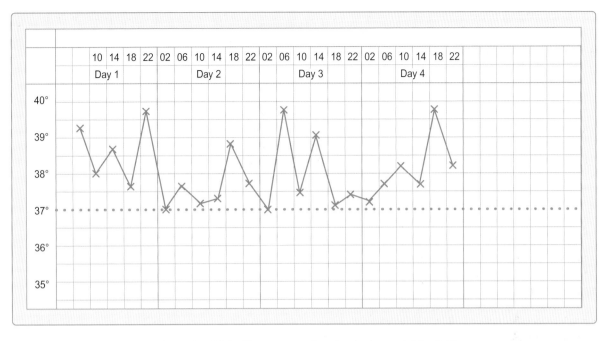

Fig. 33.2 **Typical temperature chart of a child with acute-onset systemic rheumatoid arthritis**

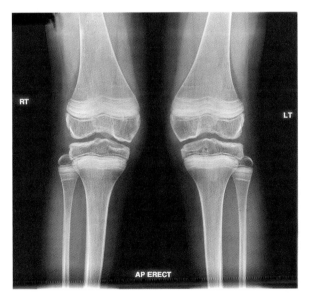

Fig. 33.3 **X-ray of knees showing periosteal osteopenia in a child with seropositive rheumatoid arthritis**

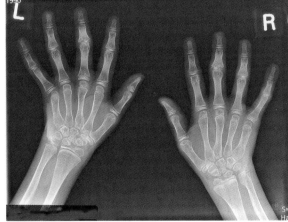

Fig. 33.4 **X-ray showing destructive changes of carpal bones in a child with polyarthritis**

Physiotherapy aims to maintain joint function, with an occupational therapist to facilitate normal living skills and provision of aids to overcome impairment. Well-fitting splints to support acutely inflamed joints are of particular importance.

NSAIDs are the first-line drug at diagnosis. Intra-articular corticosteroids are very effective at relieving pain and may prevent or reduce synovial damage and disability. Methotrexate is indicated for persistent synovitis and has been shown to be effective for all types of JIA.

Recently, anti-TNF therapy has been shown to give significant benefit to children with polyarticular JIA who failed to respond to methotrexate. It has been shown that 60–70% of children who fail to respond to methotrexate show some improvement with anti-TNF therapy. Long-term safety of these agents has not been fully assessed in children. Further drug management schedules depend on the type of JIA that the child shows. The role of systemic corticosteroids in JIA has reduced in recent years with the introduction of more effective drugs such as methotrexate. It may be valuable for inducing remission in particularly aggressive forms of the disease.

Complications

Uveitis occurs in 10% of children with JIA. Acute painful iritis is rare but is seen particularly in children with enthesitis. Painless anterior uveitis is more insidious, and if unrecognized, may cause severe visual impairment, particularly in school-age children with oligoarthritis; it is strongly associated with ANA. Regular ophthalmological assessments are necessary for recognizing and treating this condition.

The major complications of JIA are bone erosion leading to disfigurement and major mobility problems. A multiprofessional approach is required to minimize the destructive potential of this condition.

Henoch–Schönlein purpura

Henoch–Schönlein purpura (HSP, see also pp. 134 and 267) is a vasculitic disorder affecting joints, bowel and kidneys (p. 203). The cause is unknown but in some cases HSP is apparently triggered by an upper respiratory tract infection. It has an incidence of 10–15 per 100 000 children and usually presents in children below the age of 10 years, with a peak at 5 years.

Children present most commonly with a purpuric rash characteristically involving buttocks, lower limbs and elbows and/or arthralgia with joint swelling (see DVD 28). Abdominal pain occurs commonly with blood in the stool, but serious bleeding and bowel perforation, although recognized, are rare. Renal involvement (haematuria/proteinuria, rarely hypertension) occurs in 50% of cases, but persisting renal disease is rare and is seen in only 1% of cases. Urinalysis for proteinuria should be undertaken regularly throughout the course of the illness to identify renal involvement.

HSP is usually a relatively mild and benign condition that resolves fully within 2–3 weeks of its onset. Recurrent episodes may occur over the next few weeks or months.

Management is symptomatic, with simple analgesics for pain relief. The management of renal involvement is discussed on page 209.

Rheumatic fever

Rheumatic fever (see also p. 229) is now rarely seen in Western Europe but remains common in the developing world. It is due to a complication of infection with group A β-haemolytic *Strep. pyogenes*. The organism induces an immune-mediated reaction, resulting in vasculitis. Affected organs include joints, heart (pancarditis, arrhythmias), skin (erythema marginatum, subcutaneous nodules) and brain (Sydenham's chorea).

Major criteria
- Polyarthritis involving large joints and flitting*
- Carditis*
- Chorea (Sydenham's)
- Erythema marginatum
- Subcutaneous nodules on extensor surfaces

Minor criteria
- Fever
- Arthralgia
- Prolonged P–R interval
- Elevated ESR/CRP, leucocytosis
- Previous rheumatic fever
- Common.

* Common feature.

Clinical features

There are no specific markers of rheumatic fever, but the diagnosis is made on the basis of the presence of a number of clinical features that are described as the modified Jones criteria (Box 33.4). The diagnosis is made on the presence of two major criteria or one major and two minor criteria, together with evidence of recent group A streptococcal infection (positive throat swab, elevated antistreptolysin O titre (ASOT) or other antistreptococcal antibodies).

 http://www.arthritis.org/conditions/DiseaseCenter/jra.asp

Management
- Eradication of streptococcus with penicillin for 10 days
- Symptomatic relief of arthralgia with NSAIDs
- Steroids: reserved for pancarditis
- Prophylactic penicillin against further streptococcal infection for 5 years.

Polyarteritis nodosa (PAN)

This rare vasculitic condition in children affects medium-sized arteries and presents with non-specific symptoms including fever, malaise, rashes, and joint or muscle pain. Investigation findings are also non-specific and diagnosis is made on abnormal biopsy appearance. Management should be under the supervision of a paediatric rheumatologist.

Systemic lupus erythematosus (SLE)

This is rare in children but more common in adolescent and young female adults. It is an autoimmune condition with non-specific signs and symptoms, including facial (butterfly) rash, thrombocytopenia, arthralgia and fatigue. Rarely severe renal or neurological SLE may be life-threatening. The ESR is usually elevated and positive ANA is found in all cases, although these findings are non-specific as they may also be positive in the presence of other diagnoses. Management should be under the supervision of a paediatric rheumatologist.

Dermatomyositis (see also p. 18)

This is a very rare disorder in children and is of unknown aetiology. The diagnosis is made on the basis of a characteristic rash together with:
- Symmetrical proximal muscle weakness
- Abnormal muscle biopsy
- Elevated muscle enzymes
- Changes on electromyography.

The rash is the first feature in about 50% of cases, affecting eyelids (heliotropic rash), knuckles (Gottron's papules) and extensor surfaces of the knees and elbows (Fig. 28.5). Erythema of the nailfolds is a particular feature.

Often the muscle weakness first becomes obvious when difficulty climbing stairs or brushing hair is noticed. Muscle pain is frequently a feature and calcinosis of the muscle is well recognized. Myositis is confirmed by elevated muscle enzymes.

The mainstay of management is corticosteroid therapy. Dermatomyositis is often a remitting illness, but some children have a rapidly progressive form resulting in major disability.

Acknowledgement

We are grateful to Dr R. Arthur for permission to use the radiographs.

MODULE SIX

34

Inborn errors of metabolism

LEARNING OUTCOMES

By the end of this chapter you should:

- Understand the clinical presentation of metabolic disorders in the newborn
- Know the clinical features of metabolic disease in the older child
- Be able to administer and interpret tests of common metabolic disorders in conjunction with a specialist metabolic laboratory
- Be able to recognize, initiate diagnostic tests for and outline the management of hypoglycaemia, persistent or recurrent episodes of metabolic acidosis (including lactic acidosis), acute encephalopathy (including intractable seizures) and neurodevelopmental regression/dysmorphism.

Basic science and cell function

At a cellular level the nucleus is the centre of or major contributor to gene expression. Enzymes are proteins that are produced according to the genetic information provided by the nucleus. This production process is supported by other organelles that play a crucial part in the final functioning of the enzyme. Knowledge of the supporting organelles that are associated with disease is increasing but for simplicity the following model may help understanding.

The nucleus holds the genetic material of the ovum and sperm from the point of conception. The genetic material represents an equal contribution by both parents in most circumstances. This equal contribution explains why in most metabolic conditions carriers are not affected, as although enzyme activity will be reduced in carriers, it would still be sufficient to prevent disease. The exceptions are some X-linked diseases, in which the majority of patients will be males.

The mitochondrion has its own genetic material and is referred to as the mitochondrial genome; it represents only 1% of cellular nucleic acid material. This genome consists of 37 genes and has been fully sequenced. The mitochondria contain about 1000 proteins, of which only 13 are encoded by mitochondrial DNA; the rest are imported but under control of nuclear encoded DNA. Mitochondria are derived from maternal origin only, as the sperm does not contribute to the mitochondrial pool. Defects in the mitochondrial gene are inherited in a maternal inheritance pattern also called cytoplasmic inheritance. Great variability within families with maternally inherited mitochondrial disease can be explained by the principle of heteroplasmy. Heteroplasmy is the unequal division of mitochondria in the early developmental phase, meaning that cells and different tissues can get variable amounts of affected mitochondria. It is important to realize that not all mitochondrial disorders are maternally inherited, and each and every form of inheritance has been associated with mitochondrial disease. The unifying principle is that mitochondrial dysfunction is associated with energy deficiency and that is the cause of disease manifestations.

The lysosomes are intracellular organelles that are produced by the Golgi apparatus and are filled by enzymes (Box 34.1). These nuclear encoded enzymes that are produced in the endoplasmic reticulum only function at low pH and this is only found inside the lysosomes. They have a housekeeping function and, together with the peroxisomes, digest organisms, defective organelles or foreign particles.

Presentation of inborn errors of metabolism (IEM) in the neonate

Problem-orientated topic:

metabolic disease in the newborn

Mohammed is a 5-day-old baby who has been rushed to hospital acutely unwell. He was born at term and has been exclusively breastfeeding well. He is the second child of consanguineous Asian parents who lost their first child last year from cot death. Over the last 24 hours, Mohammed has been feeding less well, has become less responsive and now looks pale and mottled, his skin is cold to the touch. He is floppy and tachypnoeic with a respiratory rate of 82 breaths per minute but has only mild subcostal recession. A capillary blood gas taken by the admitting nurse shows pH 7.07, base excess −15 mmol/l, PCO_2 4.35 kPa, PO_2 3.85 kPa and blood glucose 1.2 mmol/l.

Q1. What are the three important groups of disorders in the differential diagnosis?

Q2. What features make an inborn error of metabolism more likely?

Q3. What further investigations are indicated?

Q4. What are the main principles of emergency management?

Q1. What are the three important groups of disorders in the differential diagnosis?

Neonates present with non-specific symptoms and hence the differential diagnosis is always wide. For an acutely acidotic neonate the three most common problems are:

- Sepsis
- Congenital heart disease
- IEMs.

Although IEMs are individually rare, they are collectively not uncommon and hence the possibility of an IEM should be considered, as many cases are amenable to early treatment that improves mortality and long-term neurological morbidity.

Q2. What features make an inborn error of metabolism more likely?

A number of factors in the history and examination may raise the suspicion of an IEM. These include:

- Parental consanguinity
- A family history of unexplained deaths in infancy
- Maternal history of HELLP syndrome (*h*aemolysis, *e*levated *l*iver enzymes and *l*ow *p*latelets) or acute fatty liver of pregnancy
- Previous miscarriages or non-immune hydrops fetalis
- Well period before deterioration (effectively dialysed by placenta)
- Encephalopathy ± seizures
- Metabolic acidosis with raised anion gap
- Raised blood ammonia
- Hypoglycaemia
- Urinary ketones
- Dysmorphic features
- Unusual odours.

Types of IEM that present in the neonate

These fall broadly into five clinical 'syndromes', as shown in Box 34.2.

BOX 34.2 Types of IEM that present in the neonate

1. Acute intoxication picture
- Organic acidaemias like propionic acidaemia, methylmalonic acidaemia and isovaleric acidaemia
- Maple syrup urine disease
- Urea cycle defects
- Fatty acid oxidation defects
- Transient hyperammonaemia of the newborn

2. Encephalopathy with seizures
- Non-ketotic hyperglycinaemia or other neurotransmitter defects
- Sulphite oxidase deficiency
- Pyridoxine- or folinic acid-dependent seizures
- Urea cycle disorders and maple syrup urine disease
- Congenital lactic acidosis

3. Neonatal liver disease and/or multi-organ failure
- Galactosaemia
- Tyrosinaemia
- Neonatal haemochromatosis
- Fatty acid oxidation disorders
- Mitochondrial disease
- Organomegaly: glycogen storage diseases and Niemann–Pick type C

4. Non-immune hydrops and/or dysmorphism
- Lysosomal storage disorders
- Sterol metabolism defects like Smith–Lemli–Opitz syndrome
- Peroxisomal disorders (can have Down's-like features)
- Red cell enzyme defects

5. Neurological deterioration and/or energy deficiency
- Mitochondrial disease
- Peroxisomal disorders

Q3. What further investigations are indicated?

Using the numbered categories shown in Box 34.2, investigations can be planned as most appropriate. Table 34.1 will provide the best-guess investigations in a neonate.

Table 34.1 Further investigations in IEM in the neonate

Investigation	Most helpful	Possibly helpful	Non-specific
Serum ammonia	1	2, 3, 5	4
Serum lactate			1–5
CSF lactate		2, 5	1, 3, 4
Acyl-carnitine profile	1	2, 3, 5	4
CSF amino acids	2		1, 3, 4, 5
Serum amino acids	1	2	3, 4, 5
Urine organic acids	1–3	5	4
Urine amino acids	2	1	3–5
Urine oligo- and polysaccharides	4		1, 2, 3, 5

(CSF = cerebrospinal fluid, see Box 34.2 for number explanation)

Q4. What are the main principles of emergency management?

Obviously each IEM has its own specific management plan, but even before a specific diagnosis is made there are several generic approaches to management that can be used:
- *Eliminate toxic precursors* likely to be protein, fats or some carbohydrates: therefore stop feeds.
- *Ensure anabolic state*: maintain hydration and supply sufficient calories in a simple form such as intravenous 10% dextrose or glucose polymer solution.
- *Remove toxic metabolites*: may need dialysis or alternative pathway stimulation. For hyperammonaemia use sodium benzoate and sodium phenylbutyrate as well as arginine. Choose carnitine in organic acidemias.
- *Give supportive treatment*: correction of hypoglycaemia with dextrose and acidosis with bicarbonate if needed. Treat shock and coagulopathy. Treat concomitant or suspected sepsis with broad-spectrum antibiotics.
- *Reintroduce appropriate feed* when diagnosis is confirmed: will need metabolic dietician's input.

Presentation of inborn errors of metabolism in the older child

It is important to consider inherited metabolic diseases in your differential diagnosis when presented with a child in the following clinical scenarios:
- Unexplained acute or chronic encephalopathy
- Progressive neurological disease or regression
- Dysmorphism
- Hypoglycaemia.

Many inherited metabolic diseases are exacerbated by metabolic stress such as a prolonged fast or intercurrent illness and so, when presented with a child who is disproportionately unwell with some of the above features, the diagnosis of a metabolic disease must be considered.

Q1. What would your initial management be?

The initial management of this girl should be as outlined in Advanced Paediatric Life Support (APLS, see also Ch. 45), with a primary survey addressing airway, breathing, circulation, disability (Glasgow coma score, pupils, posture) and exposure. These should then be addressed before going on to complete a secondary survey. Maya has signs of respiratory distress and shock. Her airway is stable but she should be given facial oxygen and an intravenous cannula should be inserted, with blood being taken for initial investigations (including blood glucose). She will then require a bolus of 0.9% saline and the response should be assessed. It is also important to correct hypoglycaemia and start some intravenous 10%

dextrose to try to reverse the catabolic state, which may make any underlying metabolic disorder worse.

Q2. What is your initial differential diagnosis?

See Box 34.3.

Early identification of encephalopathy is often difficult, and signs such as drowsiness, altered behaviour or unsteadiness of gait/ataxia should alert you to the fact that a child is encephalopathic. Associated with vomiting, this is a strong indication for investigation into an inherited metabolic disease.

Q3. What investigations would be appropriate?

First-line investigations into a child with acute encephalopathy should include those shown in Table 34.2.

Many of these investigations are also useful in identifying the cause of hypoglycaemia, but in addition blood should be taken for insulin, C-peptide, growth hormone (GH), cortisol, 3-hydroxybutyrate and free fatty acids.

BOX 34.3 Differential diagnosis for acute encephalopathy due to an IEM

- Hyperammonaemia: late-onset urea cycle disorders, organic acidaemias, liver failure
- Fatty acid oxidation defects: cause encephalopathy before hypoglycaemia in older children
- Late-onset/intermittent maple syrup urine disease
- Porphyria
- Mitochondrial disease

Table 34.2 **First-line investigations in acute encephalopathy**

Test	To detect
Blood gases	Metabolic or respiratory acidosis
Blood glucose	Hypoglycaemia
Electrolytes	Increased anion gap
Liver function tests	Raised transaminases
Urinalysis	Ketones and reducing substances
CSF lactate	
Blood ammonia	Hyperammonaemia
Urinary organic and amino acids	
Plasma amino acids	
Plasma carnitine and acyl-carnitines	

Results of investigations in Maya are.

- H^+ 72 nmol/l
- PCO_2 3.0 kPa
- HCO_3 16.2 mmol/l
- Lactate   2.8 mmol/l
- NH_4^+ 116 umol/l
- Na^+ 132 mmol/l
- K^+ 3.8 mmol/l
- Urea   6.8 mmol/l
- Cl^- 92 mmol/l
- Glucose   2.2 mmol/l.

There are a number of abnormalities in these results and this can sometimes cause some confusion. This child has a metabolic acidosis, with decreased bicarbonate, raised ammonia and hypoglycaemia. At this stage it is helpful to calculate the anion gap, as the pH is low and you do not know whether this is because the bicarbonate buffer is saturated due to reduced bicarbonate with increased renal or gastrointestinal losses (i.e. renal tubular acidosis or gastrointestinal losses with diarrhoea), or whether other unmeasured anions are contributing. Albumin is a major anion (buffer) but unmeasured anions, such as lactate, ketones (aceto-acetate, β-hydroxybutyrate), phosphate, sulphate or other organic acids, may contribute. The anion gap can be calculated as follows:

Anion gap $= [Na^+] - ([Cl^-] + [HCO_3])$
normally 10–15 mmol/l
$\qquad = 132 - (92 + 16.2)$
$\qquad = 23.8$ mmol/l

In this case there was an increased anion gap and this was due to a previously undiagnosed organic acidaemia. Maya's condition decompensated at this time of metabolic stress when she had an intercurrent illness and entered a catabolic state.

Q4. What features of this presentation should make you suspect a potential inherited metabolic disease?

- Inappropriately ill for history given
- Unexplained acidosis with increased anion gap
- Hypoglycaemia
- Abnormal movements, which may point towards involvement of the basal ganglia that is frequently associated with IEMs.

Q5. What conditions cause hypoglycaemia?

Although hypoglycaemia is frequently associated with IEMs, it is infrequently the presenting sign. The following conditions may present with hypoglycaemia:

Ketotic hypoglycaemia

This is the collective term for the most frequently seen cause of hypoglycaemia. It is a poorly understood condition but seems to represent decreasing fasting tolerance in the young child. It is frequently associated with babies who were intrauterine growth retarded or small for dates. This diagnosis is made by exclusion of other causes and children should never be fasted to make this diagnosis before other causes have been excluded. Treatment is by use of an emergency feeding plan during episodes of illness and prevention of prolonged fasting. Use of a glucose polymer is encouraged, and when vomiting is present, there should be early use of intravenous 10% dextrose with added electrolytes.

Medium-chain acyl-CoA dehydrogenase deficiency (MCADD) and other disorders of fatty acid oxidation

These are usually preceded by encephalopathy, and hypoglycaemia is a late sign of decompensation. The most common disorder in this group is MCADD. It is possible to screen for this condition in the neonatal period by either cord blood analysis or blood collected to measure carnitine and acyl-carnitine. Typical abnormalities of urine organic acids are also seen and are more pronounced during times of intercurrent illness or fasting. Management is by emergency feeding plan. This is a condition with a very good outcome if managed correctly, but a very poor outcome if missed in the presenting phase. Adolescents may present with acute encephalopathy after experimenting with alcohol.

Glycogen storage disorders

These can present at any age but the most common form usually presents within a few months of life with severe hypoglycaemia, high serum lactate, urate and palpable liver. Milder variants may present with hypoglycaemia only but hepatomegaly is fairly universal.

Hyperinsulinism and hyperammonaemia

These are rare metabolic causes of hypoglycaemia but can be treated easily. This is the reason for measuring ammonia in children during episodes of hypoglycaemia. It is due to a defect of the glutamate dehydrogenase enzyme.

Multi-organ failure

This causes hypoglycaemia and is associated with tyrosinaemia, galactosaemia and mitochondrial disorders.

Q6. What investigations should be performed before children are fasted for diagnostic purposes?

- Measurement of glucose by laboratory method, as glucose meters are poor at recording hypoglycaemia
- Good clinical history and examination
- Acyl-carnitine and carnitine measurement
- Serum lactate and uric acid
- Urine for organic acids and amino acids
- Pre- and postprandial 3-hydroxybutyrate and free fatty acids.

A fasting test is generally more useful to diagnose endocrine abnormalities. It should be done by professionals who are experienced in performing it and have access to a specialized laboratory.

Presentation of dysmorphism and IEM

Problem-orientated topic:

dysmorphism and progressive neurological disease (neurodevelopmental regression)

Laurie, a 4-year-old boy, presents with a history of global developmental delay and aggressive challenging behaviour. His parents report that he had apparently normal development and behaviour up until 18 months of age, but they then became concerned that his developmental progress slowed and he even lost some skills that he previously had. His parents are double first cousins and they have one other normal child. On examination Laurie has soft dysmorphic features with mild coarsening of his facial features. He has chronic diarrhoea and has been diagnosed with Perthes' disease of his left hip.

Q1. What features in the history and examination might suggest an inherited metabolic disease?

Q2. In what types of inherited metabolic diseases would you expect dysmorphism to be present?

Q3. What metabolic studies would you carry out to investigate this child's condition?

Q4. What other features should you look for on examination?

Q1. What features in the history and examination might suggest an inherited metabolic disease?

The history of a period of normal development followed by later onset of neurodevelopmental regression or slowing associated with facial coarsening/dysmorphism and skeletal abnormalities should alert you to the fact that this boy may have an inherited metabolic disease.

Q2. In what types of inherited metabolic disease would you expect dysmorphism to be present?

- Lysosomal storage disorders
  - Mucopolysaccharidoses
  - Mucolipidoses
  - Sphingolipidoses
- Peroxisomal disorders
- Mitochondrial disorders
- Abnormalities of sterol metabolism.

Q3. What metabolic studies would you carry out to investigate this young man's condition?

Often clinicians talk about doing a metabolic screen, but this is not useful and the investigations that are performed need to be carefully chosen depending on the most likely diagnosis based on the clinical picture. It is thus important to discuss the most appropriate investigations with your local laboratory.

For this child an initial list of investigations might include:
- Urine glycosaminoglycans: mucopolysaccharidoses
- Urine oligosaccharides: oligosaccharidoses
- Very long chain fatty acids (VLCFA): peroxisomal disorders
- MRI brain: distinguish between grey and white matter disease
- Skeletal survey: dysostosis multiplex
- Ophthalmology review: clouding/cherry-red spot
- Electroretinogram: retinopathy
- Visual evoked potentials: brainstem dysfunction.

Q4. What other features should you look for on examination?

- Eyes: corneal clouding, cataract
- Skeletal deformity: gibbus, kyphosis, macrocephaly
- ENT: recurrent otitis media, persistent nasal discharge
- Face: puffiness of eyelids, coarsening of features, broad nasal bridge and prominence of brow/tongue

- Teeth: small, widely spaced teeth
- Abdomen: umbilical/inguinal hernia and hepatosplenomegaly.

Peroxisomal disorders

Although there are many varied disorders in this group (e.g. Zellweger spectrum disorders), they have very similar presentations, including dysmorphism (characteristic facies), psychomotor retardation, profound hypotonia/weakness, intractable seizures, leucodystrophy (on MRI), impairments of vision and hearing and hepatocellular dysfunction. They represent a spectrum of disease from an early-onset severe disorder to milder older-onset disease.

Lysosomal storage disorders

Broadly speaking, this group of disorders presents with a number of similar features, although they may vary slightly for each individual group:
- Severe hyperactivity and poor sleeping pattern
- Skeletal abnormalities: gibbus and kyphosis
- Recurrent hernias
- Gargoylism or dysmorphic dwarfism (skeletal dysplasia)
- Increasing hepatosplenomegaly
- Gingival hypertrophy
- Degenerative disease of the central nervous system
- Clouding of the cornea
- Changes in retinal pigmentation.

Mucopolysaccharidoses

Mucopolysaccharidoses are caused by a deficiency of lysosomal enzymes that degrade glycosaminoglycans, with a variable degree of progressive mental and physical deterioration. The clinical features of these individual conditions vary depending on the normal rate of enzymatic activity within each tissue. All are inherited in an autosomal recessive manner, except Hunter's syndrome, which is X-linked.

Oligosaccharidoses

These resemble the mucopolysaccharidoses but are less common and the age of presentation tends to be earlier. Main features are skeletal dysplasia, developmental delay, coarse facial features and progressive neurological deterioration. Examples are fucosidosis, alpha-mannosidosis and sialidosis.

Sphingolipidoses

Sphingolipids are present throughout the body but are particularly important in nervous tissue, where they are components of myelin sheaths. Abnormal sphingolipids frequently accumulate in the reticuloendothelial system. They are commonly diagnosed after an incidental finding of an enlarged liver or spleen. Examples are Gaucher's disease, Fabry's disease and Niemann–Pick type A and B. Others present with severe developmental regression, a leucodystrophy picture and cherry-red spot of retina.

Mucolipidoses

These have a combination of features of the mucopolysaccharidoses and sphingolipidoses.

Lipidoses (e.g. Niemann–Pick type C)

The lipidoses or lysosomal lipid storage diseases are a diverse group of conditions that lead to accumulation of the enzyme's substrate. Presentation is either as neonatal cholestasis, as splenomegaly or with ataxia and vertical gaze palsy.

Mitochondrial respiratory chain disorders

Mitochondrial disorders can also present in a very non-specific manner affecting any organ in the body. The classical clinical picture is of failure to thrive, associated with renal tubular leak or specific constellations that give raise to the names: e.g. MELAS — *m*yoclonic *e*pilepsy, *l*actic *a*cidosis and *s*troke-like episodes, or MERRF — *m*yoclonic *e*pilepsy and *r*agged *r*ed *f*ibres.

Specific disorders

There are many IEMs that present in childhood, most of which are very rare. Only the more classical disorders are discussed here.

 More information about some others (Box 34.4) is available on the MasterCourse website.

> **BOX 34.4 Specific disorders discussed on the MasterCourse website**
>
> - Propionic, methylmalonic and isovaleric acidaemias
> - Homocystinuria
> - Glutaric aciduria type 1
> - Urea cycle disorders
> - Glycogen storage disorders
> - Porphyrias
> - Wilson's disease

Phenylketonuria

This is a disorder of amino acid metabolism where deficiency of the phenylalanine hydroxylase enzyme causes a deficiency of tyrosine and an increase in phenylalanine. Its incidence is 1:10 000–20 000. Persistently elevated levels of phenylalanine are associated with microcephaly and mental retardation. Acute elevations are not significant and no special precautions are needed during illness or surgery.

Presentation

Presentation is normal at birth and the condition should be diagnosed from screening:
- Measurement of phenylalanine from blood collected within the first 10 days of life is part of UK screening programme.
- Children arriving from other parts of the world may not have been screened and may present with developmental delay, eczema and microcephaly.

Diagnosis
- There is an elevated level of phenylalanine but decreased tyrosine.
- Biopterin metabolism is normal.
- Enzyme activity can be measured from liver tissue but is hardly ever justified.
- Mutational analysis is possible but expensive and is unlikely to influence management.

Management
- Phenylalanine-restricted diet
- Supplementation of tyrosine and other essential amino acids with special protein substitutes
- Monitoring blood levels and checking for nutritional deficiencies
- Avoidance of aspartame-containing foods
- Pregnancy counselling for adolescents, as control needs to be much tighter during pregnancy. Uncontrolled phenylalanine levels in pregnancy are associated with a high incidence of fetal abnormalities.

The organic acidurias

The organic acidaemias are a group of conditions arising from defects in the breakdown of amino acids further down the pathway from that seen in maple syrup urine disease. They include:
- Propionic acidaemia
- Methylmalonic acidaemia
- Isovaleric acidaemia (rarer than the two above).

All three conditions present and are broadly managed in similar ways.

Presentation
Children are normal at birth but usually present in the first week with:
- Acute encephalopathy
- Marked metabolic acidosis: raised lactate
- Hyperammonaemia (organic acids inhibit urea cycle)
- Dehydration/shock
- Bone marrow suppression: neutropenia, thrombocytopenia
- Sweaty odour (isovaleric acidaemia)
- Neurological complications: metabolic stroke, basal ganglia involvement
- Cardiomyopathy (propionic acidaemia)
- Pancreatitis

These disorders are triggered by sepsis, fasting or surgery.

Diagnosis
- Marked metabolic acidosis with ketosis
- Hyperammonaemia
- Urinary organic acid pattern is usually diagnostic and supported by acyl-carnitine profile
- Confirmation by enzyme analysis on fibroblasts.

Management
- Acute management is as described above, including stopping protein feeds and using 10% dextrose to prevent catabolism.
- Correct dehydration with intravenous fluids.
- Correct acidosis with sodium bicarbonate.
- Remove ammonia; may need dialysis.
- Remove organic acids:
  - Carnitine for propionic and methylmalonic acidaemia
  - Glycine for isovaleric acidaemia.
- Metronidazole reduces gut bacterial production of propionic acid (for propionic and methylmalonic acidaemia).
- Co-factor supplementation (biotin for propionic acidaemia and vitamin B_{12} for methylmalonic acidaemia); some variants may be due to co-factor deficiency alone.
- Long-term treatment involves low-protein diet with long-term oral bicarbonate, carnitine, metronidazole and co-factor, if needed.

Lactic acidosis

Lactic acid is produced by the anaerobic respiratory pathways and can be raised in two general situations.

Table 34.3 Conditions in which raised lactate is seen

Condition	Defect	Examples
Hypoxia	Increased pyruvate production	Poor perfusion, systemic disease, cardiac disease
Impaired glucose production	Increased pyruvate production	Glycogen storage disease I, hereditary fructose intolerance
Impaired NADH metabolism		Mitochondrial disorders of electron transport chain
Impaired pyruvate breakdown		Pyruvate dehydrogenase deficiency, pyruvate carboxylase deficiency, biotinidase deficiency
Impaired acetyl-CoA production	Impaired pyruvate breakdown	Fatty acid oxidation disorders
Other		Organic acidaemias

NADH = nicotinamide adenine dinucleoide.

By far the most common of these (type A) is in states of tissue hypoxia that can arise from shock, cardiac failure or other organ failure or from severe disease. A raised lactate is also seen in some metabolic conditions.

Lactate is formed from the reduction of pyruvate. Therefore a raised lactate can be seen in the conditions listed in Table 34.3.

Sabah Alvi   Paul Arundel

Sabah Alvi   Paul Arundel

CHAPTER

35

Endocrinology and diabetes

LEARNING OUTCOMES

By the end of this chapter you should:

- Understand the basic physiology of the endocrine system
- Know what constitutes normal growth and puberty
- Be able to recognize when patterns of growth and puberty are abnormal, and construct a differential diagnosis for the child with short stature
- Be able to plan investigations of disorders of growth and puberty
- Know the common causes of thyroid and adrenal abnormalities
- Know the pathophysiology of diabetes mellitus and its long term complications
- Understand the principles of management of diabetes, including diet, insulin regimens and home monitoring
- Understand the pathophysiology of diabetic ketoacidosis and its acute management.

MODULE SIX

Introduction

An understanding of normal growth and development is fundamental to the concept of paediatric medicine. Poor growth can be the first sign of a significant clinical problem and in most instances will not be due to an endocrine abnormality. However, to recognize abnormal growth, it is essential to understand what constitutes normal growth with its variants and determinants. Growth and its disorders are discussed fully in Chapter 22 (Volume 1). The aim of this chapter is not to provide a comprehensive text on endocrinology and diabetes, but to focus on the essentials of hormone disorders along with the basic science underlying the physiology and pathology of the endocrine system.

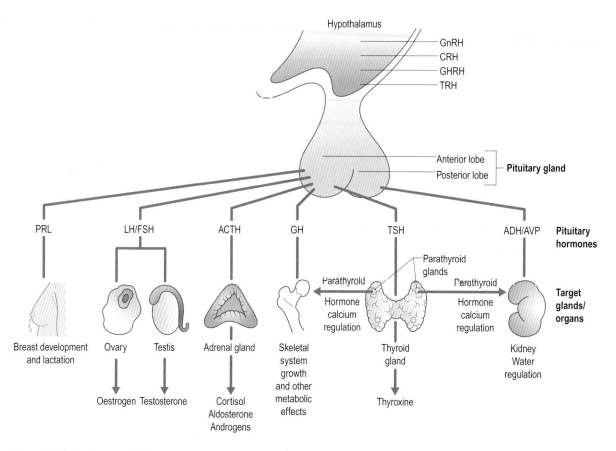

Fig. 35.1 Endocrine regulation.
(ACTH = adrenocorticotrophin; ADH/AVP = antidiuretic hormone/arginine vasopressin; CRH = corticotrophin-releasing hormone; FSH = follicle-stimulating hormone; GH = growth hormone; GHRH = growth hormone-releasing hormone; LH = luteinizing hormone; GnRH = gonadotrophin-releasing hormone; PRL = prolactin; TRH = thyrotrophin-releasing hormone; TSH = thyroid-stimulating hormone)

The endocrine axis and hormonal regulation (Fig. 35.1)

Basic science

The hypothalamo-pituitary axis is fundamental to the exchange of hormonal information. Hormonal control is dependent upon pulsatility of secretion and responds to circadian rhythms, as well as to environmental factors and higher neural centres. Knowledge of the structure and function of this intricate communication system is essential to the understanding of endocrine function, investigation and treatment. Faults at any level can disrupt the finely balanced feedback system.

The hypothalamus

The hypothalamus lies above the pituitary gland and has connections with other parts of the brain, such as the cerebral cortex, as well as the pituitary itself. The hypothalamus secretes corticotrophin-releasing hor-mone (CRH), thyrotrophin-releasing hormone (TRH), gonadotrophin-releasing hormone (GnRH) and growth hormone-releasing hormone (GHRH), all of which act on their corresponding pituitary hormones. Somatostatin and dopamine, which have inhibitory effects, are also secreted by the hypothalamus. All these hypothalamic hormones are carried to the anterior pituitary by the portal blood system.

The pituitary

The pituitary gland plays a critical role in growth, reproduction and homeostasis. It integrates complex feedback mechanisms, receiving information from the brain via the hypothalamus and signalling to peripheral endocrine organs such as the adrenals, thyroid and gonads. The pituitary gland lies within the sella turcica at the base of the brain and consists of two main lobes. The anterior lobe, the adenohypophysis, develops from the oral ectoderm, whilst the posterior lobe, the neurohypophysis, develops from the neural ectoderm.

The anterior pituitary produces six main hormones: growth hormone (GH), thyroid-stimulating hormone (TSH), adrenocorticotrophin (ACTH), luteinizing hormone (LH), follicle-stimulating hormone (FSH) and prolactin (PRL). The posterior pituitary is responsible for release of the antidiuretic hormone, vasopressin, which regulates water balance, and oxytocin, which is instrumental at parturition and lactation.

The stimulatory and inhibitory releasing hormones that are secreted by the hypothalamus regulate the hypothalamo-pituitary axis via the pituitary stalk.

Disorders of the pituitary gland and growth

Disorders of growth are the most common presenting problem in a general endocrine clinic. To recognize normal and abnormal growth you must be able firstly to measure and plot accurately on the most up-to-date centile charts, calculate mid-parental heights and then recognize when to be concerned. This topic is discussed in detail in Chapter 22 and only aspects of growth that may be referred to a more specialist clinic are discussed here.

Problem-orientated topic:

short stature

Lydia, a 6-year-old girl, is brought to clinic by her mother who is concerned that her 4-year-old sister is almost as tall as Lydia. The child is wearing out all her clothes and shoes, rather than outgrowing them. She has never been to the hospital before, but she has had several ear infections and glue ear. She has mild asthma and has been on treatment with 'a brown and a blue inhaler when she needs them', but she has not been using either recently.

Q1. What are the possible causes of this problem?
Q2. How would you assess this child?
Q3. How would you manage this condition?

Q1. What are the possible causes of this problem?

There are many reasons a child may be short (Box 35.1), but to determine which of these is the cause it is essential to take a systematic history and have a sensible differential diagnosis and investigation plan. Always remember that there may not be an endocrine cause and you must not

BOX 35.1 Causes of short stature

Normal variation
- Familial
- Idiopathic

Intrauterine growth retardation
- Infections
- Poor placental function

Genetic/congenital/chromosomal conditions
- Turner's syndrome, Noonan's syndrome, Down's syndrome
- Septo-optic dysplasia
- Skeletal dysplasias

Chronic systemic disorders
For example:
- Gastrointestinal disorders: inflammatory bowel disease, coeliac disease
- Respiratory diseases: cystic fibrosis, severe asthma
- Chronic renal failure

Endocrine abnormalities
- Hypopituitarism
- Hypothyroidism
- Cushing's syndrome

Emotional/psychosocial
- Can result in reversible growth hormone deficiency

miss other problems, especially chronic illnesses or their treatments. Familial and idiopathic short stature are very common, and it is essential to recognize this fact so that parents and children can be appropriately reassured and not inappropriately investigated.

Hypopituitarism
- *Congenital.* Growth hormone deficiency (GHD) can be inherited due to mutations in the genes responsible for regulating growth, or may be due to developmental defects in the pituitary gland (pituitary aplasia or hypoplasia). It can occur in isolation or combined with other pituitary hormone deficiencies (ACTH, TSH etc.) and may present with hypoglycaemia or jaundice in the neonate.
- *Acquired.* This is due to damage to the pituitary or hypothalamus, e.g. intracranial tumours, surgery, radiotherapy, infections or trauma.

Q2. How would you assess this child?

History
- Gestation, birth weight, perinatal problems
- Duration of concern: always been short or recently falling away from centiles?

- Family history, consanguinity, growth problems in family, (biological) parental heights
- Past medical history: chronic illnesses/operations
- Medication: corticosteroids can cause significant growth suppression
- Full systems enquiry.

Measurements

- Parental heights where possible
- Accurate measurements of height and weight
- Accurate plotting of all measurements on decimal centile charts
- Past measurements, e.g. from the child's 'red book'
- Repeated measurements, height velocity calculated over 6–12 months
- In specialist clinics, sitting height and span should also be measured.

Examination

- Any dysmorphic features, e.g. neck webbing
- Signs of chronic illness, e.g. abdominal distension, buttock wasting, pectus excavatum
- Nutritional status
- Systematic examination
- Pubertal staging (p. 105).

Investigations: blood tests

- Haematology: iron deficiency, erythrocyte sedimentation rate (ESR)
- Biochemistry: urea and electrolytes (U&E), calcium and bone profile, liver function
- Immunology: coeliac, thyroid antibodies
- Karyotype: Turner's, Down's, Klinefelter's
- Specific endocrine tests: thyroid function tests, dynamic GH secretion tests, LHRH, TRH tests.

Investigations: radiology

- X-rays:
  - Bone age (Ch. 22): this is *not* a diagnostic tool; it helps you to assess growth reserve (or limitation) by scoring the maturity of certain bones of the hand and wrist. You would not be expected to know how to calculate a bone age.
  - Skeletal survey: if considering a skeletal dysplasia such as achondroplasia.
- Ultrasound scans: renal, if any suggestion of renal disease; pelvic, e.g. ovaries for Turner's syndrome.
- Echocardiogram: heart symptoms/signs.
- CT/MRI scans: brain (intracranial space-occupying lesions, structural abnormalities of hypothalamus or pituitary); adrenal (tumours of the adrenal gland).

Of these radiological investigations, only a wrist X-ray for assessment of skeletal maturity (bone age) should be considered a baseline test.

Q3. How would you manage this condition?

For familial short stature or constitutional delay of growth, only reassurance is required. For underlying diseases, these must be corrected first; adverse psychosocial conditions may need to be addressed by removing the child from the inappropriate environment. Recombinant human growth hormone is available as a daily subcutaneous injection and this is currently licensed for use in children with:

- GH deficiency
- Turner's syndrome
- Chronic renal failure
- Prader–Willi syndrome
- Intrauterine growth restriction (small for gestational age)

Growth hormone will not usually make children grow taller than they are genetically programmed to be; however, it will help children to catch up much of their lost growth and will enable them to attain a normal growth velocity.

Septo-optic dysplasia

This is a congenital condition comprising:
- Absent septum pellucidum
- Optic nerve aplasia/hypoplasia
- Pituitary gland hypoplasia dysfunction.

Children with this condition may be visually impaired and have multiple pituitary hormone deficiencies.

Growth hormone insensitivity syndrome (GHIS; Laron's syndrome)

Children with GHIS have a genetic defect of the growth hormone receptor, which means that they cannot respond to growth hormone. Endogenous levels of GH are frequently very high. At present these children are untreatable and have an adult height of about 120–130 cm. This condition is very rare.

Hypothyroidism (p. 108)

Slowing of growth rate may be the only sign.

Cushing's disease or syndrome (p. 110)

Along with obesity, poor growth is the most consistent feature in paediatric Cushing's, and helps differentiate

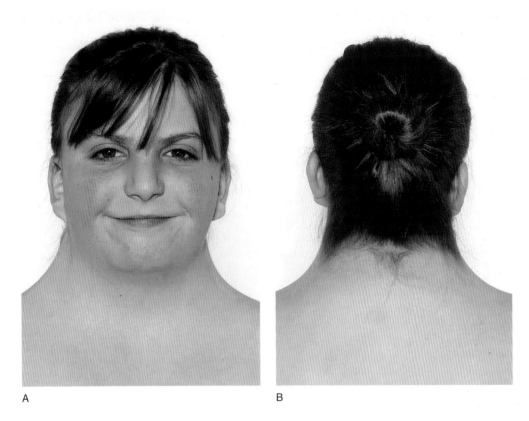

A   B

Fig. 35.2 **Turner's syndrome.**
(A) Note the neck webbing and low-set ears; (B) low posterior hairline.

the weight gain of exogenous obesity from that seen in conditions of excess glucocorticoids.

Turner's syndrome (Fig. 35.2)

Turner's syndrome results from a chromosome anomaly that affects expression and/or regulation of genes located on the X chromosome (Ch. 9). It arises in 1 in 2500 live-born girls but many affected pregnancies do not reach term. The most common karyotype is 45X but variants such as 45X/46XX, 45X/46XY or 45X/47XXX can all occur (mosaicism). The most consistent features of Turner's syndrome are short stature and gonadal dysgenesis (failure of development of the ovaries, which may be completely absent, or present just as 'streaks' of tissue), resulting in absence of secondary sex characteristics (Box 35.2). All short girls should have their karyotype checked, even if no other clinical features are present.

Although they are not GH-deficient, girls with Turner's syndrome are usually treated with GH, as untreated adult height is in the range of 142–147 cm. Almost all girls will require induction of puberty with oestrogen.

Any girl whose karyotype contains Y material must have a gonadectomy, as there is a small risk of developing a gonadoblastoma.

BOX 35.2 Clinical findings in Turner's syndrome

- Short stature
- Cubitus valgus
- Hypertelorism
- Low-set ears
- Low posterior hairline
- Multiple naevi
- Lymphoedema
- Dysplastic nails
- Broad chest
- Inverted nipples
- Neck webbing
- High-arched palate

Associated features

- Hypertension
- Renal anomalies (horseshoe kidney)
- Cardiovascular abnormalities (e.g. aortic coarctation or stenosis)
- Recurrent ear infections
- Autoimmune thyroiditis

Noonan's syndrome

This is usually an autosomal dominant condition, with short stature, cardiac abnormalities (usually pulmonary stenosis) and cryptorchidism.

Key points: short stature

- Not everything that is short is abnormal.
- The most common causes of short stature are non-endocrine in nature.
- All girls with short stature should have a karyotype, as many girls with Turner's syndrome do not have the classical phenotype.
- Chronic disease can cause severe growth failure and only appropriate management of the underlying disease will resolve the growth problem.
- Always measure and plot accurately.
- Always obtain parental heights and calculate the mid-parental height centile (Ch. 22).
- Height velocity over at least a 6-month period is of greater value than a single height measurement.
- Random GH levels are of no value in assessment of short stature.

Tall stature

This is described in Chapter 22.

Disorders of the posterior pituitary

The posterior pituitary gland secretes the antidiuretic hormone vasopressin (to regulate salt and water balance) and oxytocin. For all practical purposes in paediatrics, you need only know about disturbances in the secretion of vasopressin.

Diabetes insipidus (DI)

This results from either lack of vasopressin (cranial DI) or renal tubular unresponsiveness to vasopressin (nephrogenic DI). It must be differentiated from habitual water drinking, which will also present with polyuria and polydipsia.

Cranial DI

Congenital absence of the posterior pituitary (e.g. septo-optic dysplasia) is rare. Cranial DI usually results from mechanical damage such as surgery or radiation to the pituitary stalk, or is due to infiltrative disease such as histiocytosis. Children develop polyuria and intense polydipsia, and become dehydrated. Treatment is with the antidiuretic hormone analogue, DDAVP.

Nephrogenic DI

This is usually genetic (X-linked or autosomal recessive).

Disorders of puberty

Basic science

Normal puberty

- Follows a set sequence of hormonal and clinical events but tempo varies.
- Centrally initiated by pulsatile release of hypothalamic hormone (GnRH).
- Acts on anterior pituitary to produce luteinizing and follicle-stimulating hormones (LH and FSH).
- LH/FSH stimulate oestrogen and testosterone production; assisted by adrenal steroids, these stimulate development of physical sex characteristics.

Physical changes of puberty (see also Ch. 5)

In girls
- The first change is breast budding.
- Periods start after breast stage 3 has been reached.
- Peak height velocity occurs at the end of puberty, just before menarche.
- Menarche is the last event of puberty.
- After menarche there is very little growth left.

In boys
- The first sign of puberty is enlargement of the testes.
- Growth spurt occurs about 2 years later than in girls (14 years vs 12 years).
- Peak height velocity occurs mid-puberty.

Effects of pubertal hormones
- Testosterone:
  - Testicular enlargement
- Oestrogen:
  - Breast development
  - Uterine enlargement
  - Endometrial thickening
- Adrenal hormones:
  - Acne/greasy skin
  - Body odour
  - Pubic and axillary hair

Table 35.1 Staging of puberty (see also Fig. 5.5)

| Stage | Girls | | Boys | |
	Pubic hair	Breasts	Pubic hair	Genitalia
1	None	Pre-adolescent, elevation of papilla only	None	Pre-adolescent; testes, scrotum and penis are about same size and proportion as early childhood
2	Sparse growth of long, slightly pigmented, downy straight hair, chiefly along labia	Breast bud stage; elevation of breast and papilla as a small mound, enlargement of areolar diameter	Sparse growth of long, slightly pigmented, downy straight hair, chiefly at base of penis	Scrotum and testes have enlarged, with reddening and change of texture of scrotal skin
3	Considerably darker, coarser and more curled. The hair, spreads sparsely over the junction of the pubes	Further enlargement of breast and areola, with no separation of their contours	Considerably darker, coarser and more curled. The hair spreads sparsely over the junction of the pubes	Growth of penis in length and breadth; further growth of testes and scrotum
4	Hair adult in type, but smaller area covered; no spread to medial surface of thighs	Projection of areola and papilla to form a secondary mound above the level of the breast	Hair adult in type, but smaller area covered; no spread to medial surface of thighs	Further enlargement of penis with development of glans. Further growth of scrotum and testes
5	Adult in quantity and type, forms inverse triangle and spreads to medial surface of thighs	Mature stage; projection of papilla only, due to recession of the areola to the general contour of the breast	Adult in quantity and type, forms inverse triangle and spreads to medial surface of thighs	Adult in size and shape

Source: after Marshall and Tanner, with permission from the BMJ Publishing Group.

Puberty is staged using the Tanner system (Table 35.1).

Normal variants (Box 35.3)

Tempo

This is the timing of puberty. It can be slower or faster than the average in certain groups, e.g.:

- *Familial*: children with delayed or early puberty often have parents with the same.
- *Ethnicity*: earlier in Asian and African–Caribbean girls.
- *Psychosocial*: e.g. adopted girls may have early puberty.

- *Secular trends*: trend towards earlier age of onset since war years — probably related to better nutrition.

Premature adrenarche

- Pubic and axillary hair
- Body odour
- Acne
- No other signs of puberty.

Premature thelarche

- Isolated breast development
- Commonly infants/pre-school children
- No other signs of precocity.

Problem-orientated topic:

disorders of puberty

A mother brings her 7-year-old son, David, to see you, worried that he has developed pubic hair and has a strong body odour. He has been a bit more aggressive lately and seems to be going through a growth spurt; he is the tallest in the class but 6 months ago, when a class photograph was taken, he was about average height.

Continued overleaf

Table 35.2 Investigations in disorders of puberty

Test	Significance
Bone age	Usually advanced because of effect of high oestrogen and androgens
GnRH test	Will show rise in gonadotrophins if puberty imminent
Thyroid function tests	Hypothyroidism can cause raised FSH as well as TSH and can stimulate gonadal activity
Adrenal androgens	Very high if pubertal signs are due to an adrenal tumour
Synacthen test	To exclude congenital adrenal hyperplasia
Pelvic ultrasound scan	To look for ovarian cysts and maturation of the uterus and ovaries
Adrenal scan	Adrenal tumours
Cranial MRI	Intracranial tumours or malformations: mandatory in all boys with central precocious puberty

(FSH = follicle-stimulating hormone; GnRH = gonadotrophin-releasing hormone; TSH = thyroid-stimulating hormone)

Q1. What further information do you require?

Q2. What investigations will you request?

Q3. What is your management plan?

Q1. What further information do you require?

When you are presented with a child who displays symptoms or signs of puberty, ask yourself the following questions:

- Is this a normal sequence of puberty but happening at an abnormally early age, i.e. is it consonant? This is true or central precocious puberty and is gonadotrophin-dependent.
  OR
- Is the normal sequence disrupted and are there signs of peripheral development without activation of the hypothalamus and pituitary, i.e. is it non-consonant? This is peripheral or pseudo-precocious puberty and is gonadotrophin-independent.

As with assessment of stature, when possible disorders of puberty are presented to the clinician, it is essential to know the normal sequence of pubertal changes.

Q2. What investigations will you request?

See Table 35.2. Not all of these will be necessary; the tests selected will depend on the clinical picture.

Q3. What is your management plan?

Medical treatment is available to arrest idiopathic central precocious puberty and ameliorate the psychosocial problems that often accompany it. Rapid progression through puberty can cause early epiphyseal fusion and arresting precocious puberty may prevent height limitation.

Treatment for puberty that is not idiopathic (e.g. adrenal tumour) is directed at the underlying cause.

Central precocious puberty: gonadotrophin-dependent

Definition

Central precocious puberty is the onset of pubertal signs before age of 8 years in girls and 9 years in boys. It is often accompanied by rapid growth and skeletal maturation. LH, FSH and oestradiol/testosterone levels are raised. In girls, precocious puberty is usually idiopathic. In boys, it is usually pathological and must always be fully investigated

Causes

- Idiopathic — majority in girls:
- Central nervous system lesions:
  - Tumours
  - Hamartoma of hypothalamus
  - Infections
  - Vascular lesions
  - Hydrocephalus
  - Trauma
  - Irradiation or surgery
- Hypothyroidism
- Following pseudo-precocious puberty, e.g. in congenital adrenal hyperplasia.

Peripheral (pseudo-)precocious puberty: gonadotrophin-independent

In this there will be changes of puberty but they are not consonant, i.e. there will be no central activation, so that in a boy you may see pubic hair and enlargement of genitalia, but no enlargement of testes, which would normally be the first sign of onset of true puberty. Gonadotrophins are not raised.

Causes

- Tumours:
  - Adrenal
  - Gonadal
- Congenital adrenal hyperplasia
- Hypothyroidism
- McCune–Albright syndrome:
  - Usually affects girls
  - Non-consonant puberty — often due to ovarian cysts
  - Bony dysplasia, seen on X-rays
  - Patchy hyperpigmentation.

Delayed puberty (Box 35.4)

Delayed puberty is the absence of secondary sex characteristics at the age of 13 years in girls or 14 years in boys.

Causes

See Box 35.5.

Klinefelter's syndrome

- Most common cause of male hypogonadism.
- Between 1 in 300 and 1 in 1000 male births.
- Most common karyotype 47XXY, but variants reported.
- There may not be any problems before puberty, which may be delayed.
- At puberty, pubic hair is usually normal but testes remain small.

BOX 35.4 Causes of delayed puberty

With low gonadotrophins
- Constitutional (p. 105):
  - Often familial
- Hypothalamo-pituitary problems:
  - Panhypopituitarism
  - Tumours: e.g. craniopharyngioma; prolactinoma
  - Hypothyroidism
  - Kallmann's syndrome (anosmia, hypogonadism, colour blindness)
- Systemic disease:
  - Severe chronic illness, e.g. Crohn's disease, renal failure
  - Malnutrition/anorexia/nervosa athleticism

With high gonadotrophins
- Gonadal dysgenesis:
  - Turner's syndrome
  - Klinefelter's syndrome
- Primary gonadal failure:
  - Testicular torsion
  - Gonadal irradiation

BOX 35.5 Causes of abnormal pubertal development

- Familial/constitutional
- Chronic ill health
- Intracranial lesions: germinoma, prolactinoma
- Adrenal/gonadal abnormalities: congenital adrenal hyperplasia (CAH), tumours
- Undernutrition: anorexia, athleticism
- Iatrogenic: surgery/radiotherapy to pituitary
- Syndromes: Turner's, Klinefelter's

- Child is often tall; may develop gynaecomastia.
- Infertile.

Amenorrhoea

Primary: never had periods

- Anatomical abnormalities, e.g. absence of uterus/ovaries
- Turner's syndrome
- Androgen insensitivity syndrome (46XY girl).

Secondary: cessation of established periods

- Can be due to anorexia, systemic disease or damage to hypothalamo-pituitary-ovarian axis after puberty is complete.

Remember, even in paediatric medicine, pregnancy can be a cause of secondary amenorrhoea.

Disorders of the thyroid gland

Basic science

The function of the thyroid gland is to concentrate iodide from the blood and to return it to peripheral tissues via the thyroid hormones, thyroxine (T_4) and tri-iodothyronine (T_3). These hormones play a vital role in cellular metabolism and have profound effects on growth and differentiation of most organs, including the brain. Consequently a deficit in thyroid hormones and/or iodine during early life will result not only in general reduction in metabolism, but also in severe intellectual deterioration.

The human fetal thyroid gland develops in two parts. A midline out-pouching of the endoderm in the floor of the primitive buccal cavity is first visible by 16–17 days of gestation. At the same time two lateral structures derived from the fourth pharyngeal pouches appear and develop. By 24 days the gland is still attached to the buccal cavity. By 50 days of gestation the gland descends to the lower part of the neck. It is able to accumulate iodine by 10–12 weeks of gestation. T_4 and T_3 are present at the end of the first trimester.

The thyroid gland grows progressively and thyroid hormones accumulate during the second and third trimesters.

Regulation of thyroid hormones

- Thyrotrophin-releasing hormone (TRH) is secreted by the hypothalamus.
- This stimulates the anterior pituitary to secrete thyroid-stimulating hormone (TSH). TSH binds to its specific receptor on the thyroid cell and triggers off intracellular processes that result in the synthesis of thyroid hormones.
- Iodine is essential in the synthesis of thyroid hormones and this is actively taken up from dietary sources.
- Formed thyroid hormones are released into the circulation, mainly bound to thyroid-binding globulin (TBG).
- Free hormone is released at target tissues.

Classification of thyroid disorders (Box 35.9)

Congenital hypothyroidism (CHT)

- Incidence is 1 in 3500–4500 births.
- Children in developed countries have been screened since the early 1980s.
- Thyroid dysgenesis is the most common cause (~85%) in the UK.
- Heel prick sample at day 5–7 (Guthrie card) measures TSH.
- It is easy to treat with daily oral thyroxine.
- It is essential to start treatment as soon as diagnosis is made (and definitely within 2 weeks) to prevent/minimize developmental delay.
- Treatment required is life-long.
- There is a good long-term prognosis if treatment is started early enough, if there is good compliance and if the appropriate dose is given.
- Higher doses are required in infancy and puberty.

Clinical features (Box 35.6)

As the neonatal screening system is so successful, it is rare to see the developed picture of congenital hypothyroidism, but in a sleepy lethargic baby with a history of poor feeding and prolonged jaundice, you should always consider a missed diagnosis.

BOX 35.6 Presentation of congenital hypothyroidism

Signs
- Jaundice
- Macroglossia
- Umbilical hernia
- Wide posterior fontanelle
- Hypotonia

Symptoms
- Poor feeding
- Lethargy
- Sleepiness
- Constipation

Screening for congenital hypothyroidism

Screening for this condition started in the UK in the early 1980s. Examiners are fond of asking about screening (Ch. 15), and congenital hypothyroidism fulfils all the characteristics of a disease for which screening is justified:

1. It is a common condition.
2. Serious problems (neurodevelopmental delay) can only be prevented when the diagnosis is made very early, ideally during the first few days of life.
3. Clinical recognition of the disease at that early age is difficult as the signs and symptoms are non-specific.
4. Screening tests are available with high sensitivity and specificity.
5. Cost-effective treatment is readily available.

Acquired hypothyroidism (Box 35.7)

- Iodine deficiency most common reason world-wide.

BOX 35.7 Main features of acquired hypothyroidism

Signs
- Full, puffy face
- Short stature
- Dry skin
- Obesity
- Goitre

Symptoms
- Fatigue
- Weight gain despite reduced appetite
- Poor growth
- Cold intolerance
- Constipation

- Autoimmunity (Hashimoto's thyroiditis) most common in the West.
- More common in girls.
- Can present at any age but most commonly does so in adolescence.
- Often there is a family history of autoimmune thyroid disease or other autoimmune conditions.
- Can be secondary to pituitary or hypothalamic disease/damage.
- Treatment is with thyroxine.

Hyperthyroidism

Problem-orientated topic:

goitre

Janine, a 14-year-old girl, presents with a neck swelling and a history of weight loss and restlessness.

Q1. What features of her history do you want to explore?

Q2. What other clinical features will you look for on examination?

Q3. How would you manage this problem?

Q1. What features of her history do you want to explore?

A goitre is an enlargement of the thyroid gland and is not indicative of aetiology. The child/adolescent with a goitre may be euthyroid, hypothyroid or hyperthyroid (see Box 35.9 below).

The main causes are:
- Simple colloid goitre: usually pubertal, euthyroid
- Hashimoto's thyroiditis: hypothyroid
- Graves' disease: hyperthyroid
- Viral thyroiditis
- Congenital hypothyroidism due to inborn errors of thyroid hormone metabolism (dyshormonogenesis).

In this case the most likely cause is Graves' disease, which accounts for more than 90% of childhood hyperthyroidism. The main features of Graves' disease are:
- Autoimmune condition in genetically susceptible individuals.
- Affects girls about seven times more often than boys.
- Can develop at any age but adolescence most common time for presentation.
- Presentation often insidious (see below).
- Caused by TSH receptor antibodies that mimic action of TSH.

BOX 35.8 Main features of Graves' disease

Signs
- Diffusely enlarged thyroid gland
- Thyroid and/or carotid bruits
- Tachycardia
- Ophthalmopathy: often 'staring' eyes rather than ophthalmoplegia
- Warm moist hands with fine tremor
- Restlessness

Symptoms
- Heat intolerance
- Anxiety and palpitations
- Weight loss despite increased appetite
- Deteriorating school performance and behaviour
- Menstrual irregularities
- Rapid growth

- Diagnosis made on history, examination and raised T_4 and T_3 but suppressed TSH levels.

Q2. What other clinical features will you look for on examination?

 See Box 35.8.

Q3. How would you manage this problem?

There are three therapeutic options:
1. *Medical*: with carbimazole or propylthiouracil (PTU), usually for 2–3 years; beware of idiosyncratic bone marrow suppression. High rate of relapse on discontinuing treatment.
2. *Radioactive iodine ablation*: little experience in children; fear of inducing malignancy. Permanent ablation, lifelong thyroxine required.
3. *Surgery*: should only be performed by experienced surgeons: risk to recurrent laryngeal nerve. If total thyroidectomy, will require lifelong thyroxine replacement and may result in hypoparathyroidism.

Neonatal thyrotoxicosis

This is a rare condition but can be an emergency when it arises. It occurs because of transplacental transfer of maternal antibodies — from a mother with Graves' disease — which stimulate the fetal thyroid gland, and symptoms will often develop in the first few days of life. It is a self-limiting condition, as the antibodies will clear from the infant circulation by about 3 months of age. Goitre, irritability, weight loss, tachycardia, arrhythmias and heart failure are features of neonatal thyrotoxicosis. Treatment is with antithyroid drugs

Hypothyroidism

- Congenital:
  - Agenesis/hypoplasia/ectopic
  - Dyshormonogenesis
- Acquired:
  - Primary: autoimmune
  - Secondary: hypothalamic/pituitary defects

Hyperthyroidism

- Neonatal: transient
- Autoimmune: Graves' disease

  Both hypo- or hyperthyroidism can be associated with Down's syndrome, Turner's syndrome or type 1 diabetes mellitus and other autoimmune conditions.

(carbimazole or PTU), and may also require iodine and propranolol until symptoms have diminished. The condition will usually respond to these manoeuvres within a week to 10 days, but antithyroid drugs may be necessary for up to 3 months.

Disorders of the adrenal gland

Basic science

The adrenal gland is encapsulated and developed by the ninth week of gestation and is clearly associated with the upper pole of the kidney, which is much smaller at this stage. It is composed of an outer cortex that accounts for about 90% of the gland and is derived from the mesodermal urogenital ridge; this synthesizes steroid hormones. The inner medulla is derived from the neural crest, from ectodermal tissue, and synthesizes catecholamines.

The adrenal cortex is divided into three zones (Fig. 35.3):

- *The zona glomerulosa*, the outer zone, produces aldosterone and is under control of the renin–angiotensin system
- *The zona fasciculata* secretes glucocorticoids under hypothalamo-pituitary control via corticotrophin-releasing hormone (CRH) and ACTH (adrenocorticotrophin).
- *The zona reticularis* is largely inactive until puberty and secretes predominantly adrenal androgens (dihydroepiandrosterone, DHEAS).

These three types of steroid are synthesized from a common precursor, cholesterol, and there are many pathways involved in their production. In practice you will need to know about the effects of too much or too little corticosteroid and about the most common problem of steroid synthesis, congenital adrenal hyperplasia.

Glucocorticoid excess: Cushing's syndrome

Primary Cushing's disease, caused by an ACTH-secreting pituitary adenoma (Fig. 35.4), is very rare in childhood, but Cushing's syndrome is more commonly seen and most often will be iatrogenic in origin.

Causes of Cushing's syndrome

The main causes are:

- Iatrogenic : oral, inhaled or topical steroids
- Adrenal adenoma.

Clinical features of Cushing's syndrome

- Central obesity
- Moon face
- Poor growth/short stature

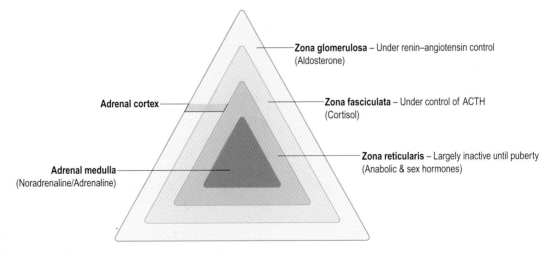

Fig. 35.3 **Structure of the adrenal glands**

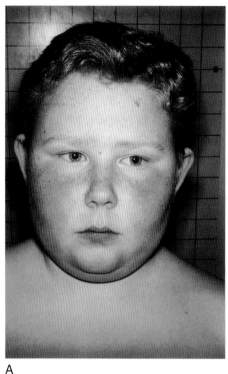

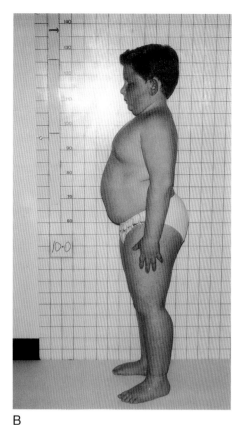

Fig. 35.4 **Cushing's disease.**
(A) Note the central obesity, striae and plethoric facies; (B) this boy is also short.

- Hirsutism
- Striae
- Acne
- Hypertension
- Thin skin.

The history of poor growth in the presence of obesity is fundamental in this diagnosis, as exogenous obesity is almost never accompanied by slowing of linear growth; indeed, these children are usually tall compared with their peers. Always ensure you have a couple of measurements so that you can assess the child's height velocity. If this is normal and there are no other worrying features, Cushing's is highly unlikely.

In paediatrics, you are more likely to see children with iatrogenic Cushing's in respiratory, rheumatology and renal clinics, when high-dose steroids have been used for their immunosuppressive activity.

Adrenal insufficiency

Primary adrenal insufficiency is due to inadequate secretion of adrenal steroids; secondary deficiency is usually due to lack of ACTH (Box 35.10).

BOX 35.10 Some causes of adrenal insufficiency

Primary
- Congenital:
  - Congenital adrenal hyperplasia
  - Adrenal hypoplasia congenita
- Acquired:
  - Autoimmune: Addison's disease
  - Adrenoleucodystrophy

Secondary
- Congenital:
  - Congenital hypopituitarism
  - Septo-optic dysplasia
- Acquired:
  - Cranial surgery or irradiation
  - Steroid therapy/withdrawal

Congenital adrenal hyperplasia (CAH)

Basic science

There is a group of disorders of steroid synthesis collectively called the adrenal hyperplasias, and each is caused by a particular enzyme defect. The resultant clinical picture

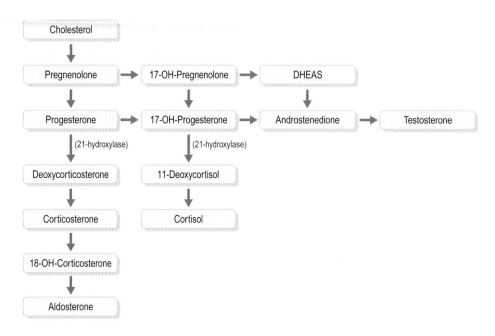

Fig. 35.5 Deficiency of the 21-hydroxylase enzyme

depends on the specific enzyme deficiency. Although the biochemical pathways are quite complicated, the simplified summary in Figure 35.5 can help you to understand the most common enzyme problem, deficiency of the 21-hydroxylase enzyme (Box 35.11).

This single enzyme defect results in three major (and potentially fatal) clinical problems:

1. Block in the mineralocorticoid pathway means the child is unable to synthesize aldosterone, which helps to conserve sodium. Absence of this hormone results in renal salt-wasting (salt-losing crisis) and retention of potassium.

2. Block in production of cortisol causes hypoglycaemia and a classical 'adrenal crisis'. The child therefore typically presents with a short history of lethargy, poor feeding, abdominal pain and vomiting, and is usually found to be dehydrated and hypotensive. There is hyponatraemia, hyperkalaemia and hypoglycaemia, and there may be a profound metabolic acidosis if the process continues unchecked. (This situation can be fatal; it is necessary to recognize it as an acute medical emergency. Intravenous access should be obtained at once; the child should be resuscitated with saline and dextrose and given intravenous hydrocortisone).

3. There is a build-up of precursors proximal to the block, i.e. 17-hydroxyprogesterone. As this cannot be converted to the next stage in the glucocorticoid pathway, it is diverted into an alternative pathway

BOX 35.11 21-hydroxylase deficiency

- Most common adrenal disorder in childhood
- 1 in 15 000 births in the UK
- Causes ~90% of all CAH
- Autosomal recessive: gene mutation on chromosome 6

Presentation
- Females: virilized; genital ambiguity at birth
- Males: salt-losing/adrenal crisis at age 7–14 days

Investigations
- Day 1: karyotype, pelvic ultrasound scan
- Day 3: 17-hydroxyprogesterone/urea and electrolytes

Management
- Hydrocortisone (glucocorticoid replacement)
- Fludrocortisone (mineralocorticoid replacement)
- Salt supplements in infancy
- Virilized female may require surgery

Long-term problems (often relate to level of compliance)
- Short stature
- Virilization
- Precocious puberty
- Subfertility

Antenatal diagnosis and treatment (dexamethasone) possible in subsequent pregnancies.

and is converted into androstenedione and testosterone. It is these androgens that cause virilization.

Congenital adrenal hypoplasia

- Rare autosomal or X-linked recessive condition.
- Presentation similar to CAH, but 17-hydroxyprogesterone levels will be low or normal.
- Treatment identical to CAH, but virilization not an issue.
- Can be associated with hypogonadism in some boys.

Acquired adrenal deficiency

- Most common cause is autoimmune: Addison's disease.
- Can be isolated or found in association with other autoimmune disorders such as Hashimoto's thyroiditis, or diabetes mellitus.
- Can be part of autoimmune polyglandular syndromes.

Features of Addison's disease
- Pigmentation in areas not exposed to sun
- Lethargy
- Weakness
- Weight loss
- Abdominal pain
- Vomiting.

Other causes of adrenal insufficiency
Although the development of Cushing's syndrome is a possibility in children who have been on long-term steroid therapy, adrenal deficiency can result from prolonged suppression of endogenous cortisol production, and therefore sudden withdrawal of therapy can result in an adrenal crisis. Although this usually occurs in those who have been on prolonged courses of oral steroids, more cases are coming to light in children who have been on high doses of inhaled steroids and therefore it is vital to remember *all* forms of steroid treatment when faced with a possible adrenal crisis.

All children who are dependent on steroid treatment must carry steroid cards, wear some form of SOS talisman and be given instructions to double their maintenance dose of oral hydrocortisone during intercurrent illness. If they are unable to tolerate oral medication, they must seek immediate medical help, as they may need parenteral treatment. Patients undergoing surgery must be given intravenous steroid cover.

Disorders of sexual development/genital ambiguity

Basic science

Sexual determination and differentiation are quite complicated and are set early in life. It is important to have a basic understanding of the processes involved, as occasionally children will be born whose sex is not immediately clear.

There are three main components to gender:
- *Genetic sex*: the genotype, determined at the time of conception
- *Sex differentiation*: the development of the internal and external genitalia under the influence of genes and hormones
- *Sexuality*: gender identity under the influence of genes, hormones and psychological/environmental factors.

Fetal sex differentiation

Basic science of embryology (Fig. 35.6)

The main events are as follow:
- Gonadal development is apparent from week 5 of gestation.
- The thickened area of the genital ridge develops into an undifferentiated (bipotential) gonad.
- Under the influence of a Y chromosome, the gonad develops into a testis and secretes testosterone and a substance called anti-Müllerian hormone. These cause regression of the female system, and the Wolffian ducts develop into epididymis, vas deferens and seminal vesicles.
- In the absence of a Y chromosome, a testis is not formed, the gonad develops into an ovary, the Wolffian ducts involute and the Müllerian system develops into the Fallopian tubes, uterus and upper third of the vagina. The urogenital sinus develops into the lower two-thirds of the vagina and urethra.

Genital ambiguity

This is a very traumatic situation for both parents and professionals and must be handled with extreme sensitivity. Always ask for senior help immediately. Explain to parents that, although there is something the matter with the way the baby's genitals have developed, this does arise from time to time, and some tests will need to be done before it will be possible to say whether baby will be brought up as a boy or girl. Reassure the

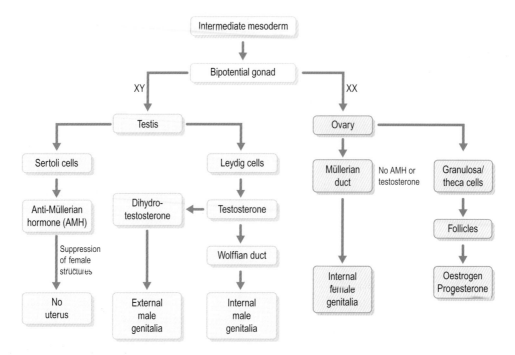

Fig. 35.6 **Sex differentiation**

parents that the baby will definitely be assigned a single gender and will not be 'something in between'.

The vignette below shows how to manage a newborn baby with genital ambiguity.

Problem-orientated topic:

ambiguous genitalia

The midwife on the delivery suite calls you because a baby has been born whose gender is unclear. She wants you to explain to the distraught parents what is wrong and what you are going to do.

Q1. What are the causes of genital ambiguity?

Q2. How do you approach this problem?

Q1. What are the causes of genital ambiguity?

- Virilized female (karyotype 46XX, ovaries present on pelvic ultrasound):
  - Almost always will be a girl with CAH.
- Undervirilized male (karyotype 46XY, testes present):
  - Defective testis differentiation: agenesis or dysgenesis

- Defective testosterone synthesis: e.g. rare forms of CAH; 5-alpha-reductase deficiency (very rare)
- Defective response to male hormones: partial androgen insensitivity syndrome.

Q2. How do you approach this problem?

- Seek senior help.
- Do not refer to the baby as 'he', 'she' or 'it'.
- Reassure parents that gender will be assigned but tests will be necessary and results may take some time.

History
- Obstetric history
- Maternal virilization
- Family history (e.g. androgen insensitivity syndrome).

Examination
- Virilized female or undervirilized male?
- Are gonads present? Appearance of labioscrotal folds
- Size of clitoris/phallus; how many urogenital openings?
- Other abnormalities/recognizable syndrome?

Investigations
- Cord or venous blood for karyotype and DNA
- Pelvic and abdominal ultrasound:
  - Internal structures, gonads

- After 72 hours:
  - U&E
  - 17-hydroxyprogesterone
  - Urine for steroid profile
- Further investigations:
  - Discuss with paediatric endocrinologists, surgeons, geneticists, radiologists and psychologists.

Disorders of calcium and bone

Basic science of calcium homeostasis

Normal total serum calcium is 2.2–2.6 mmol/l. The vast majority of body calcium is found in bone and is fundamental to maintaining skeletal integrity. In blood, it is found in three forms: ionized, bound to proteins and as complexes with substances such as citrate. In its ionized (biologically active) form, calcium is vital to nerve conduction, muscle contraction and blood coagulation. Complexed calcium is largely insignificant, but protein-bound calcium is affected by albumin concentration and this must be taken into consideration when interpreting results. Extracellular calcium homeostasis is maintained by two main factors: vitamin D and parathyroid hormone.

Vitamin D

Vitamin D is obtained either from the diet (animal or vegetable sterols) or from the action of sunlight on skin. This circulating vitamin D is then metabolized in the liver to 25-hydroxyvitamin D, which is further hydroxylated in the kidney to the active 1,25-dihydroxyvitamin D. Vitamin D acts on intestinal epithelium to increase calcium and phosphate absorption, and increases skeletal mineralization and bone formation. Any problems in obtaining vitamin D (dietary deficiency) or metabolizing it (liver or renal disease) will therefore have consequences for calcium and bone regulation.

Parathyroid hormone

The four parathyroid glands, found behind the thyroid gland, develop from the third and fourth branchial pouches. They secrete parathyroid hormone (PTH) in response to low circulating ionized calcium. PTH regulates extracellular calcium by increasing renal calcium absorption and mobilizing calcium and phosphate from bone.

Hypocalcaemia

Problem-orientated topic:

tingling and spasms of the hands

Prika, a 14-year-old Asian girl, presents with a 6-week history of intermittent tingling and spasm of her hands. She is on the 25th centile for height and 10th centile for weight, and is in puberty. There are no abnormal findings on examination.

Q1. What is your differential diagnosis?
Q2. What investigations would you undertake?
Q3. How would you treat Prika?

Q1. What is your differential diagnosis?

In a teenager such as Prika, tetany due to hypocalcaemia is the most likely diagnosis. In practice you may also come across a baby with seizures who is found to have low calcium, or an infant with failure to thrive and features of rickets.

Clinical features of hypocalcaemia
- Infants:
  - Jitteriness
  - Poor appetite
  - Vomiting
  - Seizures
  - Apnoeic episodes
  - Stridor
  - Proximal myopathy with delayed motor development
- Older children/adolescents:
  - Tingling: fingers, perioral
  - Tetany: carpal/pedal spasm
  - Latent tetany: Chvostek/Trousseau signs.

Causes of hypocalcaemia
- In neonates:
  - Prematurity
  - Maternal vitamin D deficiency
  - Maternal hyperparathyroidism
  - Hypomagnesaemia
  - High milk phosphate
  - Congenital hypoparathyroidism
- In childhood:
  - Vitamin D deficiency
  - Hypoparathyroidism
  - Renal disease.

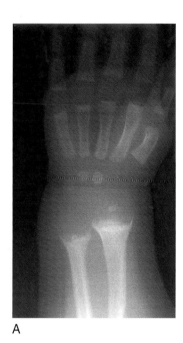
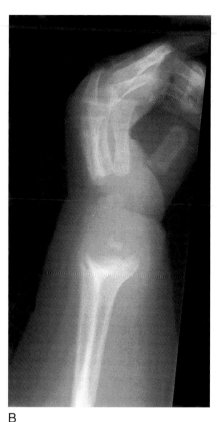

A   B

Fig. 35.7 Wrist X-rays showing changes of rickets—metaphyseal cupping and splaying. (A) Lateral view; (B) straight view.

Hypoparathyroidism
- *Congenital*: due to aplasia of the glands as part of the Di George spectrum of anomalies
- *Acquired*: can be isolated or in association with other autoimmune conditions, e.g. polyglandular syndrome 1.

Rickets
This describes the clinical picture resulting from defective mineralization of osteoid tissue. There is a resurgence of rickets in the UK, especially in infants who are exclusively breastfed or from certain ethnic minority groups. It is imperative therefore that all babies at high risk of vitamin D deficiency should have feeds supplemented with vitamin D for at least the first 2 years of life. Pregnant women (especially those of Asian origin, as they are particularly susceptible) should also receive supplements. The most common cause of rickets is vitamin D deficiency, although rarer forms are also seen.

Causes of vitamin D deficiency
- *Inadequate sunshine*: most vitamin D is converted from sterols in the skin by the action of sunlight.
- *Dietary insufficiency*.
- *Malabsorption*: as vitamin D is fat-soluble, conditions such as coeliac disease can be a cause.

- *Hepatic/renal disease*: vitamin D is converted in both liver and kidney.

Clinical features of rickets
- Craniotabes: softening of skull with delayed closure of fontanelles
- Rachitic rosary: enlargement of costochondral junctions
- Delayed dentition
- Bowing of legs in weight-bearing children
- Tetany: usually adolescents.

Q2. What investigations would you undertake?

Biochemistry
- Alkaline phosphatase: high
- PTH: high
- Calcium: low or normal
- Phosphate: low or normal
- Vitamin D: low.

X-rays
These show widening of the growth spaces between metaphyses and ossification centres, with cupping and splaying of the metaphyses (Fig. 35.7).

Q3. How would you treat Prika?

- Give oral vitamin D supplementation (ergocalciferol or cholecalciferol).
- Calcium supplements may also be required if there is hypocalcaemia.

Hypercalcaemia

This is much less common than hypocalcaemia.

Causes
- Iatrogenic: hypervitaminosis D
- Williams' syndrome:
  - 'Elfin' features
  - Supravalvular aortic stenosis
- Hyperparathyroidism.

Hypoglycaemia

Hypoglycaemia (blood glucose below 2.6 mmol/l) occurs when glucose uptake exceeds supply. Especially in the neonatal period, this can cause seizures and severe neurodevelopmental or cognitive defects if it is persistent and profound. Hypoglycaemia can be the presenting feature of hypopituitarism, and therefore it is vital that it is fully investigated before it is corrected.

Causes
(Hypoglycaemia in diabetes is discussed in the next section.)
- *Hyperinsulinism*: Persisting Hyperinsulinism of Infancy (PHI), (previously known as nesidio-blastosis), Beckwith–Wiedemann syndrome (p. 388), insulinoma (very rare)
- *Hormone deficiency*: isolated or combined growth hormone/ACTH/cortisol
- *Metabolic conditions*: e.g. glycogen storage diseases, fatty acid oxidation defects (Ch. 94)
- *Miscellaneous*: aspirin, liver failure, Reye's syndrome.

Investigations
Hypoglycaemia must be confirmed with a laboratory glucose level and the following blood tests taken before any glucose is given:
- Lactate
- Ammonia
- Insulin/C-peptide
- Growth hormone
- Cortisol
- Free fatty acids
- Beta-hydroxybutyrate/aceto-acetate
- Organic acids
- Acyl-carnitine.

Insulin should be undetectable in the presence of hypoglycaemia, and if measurable, confirms hyperinsulinism. Medical (diazoxide) or surgical (pancreatectomy) treatment may be required. Deficiency of GH or cortisol calls for replacement of these hormones. Metabolic and hepatic causes of hypoglycaemia are discussed in Chapter 34.

Diabetes mellitus
Definition

Diabetes mellitus is a chronic disorder caused by an absolute or relative deficiency of insulin that is characterized by hyperglycaemia.

Basic science
Pathophysiology

Insulin is an anabolic hormone that has a central role in the metabolism of carbohydrate, fat and protein. It is produced in the pancreas by the beta cells of the islets of Langerhans. It reduces blood glucose levels by stimulating the conversion of glucose to glycogen and enabling glucose to enter cells. It also inhibits the breakdown of glycogen, protein and fat.

The symptoms of diabetes mellitus at presentation depend upon the degree of metabolic decompensation and are generally secondary to hyperglycaemia, glycosuria and ketoacidosis. Hyperglycaemia leads to glycosuria and an osmotic diuresis. This in turn causes polyuria (often worse at night and can therefore cause enuresis in a previously continent child), increased thirst and dehydration. Other symptoms at presentation include non-specific malaise and weight loss. The latter is due to the uninhibited breakdown of fat and protein that occurs in the absence of sufficient circulating levels of insulin. Uninhibited breakdown of fat leads to the generation of ketones. At high levels these cause nausea and vomiting that can further exacerbate the dehydration, leading to shock. This is the phenomenon of diabetic ketoacidosis (DKA), which is discussed in more detail later. Other clinical signs in DKA include an abnormal pattern of breathing due to the acidosis (Kussmaul breathing) and abdominal pain that can mimic an acute surgical abdomen.

Classification and aetiology of diabetes mellitus
Type 1

Most diabetes developing in childhood is classified as type 1 diabetes, a term that encompasses cases of diabetes that are due to the destruction of pancreatic beta cells (usually leading to absolute insulin deficiency):

- Beta cell destruction is almost always caused by an environmental trigger in a genetically susceptible person.
- HLA DR3 and DR4 are associated with type 1 diabetes.
- Monozygotic twins have up to a 60% lifetime concordance for the development of type 1 diabetes.
- Viral infections (Coxsackie B, rubella) may be the most important environmental trigger, probably initiating or modifying an autoimmune process.
- Autoantibodies such as islet cell, glutamic acid decarboxylase (GAD) and insulin antibodies, are often positive at the time of presentation.
- Dietary factors are also relevant. The consumption of cow's milk per capita correlates well with the incidence of type 1 diabetes in a region.

There is a wide geographical variation in the incidence and prevalence of type 1 diabetes. The National Paediatric Diabetes Audit, using data from 2002, showed:

- Prevalence in UK (excluding Scotland) of 1.65 per 1000 children aged 0–16 years.
- Incidence in England and Wales of 14.9 per 100 000 children aged 0–16 years.

Type 2

Type 2 diabetes mellitus is a heterogeneous condition characterized by variable degrees of insulin resistance and beta cell secretory failure. Although it is predominantly a condition of the over-40 age group, it has now been described in children, and the increasing prevalence of obesity in children and adolescents means that it is becoming more common.

Common characteristics
- Overweight
- Strong family history of type 2 diabetes
- Female preponderance
- Asian or Arabic origin (although has been reported in white children).

Management
Management of type 2 diabetes involves the stepwise introduction of dietary intervention with exercise promotion, oral hypoglycaemic agents and, if necessary, insulin therapy.

Maturity-onset diabetes of the young (MODY)

- Autosomal dominant inheritance
- Strong family history of early-onset diabetes (< 25 years)

- Rare (only 1–2% of cases of diabetes mellitus in childhood)
- Mild presentation.

A number of specific genetic defects in beta cell function have been identified that explain most cases of MODY. One important reason for making the diagnosis is that some forms of MODY will not require treatment with insulin.

Other types of diabetes mellitus

Diseases of the exocrine pancreas
- Cystic fibrosis
- Pancreatectomy, e.g. for PHI (p. 117)
- Pancreatitis
- Trauma
- Haemochromatosis.

Genetic syndromes associated with diabetes
- Turner's syndrome
- Bardet–Biedl syndrome
- Prader–Willi syndrome
- Wolfram's syndrome — *d*iabetes *i*nsipidus, *d*iabetes *m*ellitus, *o*ptic *a*trophy, *d*eafness (DIDMOAD).

Problem-orientated topic:

diabetes mellitus

Thomas, a 4-year-old boy, is referred urgently to the accident and emergency department by his GP with a provisional diagnosis of diabetes mellitus. He has a 2-week history of weight loss and polyuria. The GP had tested the boy's urine and found it to contain large amounts of glucose and a small amount of ketones.

Q1. How do you establish whether this child has diabetes mellitus?

Q2. What are the principles of management?

Q1. How do you establish whether this child has diabetes mellitus?

The World Health Organization (WHO) diagnostic criteria for diabetes mellitus are:

- Fasting plasma glucose ≥ 7.0 mmol/l (whole blood glucose ≥ 6.1 mmol/l)
  or
- A plasma glucose level taken 2 hours following an oral glucose tolerance test (oGTT) ≥ 11.1 mmol/l.

BOX 35.12 Members of the diabetes team

- Paediatrician
- Children's diabetes nurse specialist
- Specialist dietician
- Psychologist or psychiatrist
- Social worker

The diagnosis of type 1 diabetes in children is usually straightforward and made on the basis of:

- A typical history of polyuria, polydipsia, weight loss
- Hyperglycaemia
- Marked glycosuria
- Ketonuria.

A single blood glucose measurement in excess of 11 mmol/l establishes the diagnosis in such cases. An oGTT is not often required in childhood.

Once the diagnosis of diabetes mellitus has been made, care and education of the child and family by a specialist multidisciplinary team must begin immediately.

Q2. What are the principles of management?

The long-term successful management of a child and the family with diabetes depends on effective team work (Box 35.12).

The majority of children who present with diabetes mellitus are not acutely unwell and much of the initial management of diabetes mellitus can be outpatient-based. Many teams do not routinely admit children to hospital to initiate insulin therapy unless they are unwell. It is essential to have a clear understanding of the principles underpinning the management of diabetes mellitus and the skills required.

Principles and practice of insulin therapy

Starting treatment

The first subcutaneous injection can have tremendous significance for children and their families. It should be taught or administered by someone experienced and confident with injections. A dose of 0.5–0.7 units of insulin per kilogram body weight per day is usually required but will be tailored to individual needs. Insulin injection sites must be varied because repeated injections into the same site can cause lipohypertrophy; as well as being unsightly, this can lead to poor glycaemic control, as absorption from such sites is unpredictable.

Remission ('honeymoon') phase

Type 1 diabetes presents with symptoms when approximately 90% of the beta cells have been destroyed. This means that most children will still have some functioning beta cell mass for a period after the time of diagnosis. This is reflected in the low insulin requirements from a short time after diagnosis and during the remission phase. This phase usually lasts only a few months but can last for over a year.

Insulin types

Basic science

Insulin is a protein consisting of two peptide chains linked by two disulphide bonds. It cannot be absorbed intact (in its bioactive form) from the gastrointestinal tract and therefore at present is only routinely administered via subcutaneous injection. However, this suboptimal simulation of physiology results in many of the difficulties and complications of diabetes.

Until recently, most prescribed insulin was human insulin produced by recombinant technology. Pure insulin is short-acting and appears clear in solution. Various additives prolong the release of insulin into the blood stream (e.g. NPH-lente) and produce intermediate or long-acting insulins that have a cloudy appearance. However, in the last few years, a number of so-called insulin analogues have become available. These are modified forms of human insulin that have a more favourable profile than the traditionally used insulins. Now both rapid-acting and long-acting (or basal) insulin analogues are widely used in paediatric practice.

An inhaled insulin preparation has recently been licensed in the UK, but at present is not recommended treatment.

Insulin regimens

Traditionally children have most commonly been managed on twice-daily injections of mixtures of short- and intermediate-acting insulins (e.g. 30% short-acting and 70% intermediate-acting): one before breakfast and one before the evening meal. Typically around two-thirds of the total daily dose is given as the morning dose. Glycaemic control, however, is often limited by disabling hypoglycaemia. There are three main problems with this regimen:

1. Control of postprandial hyperglycaemia is difficult without a short-acting insulin bolus at lunchtime.
2. 'The dawn phenomenon' — the profile of the intermediate-acting component of the evening insulin results in a decline in insulin levels in the early hours before breakfast, leading to

(a)

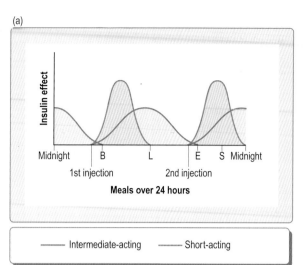

(b)

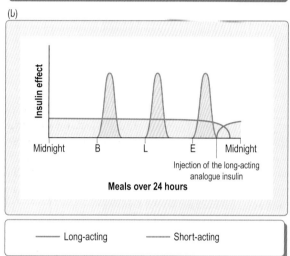

Fig. 35.8 Insulin action.
(a) Insulin effect of traditional regimen of twice-daily mixed short- and intermediate-acting insulin; (b) Insulin effect of multiple daily injection regimen of once-daily long-acting analogue insulin with rapid-acting insulin given at mealtimes. (B = breakfast; L = lunch; E = evening meal; S = supper)

hyperglycaemia that is exacerbated (particularly in adolescents) by the coincident surge in hormones that oppose the effects of insulin.

3. A snack is usually necessary to avoid hypoglycaemia mid-morning due to the profile of the intermediate-acting insulin.

Multiple daily injection (MDI) regimens using insulin analogues can overcome some of the above problems and this has led to their increasingly widespread adoption in paediatric practice. Such regimens usually consist of the administration of a dose of a long-acting insulin analogue once daily (usually at night) and doses of a rapid-acting insulin analogue to cover mealtimes (Fig. 35.8). The required dose of mealtime insulin depends on the carbohydrate content of a meal and the individual's sensitivity to insulin. Dose adequacy (and also sensitivity to insulin) can be judged by checking

blood glucose levels before and between 2 and 4 hours after a meal whose carbohydrate content is known.

Continuous subcutaneous infusion of rapid-acting insulin ('the insulin pump') is becoming increasingly used in paediatric practice but should only be initiated by a trained specialist team. It offers the ability to achieve a much more physiological profile of insulin delivery. According to the National Institute of Clinical Excellence (NICE), it is recommended as an option for people with type 1 diabetes provided that:

• MDI therapy has failed — meaning when it has been impossible to maintain an HbA_{1c} level at less than 7.5% without disabling hypoglycaemia, despite a high level of self-care
• Those receiving the treatment have the commitment and competence to use the therapy effectively.

http://www.nice.org.uk

Patient and parent education

An understanding of insulin therapy is crucial to the management of diabetes mellitus. But in order to maintain good glycaemic control without problematic hypoglycaemia, children and their families must understand the effect of diet and exercise and be able to monitor blood glucose levels.

Diet

The emphasis is on 'healthy eating'. Any diet should provide sufficient energy and nutrients to allow optimal growth and development (Box 35.13):

• Total energy intake depends on the individual's particular needs.
• Appropriate snacks, such as those before bedtime, are to be encouraged.
• The dose of insulin should be adjusted according to the food being consumed.
• The increased use of MDI regimens means that some individuals must learn how to estimate the carbohydrate content of their meals.

Exercise

Children with diabetes should be encouraged to undertake regular exercise and understand how to adjust diet and insulin in order to maintain good glycaemic control both during and after different types of exercise. In particular, children should be aware that exercise can lead to hypoglycaemia, sometimes several hours after the exercise, and that they will require extra carbohydrate before and after a bout of intensive exercise. They also should be encouraged to monitor their blood glucose levels before and after exercise.

Education

The amount of explanation required at diagnosis will vary according to the circumstances of the admission and the family involved. Prior to discharge there are several areas that ought to be covered in discussion with the family:
- Pathophysiology, including explanation of symptoms
- Lifelong need for insulin
- Methods of insulin administration
- Hypoglycaemia: how to identify and treat
- Importance of good control
- Details of support groups (e.g. Diabetes UK).

Education of the child and family is an ongoing process involving all members of the multidisciplinary team. Education should also be offered to other carers, such as teachers. It is particularly important that these people be able to recognize and manage hypoglycaemia.

 http://www.diabetes.org.uk

Blood glucose monitoring

Monitoring of blood glucose levels at home with hand-held meters allows short-term monitoring of glycaemic control and is associated with reduced levels of HbA_{1c}. HbA_{1c} is a derivative of glycosylated haemoglobin. It correlates well with average glucose concentrations over the preceding 8–10 weeks and thereby provides an important measure of glycaemic control. The Diabetes Control and Complications Trial (1993) clearly showed a direct correlation between HbA_{1c} and long-term complications. The aim of treatment is to achieve an HbA_{1c} of less than 7.5% but this is often difficult to achieve, especially because of fear of hypoglycaemia. HbA_{1c} should be checked every 3–6 months. Optimal targets for short-term glycaemic control are a preprandial blood glucose level of 4–8 mmol/l and a postprandial blood glucose level of no more than 10 mmol/l.

Hypoglycaemia

Hypoglycaemia is commonly due to inadequate carbohydrate, too much insulin or physical activity. It is a particular concern in preschool children because repeated episodes of hypoglycaemia may lead to intellectual impairment.

For diabetes control hypoglycaemia is generally defined as blood glucose below 4 mmol/l. Symptoms depend on the absolute blood glucose value, the rate of fall of glucose levels and the background glycaemic control. Early (autonomic) symptoms include:
- Hunger
- Feeling shaky
- Sweating
- Pallor.

If these are ignored, then more profound symptoms of neuroglycopenia may develop, including:
- Disorientation
- Aggression
- Difficulty with speech
- Poor concentration
- Changes in vision
- Loss of consciousness.

At clinic visits it is important to enquire about hypoglycaemia unawareness, i.e. the onset of neuroglycopenic symptoms without the warning of autonomic symptoms.

Children should be encouraged always to have access to an immediate source of carbohydrate (glucose or sucrose) and to wear some form of medical identification.

Symptomatic proven hypoglycaemia should always be treated immediately. Parents should know how and when to administer oral glucose gel or glucagon. Choice of treatment depends on the affected child's compliance and level of consciousness.

In hospital, intravenous treatment with 5 ml/kg 10% dextrose is usually sufficient to correct hypoglycaemia. There is no place for high-concentration glucose solutions.

Illness and hyperglycaemia

During periods of illness it is essential that insulin therapy is not interrupted and that blood glucose is checked frequently. Urine or blood should be regularly tested for ketones. The child should be encouraged to drink, and if food cannot be tolerated, then it should be replaced by small amounts of sugar-containing fluids. If the child is vomiting, develops ketones or otherwise deteriorates, then the family should seek medical help.

Long-term complications

Long-term complications such as nephropathy and retinopathy arise as a result of chronic hyperglycaemia.

At every clinic visit

- Height and weight
- HbA_{1c}
- Check injection sites

Once a year

- Check for retinopathy, microalbuminuria and blood pressure from 12 years
- Screen for thyroid disease
- Review foot care

Every 3 years

- Screen for coeliac disease

Their incidence is related to the duration of diabetes and the level of glycaemic control. Such complications are rare in childhood, but a young adult who was diagnosed in childhood will have already been exposed to the effects of hyperglycaemia for long enough to develop complications. There is therefore a particular onus on the paediatric diabetes team to enable the family to achieve sustained good control of their child's diabetes. Screening for complications should begin in adolescence.

Clinics and screening

Clinic visits are a convenient vehicle for the diabetes team to be able to review a child's insulin therapy, blood glucose control and diet. They also allow regular screening for complications and associations of diabetes mellitus to take place.

Finally, the annual review is an opportunity to consider aims and objectives for the 12 months ahead (Box 35.14).

Immunizations

The Department of Health recommends immunization against influenza for children over the age of 6 months.

Problem-orientated topic:

diabetic ketoacidosis

Donna, a 15-year-old girl, presents to the accident and emergency department with a history of abdominal pain and vomiting. She has a reduced level of consciousness and her breathing is laboured. Her capillary blood sugar is 35 mmol/l and blood gas analysis shows: pH 7.09, base excess −17 mmol/l. This is the third time that she has presented to hospital in a similar way over the last 12 months.

Q1. What is the diagnosis?

Q2. How would you approach Donna's management?

Q3. Why do you think this has happened?

Q4. What are the complications of this condition?

Q1. What is the diagnosis?

This is a typical picture of DKA and is caused by insufficient circulating insulin associated with increases in counter-regulatory hormones. It has been reported to be present at diagnosis in 15–67% of new cases. The risk in established cases of type 1 diabetes is 1–10% per patient per year.

Q2. How would you approach Donna's management?

The British Society for Paediatric Endocrinology and Diabetes (BSPED) has produced detailed guidelines for the management of DKA. Any prospective MRCPCH candidate should be familiar with these and have some practical experience of managing DKA. Therefore only the basic principles that underpin the management of DKA and the potential pitfalls have been highlighted.

Initial management consists of assessing and providing support to the airway, breathing and circulation. A nasogastric tube should be used to decompress the stomach and reduce the risk of aspiration. Administer 100% oxygen and place the patient on a cardiac monitor. If the child is shocked, restore circulating volume with normal saline then rehydrate slowly over 48 hours. Start an intravenous infusion of short- or rapid-acting insulin to switch off ketogenesis and aim to achieve normoglycaemia gradually.

 http://www.bsped.org.uk

Q3. Why do you think this has happened?

Major reasons for recurrent DKA are insulin omission and acute illness. Education and other steps such as adult supervision of insulin administration have been shown to help prevent DKA.

Q4. What are the complications of this condition?

DKA has reported mortality rates of 0.15–0.31%. Be aware that some of the risks of DKA are associated with the period of stabilization when treatment has already begun. Although serum potassium levels are often high at presentation, they will fall once insulin has been started and this must be taken into consideration during the prescription of fluids and electrolytes as the consequent hypokalaemia may result in dangerous cardiac dysrhythmias. Hypoglycaemia can occur if the rate of insulin infusion is not reduced or glucose is not added to the intravenous fluids in a timely fashion. Cerebral oedema (which accounts for 57–87% of all DKA deaths) may develop as a result of rapid fluid replacement with hypotonic fluids but can occur even before the initiation of any treatment. Therefore, once the patient is no longer in shock, it is important that fluid and electrolyte replacement is not carried out in haste.

Monitoring to prevent further episodes of DKA

One of the key messages about the management of DKA is the importance of monitoring and frequent review:

- Frequent blood gases and electrolytes
- Cardiac monitoring
- Regular assessment of the Glasgow Coma Score
- Prompt reporting of any symptoms or signs that might indicate cerebral oedema.

Social and psychological aspects of diabetes

Type 1 diabetes is a lifelong condition. The implications of the diagnosis affect the entire family, as well as the child or young person. Anxiety, depression and eating disorders are well described in children and young people with diabetes. Good psychosocial support is vital if young people are to comply with treatment and maintain high self-esteem. In particular specific support strategies should be offered that reduce conflict within the family. In some cases child mental health teams may need to be involved. It is important to remember that a child's level of understanding changes with time and the condition and treatment must be explained regularly in terms that are age-appropriate.

Adolescence

During puberty, changes in GH and sex steroid secretion can increase insulin requirements and make good glycaemic control more difficult to achieve. However, a major cause of poor glycaemic control in adolescence is poor compliance. Young people must be clearly but sensitively informed of the dangers of administering inadequate amounts of insulin, as the relationship between an individual and the diabetes team must not break down.

Adolescents should be warned of the specific effects of alcohol on glycaemic control, in particular the risk of nocturnal hypoglycaemia. They should be discouraged from cigarette smoking and be warned of the health problems associated with it, especially the risks of developing vascular complications. They should also receive education about sexual health and pregnancy planning.

Disability Living Allowance

Families may apply for the Disability Living Allowance, in particular the care component.

Driving

The Driver and Vehicle Licensing Agency (DVLA) must be informed of the diagnosis of diabetes. If the individual is considered safe to drive (well-controlled without frequent, unexpected hypoglycaemic episodes), a licence can be issued, but only for a limited period at a time.

Employment

Diabetes UK regularly publishes an up-to-date guide ('Employment and Diabetes') about the restrictions to employment faced by individuals with diabetes.

Richard B. Warren   Julian L. Verbov

Skin disorders in children

LEARNING OUTCOMES

By the end of this chapter you should:

- Be able to make an initial assessment of a child with a skin complaint
- Be able to describe skin lesions using the appropriate nomenclature
- Be able to recognize a number of common disorders of the skin
- Be able to construct a reasonable differential diagnosis
- Be able to implement a management plan.

Introduction

In this chapter we will discuss commonly encountered conditions based on the very common symptom of itching, and will consider a chronic eruption. Important disorders not covered in this format will also be briefly discussed.

Basic science

A basic understanding of skin anatomy is desirable and is best understood from a cross-section (Fig. 36.1). The skin is the largest organ in the body and has a mean thickness of 2 mm, of which the outermost portion, the epidermis, is 0.2 mm thick and the dermis is 1.8 mm thick. The epidermis is mainly cellular whereas the dermis is vascular and contains collagen and elastic tissue, glands (sweat and sebaceous) and hair follicles. Beneath the skin lies the subcutaneous fat. Basic cells within the skin include keratinocytes (responsible for skin reproduction), melanocytes (for pigment production), Langerhans' cells (with an immunological function) and numerous adnexal structures such as sweat and sebaceous glands. The epidermis originates from the ectoderm whereas the dermis originates from the mesoderm. Melanocytes originate from the neural crest. Fetal skin development occurs mainly between 4 and 6 months of gestation.

The skin has a number of basic functions (Box 36.1). It is important to appreciate the special needs of the preterm infant, who has high transepidermal fluid loss because the skin is very thin and poorly keratinized and lacks subcutaneous fat. This has clear implications for both fluid balance and temperature control (p. 327). Absorption of noxious substances across the skin is also possible in the preterm infant. To some extent this situation is replicated in diseased skin if there is epidermal loss.

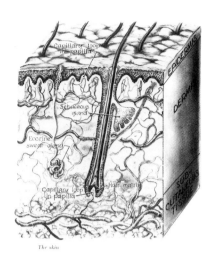

Fig. 36.1 **Normal skin.**
Diagrammatic cross-section.

Description of terminology

See Box 36.2.

Itching

Problem-orientated topic:

itching

Tom, a 1-year-old boy, attends clinic with a 12-week history of an increasingly itchy rash. The rash, which began over the face, is spreading over much of his body, including the antecubital and popliteal fossae, and is described by the GP as weeping around the neckline. He has been given 1% hydrocortisone cream by his GP with little effect. Tom has an older sister who has had mild itching over her arms.

Q1. What is your differential diagnosis of a child with pruritus?

Q2. What further history would you like to know?

Continued overleaf

BOX 36.1 Basic skin functions

- Protective barrier
- Temperature regulation and fluid regulation
- Immunological function

BOX 36.2 Glossary of basic dermatological terms

Macule	Indicates a change in colour of skin, either localized or widespread, e.g. freckles or measles
Papule	A circumscribed solid raised lesion less than 0.5 cm in diameter, e.g. molluscum contagiosum
Pustule	An elevated fluid-containing lesion, the fluid being pus, e.g. impetigo
Vesicle	An elevated fluid-containing lesion less than 0.5 cm in diameter, e.g. varicella
Bulla	An elevated fluid-containing lesion greater than 0.5 cm in diameter, e.g. epidermolysis bullosa
Weal	A localized area of dermal oedema, e.g. urticaria
Plaque	A well-defined elevated area of skin that may or may not show scaling, e.g. psoriasis
Purpura	Bleeding into the skin or a mucosal surface. Small areas of purpura are termed petechiae and larger areas ecchymoses, e.g. Henoch–Schönlein purpura
Naevus	A localized malformation of tissue structures, e.g. moles (pigmented naevi)
Erythema	Redness
Annular	Ring-shaped
Atrophy	Tissue loss that may affect all levels of skin and subcutaneous fat
Dermatitis/eczema	In general the terms can be considered synonymous — an inflammatory condition of the skin characterized by papules and vesicles on an erythematous (red) base. Because of the irritation, excoriations and secondary infection (impetiginization) are common
Lichenification	A peculiar skin change with accentuated markings, usually as a consequence of prolonged rubbing of the skin in localized areas of atopic eczema
Pruritus	Itching
Excoriation	Loss of the epidermal surface (partial or complete) due to scratching, e.g. in eczema
Ulcer	A break in the continuity of the skin that can involve loss of the whole thickness of the epidermis and upper dermis
Fissure	A small narrow ulcer, e.g. in the perianal region

Q3. On examining the child, what features may help you to decide on appropriate investigations?

Q4. What is the most likely diagnosis in this child?

Q1. What is your differential diagnosis of a child with pruritus?

See Box 36.3.

Q2. What further history would you like to know?

Commonly in a child with a rash the details are sparse with little history. It is, however, very important that due attention is applied to the history, as in any other medical case. A basic knowledge of descriptive terms for skin disorders is essential (Box 36.2). In this particular instance the differential diagnosis includes both inflammatory and infective conditions.

Distribution

Focusing on the distribution of the rash can be extremely helpful. Atopic dermatitis commonly affects the face or scalp initially (Fig. 36.2). Common eruptions, such as atopic dermatitis and psoriasis, are classically distributed on the flexor and extensor surface of the limbs respectively (Figs 36.3 and 36.4). Particular focus on the palms and soles may reveal scabietic burrows that can easily be missed and confused with eczema, as the itching invoked by the mite may cause eczema (and often bacterial infection) as secondary phenomena.

Duration

Duration of the rash may prove helpful; if the rash clears quickly within hours to days, this may for example suggest a diagnosis of urticaria. In addition, pityriasis

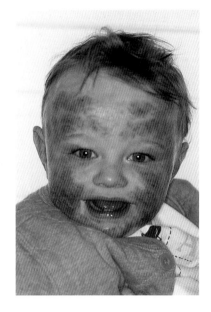

Fig. 36.2 Atopic dermatitis.
A 1-year-old boy with severe facial eczema. With treatment other affected body areas cleared rapidly but his face was slow to respond.

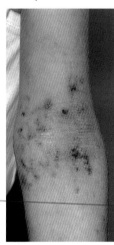

Fig. 36.3 Atopic dermatitis.
Left cubital fossa showing excoriated and infected eczema. Lichenification is also visible in this 5-year-old boy.

BOX 36.3 Differential diagnosis of pruritus

- Eczema/dermatitis
- Psoriasis (p. 127)
- Scabies
- Varicella
- Head lice infestation
- Fungal infection
- Pityriasis rosea
- Urticaria
- Papular urticaria
- Urticaria pigmentosa
- Drug eruption

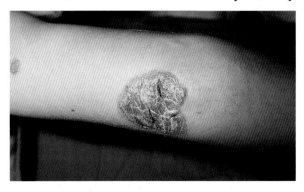

Fig. 36.4 Psoriasis.
Typical well-defined plaque over elbow.

rosea can be diagnosed from the history, as there may have been an initial lesion, known as the herald patch, prior to the evolution of a more widespread rash.

Family history/contacts

Scabies, lice infestation and fungal infection may all be spread by contact; others in close contact who itch should be actively sought. The genetics of atopic eczema and psoriasis is complex, but this clearly plays a role and a knowledge of family history is essential. In this case we have details of another family member being itchy; examination of the second case would therefore be useful and desirable.

Systemic upset

In this history the neck has been described as weeping. An early sign of skin infection may be 'breaks' in the skin surface with weeping from the lesion. The child's general well-being should be established. If there is systemic upset a parenteral antibiotic may be indicated. In addition, rare conditions such as urticaria pigmentosa (a form of mast cell disorder) may be associated with systemic symptoms such as flushing or wheezing.

Compliance/understanding

Two of the major reasons for failure of therapy in eczema or psoriasis are lack of understanding of how and when to apply topical therapy, and fear of the consequences of topical steroids. It is extremely important that support is offered to parents and children, with initial practical supervision being invaluable.

Q3. On examining the child, what features may help you to decide on appropriate investigations?

Investigations will be guided by the appearance and history of the eruption but the following should be considered.

In the case of atopy, IgE level is often elevated. As patients with dermatitis are susceptible to infection, they may also have a neutrophilia.

Skin scrapings can be sent for mycological examination for confirmation of a ringworm fungal infection. If scalp ringworm is suspected, plucked scalp hairs can be sent for mycological analysis. Scraping of a scabietic burrow can isolate the mite *Sarcoptes scabiei* var. *hominis*, larvae, empty egg cases or faecal material.

In most cases in children, skin biopsy can be avoided with an accurate history and examination. This investigation is usually reserved for, and is more appropriate to the diagnosis of puzzling lesions.

Allergy testing can take several forms (Ch. 44) but is usually neither indicated nor useful in young children with atopic eczema. If a child appears to be reacting to a topical product, then patch-testing may be useful. This, however, is more often useful in adults. If the history has revealed urticaria/angioedema, then radioallergosorbent testing (RAST) against a diverse range of dietary products is available in some laboratories. These tests are of low specificity, however, and their role can be overstated. Anxious parents will express a desire for 'allergy' testing, believing that this holds the answers to their child's problems; it is very important to explain that there is little evidence for a role of dietary allergy in the pathogenesis of most dermatological conditions. However, negative skin prick tests or RAST for food and environment allergens may sometimes be useful in older children with atopic dermatitis.

Q4. What is the most likely diagnosis in this child?

The vignette suggests that atopic dermatitis is the cause of the itching in this particular child. Atopy refers to an inherited tendency to develop one of several related conditions (asthma, eczema of atopic type, allergic rhinitis and urticaria of allergic type) but it is also subject to environmental influence. It is a very common condition affecting up to 20% of children; in most cases onset is in the first year of life, but its severity varies widely. The skin is usually dry in atopic eczema. This condition, like asthma, has shown an increased incidence with no clear indication of why this should be. In this child there may have been fear over the use of topical steroids by his GP, which allowed the condition to flare. In some instances a stronger steroid is required for a short time to regain control.

Management of atopic eczema is shown in Box 36.4.

Chronic eruptions

Problem-orientated topic:

chronic eruptions

An 11-year-old boy, Martin, is referred from his GP with a persistent rash consisting of discrete small reddish lesions with scaling over much of the trunk. A week or two before the onset of the eruption he had a sore throat. The eruption has been

Continued overleaf

BOX 36.4 Management of atopic eczema

Education
- Although not a curable condition, it can be managed well and tends to be self-limiting
- 50% of children with eczema will clear by the age of 12 years

Emollients
- Liberal and regular use is essential
- Wet wraps are sometimes useful in the short term

Steroid preparations
- Mildly potent, e.g. hydrocortisone (may be used on the face)
- Moderately potent, e.g. clobetasone
- Potent, e.g. mometasone (short-term use, avoid the face)
- Education on when and where to apply each type of steroid preparation

Topical immunomodulators
- Examples are pimecrolimus and tacrolimus
- Novel mechanism of action
- No skin atrophy
- Maintenance therapy if steroid use is excessive and potentially damaging
- For longer-term use more data are needed

Antibiotics
- Topical or parenteral
- Fears of resistant *Staphylococcus aureus* due to over-prescribing

Oral antihistamines
- Chlorpheniramine maleate
- Hydroxyzine hydrochloride (also has anti-anxiety action)
- Alimemazine tartrate at night can be useful

Oral steroids
- Very occasional use for severe flares may be indicated

Ultraviolet light
- May have a place

treated with emollients but is unresponsive. It has now been present for over 3 months. All other family members are fit and well. Martin was treated for congenital hip dislocation in infancy, but otherwise is fit and well.

Q1. What is your differential diagnosis in this child?

Q2. What is the basic abnormality in the skin in psoriasis?

Q3. How would you manage this patient?

Q1. What is your differential diagnosis in this child?

Psoriasis seems the most likely diagnosis here. Psoriasis usually presents at a later age than eczema, with onset before the age of 2 years being rare. It is subject to exacerbations and remissions. The genetic links with this condition are stronger than with atopic eczema, and it is now clear that psoriasis is an immunologically driven disorder. This condition is not usually as pruritic as eczema. The plaque type of psoriasis typically affects bony prominences but in children guttate (raindrop-like) lesions (Fig. 36.5) often follow a streptococcal or viral ear or throat infection. In both types the lesions show overlying silvery scales. In active psoriasis the Köbner phenomenon may be found, with lesions occurring at the sites of trauma. Nail changes such as pitting and separation of the free end of the nail from the nail bed (onycholysis) may also be seen. Psoriatic arthritis is uncommon in children.

Other chronic eruptions include eczema, of which there are many types, although in children atopic eczema is the most common. Eczema can be excluded by assessing the morphology of the rash, as can chronic

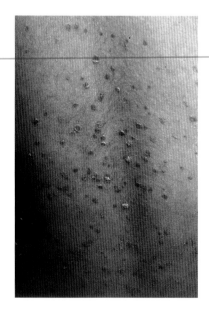

Fig. 36.5 Psoriasis.
A 5½-year-old boy with guttate psoriasis over the back. An attack of guttate psoriasis often follows a streptococcal tonsillitis or other infection.

urticaria. In some instances of chronic eruption a skin biopsy may be required: for example, in suspected urticaria pigmentosa.

Q2. What is the basic abnormality of the skin in psoriasis?

Examination of a psoriatic plaque allows a basic understanding of the abnormalities that occur in psoriasis. There is increased thickness of the outer layer of the skin (the epidermis), resulting in a raised scaly surface. In addition gentle removal of superficial scale will often reveal visible pinpoint capillary bleeding (the Auspitz sign). Historically psoriasis was thought to be due to an abnormality in keratinocytes (the reproductive cell in the skin), with division of these cells being too rapid and not allowing adequate differentiation of the skin. It is now clear that psoriasis is a T cell-mediated condition, with the increased epidermal turnover being immunologically driven. In many ways it is analogous to other autoimmune diseases in which antibodies are interacting with a self-antigen leading to inflammation, the end result in this case being over-activity of the keratinocyte. What is not clear in psoriasis is what may be acting as the antigen.

Q3. How would you manage this patient?

See Box 36.5.

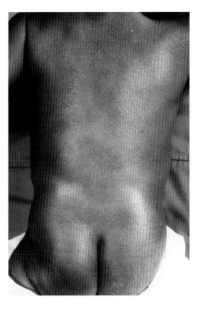

Fig. 36.6 Mongolian patches.
Nigerian infant with macular black patches over trunk.

Specific skin disorders

Brief notes

Mongolian patches (Fig. 36.6)

These lesions are congenital macular slate-grey or black patches; they are generally found over the lumbosacral areas and buttocks but can occur anywhere. Most black and oriental babies show them but they are present in less than 10% of white Caucasians. They usually disappear by the end of the first decade. It is important to distinguish them from bruises.

Capillary haemangioma (strawberry naevus) (Fig. 36.7)

Capillary haemangiomas are common vascular naevi that may present at birth or in the first month of life. They appear as well-defined small areas that grow to become raised red lobulated tumours, with capillaries sometimes visible over the surface. They grow rapidly with the child in the first 8–18 months of life and then become static, involuting over the next 5–8 years.

Port-wine stain (naevus flammeus)

This is a vascular malformation present at birth. Port-wine stains do not involute but some may fade in colour with time. An association of facial port-wine stain with congenital glaucoma should be appreciated, as the glaucoma is usually asymptomatic early in life. Port-wine stains involving the supraorbital region are particularly likely to be associated with similar lesions

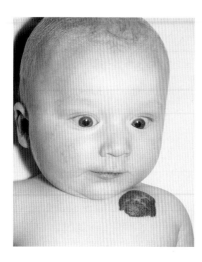

Fig. 36.7 Capillary haemangioma (strawberry mark).
Strawberry mark over left clavicular region.

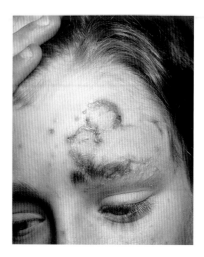

Fig. 36.8 Impetigo.
Close-up of crusted forehead lesions.

involving the meninges on the same side, constituting the Sturge–Weber syndrome (p. 10). Manifestations of the latter include epilepsy and hemiplegia.

Pigmented naevi (moles)

These benign lesions are common and it is normal for them to grow as the child grows. It is change in shape and colour, or in size other than with growth of the child, that should raise the possibility of malignant melanoma. However, malignant melanoma is rare in children under 14 years of age.

Infantile seborrhoeic dermatitis

Classically this self-limiting condition involves the napkin area, axillae and scalp, with erythema, maceration and scaling often confluent in the skin folds. A yellowish, greasy scalp (cradle cap) may be the only sign in some infants. Candida infection may sometimes complicate this eruption in the napkin area. It typically occurs in the first 3–4 months of life.

Epidermolysis bullosa (EB)

EB indicates a group of inherited non-inflammatory disorders in which blisters and erosions occur with mechanical, often minor, trauma. There are both scarring and non-scarring types. Recessive forms tend to be much more severe.

Impetigo

 This is usually due to *Staph. aureus* but can be complicated by streptococci. It is very contagious and often associated with poor hygiene and

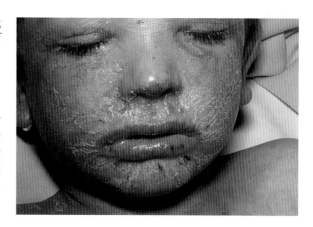

Fig. 36.9 Staphylococcal scalded skin syndrome.
Close-up of face of a 4½-year-old boy admitted as an emergency, unwell with a widespread scalded skin appearance and crusting around the mouth. Four days later, following flucloxacillin, he was fine.

overcrowding. In the infant it can often present in bullous form. In older children blisters occur but rapidly burst, dry and crust (Fig. 36.8).

Staphylococcal scalded skin syndrome

This is due to a staphylococcal exotoxin and usually occurs in the under-5 year age group. The scald-like appearance often involves much of the skin but not the mucosal surfaces. Crusting around the mouth is typical (Fig. 36.9). The condition is often preceded by a purulent conjunctivitis, otitis media or upper respiratory infection. Another family member, such as a sibling, may have ordinary impetigo. Treatment is with a penicillinase-resistant penicillin, fusidic acid, erythromycin or appropriate cephalosporin, with recovery in 5–7 days without scarring.

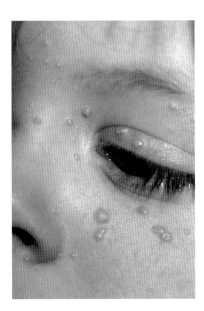

Fig. 36.10 **Molluscum contagiosum.**
Some of the pearly lesions show umbilication.

Cellulitis

Acute cellulitis (erysipelas) is due to group A haemolytic streptococci entering through a break in the skin, usually near the eye, ear, nostril or mouth. Treatment is with benzylpenicillin or oral phenoxymethylpenicillin (or erythromycin or other macrolide if child is penicillin-allergic). Low-grade cellulitis is more common and may be recurrent. Although usually due to haemolytic streptococcal infection, cellulitis can also be caused by other organisms such as *Staph. aureus* (which can be treated with phenoxymethylpenicillin (or benzylpenicillin) plus flucloxacillin), *Streptococcus pneumoniae* and *Haemophilus influenzae*. Before young children began to be immunized with conjugate *H. influenzae* type b vaccine, buccal cellulitis, due to *H. influenzae* type b, was responsible for up to 25% of cases of facial cellulitis in children of 3–24 months of age. Now such cellulitis is rare. Infection originated in the upper respiratory tract.

Perianal cellulitis

This occurs mainly in young children and is generally caused by group A streptococci. Manifestations include perianal pruritus and erythema, anal fissures, pus and rectal bleeding. Treatment is with oral phenoxymethylpenicillin. Child abuse may sometimes be suspected but can usually be excluded by history and clinical findings.

Molluscum contagiosum (Fig. 36.10)

This infection is caused by a poxvirus and typically there are small discrete pearly lesions with umbilication.

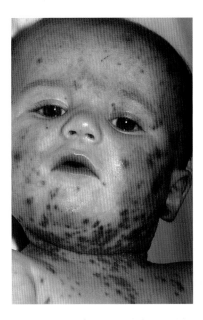

Fig. 36.11 **Eczema herpeticum.**
This 6-month-old infant with atopic eczema was admitted as an emergency. He was unwell with fever. He has primary herpes simplex with profuse lesions, some showing umbilication. He rapidly improved following administration of intravenous aciclovir.

It is most common in infants and younger children. It can be mildly itchy and may complicate atopic eczema, making treatment more difficult. Steroids used to suppress the eczema appear to encourage the lesions, so eczema treatment should be restricted to emollients or other non-steroidal applications if these conditions occur together. Molluscum contagiosum is self-limiting, but secondarily infected lesions require topical antiseptic/antibiotic treatment. Problem lesions can sometimes be treated with gentle cryotherapy with liquid nitrogen.

Viral warts

Viral warts, which are common in children, are caused by the human papillomavirus, of which there are many types. The virus is spread by direct contact from person to person. Generally warts are self-limiting in the immunocompetent child, but problem warts can be treated with a variety of topical treatments (e.g. salicylic acid-based preparations) and liquid nitrogen cryotherapy, which may speed up their resolution.

Eczema herpeticum

This acute, sometimes disseminated, herpes simplex infection appears most commonly against a background of atopic dermatitis (Fig. 36.11). Usually there will be a sudden decline in control of the child's eczema, with vesicles and oozing from the sites involved. Often the child will

131

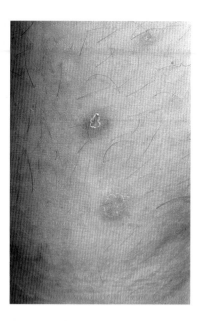

Fig. 36.12 **Pityriasis rosea.**
Close-up to show scaling lesions in the popliteal fossa.

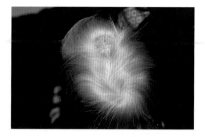

Fig. 36.13 **Scalp ringworm (tinea capitis).**
Kerion on scalp. The father had active ringworm over the neck.

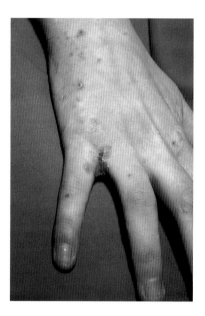

Fig. 36.14 **Scabies.**
Finger web involvement.

be systemically unwell. Treatment is usually with intravenous aciclovir and skin swabs should be taken to exclude the presence, of a secondary bacterial infection. In practice, systemic antibiotic treatment for secondary bacterial infection is often required. Topical steroids should be discontinued because their use may encourage spread of the virus.

Varicella

This eruption can be itchy at the outset and, as it evolves, the diagnosis will become clear from the typical erythematous vesicular rash. Varicella is most common in young children and systemic symptoms are mild. Secondary bacterial infection of the lesions is the most frequent complication of varicella, occurring in 5–10% of children. Healthy children rarely develop more serious side-effects such as pneumonitis, encephalitis and cerebellar ataxia. In patients with atopic eczema the eruption may resemble eczema herpeticum.

Pityriasis rosea (Fig. 36.12)

This is commonly mildly itchy, particularly after a bath, and can be mistaken for psoriasis. It is more common in the winter months (November to February) and affects adolescents more than infants. The rash is concentrated on the trunk; the lesions are red and 1–2 cm in diameter, with fine scales. This rash is self-limiting and therefore requires non-specific treatment. The cause is unknown but it is thought to be due to an infective agent.

Ringworm

Ringworm may affect the hair, skin and nails. Scalp ringworm (tinea capitis) can lead to marked inflammation with pustule formation, termed a kerion (Fig. 36.13). Scalp infection often requires oral antifungal agents.

Scabies (Fig. 36.14)

This infestation follows an incubation period of 2–6 weeks after contact with the mite *Sarcoptes scabiei* var. *hominis*. It affects areas below the neck, including finger and toe web spaces, palms, elbows, soles, wrists, breasts and penis. Severe irritation tends to be worse at night. Treatment must include all family contacts, whether symptomatic or not. Options include application of permethrin cream (5%) from the neck down, with washing 8–12 hours later and malathion (0.5%) in an aqueous base.

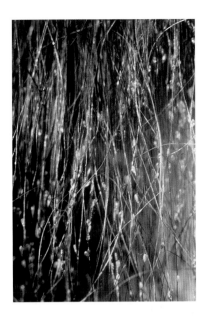

Fig. 36.15 Head lice infestation (*Pediculosis capitis*). Numerous 'nits' can be seen on hairs.

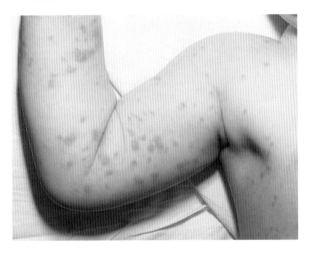

Fig. 36.16 Urticaria. Typical pink weals over an upper limb.

Head lice infestation (pediculosis capitis)

(Fig. 36.15)

This usually presents with scalp and nape irritation, and secondary bacterial infection over the neck (impetiginization) is common. Nits (empty egg cases) and live lice should be looked for. Pubic lice infestation is occasionally seen affecting the pubic area and sometimes eyelashes. Treatment options are similar to scabies.

Urticaria

Ordinary urticaria or 'hives' is an itchy erythematous eruption characterized by flesh-coloured weals (Fig. 36.16). These are due to a local increased permeability of capillaries and small venules. It may be associated with angioedema, in which swelling of the lips, eyelids, genitalia, tongue or larynx can occur. It is very common and important causes are drugs, food, inhalants or infections, although many cases are of unknown cause.

Papular urticaria

This represents a hypersensitivity reaction to a bite from a flea, bed bug, mosquito or dog louse. Irritation, vesicles, papules and weals appear over buttocks and limbs but distribution can be wide in chronic cases.

Urticaria pigmentosa

This is the most common of a group of uncommon conditions in which there is accumulation of mast cells in the skin. It is, however, an important condition to recognize, as occasionally there may be involvement of other tissues, most notably the bone marrow. The initial presentation is a widespread orange–red maculopapular rash, some lesions of which may urticate with rubbing. The condition can appear in infancy and may occasionally be associated with severe itching, flushing and wheeze. Lesions tend to become pigmented with time. Treatment is with oral antihistamines and sometimes in severe disease sodium cromoglicate can be added as a mast cell stabilizer.

Sunburn (acute solar dermatitis)

Sadly this is a very common entity. Proper preventive measures, such as covering up with loose cool clothing, hats and sunscreen lotion/cream of sun protection factor (SPF) 15 and above, are most important, particularly in infants and fair-skinned children. Parents must be educated.

Drug eruptions

Drug eruptions are uncommon in young children. However, widespread maculopapular eruptions and urticaria are the most frequently seen presentations. More extreme reactions with marked mucosal involvement and skin loss can occur as part of the Stevens–Johnson syndrome, in which drugs such as sulphonamides and anticonvulsants (carbamazepine and phenytoin) may be implicated.

Alopecia

There are a number of causes of scalp hair loss, which in the child can cause significant concern. The four most common are discussed below.

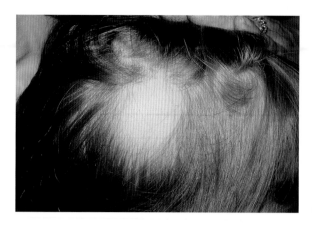

Fig. 36.17 Alopecia areata.
Patch of scalp hair loss showing a well-defined area of complete hair loss without inflammation.

Alopecia areata

This is a common cause of hair loss in childhood. Typically smooth areas of skin with exclamation mark hairs (broken hairs at the edge of active patches) occur (Fig. 36.17). Although most commonly seen as patches on the scalp, this condition can progress to involve the whole scalp or, more rarely, all body hair. The prognosis tends to be worse, the more widespread the condition. It is linked to other autoimmune conditions such as vitiligo (a condition with primary loss of skin melanin pigment).

Traumatic alopecia

This can be intentional or unintentional. Typically traction from ponytails or other similar hairstyles may cause patchy alopecia. Intentional hair loss can be much more difficult to manage and used to be termed trichotillomania. Underlying triggers such as social deprivation in the home environment should be actively sought. In severe cases the appearance of the hair is often bizarre, with unusual patterns. It is interesting to note that trichotillomania may follow alopecia areata, possibly as a consequence of the attention the child has been receiving for the original complaint.

Scarring alopecia

Any cause of scarring to the hair follicle will result in an area of alopecia. This can be difficult to distinguish from other causes.

Systemic disease

Endocrine abnormalities, such as hypothyroidism or diabetes, can produce hair loss.

- Streptococcal infection
- Tuberculosis
- Sarcoidosis
- Drugs
- Inflammatory bowel disease
- Idiopathic

Erythema nodosum (EN)

Typical EN presents with discrete red painful nodules over the anterior shins that may later become confluent. In around 30% of cases no cause is found but the differential diagnosis is wide (Box 36.6). Lesions may involve other sites, including thighs, arms and even the face. Resolution takes around 5–6 weeks and typically the lesions become bluish in colour as they resolve.

Henoch–Schönlein purpura

This is the most common childhood vasculitis (Fig. 36.18) and is discussed in detail on page 267. In around one-third of children an upper respiratory infection precedes the eruption, with purpura predominantly over the extensor surfaces of the limbs. It is usually self-limiting but can involve gastrointestinal vessels causing colic and, although renal involvement is usually transient, glomerulonephritis can occasionally occur.

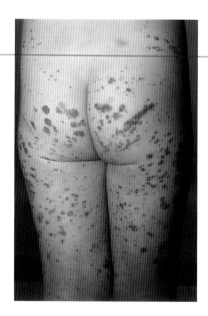

Fig. 36.18 Henoch–Schönlein purpura.
A 6-year-old girl with purpura over buttocks and lower limbs.

What is the likely diagnosis?

Acute urticaria is most likely. Certain foods are one of the common causes of acute urticaria.

What is your diagnosis?

Pityriasis rosea seems most likely. The description of the first or so-called herald patch and the trunk distribution is suggestive of this self-limiting condition.

Malcolm Levene   Neela Shabde   Martin Samuels

37

Child abuse and neglect: the hospital perspective

LEARNING OUTCOMES

By the end of this chapter you should:

- Know and understand the role and responsibilities of the paediatrician in recognizing and managing abuse and neglect
- Know and understand the importance of awareness of abuse and neglect
- Know and understand which children and families are most of risk of abuse and neglect
- Know and understand the legal aspects and the rights of the child
- Understand multi-agency working and confidentiality
- Know and understand the diagnosis of physical and child sexual abuse and appreciate that a multi-agency approach is essential
- Know and understand the importance of discharging the child to a safe place.

Introduction

Protecting children from intentional harm is the role and duty of every paediatrician. There is a basic level of knowledge that all such doctors must possess in order to be able to fulfil this function. This chapter describes the basis of child protection from the point of view of a trainee in paediatrics and Chapter 21 describes this from a primary care doctor's perspective.

Table 37.1 Types of ill treatment and examples

Form of abuse	Example
Physical abuse	Fractures, burns, cerebral and abdominal injuries
Sexual abuse	Unlawful sexual intercourse, buggery, participation in pornographic media
Emotional abuse (Ch. 21)	Demeaning, critical and unloving behaviour, verbal abuse
Neglect (Ch. 21)	Failure to thrive, missed healthcare and/or educational opportunities
Induced illness (Ch. 21)	Suffocation, poisoning, inappropriate interference with feeding tubes and intravenous lines
Fabricated illness (Ch. 21)	Falsifying histories, exaggerating handicap, interfering with tests

The basic principles involved in child protection are:

- Recognition of the problem
- Reporting the doctor's suspicions
- Investigation and management of the problem.

These two chapters give an overview of child protection, but in Britain it is a requirement that all paediatric trainees undergo a formal child protection educational programme for doctors, including a training day developed by the Royal College of Paediatrics and Child Health (RCPCH) in conjunction with the National Society for Prevention of Cruelty to Children (NSPCC) and the Advanced Life Support Group (ALSG). 'Recognition and Response in Child Protection — an Education Programme for Doctors in Training' will be delivered by ALSG. These chapters are not intended as a substitute for this training but give an overview and précis of material that is available on this course.

Child abuse can be defined under six categories, which are not mutually exclusive and often form a spectrum of abuse (Table 37.1). A child suffering one form of abuse is often subjected to other forms as well.

Many of these forms of maltreatment present to healthcare providers in either primary or secondary care, usually in the form of apparently accidental injury or genuine illness. The health professional has the opportunity to recognize these forms of maltreatment, and in so doing, will have to document why maltreatment explains the child's condition. This may need further investigation and the opinions of other medical specialties, e.g. in radiology, orthopaedics or neurosurgery. It is important to note that a child with chronic illness or disability can also be subjected to fabricated and induced illness so there is a need for awareness and recognition of this form of abuse.

Child abuse is commonly considered to result from a pattern of behaviour by an adult that is apart from other human behaviour. Whilst the most severe abuse results from behaviour that is clearly abnormal (cigarette burns, sadistic beatings, sexual abuse and physical isolation), there is some behaviour where the definition of abuse is dependent on the culture in which it occurs. The whole range of maltreatment of children, therefore, is best considered part of a spectrum of behaviour, ranging from that which is often part of normal behaviour (the 'reflex' smack, frustrated aggressive shout or derogatory remark; conscious 'disciplinary' acts accepted in some societies) through to very disturbed patterns of behaviour that result in conscious sadistic acts by an adult.

Role of the paediatrician

Paediatricians are *not* expected to deal with the maltreatment of children and young people alone; their role is to recognize and report when abuse may be occurring in the many different clinical presentations and to assist statutory agencies in the investigation of possible significant harm to a child. This would include establishing the likelihood of non-intentional injury or organic disease versus deliberate harm to the child. Such distinction is not often easy or possible, as some children with chronic disease or disability may also be subjected to child abuse and neglect; indeed, research confirms that they are at increased risk. The paediatrician therefore must liaise with the statutory agencies for child protection. It is the statutory agencies, including social services, the NSPCC and the police, that have a legal responsibility for protecting children and investigating child protection concerns. Current government guidance and law (Children Act 1989) in the UK places professional responsibility on health professionals to recognize and respond to child protection concerns and work within an inter-agency framework (colleagues), cooperating with statutory agencies in the best interest of the child. Paediatricians usually refer to social services in keeping with the local procedures and protocols.

Thus the key tasks of the paediatrician are to:

- Take a detailed history and perform a full physical examination
- Document the findings accurately and legibly in the medical records
- Consider whether child protection concerns exist*
- Check the child's name against the Child Protection Register (this will disappear in name with the new working together arrangements); also, to check whether the child is the subject of a child protection plan (held by the local social services or the NSPCC)

- Communicate with other professionals who have seen the child
- Undertake further medical investigation or obtain specialist opinion, where appropriate*
- Decide on the likelihood of accidental versus non-accidental injury, or organic versus non-organic illness*
- Report any child protection concerns to the statutory agencies for child protection, both verbally and in writing
- Carefully and contemporaneously document what actions are being taken, including discussions with social services/police and the plan arising from these
- Explain any findings and concerns to the parents (unless to do so would increase the risk to the child). Parents should be shown respect.*

(* These tasks should be undertaken in consultation with senior colleagues, including the named or designated doctor or nurse for child protection.)

The investigation and management of a case of maltreatment of a child must be approached in the same systematic and rigorous manner as would be appropriate to the investigation and management of any other potentially fatal disease (as suggested by Lord Laming in the Victoria Climbié inquiry). When a child is admitted to hospital, a clear decision must always be made and documented as to which consultant is responsible for the child protection aspects of the child's care. The child must *not* be discharged from hospital until child protection concerns have been resolved.

Importance of awareness of abuse

In cases where professionals who deal with children know of or suspect abuse there is the opportunity for intervention, including either family support or protection of the child by removal from home, but only if this is reported to child protection agencies. Failure to report concerns or knowledge of maltreatment can have substantial long-term consequences for the child, who may remain the victim of abuse.

The long-term effects of child abuse and neglect include:

- *Emotional harm*, e.g. low self-esteem, depression, unresolved anger and aggression, anorexia, self-harm and suicide
- *Physical harm*, e.g. brain injury, organ damage, deformities, scars (e.g. burns) and handicap
- *Educational problems*, e.g. learning difficulties, failed schooling, employment difficulties

---

BOX 37.1 Examples of severe or life-threatening child abuse

Direct
- Asphyxia or suffocation
- Non-accidental head injury
- Poisoning and other induced illness, e.g. septicaemia
- Abdominal injury
- Spinal injury, including cervical spine
- Rib cage and long bone fractures
- Drowning
- Burns

Indirect
- Sexual abuse
- Severe emotional abuse (through later deliberate self-harm or other suicidal acts)
- Neglect, e.g. accidents, lack of supervision, severe untreated infections, malnutrition, severe anaemia (secondary to scratching from head lice)

- *Social and relationship difficulties*, e.g. family violence, promiscuity and prostitution, drug and alcohol abuse, parenting difficulties.

Each year, substantial numbers of children suffer long-term morbidity or death (50–100 cases per year) as a result of maltreatment. In large numbers of these cases, earlier detection and intervention can avoid the serious consequences of abuse. Some of the most serious abusive injuries, including those that are life-threatening, are listed in Box 37.1.

Children at risk of abuse

Following any childhood injury, it is important to consider the circumstances of the injury and to obtain a clear history of what is alleged to have happened. If an explanation is absent, inconsistent or otherwise unsatisfactory, then the possibility of maltreatment must be considered. The same applies to illness that persistently defies explanation or is not consistent with usual medical experience. Child abuse/maltreatment occurs in all social classes. However, features that are known to occur more frequently in families who abuse their children, in comparison to families who do not, include:

- Where the relationship between the parent and child does not appear loving and caring
- Where one or both parents have been abused themselves as children
- Parents who are young, single, unsupported or substitutive

- Parents with learning difficulties
- Parents who have a poor or unstable relationship
- Situations where there is domestic violence, or drug or alcohol dependence/misuse
- Parents who have mental illness or personality disorders
- Situations of poverty and deprivation, although most poor families do not abuse their children.

Factors in the child that are associated with vulnerability to abuse and neglect include:
- Prematurity and/or separation in the neonatal period
- Chronic illness, with frequent or prolonged hospitalizations
- Physical or mental handicap
- Poor maternal attachment
- Behavioural problems, e.g. soiling and wetting, challenging behaviour and hyperactivity
- Difficult temperament
- Screaming, crying interminably and inconsolably
- Looked-after children, i.e. those in the care of the local authority.

The above may reflect both an increased susceptibility to and a consequence of maltreatment, but their presence does not mean abuse has occurred. Children in all circumstances may be subjected to abuse and have a right to be protected from it.

Legal aspects and rights of the child

Child protection in Britain is guided by a legal framework set out in the Children Act (1989). The new Children Act (2004) incorporates principles within the United Nations Convention on the Rights of the Child and the European Convention on Human Rights. Children are protected from abuse and neglect by multi-agency working and by both voluntary and legal intervention. The new act also emphasizes the promotion of children's welfare and their protection from abuse and neglect. The Department of Health (1999) and new Working Together (2006) document, 'Working Together to Safeguard Children', incorporates all the legislation and sets out principles for professionals working with children. The main features are as follows:
- The welfare of children is paramount.
- Children must be listened to.
- Children should have the right to grow up within their families in an environment that promotes their health and safety.
- Look at the child and family rather than the injury.
- Describes roles and responsibilities of different agencies and practitioners.

- Places child protection procedures within the remit of a local Area Child Protection Committee (ACPC) — to be replaced by Local Safeguarding Children Boards (LSCB; emphasis on safeguarding) — which describes inter-agency working.
- Describes processes to be followed when there are concerns about a child and actions to be taken to safeguard and promote the welfare of children suffering, or at risk of suffering, significant harm.
- Provides guidance on child protection for 'looked-after' children who are in care of the local authority.

The United Nations Convention on the Rights of the Child (1989) provides an internationally accepted set of principles and standards to ensure that children everywhere — without discrimination — have the right to survival; to develop to the fullest; to protection from harmful influences, abuse and exploitation; and to participate fully in family, cultural and social life. The rights apply to the practice of children's healthcare for all children and young people up to the age of 18 years. All but two countries in the world (USA and Somalia) have ratified the Convention.

Article 3 provides that any decision or action affecting children either as individuals or as a group should be taken with 'their best interest' as the most important consideration.

Article 9 holds that children have a right not to be separated from their parents or carers unless it is judged to be in the child's best interest.

Article 12 places an obligation on health professionals to seek a child's opinion before taking decisions that affect her or his future.

Article 19 states that legislative, administrative, social and educational measures should be taken to protect children from all forms of physical or mental violence, injury or abuse, neglect or negligent treatment, maltreatment or exploitation, including sexual abuse, while in the care of parent(s), legal guardian(s) or any other person who has the care of the child.

Article 37 states that no child shall be subjected to torture or other cruel, inhuman or degrading treatment or punishment.

Reporting of child protection concerns

Any person who has knowledge or a suspicion that a child is suffering significant harm, or is at risk of significant harm, should refer that concern to one or more of the agencies with statutory duties and/or powers to investigate and intervene: the social services department, the police or the NSPCC. All referrals to statutory authorities are taken seriously and considered with an open mind. Professionals should be able to refer to child protection agencies in good faith without fear that this will lead to uncoordinated and/or premature action or any adverse consequences to themselves.

At present, there is no mandatory requirement for healthcare professionals in the UK to report suspicions of child maltreatment to the statutory agencies. However, there is a professional duty to do so; the General Medical Council (GMC) good medical practice guidelines stipulate that patients must be able to trust doctors with their lives and wellbeing. In the practice of paediatrics, this applies to infants, children and young people up to age 18 years. Paediatricians must make the care of their patient their first concern. The GMC stipulates:

If you believe a patient to be a victim of neglect or physical, sexual or emotional abuse and that the patient cannot give or withhold consent to disclosure, you must give information promptly to an appropriate responsible person or statutory agency, where you believe that the disclosure is in the patient's best interest. If, for any reason, you believe that disclosure of information is not in the best interest of an abused or neglected patient, you must discuss the issues with an experienced colleague. If you decide not to disclose information, you must be prepared to justify your decision.

Whilst any health professional may report concerns or suspicions of child abuse to the statutory child protection agencies, more commonly general practitioners, community nursing staff and doctors in accident and emergency departments choose in the first place to refer such cases to paediatricians (either community or hospital-based paediatricians). In these circumstances, it is the consultant paediatrician who will then decide whether or not to refer a child to the statutory agencies. Nevertheless, the GMC recognizes that 'health care is increasingly provided by multi-disciplinary teams' and

if you disagree with your team's decision, you may be able to persuade other team members to change their minds. If not, and you believe that the decision would harm the patient, tell someone who can take action. If there are difficulties or disagreements about if and when to refer a child, then discussion with a named or designated doctor or nurse is strongly advised.

Critical threshold

Professionals need to be aware of the manifestations of maltreatment or abuse to ensure children are protected from harm. However, the detection of abuse is sometimes far from simple and requires the building up of a jigsaw of information; some of the pieces may be from a medical assessment (history, examination,

---

BOX 37.2 The child at risk of significant harm

The Children Act 1989 (together with Children Act 2004) introduced the concept of 'significant harm' as the legal threshold for compulsory intervention in child protection cases. Where social services have reasonable cause to suspect that a child is suffering or is likely to suffer significant harm, they are under a duty to investigate the claim. Furthermore, courts can only make a care or supervision order if they are satisfied that:

- The child is suffering, or is likely to suffer, significant harm, and
- The harm or likelihood of harm is attributable to a lack of adequate parental care or control.

There are no absolute criteria by which significant harm can be judged; decisions take into consideration the effect of any ill treatment on the child's overall physical and psychological health and development. The Children Act 1989 introduced the concept of significant harm as the threshold that justifies compulsory intervention in family life in the best interests of children, and gives local authorities a duty to make enquiries to decide whether they should take action to safeguard or promote the welfare of a child who is suffering or is likely to suffer significant harm.

BOX 37.3 The child in need

A child should be taken to be in need if he/she is unlikely to achieve or maintain, or to have the opportunity of achieving or maintaining, a reasonable standard of health or development without the provision of services by a local authority, or his/her health or development is likely to be significantly impaired or further impaired without the provision of such services, or he/she is disabled.

A child in need who is not receiving services may be at risk of significant harm.

---

investigations, subspecialty opinions) and some from information from other professionals or agencies. Sometimes the critical information — for example, a parent's past history of abusing a child — is held by the statutory agency and failure to share information with that agency may delay protection of the child. The clinician must make a decision when to liaise or refer to the statutory agencies. This is usually when the case has reached the 'critical threshold' (Boxes 37.2 and 37.3).

The 'critical threshold' is the point where the professional's concerns that the child may be being harmed cannot be satisfactorily resolved. Certainly in some cases it may fall short of clinical certainty or confirmation of diagnosis. The professional will be assisted by discussion with others, including a designated or named doctor or nurse. This critical threshold is the point when concerns need to be referred to the statutory authorities for child protection. Sometimes this critical threshold may be immediately apparent, e.g. an infant who has suffered a skull fracture and intracranial haemorrhage without adequate explanation. In other circumstances, a combination of history and non-specific signs suggests that there may be a problem. If there is any doubt about whether to report, consultation with a senior colleague or the named/designated doctor for child protection is recommended. As a rule, if in doubt after appropriate discussion and consultation, it is better for a report to be made to social services so that an assessment of the child and family can be made. This may identify that the child either is 'at risk' of significant harm, or may still be 'in need of services'. Both approaches should allow for the institution of appropriate family support and/or protection for the child and other measures as considered appropriate.

Child protection register

This is soon to be replaced by a list of children who are subject to a child protection plan. In each area covered by a social services department, a central register is kept, listing all the children in the area who have been abused or who are considered to be at risk of abuse and are therefore the subject of an inter-agency plan to protect them. The register is more concerned with the future protection of the child rather than past abuse. Children in the UK are placed on the Child Protection Register in one of four categories: neglect, physical abuse, sexual abuse or emotional abuse.

The decision for a child's name to be entered on to the Child Protection Register usually follows the sharing of information and discussion at a Child Protection Conference, and where an inter-agency agreement is made to work cooperatively with the family to protect the child. Similarly, a Child Protection Conference is required normally to make the decision to remove a child's name from the Child Protection Register. The register provides a central point of speedy enquiry for professional staff who are worried about a child and want to know whether the child is already the subject of an inter-agency protection plan. The Child Protection Register is maintained by social services departments and can be accessed by any health professional who has concerns about a child. It is important to note whether a child is the subject of a child protection plan.

Inter-agency working/ working together

Child protection mostly involves working in partnership with the family and with professionals from other agencies. With regard to the former, there are some essential principles that the clinician should be aware of:
- Treat all family members as you would wish to be treated — with dignity and respect.
- Ensure family members know that the child's safety and welfare must be given first priority.
- Be clear with yourself and family members about the purpose of your professional involvement.
- Listen to the concerns of the child and his or her family.
- Respect confidentiality.
- Be open and honest about your concerns and responsibilities.
- Take care to distinguish between your professional role and responsibilities and your personal feelings, values, prejudices and beliefs.

It is not always possible to work in partnership with parents. In these circumstances, the best you can do is to keep the parents informed, whilst liaising with senior colleagues and the statutory authorities. If there is an immediate danger to the child's life, the police should be called.

Inter-agency working demands that agencies and professionals:
- Share information
- Collaborate and understand each other's position
- Work in partnership with each other and children and their families to plan comprehensive and coordinated services
- Recognize those most vulnerable children and coordinate services from various appropriate agencies, including the voluntary sector
- Work with adult services, particularly mental health
- Participate in joint working to safeguard children and where necessary to help bring to justice the perpetrators of crime against children.

All trusts should have a named doctor and a named nurse for child protection, who take a professional lead within the trust on child protection matters. Their responsibilities include education, support and supervision. Each local area must have a designated doctor and nurse for child protection who work closely with the named professionals in supporting activities within trusts.

Health professionals are expected to work in partnership with local authorities following government guidelines identifying clear roles and responsibilities for commissioners and providers within the health service.

Confidentiality

Issues around confidentiality often appear to be more complicated in child protection than in other areas, but it should always be recognized that the needs and the welfare of the child are paramount. Key issues highlighted in recent guidance from the RCPCH are as follows:

- The doctor's primary duty is to act in the child's best interest. If there is conflict between the doctor and parents or parents and child, then the child's needs are paramount.
- When there are reasonable grounds to believe a child is at risk of significant harm, the facts should be reported to social services in England, Wales and Northern Ireland, whereas in Scotland, the key test for reporting to the Reporter to the Children's Panel is a perceived need for compulsory measures of supervision.
- Health trusts and their employees have a statutory duty to assist social services departments making enquiries under the Children Act 1989.
- Consent to disclosure of relevant information about the child and other family members as a result of these enquires should normally be sought from a competent child and carer, unless doing so would place the child or a sibling at greater risk or hinder enquiries by provoking interference with verbal evidence.
- Medical practitioners should disclose information about a non-competent child if they can justify doing so as essential to their patient's medical interest. Disclosure without consent may also take place where failure to do so may place a child at risk of death or serious harm, or where the information would help prevent, detect or prosecute a serious crime.
- Where there is uncertainty as to whether there is a risk of death or serious harm and an apparently competent child or parent refuses permission for disclosure, the doctor is obliged to act when a child is in danger.
- The doctor should document thoroughly all decisions and the reasoning behind them and should always separate details of fact from those of speculation and opinion.

The doctor–parent–child relationship is founded on mutual trust and respect, as well as a common aim to benefit the child. Where the child presents with symptoms or signs suggesting he or she has been a subject of abuse, it may no longer be possible to regard parent and child as a single unit. In this situation, it is the moral duty of the doctor to act in the best interest of the child.

Department of Health best practice guidance (May 2003) states:

A decision whether to disclose information may be particularly difficult if you think it may damage the trust between you and your patient or client. Wherever possible you should explain the problem, seek agreement and explain the reasons if you decide to act against a parent or the child's agreement.

A sensible safeguard, before dispensing with parental consent, is to seek advice and a further opinion from a more experienced colleague.

Lord Laming chaired a major inquiry following the death of Victoria Climbié. Amongst his wide-ranging recommendations he stated that difficulties in seeking or refusal of parental permission must not restrict the initial information gathering and sharing, e.g. between health and social services, and this should if necessary include talking to the child. He stated:

When the deliberate harm of a child is identified as a possibility, the examining doctor should consider whether taking a history directly from the child is in that child's best interests. When that is so, the history should be taken even when the consent of the carer has not been obtained, with the reason for dispensing with consent recorded by the examining doctor. In those cases in which English is not the first language of the child concerned, the use of an interpreter should be considered.

Civil and criminal proceedings

Significant harm to children gives rise to both child welfare concerns, dealt with in civil proceedings by social services (local authorities), and law enforcement issues, dealt with in criminal proceedings. The police have a duty to carry out thorough and professional investigations into allegations of crime, and the obtaining of good evidence is often in the best interests of a child, as it may make it less likely that a child will have to give evidence in court. It also contributes to the development of a good evidence base upon which to develop future support and help for the child and family.

Health professionals need to keep in mind that child protection work can lead to criminal proceedings. However, children should not be exposed to multiple intimate examinations simply to provide evidence for court proceedings. Furthermore, leading or suggestive communication with children or other members of the family should always be avoided. Further advice should be sought from either the police or the trust legal team when a doctor believes that criminal offences may have been committed.

Key points

- Be aware of the range of presentations of child maltreatment/abuse.
- Take a detailed history and perform a full physical examination.
- Document your findings accurately in the medical records; note what was explained to the parents and what actions you are taking.
- If there are child protection concerns, check the Child Protection Register to see if the child is the subject of a child protection plan.
- Discuss your concerns with senior colleagues or the named/designated doctor/nurse for child protection.
- Consider the need to communicate with other health professionals who have seen the child.
- Undertake further investigation or obtain specialist opinion, where appropriate.
- Explain any concerns to the parents and what you intend to do as a result.
- Refer child protection concerns to the statutory agencies for child protection.
- Document any discussions, including referrals to social services and what actions will be taken.
- Do not discharge home until child protection concerns have been resolved.
- Always involve a senior colleague. A consultant will ultimately have responsibility for the patient.

Physical abuse

Although serious cases of physical abuse may be obvious, the range and incidence of physical abuse varies depending on cultural practices. In some countries legislation has been established against smacking, which is considered abusive, but this is not the case in the UK and it remains legal to use reasonable force to discipline a child. Most people would, however, agree that any force that causes an injury to a child, such as bruising, represents unacceptable force. Bullying at school may also be a cause of physical or emotional abuse and it is estimated that 450 000 children are bullied at school at least once per week.

It has been shown that 14% of children in the UK suffered the effects or severe effects of physical punishment, including babies who are regularly smacked or hit. Mothers hit their children more often than fathers, but severe injury is most commonly inflicted by a man in the household.

Abuse may be severe and result in the child's death. Fatal outcome may be due to:

> **BOX 37.4 Common types of injury that result from physical abuse**
>
> - Bruising from blows
> - Fractures from grabbing limbs and direct blows
> - Bites (distinguish between dog and human dental patterns)
> - Burns from being held in direct contact with hot objects or scalds from forced immersion
> - Intra-oral injuries suggesting forcible insertion of bottles or spoons

---

> **BOX 37.5 Features that should arouse suspicion of physical abuse**
>
> - Repeated injuries
> - No consistent explanation for how the injury occurred
> - Patterns of injury
> - Evasive or uncooperative history from a parent or caregiver
> - Inappropriate child response (e.g. 'didn't cry', 'felt no pain')
> - Signs of other abuse (neglect, failure to thrive, sexual abuse)
> - The child's age too young to be consistent with the history of how injury occurred
> - Unreasonable delay in presentation
> - Parental aggression

- Shaking injury
- Blunt injury causing severe damage to brain or abdominal organs
- Suffocation (may present as recurrent apnoea or sudden unexplained death in infancy)
- Poisoning (see also Ch. 21).

Box 37.4 lists the more common types of injury that result from physical abuse.

The doctor must be alert to the varied ways in which physical abuse may present. Important features are listed in Box 37.5. A thorough medical examination (top-to-toe surface examination), including assessment of growth and development, is essential in all cases of suspected child abuse.

Bruising

There is no pathognomonic site of bruising that indicates child abuse. It is essential to document the number, distribution and pattern of all bruising carefully. Up to a half of all mobile children have at least one bruise and many have more than one, although more than ten are suspicious. An important clue to a potentially abusing family is if consent is not given to undress and

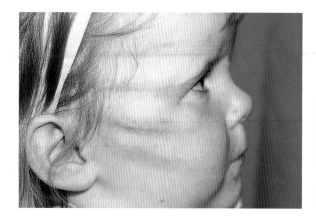

Fig. 37.1 Bruising to cheek — adult hand slap in a female aged 3 years
(Courtesy of Dr C Hobbs)

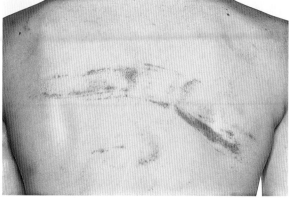

Fig. 37.3 Bruising to back as a result of belt marks in a male child aged 13 years
(Courtesy of Dr C Hobbs)

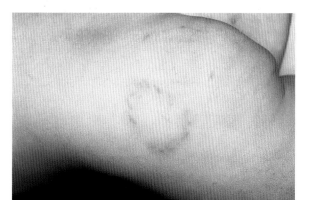

Fig 37.2 Bite marks in a male aged 3 years
(Courtesy of Dr C Hobbs)

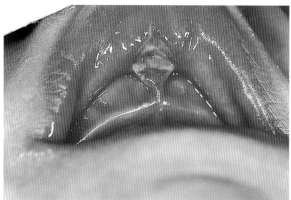

Fig. 37.4 Torn frenulum in a male aged 3 months
(Courtesy of Dr C Hobbs)

examine the whole child. Describe how many bruises and illustrate distribution with a simple diagram on the body chart. (Those on shins, bony prominences and forehead are more likely to be accidental.) Attempting to age bruises is unreliable and should not be done, not being based on good evidence. Is there a consistent history for the site of the bruising?

Particularly suspicious bruising includes:

- Unusual sites such as ears, cheeks (Fig. 37.1), eyes, mouth, trunk, genitalia, upper or unexposed parts of limbs, buttocks and neck
- Unusual patterns suggestive of grip marks, bites (Fig. 37.2), marks consistent with a stick, belt (Fig. 37.3), buckle or shoe
- Injuries in the mouth (Fig. 37.4)
- Two black eyes.

The differential diagnosis of excessive bruising includes:

- Coagulation disorders
- Henoch–Schönlein purpura (p. 267)
- Collagen disorders (rare)
- Asphyxia
- Mongolian blue spots (p. 129)
- Artefacts such as dirt, felt tip marks or dye from clothes.

Fractures

Fractures due to child abuse are most common in babies below the age of 2 years. In the first 18 months 85% of fractures are due to abuse and in premobile children (<9 months) fractures should always be treated as highly suspicious.

In all children certain fractures should lead to suspicion of abuse. These include:

- Rib fractures, which are highly specific for abuse (fresh fractures may be difficult to recognize on X-ray). Cardiopulmonary resuscitation rarely causes rib fracture and does not cause posterior rib fractures.
- Fractures involving a long bone metaphysis (Fig. 37.5).
- Any fracture of femur or humerus in infants.

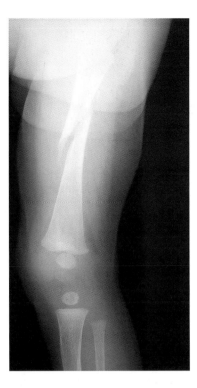

Fig. 37.5 Femoral shaft fracture in a girl of 6 months
(Courtesy of Dr C Hobbs)

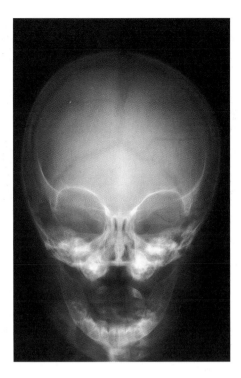

Fig. 37.6 Bilateral linear parietal skull fractures in a girl of 6 months
(Courtesy of Dr C Hobbs)

- Multiple fracture sites.
- A fracture that occurs as the result of minor trauma, e.g. an infant falling off a sofa.
- Evidence of fractures of different ages on X-ray examination.
- An inadequate or absent explanation for how the fracture occurred.
- Skull fractures, which do not occur without considerable force. Is the explanation appropriate? Particularly concerning are those involving the occipital bone, depressed fractures, wide (> 3 mm) fractures and multiple fractures, particularly if crossing a suture line (Fig. 37.6).
- Spinal fractures. Cervical fractures occasionally occur with non-accidental shaking injury.

Differential diagnoses for the cause of fractures include:
- Accident
- Abuse
- Birth injury (e.g. clavicle, humerus)
- Osteopenia (rickets) of prematurity (p. 376)
- Osteogenesis imperfecta
- Copper deficiency (very rare)
- Structural variant, e.g. aberrant cranial suture.

Investigations

A skeletal survey is mandatory when there is a fracture suggestive of abuse. It is also recommended for any child under the age of 2 years who is suspected of being physically abused. Repeating the survey (a chest X-ray and films of other suspicious areas) after 2 weeks may reveal previously undiagnosed fractures and can help in the dating of the onset of the fracture. Computed tomography (CT) head scans and bone scans may be indicated but require discussion with a senior colleague.

Thermal injuries

These occur commonly in childhood and often present to primary care doctors. A relatively small number are due to child abuse but are known to be under-recognized. Thermal injuries include burns and scalds. These include scalds from hot water, food or steam. Burns may follow contact from hot metal objects such as an iron or radiator, cigarettes, matches or flames, friction from being dragged across a carpet, and from electrical and chemical sources.

In evaluating a burn the following features are important:
- Inconsistent history as to how the injury occurred
- Denial that the injury is a burn
- Repeated burns
- Site or multiple sites (lesions on the feet and backs of hands are commonly due to abuse)

145

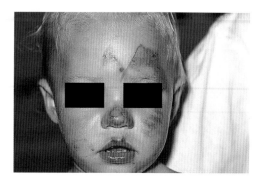

Fig. 37.7 Contact burns from an iron in an 18-month old girl)
(Courtesy of Dr C Hobbs)

- Shape:
  - Is it consistent with the history?
  - Are demarcation lines suggestive of a particular object (Fig. 37.7)?
  - Cigarette burns cause deep circular craters 0.5–1 cm in diameter, which scar (Fig. 37.8). Accidental brushed contact causes superficial injury roughly circular but with a tail.

Immersion scalds should be particularly evaluated for evidence of:

- Tide marks indicating that limb or buttocks were forcibly immersed (Fig. 37.9)
- Absent splash marks suggestive of removal from the hot water.

The differential diagnosis of burns includes:

- Impetigo (p. 130)
- Nappy rash (Ch. 27)
- Staphylococcal scalded skin (p. 130)
- Ringworm infection (p. 132).

Head injury

This form of abuse carries the highest mortality rates and is particularly common in infants. Isolated severe head injury

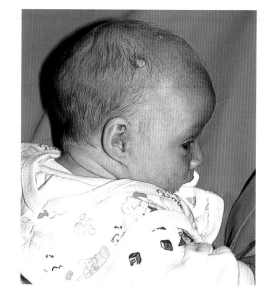

Fig. 37.8 Cigarette burn in a 8-week-old male
(Courtesy of Dr C Hobbs)

suggests either shaking or impact injury or both. Shaking injury resulting in combinations of subdural haemorrhage, brain injury and retinal haemorrhage is most common at around 3–6 months of age. Subdural haemorrhage may follow birth or accidental trauma. Small asymptomatic bleeds may be seen with imaging performed after birth, but resolve within the first 4 weeks of life.

The main clinical features of non-accidental head injury (NAHI) include:

- *Delay in presentation*: e.g. child may be well with enlarging head
- *Inconsistent explanation*: e.g. history of a minor fall, severe injury
- *Sudden collapse* in an otherwise well child
- *Presence of other injuries* (bruises, skull, rib or long bone fractures)
- *Retinal haemorrhages* in one or both eyes.

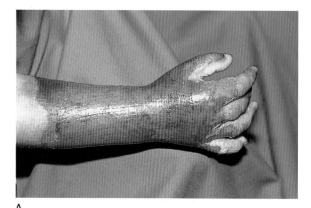

A

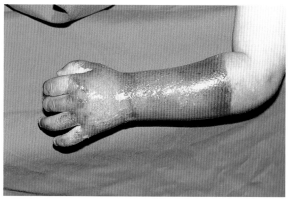

B

Fig. 37.9 Forced immersion scalds in male 18 months old
(A and B) (Courtesy of Dr C Hobbs)

N.B. The absence of one or more of fractures, bruises or retinal haemorrhages does not exclude abuse.

All children suspected of having non-accidental or other head injury should have a magnetic resonance (MR) or CT head scan to confirm the presence of subdural haemorrhage. Skeletal survey may reveal other bony injuries. An experienced ophthalmologist should be asked to examine the child's eyes as soon as possible after admission to look for retinal haemorrhages. These are a common feature after birth but usually disappear within days. They may occur after severe accidental injury (e.g. car accident).

Child sexual abuse

Sexual abuse in children will not be recognized if it is not considered by the clinician. A high index of suspicion must exist and healthcare professionals must acknowledge that child sexual abuse may occur in any family. One study found that in the UK 12% of girls and 8% of boys have suffered sexual abuse at some time in their childhood. Other studies have suggested higher figures. Boys are less likely to disclose abuse than girls. The abuser is most commonly a member of the household or an extended family member or friend. In the vast majority of cases the child knows the abuser, who may be either a man or a woman. Sexual abuse of children by strangers is much less common.

Abusers usually groom and manipulate children into silence over a period of time. A child who is abused by a close family member may adapt psychologically, a process that has been termed 'the child sexual abuse accommodation syndrome'. The components of this comprise:
- Secrecy
- Entrapment and helplessness
- Accommodation, in which the child takes responsibility and feelings of guilt for the abuse
- Delayed unconvincing disclosure and later retraction of disclosure.

Child sexual abuse has both short- and long-term effects. Short-term (childhood) effects include:
- Emotional, behavioural and psychosomatic disorder
- Difficulties forming friendships and trusting relationships
- School underachievement and truancy or excellent school performance and attendance
- Pregnancy, sexually transmitted infection (STI)
- Abusive behaviour towards younger children.

Long-term effects include:
- Sexual relationship difficulties
- Mental health problems, e.g. depression, eating disorder
- Social dysfunction
- May become a perpetrator.

Problem-orientated topic:

a girl with blood-stained underwear

Jane is 3 years old and her preschool teacher has noted blood staining on her knickers three times in the last month. Jane is an aggressive child who frequently hits other children in the nursery. She uses swear words, which the teacher thinks she can only have heard at home. Her teacher is concerned but does not want to upset Jane's mother and notifies the health visitor, who in turn informs the GP. The GP refers the case to hospital.

Q1. What should the paediatrician do?

Q2. What investigations should be performed?

Q3. How should the child and family be managed?

Q1. What should the paediatrician do?

There are very few signs that are diagnostic of sexual abuse in themselves. The diagnosis is usually made by piecing together a jigsaw of information from many sources. The major clues to diagnosis are as follows.

Disclosure

This is the most common way in which sexual abuse is diagnosed. Children rarely fabricate disclosure of sexual abuse and their account should always be taken seriously and investigated. The child should be told that the disclosure will be passed on to social services and the police. The doctor to whom the child discloses should not interrogate the child, as this may compromise the subsequent legal process. The doctor may, however, gently question the child in open and non-leading ways to find out, for example, what it is that makes them sore between their legs. If a child discloses in confidence he or she must be told that the information will be passed on for his or her protection, as well as for the protection of other children. The doctor should have no ethical dilemma as to whether this information should be disclosed, as the GMC acknowledges that protection of the patient overrides the duty of confidentiality to the patient.

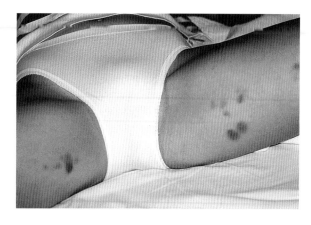

Fig. 37.10 Fingertip thigh bruises in sexual assault in female aged 9 years
(Courtesy of Dr C Hobbs)

Never promise to keep a child's secret, especially in advance of knowing what it is.

Vaginal discharge or urinary symptoms

These are non-specific symptoms in prepubertal girls but should arouse suspicion of sexual abuse. Many girls who have been rubbed or fondled may develop vulvovaginitis, but only a proportion of girls with vulvovaginitis have been sexually abused. Vaginal discharge in one case control study was found significantly more often than in non-abused controls. The differential diagnosis of vulvovaginitis is discussed in Volume 1 on page 331.

A vulval swab and urine culture should be taken. Do not insert the swab into the vagina but take the specimen from the labia.

Rectal or vaginal bleeding

Vaginal bleeding in a prepubertal child is usually due to trauma and as such is strongly linked to sexual abuse. Differentiating abuse from non-abusive genital trauma, such as a straddle injury, is not always simple. Even with a clear history, repeated by the child, caution is required. Injury to the hymen, posterior genital injury and bruising elsewhere should raise concerns and prompt a thorough assessment and referral to social services. Rectal bleeding may occur as the result of a fissure, rectal polyp, inflammatory bowel disease or gastroenteritis. The presence of either of these symptoms in a prepubertal child without an obvious unambiguous history demands rapid referral to a child protection team (Fig. 37.10).

Behavioural disturbance

Emotional and behavioural disturbance following child sexual abuse is common and may include self-harm, mutilation, aggression and sexualized behaviours. More often, however, the parents describe non-specific symptoms including anxiety, interrupted sleep, bad dreams, naughtiness, disobedience or just a non-specific subtle change in the child's behaviour. Psychosomatic symptoms are common and include abdominal pains and headaches. Secondary wetting and soiling are also important symptoms.

Pregnancy

This is clear evidence of sexual activity! It is obviously important to distinguish between consensual intercourse with a teenage boyfriend, which is not abusive, and pregnancy resulting from an abusive exploitative relationship with an older adult. The issue of consent in the latter situation is one of whether this can in reality be meaningful and given on an equitable basis or whether the girl has been groomed and exploited/corrupted.

Examination

There may be evidence of force during the assault, as seen in physical injuries such as bruising of the lower abdomen, genital area, thighs, buttocks, breasts and grip mark bruising around the knees or on the upper arms. Examination of the genitalia may reveal either supportive or diagnostic findings of abuse. For example, a fresh tear of the hymen with fresh bleeding or an old healed transaction of the hymen are both strong evidence of penetrating trauma. An anal laceration or scar is a diagnostic sign of anal penetration and reflex anal dilatation is one of a number of other findings supportive of anal abuse.

Q2. What investigations should be performed?

If a vulval swab identifies a sexually transmitted infection (STI), immediate referral to a child protection team should be made. The incidence of STI in abused children is about 5% and the most commonly encountered are gonorrhoea, genital or anal warts and chlamydia. *Trichomonas vaginalis* infection (usually asymptomatic) in a child over 12 months suggests recent sexual contact. Other infections that can be sexually transmitted include genital herpes simplex, human immunodeficiency virus (HIV), syphilis and pubic lice. Very often children with STI show no sign of injury to the genital or anal areas.

Q3. How should the child and family be managed?

If a doctor has evidence causing him or her to suspect child sexual abuse, this information must be passed on to the social services. Discussion with a named or designated paediatrician may be useful if further advice is required. The primary caregiver should be informed of the referral unless there is any concern that the abuser may be warned and evidence may be destroyed or pressure put on the child to withdraw the disclosure or change the story.

The doctor must keep careful and accurate contemporaneous notes of the interview, including who said what to whom and any examination findings. All paediatricians should be familiar with the Royal College of Physicians (RCP) document, 'The Physical Signs of Sexual Abuse in Children'.

Once the social services have been informed, a child protection investigation occurs. If the child is making a disclosure or allegation of abuse, he or she is usually interviewed jointly by an experienced social worker and police officer and the interview is videotaped as evidence for any later court hearing.

The child should be examined by a paediatrician trained in examination and assessment of child sexual abuse either alone or jointly with an experienced police surgeon. The key issue is whether the doctor has the necessary skills. Remember that no physical evidence may be found, even in cases with a clear allegation of penetrative sexual abuse. The purpose of this examination is to:

- Assess the nature of any abuse
- Collect forensic evidence of sexual abuse (e.g. semen or spermatozoa in the vagina, rectum, mouth or elsewhere)
- Screen for STIs and pregnancy
- Provide reassurance that there is no permanent physical damage
- Arrange a treatment plan for identified medical, psychological and emotional problems

- Offer emergency contraception to postmenarchal girls presenting within 72 hours of a sexually abusive event.

The main aim of management is to prevent further abuse and provide support for the child and family as necessary. Referral to a therapeutic service, e.g. Child and Adolescent Mental Health, may be required.

 http://www.bma.org.uk/ap.nsf/Content/childprotection

British Medical Association: Doctors' Responsibilities in Child Protection Cases, June 2004

 http://www.gmc-uk.org/guidance/good_medical_practice/index.asp

General Medical Council: advice on good medical practice and confidentiality

Acknowledgments

We are very grateful to Dr Chris Hobbs for advice about the manuscript and for allowing us to use his illustrations.

Further reading

Hobbs CJ, Wynne JM 2001 Physical signs of child abuse: a colour atlas, 2nd edn. WB Saunders, Philadelphia
Report of a working party of the Royal College of Physicians 1997 Physical signs of sexual abuse in children. RCP, London

Anthony Costello   Therese Hesketh   David Osrin   Andrew Tomkins

Child health in developing countries

LEARNING OUTCOMES

By the end of this chapter you should:

- Know and understand definitions of key statistics
- Know and understand the UN Millennium Development Goals
- Be familiar with the major infectious illnesses of developing countries: malaria, HIV/AIDS and tuberculosis
- Understand why neonatal mortality is so high in developing countries and methods to reduce it
- Understand malnutrition: its dietary, social, environmental and disease causes; diagnosis — clinical and biochemical; its impact on child health; prevention and treatment
- Understand the concept and the global importance of children in difficult circumstances.

MODULE SIX

Introduction

A third of global deaths occur in children under 5 years. This equates to almost 11 million deaths per annum, of which almost all (98%) take place in poor countries.

Beneath the classification of cause of death lies a raft of influences, in which poverty, gender, governance, macroeconomics and malnutrition all play a part. It remains a fact that, of the 4.4 billion people living in poor countries, 60% lack access to sanitation, 33% lack clean water, 20% have no healthcare, and 20% do not have enough dietary energy and protein.

Child international health

Problem-orientated topic:

a presentation on child public health

You are invited to make a presentation on child public health in your area of the UK at an international meeting. The audience will include health professionals from a number of countries, with representation from Africa and South Asia. You feel that it would be productive to set your discussion in the context of global child health, and to highlight the areas in which your practice is similar to and differs from that of your international colleagues. You will have to deal with questions about common international child health concerns.

Q1. Which child survival statistics will you use in the introductory discussion?

Q2. Against which international goals might you frame the discussion?

Q3. What are the world's top three causes of child mortality?

Q4. Can you name and summarize three international child health programmes that are relevant to both your practice in the UK and your colleagues' practice in developing countries?

Q5. What are the immunization schedules likely to be in your colleagues' countries?

Q6. What is your opinion of the WHO strategy for the Integrated Management of Childhood Illness (IMCI) as a model for ambulatory paediatric clinics in the UK?

Q1. Which child survival statistics will you use in the introductory discussion?

Although rough figures are available, we do not have accurate data on the numbers and causes of child deaths in developing countries, particularly at the younger end of the scale. Ideally, statistics would be based on vital registration — as they are in the UK — and death certification would be used to monitor mortality patterns and document leading causes of death. Unfortunately, vital registration systems are not fully functional in most poor countries, and we have to rely on either small sentinel registration initiatives or sample surveys. One well-known source of figures is the Demographic and Health Survey (DHS), which collects information on a range of family issues from a national sample and is organized to be comparable between countries.

The most common child health indices used to compare different areas or progress over time are the under-5 mortality rate and the infant mortality rate. Although child mortality does have a technical meaning, it is often used as shorthand for under-5 mortality.

Definitions

Definitions of terms are given in Table 38.1 and Figure 38.1.

Q2. Against which international goals might you frame the discussion?

Child survival is addressed in the Millennium Development Goals set by the UN. Although there is a specific

Table 38.1 Definitions

Term	Definition	Related term	Definition
Stillbirth*	A fetus born after 28 complete weeks of gestation, who has died before delivery	Stillbirth rate (SBR)	Stillbirths per 1000 births, live and still
Early neonatal death	Death of a live-born infant within 7 complete days postpartum	Early neonatal mortality rate (ENMR)	Early neonatal deaths per 1000 live births
Late neonatal death	Death of a live-born infant between 8 and 28 complete days postpartum	Late neonatal mortality rate (LNMR)	Late neonatal deaths per 1000 live births
Perinatal death	Stillbirth or early neonatal death	Perinatal mortality rate (PMR)	Stillbirths and early neonatal deaths per 1000 births, live and still
Neonatal death	Early or late neonatal death	Neonatal mortality rate (NMR)	Early and late neonatal deaths per 1000 live births
Post-neonatal death	Death of a live-born infant between 28 days and 12 complete months postpartum	Post-neonatal mortality rate (PNMR)	Post-neonatal deaths per 1000 live births
Infant death	Neonatal or post-neonatal death	Infant mortality rate (IMR)	Infant deaths per 1000 live births
Under-5 death	Death of a live-born infant within 5 complete years postpartum	Under-5 mortality rate (U5MR)	Under-5 deaths per 1000 live births

* This is a working definition, which accords with the International Statistical Classification of Diseases — 9th revision (ICD-9). In view of the fact that newborn infants of lower gestations now routinely survive in industrialized countries, the definition has been revised in ICD-10 to take in gestations as low as 22 complete weeks.

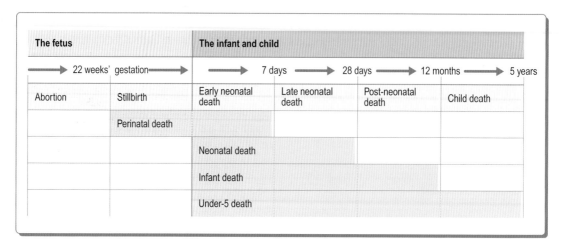

Fig. 38.1 **Definitions**

Table 38.2 **Millennium Development Goals**

Goal/target	Description
Goal 1	**Eradicate extreme poverty and hunger**
Target 1	Halve, between 1990 and 2015, the proportion of people whose income is less than US $1 a day
Target 2	Halve, between 1990 and 2015, the proportion of people who suffer from hunger
Goal 2	**Achieve universal primary education**
Target 3	Ensure that, by 2015, children everywhere, boys and girls alike, will be able to complete a full course of primary education
Goal 3	**Promote gender equality and empower women**
Target 4	Eliminate gender disparity in primary and secondary education, preferably by 2005 and to all levels of education no later than 2015
Goal 4	**Reduce child mortality**
Target 5	Reduce by two-thirds, between 1990 and 2015, the under-5 mortality rate
Goal 5	**Improve maternal health**
Target 6	Reduce by three-quarters, between 1990 and 2015, the maternal mortality ratio
Goal 6	**Combat HIV/AIDS, malaria and other diseases**
Target 7	Have halted by 2015, and begun to reverse, the spread of HIV/AIDS
Target 8	Have halted by 2015, and begun to reverse, the incidence of malaria and other major diseases
Goal 7	**Ensure environmental sustainability**
Target 9	Integrate the principles of sustainable development into country policies and programmes and reverse the loss of environmental resources
Target 10	Halve, by 2015, the proportion of people without sustainable access to safe drinking water
Target 11	By 2020, to have achieved a significant improvement in the lives of at least 100 million slum dwellers

goal for improving child survival, all the goals are intimately linked with child health (Table 38.2).

Q3. What are the world's top three causes of child mortality?

Global causes of childhood death, in order of magnitude, are:

- Perinatal and neonatal disorders
- Diarrhoeal disease
- Respiratory infection
- Malaria
- Human immunodeficiency virus/acquired immune deficiency syndrome (HIV/AIDS)
- Measles.

Q4. Can you name and summarize three international child health programmes that are relevant to both your practice in the UK and your colleagues' practice in developing countries?

Child health is affected by improvements in education, infrastructure, health service systems, sanitation and nutrition. However, a number of programmes specifically target health issues. Some of these programmes are limited to one type of disease (vertical) and some attempt to address a range of problems (integrated).

Three international programmes that are directly relevant to developing countries are discussed below (Box 38.1). These also have relevance in the UK.

BOX 38.1 International Child Health Programmes

- Expanded Programme on Immunization (EPI)
- Control of Diarrhoeal Disease (CDD)
- Acute Respiratory Infection (ARI)

Q5. What are the immunization schedules likely to be in your colleagues' countries?

Expanded Programme on Immunization (EPI)

The EPI is the basis for all global immunization programmes (Table 38.3), with varying support from international organizations depending on a country's needs. World-wide coverage is roughly 80% overall, but there are wide variations, especially in receipt of all three diphtheria/tetanus/pertussis (DTP) doses.

The campaign to eradicate polio began in 1988 and has achieved over 99% reduction in disease incidence through a strategy based on:

- High routine infant immunization
- Supplementary doses to all children under 5 years during national immunization days
- Surveillance for wild poliovirus through reporting and testing of all cases of acute flaccid paralysis in children under 15 years
- Targeted mop-up campaigns once wild poliovirus transmission is focal.

Presently, polio remains endemic in seven countries, and six countries have been labelled as susceptible to reintroduction. Attention has now shifted to the endgame. In order to be certified polio-free, a country must have had at least 3 years of no cases of wild polio, demonstrate a capacity to detect, report and respond to imported cases, and have contained laboratory virus stocks. Likewise, sufficient stocks of vaccine must exist to cover potential outbreaks and routine immunization programmes must be strong. Because of the proportionately growing incidence of vaccine-derived polio, many countries are switching from oral to injectable polio vaccine.

Measles is responsible for about 10% of under-5 deaths — 800 000 deaths per year — 85% of which occur in Africa and Asia. Epidemics are particularly severe in crowded conditions such as urban slums, schools, hospitals and refugee camps. Mortality is reduced if vitamin A stores are replete, if antibiotics are given for bacterial complications, if oral rehydration therapy is used for diarrhoea, and if food intake is increased for up to 2 months after the illness. A measles eradication goal was set in 1997. Unfortunately, the necessary coverage to achieve eradication is over 90% and the current level is on average about 70%. Eradication will therefore require a series of national and local catch-up rounds of immunization, as well as very good routine immunization systems.

Control of Diarrhoeal Disease (CDD)

The discovery that oral water, salt and sugar repletion (oral rehydration solution, ORS) was a powerful tool for treating the dehydration caused by diarrhoea led to the institutionalization of oral rehydration therapy (ORT) and its inclusion in the child survival initiatives of the 1980s. Many healthcare facilities now have ORT areas, and outreach workers are routinely trained to assess degrees of dehydration and manage diarrhoea at home or refer appropriately.

Acute Respiratory Infection (ARI)

Outreach workers are also central to efforts to reduce the toll of lower respiratory tract infection. Pneumonia is responsible for 20% of child deaths, about 2 million annually. Current initiatives are based on the idea that:

- Most fatal pneumonias are bacterial (particularly *Streptococcus pneumoniae* and *Haemophilus influenzae*).
- Timely antibiotic treatment reduces case fatality.
- Simple algorithms based on counting respiratory rates are sensitive and adequately specific to identify children who require antibiotics.
- Health workers can use the algorithms, select appropriate treatment, administer antibiotics in

Table 38.3 **Immunization programmes**

Age	Vaccines	Where hepatitis B transmission common	Where hepatitis B transmission less common
Birth	BCG	HB1	
6 weeks	DTP1, OPV1	HB2	HB1
10 weeks	DTP2, OPV2		HB2
14 weeks	DTP3, OPV3	HB3	HB3
9 months	Measles, yellow fever*		

* Where yellow fever is a risk.
(BCG = bacille Calmette–Guérin; DTP = diphtheria, tetanus and pertussis vaccine; OPV = oral polio vaccine; HB = hepatitis B)

the community, counsel parents, follow children up and refer in case of complications. The World Health Organization (WHO) algorithm classifies a respiratory illness as pneumonia if the respiratory rate is greater than 50 per minute in a child older than 3 months. This model is being introduced in a number of countries but has yet to be rolled out world-wide.

Q6. What is your opinion of the WHO strategy for the Integrated Management of Childhood Illness (IMCI) as a model for ambulatory paediatric clinics in the UK?

A strategy adopted by the WHO, IMCI grew out of the knowledge that most childhood deaths occurred as a result of five conditions: pneumonia, diarrhoea, measles, malnutrition and malaria. A sick child may be suffering from more than one condition, individual symptoms and signs can arise from a number of conditions, and there is an opportunity to integrate programmes such as CDD and ARI into a more holistic package. The IMCI strategy has three components:

- Improving the skills of health personnel in the prevention and treatment of childhood illness
- Improving health systems to deliver quality care
- Improving family and community practices in relation to child health.

The introductory phase involves orientation of country decision-makers, creation of the necessary management structure, and extensive discussions with ministries of health. A national strategy is devised, IMCI guidelines are adapted for local use, and activities begin in a number of districts. These activities generally involve training of healthcare workers, health system strengthening and dialogue with communities about child health problems.

From a clinical point of view, health workers are trained to approach the sick child systematically: to check initially for danger signs, assess the main symptoms, assess nutrition and immunization status and feeding problems, and check for other problems. This allows classification into one of three groups: children who need urgent referral, children who can be managed at an outpatient health facility and children who can be managed at home. The first dose of treatment is given on site and the health worker counsels the family on subsequent treatment and follow-up. This systematic approach improves the quality of care, provider morale and client satisfaction. It also leads to more rational drug use.

http://www.who.int/child-adolescent-health/integr.htm

IMCI integrated approach to the management of childhood illness

Major infections

Malaria

Around 90% of the 1 million annual deaths from malaria occur in sub-Saharan Africa, mostly in pregnant women and children under 5. Malaria morbidity and mortality have actually increased over the last decade. In areas of low endemicity where immunity is not usually acquired, malaria during pregnancy doubles or triples the risk of death. In areas of high endemicity, infection during pregnancy tends to exacerbate anaemia and is associated with low birth weight in infants. About 500 000 African children develop cerebral malaria each year, of whom up to 20% die and about 7% are left with permanent neurological damage.

The 'Roll Back Malaria' campaign, launched in 1998, aims to halve the deaths from malaria by 2010. The key interventions for reducing malarial deaths are preventive — bed nets, particularly when treated with insecticides, household insecticide spraying — and therapeutic — treatment with standard drugs, and particularly artemisinin derivatives for resistant strains of *Plasmodium falciparum*. Although insecticide-treated bed nets are effective, increasing their usage has been problematic. At present, less than a fifth of children in Africa sleep under a net and as few as 2% sleep under a net that has been impregnated with insecticide. A growing threat is that of resistance in the *P. falciparum* parasite. Chloroquine resistance is now the norm in much of Africa and resistance to sulfadoxine–pyrimethamine is increasing. Combination therapy, including artemisinin derivatives, is likely to be the best strategy, but there are serious cost issues unless it is subsidized. Pregnant women can be offered intermittent preventive treatment with at least two doses of antimalarial to reduce the burden of placental infection and low birth weight.

HIV/AIDS (see also p. 277)

About 2 million children are currently living with HIV, 1.9 million of them in Africa. About half a million children die each year from complications of HIV/AIDS. Around 90% of HIV infections in children are acquired perinatally. About a third of perinatally infected children do not reach 1 year of age, and over half die before the age of 2. Progression is generally more rapid in children than in adults. Recurrent bacterial infections are common, HIV viral loads tend to be higher and opportunistic infections tend to be more aggressive. HIV/AIDS is cutting a swathe through the developing world, decimating the population of working age — including healthcare workers and schoolteachers — and leaving a growing pool of orphans in the care of overstretched communities and the elderly. Current initiatives include a drive towards having one agreed national HIV/AIDS action framework, one national AIDS authority and one country-level monitoring system.

Voluntary counselling and testing (VCT) acts as an entry point for HIV prevention and care, and is particularly important so that women can be offered treatment to prevent perinatal mother-to-child transmission (PMTCT). Untreated, the transmission rate of HIV-1 is about 35%. About half of this is explained by breastfeeding, another tranche by perinatal transmission and a smaller proportion by transmission in utero. Risk factors for PMTCT include new infection in mothers, high plasma viral loads, advanced disease, breast problems and prolonged breastfeeding. It is also possible that exclusive breastfeeding poses less of a risk than mixed feeding with breast milk and other liquids or solids.

There are four important ways to prevent MTCT. The first is to prevent a woman from ever acquiring the virus, through self-determination and safe sex. In the event of infection, MTCT can be reduced by operative delivery, by prophylactic antiretroviral therapy, and by changes in breastfeeding practice. In places where a woman receives zidovudine from 28 weeks' gestation onward, both mother and baby receive one dose of oral nevirapine and breastfeeding is avoided, transmission rates are as low as 1%.

Breastfeeding is the most controversial current issue. Attitudes vary since, on the one hand, breastfeeding may lead to around 300 000 HIV infections each year, and on the other hand, breastfeeding may prevent up to 1.5 million child deaths each year. The best analyses suggest that the risk of transmission increases by about 4% for every 6 months of breastfeeding.

Strategies to reduce PMTCT of HIV through breastfeeding in poor settings

- Exclusive breastfeeding during the first 6 months
- Shortening the duration of breastfeeding to about 6 months
- Good lactation management to avoid problems such as cracked nipples, engorgement and mastitis
- If a mother develops mastitis or abscesses, frequent expression of milk from the affected side (the mother should discard this milk, continuing feeding from the unaffected side)
- Use of condoms throughout the lactation period

- Encouragement of mothers with AIDS or low CD4 counts to replacement-feed
- Support for replacement feeding, if it is chosen.

Tuberculosis (see also p. 284)

Someone in the world is infected with *Mycobacterium tuberculosis* every second, someone dies from tuberculosis every 15 seconds and a third of all deaths are in children. The WHO declared tuberculosis a global emergency in 1993. Around 3.6 million cases are notified annually but the true prevalence may reach 10 million.

Tuberculosis is difficult to diagnose in children; symptoms and signs are less specific, sputum samples are hard to get, and tuberculin test responsiveness is diminished with malnutrition and HIV/AIDS. Induced sputum may be useful and rapid T cell antigen tests are under trial. BCG vaccine is of variable utility. It reduces the incidence of meningeal and miliary tuberculosis by about 75% in infants and children and probably protects against *M. leprae*, but does not reduce the population prevalence of infection.

The current aim is therefore to treat infected people through case-finding and treatment, which will in turn protect children from exposure. The WHO strategy relies on diagnosis via sputum smear microscopy and short-course directly observed therapy (DOTS) with a standardized regimen. In a typical case, therapy would last for 6 months: 2 months of a daily four-drug regimen followed by 4 months of a thrice-weekly two-drug regimen. Presently, about 30% of people diagnosed with tuberculosis receive DOTS management.

Two major concerns for tuberculosis control are HIV/AIDS and the development of multidrug-resistant tuberculosis (MDR-TB). Development of active tuberculosis is anything from six to 100 times more likely in the presence of HIV infection. In sub-Saharan Africa, 70% of people with AIDS develop tuberculosis, and — conversely — progression of HIV/AIDS accelerates in the presence of tuberculosis. HIV/AIDS also modifies the clinical picture of tuberculosis (the 'new tuberculosis'). Extrapulmonary disease is more common, sputum smear microscopy and tuberculin tests are more often negative, and chest X-rays often atypical. Although treatment regimens are similar, case fatality rates are higher, and drug interactions and adverse effects are more common. The rise of MDR-TB has been mapped to a number of global hot spots in which its prevalence is over 3%, although in some areas it reaches 30%. Standardization of treatment is recommended in order to:

- Reduce the exposure of *M. tuberculosis* to a wide range of drugs
- Ensure drugs are used in combination and not singly
- Optimize cure rates.

Neonatal health

neonatal health and care outside the UK

You are representing your department at an international meeting on newborn health and care at the WHO in Geneva. Before attending the meeting, you are keen to find out more about the problems of neonatal health outside the UK.

Q1. What is the burden of neonatal disease in the developing world?

Q2. What are the major causes of global newborn mortality?

Q3. What are the causes and consequences of being born with a low birth weight? What risks does a low birth weight present to an infant?

Q4. What are the essential principles of newborn care worldwide?

Q5. How might neonatal mortality be reduced in settings where resources are extremely limited and there is no access to neonatal units in hospitals? What is meant by 'levels of care'?

Q1. What is the burden of neonatal disease in the developing world?

Of the 130 million babies born every year, about 4 million die in the first 4 weeks of life: the neonatal period. A similar number of babies are stillborn, i.e. they die in the last 4 months of pregnancy. About half a million mothers also die from the complications of pregnancy and childbirth. Almost all maternal and neonatal deaths (99%) occur in low- or middle-income countries rather than the wealthy industrialized world, and about half occur at home. Three-quarters of deaths occur in the first week, and the highest risk is on the first day after birth.

Q2. What are the major causes of global newborn mortality?

Globally the three main causes of death are estimated to be preterm birth (28%), severe infections (26%) and asphyxia (23%). Neonatal tetanus accounts for a much smaller proportion of deaths but is easily preventable through maternal vaccination. Other infections include newborn septicaemia resulting from an unhygienic delivery or poor cord care, and pneumonia. Malaria

exerts a more indirect effect in pregnancy by increasing the risk of low birth weight and stillbirth.

Asphyxia refers to an impairment of exchange of respiratory gases (oxygen and carbon dioxide), leading to neurological impairment in the newborn infant. Most commonly asphyxia results from a delayed or obstructed labour, or from failure of a birth attendant to resuscitate or assist breathing adequately after birth. The best way of assessing the severity of birth asphyxia in a newborn infant is to use a clinical scoring method to grade the severity of neonatal encephalopathy (grade 1, mild; grade 2, moderate; and grade 3, severe). There have been few studies on the epidemiology of asphyxia and encephalopathy in the developing world, but these show fresh stillbirth rates are 10–20 times higher than in rich countries, that encephalopathy rates are 2–3 times higher, and that survival of moderately or severely encephalopathic infants is poor.

Prematurity, rather than growth retardation, is probably the biggest risk to a newborn infant. Being born 1 or 2 months before the due date hugely increases the risk of newborn death in communities where special nursing care for low-birth weight babies is not available. Another indirect cause of neonatal deaths is hypothermia, which occurs throughout the world and in all climates, and is due to lack of knowledge rather than lack of equipment. Less than 5% die from other causes such as jaundice and haemolytic disease of the newborn. It is important to appreciate that a death may result from multiple causes, and the assignment of cause of death in the neonatal period is extremely difficult.

Direct causes of stillbirths include hypoxia during labour, asphyxia during delivery, infections such as HIV, malaria, maternal syphilis and chorioamnionitis, and congenital anomalies.

Q3. What are the causes and consequences of being born with a low birth weight? What risks does a low birth weight present to an infant?

Amongst the indirect causes of neonatal and perinatal death low birth weight, a weight of less than 2.5 kg at birth, is the most important. Causes of low birth weight are complex and often stem from the effects of poverty in past generations. An important factor is the health and nutrition of the mother and other risk factors include untreated maternal infections, demanding physical work, the use of smoking, alcohol and drugs, and short inter-pregnancy intervals.

Low birth weight increases the risk of neonatal death and also the risk of complications later in pregnancy. More recently, researchers have identified a link between fetal and infant growth and the risk of diseases in adult life such as hypertension, ischaemic heart disease and diabetes. Programming of fetal physiology such as cortisol secretion in response to stress, insulin resistance and vascular responsiveness are thought to be some of the underlying mechanisms.

Q5. How might neonatal mortality be reduced in settings where resources are extremely limited and there is no access to neonatal units in hospitals? What is meant by 'levels of care'?

It is often believed, mistakenly, that good newborn care requires specialist units, high technology and expensive resources. In fact the principles of essential newborn care were laid down by Pierre Budin, a French obstetrician, in 1905 (Box 38.2). These principles can be implemented by mothers or health workers in the home or health centre, without access to expensive technology.

The top priority is to maintain an airway through clearance of secretions or by laying the baby on his or her side or in a prone position. Gentle stimulation of the baby may initiate breathing if there is apnoea. Some programmes have shown that primary care workers or even traditional birth attendants can be trained to conduct resuscitation of an apnoeic infant using a tube and mask or a bag and mask.

The most effective and reliable way to maintain body temperature and prevent hypothermia is to nurse the baby, skin-to-skin, on the mother's chest, the warmest part of her body. This has the added advantage of improving the chance of early breastfeeding. Skin-to-skin nursing has been shown to be more effective than incubator management in maintaining a steady body temperature, except in situations where the baby is sick or unstable.

Exclusive breastfeeding provides all nutritional needs, protects against infection, boosts passive immunity through immunoglobulins in colostrum, promotes thermal care and bonding with the mother, and guarantees excellent growth in infancy. There are serious risks in formula feeding in poor communities where

BOX 38.2 Principles of essential newborn care

Air	Maintain airway
Warmth	Keep warm
Love	Keep with mother
Food	Feed frequently, breastfeed immediately, avoid pre-lacteals
Hygiene	Avoid infection
Illness	Treat promptly

BOX 38.3 Interventions to reduce neonatal mortality

During pregnancy
- Tetanus toxoid
- Iron and folate supplementation
- Insecticide-treated bed nets and intermittent treatment for malaria
- Dietary supplements
- Birth preparedness
- Screening for sexually transmitted infections (STIs) and HIV
- Antiretroviral treatment to prevent mother-to-child transmission (MTCT) of HIV

During childbirth
- A companion
- A skilled attendant
- Caesarean for obstructed labour
- Safe delivery kits
- Tube and mask resuscitation using air not oxygen
- Nevirapine to reduce MTCT

During the newborn period
- Drying and wrapping; skin-to-skin 'kangaroo care'; avoidance of early baths
- Early breastfeeding and colostrum
- Clean cord care
- Antibiotics for infants with signs of sepsis
- Avoid separation from mother

water supplies are unsafe and illiteracy high. Failure to thrive, gastroenteritis and death are markedly increased in non-breastfed infants.

Hygiene is a critical element in reducing perinatal sepsis for both mothers and infants. A clean surface for delivery, hand-washing by birth attendants and clean cutting of the cord will prevent a large number of unnecessary deaths. A recent cluster randomized controlled trial of training traditional birth attendants in Pakistan showed a reduction in perinatal mortality and a large diminution in perinatal sepsis.

The problem in tackling newborn deaths is not that we do not know what to do. There are many potential low-cost and evidence-based interventions available to reduce newborn mortality. The challenge is how to implement these interventions on a large scale, reaching out to the families who are most at risk, particularly those where home delivery is the norm and access to obstetric and medical services is difficult (Box 38.3).

Levels of perinatal care (Box 38.4)

It is important to establish what should be the minimum standards of care at each level of a health system.

Level 1	Home/domiciliary/traditional birth attendant
Level 2	Health centre/small hospital
Level 3	Large district hospital
Level 4	Regional referral hospital

World Bank studies show that, in most developing countries, more than 90% of women living in the poorest quintile of households deliver their babies at home, usually with only a relative or a traditional birth attendant. The care provided at level 1 is therefore extremely important if neonatal mortality rates are to be reduced. In India a controlled, though not randomized, trial showed that mortality fell by 62% in villages where a home-based care package was introduced involving traditional birth attendant training, health education and the use of village women trained to detect and manage neonatal sepsis using injectable antibiotics in the home. In Nepal, a cluster randomized controlled trial of a participatory intervention involving women's groups addressed maternal and newborn health problems in a large rural population. The women's groups showed astonishing creativity and self-organizing capacity. They developed their own delivery kits, stretcher schemes, emergency funds and discussion groups using picture cards for illiterate women. After 2 years, even though health services remained weak, newborn mortality fell by one-third and maternal deaths by three-quarters. The cost of this demand-side intervention was just $0.75 per head.

 http://www.child.ich.ucl.ac.uk

UCL Centre for International Health and Development

Nutrition and malnutrition

Causes of malnutrition

Malnutrition is essentially the end result of the interaction of three factors: diet, diseases and care.

Diet

Dietary intake should be assessed for macronutrient and micronutrient content and quality. Macronutrient intake comes from carbohydrate, fat and protein; the protein:energy ratio should exceed 15%. Micronutrients come from specific foods such as green leafy vegetables and carotene-containing fruits for vitamin A, meat for iron and fish for zinc. Poor dietary intake is caused by:

- *Inadequate nutritional knowledge*: parents/carers may not know what foods children need. Peer culture and food taboos are affected by commercial pressures/advertising.
- *Poverty*: nutritional knowledge may be adequate but poverty prevents parents/carers from purchasing foods that enable satisfactory growth and health of children.
- *Political factors*: wars prevent access to food.
- *Psychological factors*: anorexia nervosa.

 http://ivacg.ilsi.org/

International Vitamin A Consultative Group

 http://www.sphereproject.org/

Sphere Project Training of Trainers courses

Disease

Illnesses such as pertussis, otitis media, inflammatory bowel disease and cystic fibrosis and infections such as tuberculosis, HIV and persistent diarrhoea are often complicated by malnutrition. There are several mechanisms:

- *Poor dietary intake*: painful mouth, cough and systemic infection (leading to elevated inflammatory cytokines that cause anorexia) prevent adequate food intake.
- *Malabsorption*: persistent diarrhoea (e.g. in coeliac disease and *Giardia* infection) causes malabsorption of fat and fat-soluble vitamins. High-lactose diets contribute to diarrhoea in clinical lactase deficiency.
- *Increased nutrient requirements*: energy expenditure is increased in systemic infection by around 10% for each degree Celsius rise in body temperature.
- *Metabolic responses*: inflammatory response causes reduction of plasma levels of micronutrients including vitamin A and zinc, and liver transport proteins such as albumin and retinol binding protein. Catabolic responses cause muscle breakdown and increased urinary nutrient loss.

Care

Lack of time and/or compassion lead to inadequate nutritional intake. A poor social environment at home where nurturing is absent, or an unsupportive feeding/nutrition culture in hospital/clinic causes malnutrition, especially if the patient has anorexia.

Diagnosis

Certain malnutrition syndromes have specific clinical signs such as severe malnutrition (previously called protein energy malnutrition) or deficiency of vitamin A, iodine or vitamin D. However, the majority of children have subclinical malnutrition.

 http://indorgs.virginia.edu/iccidd/

International Council for the Control of Iodine Deficiency Disorders

Subclinical malnutrition

Diagnosing this form of malnutrition requires the use of anthropometric measurements and blood assays. Interpretation of blood assays in subclinical micronutrient malnutrition is difficult because of the variation in plasma levels of micronutrients such as retinol or zinc that occurs in inflammation. Evidence that a micronutrient deficiency is present in a population comes mainly from trials of micronutrient interventions, which have shown the impact of vitamin A deficiency on eye disease and mortality and the impact of zinc deficiency on diarrhoeal disease and mortality. Even children with satisfactory anthropometric indices (weight and height against international standards for their age) may have subclinical micronutrient malnutrition.

Severe malnutrition (SM)

SM is defined as the presence of pedal oedema or severe wasting (below 3 SD weight for height standard or below 70% median weight/height standard). There are several clinical syndromes:

- *Marasmus* is characterized by severe visible wasting with lack of body fat and loss of muscle mass around the arms, buttocks and thighs.
- *Kwashiorkor* involves severe pedal oedema, sometimes spreading all over the body and often associated with cracking of the skin; there may be discoloration of the hair in kwashiorkor. Plasma albumin is lower in kwashiorkor than in marasmus.

Causes

- Poor dietary intake of energy, protein and micronutrients
- Precipitating infection such as measles, persistent diarrhoea, tuberculosis and HIV
- Early cessation of breastfeeding
- Psychosocial stress within family.

Clinical features

- Poor resistance to infection, especially pneumonia, diarrhoea and tuberculosis

- Hypothermia
- Hypoglycaemia
- Dehydration: often under-diagnosed in kwashiorkor because of interstitial fluid and over-diagnosed in marasmus because of loss of skin elasticity
- Metabolic problems: decreased inability to excrete sodium adequately and tendency to develop fluid overload, leading to cardiac failure.

Prevention

Improving household food security, nutrition knowledge and care in poor communities is vital, as are promoting family hygiene and sanitation, ensuring immunizations and deworming, encouraging early treatment for childhood illnesses and protecting children in adverse circumstances, including political crises, wars and famines.

Management

1. *Initial stabilization phase* (1–7 days). This involves treatment of fluid and electrolyte imbalance and sepsis, corneal ulceration due to vitamin A deficiency, severe anaemia, hypoglycaemia, hypothermia and infection. Infections are difficult to diagnose on clinical grounds, as signs are less striking in SM. All children with SM should receive a broad-spectrum antibiotic. Refeeding starts with small frequent meals of low osmolality and low lactose providing around 75 kcal/kg body weight/day until oedema clears.
2. *Catch-up growth*. This requires at least 100 kcal/kg body weight/day for at least 2–6 weeks. Avoid over-feeding, which may precipitate cardiac failure. Use low-sodium rehydration solutions (60 mmol). Multiple micronutrient supplements (WHO formula) are added to the feed. Once infection is controlled and the child is gaining weight, ferrous sulphate may be added. Oral vitamin A should be given on admission.
3. *Follow-up*. It is important to maintain an adequate dietary intake once the child is at home. Ready-to-use therapeutic feeds can be made up using local mixes of groundnuts, sugar, oil and micronutrients in heat-sealed bags, which can be given to mothers during regular visits to the nutrition unit for checking that weight gain is maintained. Sensory stimulation and emotional support are important to ensure recovery of child development. Rates of weight gain during the rehabilitation phase can exceed the normal (1 g/kg body weight/day) for children between 1 and 5 years. Weight gain of at least 5–10 g/kg body weight/day should be achieved. SM is increasingly precipitated by HIV and antiretroviral drugs may be used.

Table 38.4 Deficiency syndromes, their causes and management

Deficiency	Clinical features	Prevention/treatment
Vitamin A	Xerophthalmia in severe cases Night blindness Reduced immunity	Mango, papaya, yellow sweet potatoes, carrots, palm oil
Zinc	Subclinical deficiency common Acrodermatitis enteropathica	Fish and meat Attention to cooking methods to reduce phytate levels
Thiamine	Beri-beri (peripheral neuropathy and cardiac failure)	Thiamine i.m. for beri-beri
Riboflavin	Angular stomatitis Anaemia	Avoid over-reliance on cereals Riboflavin orally
Niacin	Diarrhoea, dermatitis and dementia	Varied diet Thiamine orally
Vitamin C	Clinical signs rare (scurvy)	Ensure fruit in diet and avoid excessive boiling of vegetables
Iodine	Goitre, intellectual loss Poor growth	Supplement with iodine to combat deficiency in soil Treat with iodized salt
Iron	Anaemia in severe cases Impaired psychomotor development	Meat eating
Vitamin D	Rickets	Ensure adequate exposure to light
Folic acid	Megaloblastic anaemia Atrophic glossitis	Treat with folic acid

Deficiency syndromes

Disease or disability may arise as a result of a number of specific deficiency syndromes or a combination of multiple deficiency disorders. Table 38.4 lists the major features of deficiency syndromes.

 More detailed information is given on the website.

 http://www.ennonline.net

Emergency Nutrition Network

 http://www.who.int/child-adolescent-health/ publications/CHILD_HEALTH/WHO_FCH_CAH_ 00.1.htm

Management of the child with a serious infection or severe malnutrition

Children in difficult circumstances (CDC)

Who are children in difficult circumstances?

The term 'children in difficult circumstances' describes a number of different categories of children who, as the name implies, live in difficult or extreme situations. The terminology in this area varies between countries and organizations, something you need to be aware of for Web searches. The other names frequently used for CDC are shown in Box 38.5.

> **BOX 38.5 Other names for children in difficult circumstances**
>
> - Children in especially difficult circumstances (CEDCs)
> - Children in special circumstances (CSCs)
> - Children in need of special protection (CNSP)
> - Children at risk
> - Vulnerable children
> - Orphans and vulnerable children, made vulnerable through HIV (OVC)

The major groups generally classified as CDC are:
- Children living and working on the street
- Child workers
- Orphans (usually now defined as having lost one or both parents)
- Children living with HIV
- Refugees and migrants
- Child soldiers
- Sexually abused and exploited children (including those involved in prostitution and pornography).

Some countries and organizations would also include:
- Children in custodial care
- Children of imprisoned mothers
- Child/adolescent mothers
- Child carers
- Children of substance-abusing parents
- Children of parents with learning difficulties.

There is, however, considerable overlap between many of these groups. For example, nearly all street children are also working children and being in one group makes a child vulnerable to other forms of exploitation. For example, orphans are more likely to end up living and working on the street or in child labour, and girls in domestic service are particularly vulnerable to physical and sexual abuse.

We should not assume, however, that difficult circumstances are always harmful to children. Children respond very differently to adverse circumstances. Some children gain strength and resilience as a result of adverse situations. For many the circumstances will be the norm in their experience. For example, many children in poor communities would expect to work throughout childhood alongside their peers.

How many children are involved?

We know that huge numbers of children around the world can be classified as CDC but it is very difficult to estimate actual figures for several reasons:

- In the countries where the numbers are greatest, information collection systems are usually very poor.
- Many of the activities of CDC are illegal and hence hidden.
- Governments are not motivated to reveal real figures, even if they had them, for fear of criticism.

Furthermore, where figures are available, they are rarely disaggregated by age and sex, which are both key determinants in terms of vulnerability, exploitation and risk of long-term damage. For example, it may be quite acceptable for a 16-year-old to work on a plantation, but it is certainly not acceptable for a 6-year-old.

So, although global and national estimates should be treated with caution, they do give some indication of the magnitude of the problems. Some official estimates, mainly sourced from UN organizations, are shown in Box 38.6.

An influential UNICEF report has helped us to understand the impact on children of war alone. The report (UNICEF 2000) looked at the effect of wars from 1986 to 1996 and found that:

- 2 m children were killed
- 6 m children were injured
- 12 m children were made homeless
- > 1 million children were orphaned or separated from their parents.

What are the causes of difficult circumstances?

Clearly the causes are multifactorial and will vary by situation and country. The major causes are:

> **BOX 38.6 Some global estimates for children in difficult circumstances**
>
> - 210 m children aged 5–14 economically active (International Labour Organization (ILO) 2004)
> - 110 m children aged 5–14 involved in hazardous or intolerable labour (ILO 2004)
> - 10–100 m street children (depending on definition) (United Nations Children's Fund (UNICEF) 1998)
> - 10 m children involved in the sex industry (UNICEF 2003)
> - 300 000 children used in armed conflict (ILO 2003)
> - 14 m children have lost one or both parents to HIV/AIDS (Joint United Nations Programme on HIV/AIDS (UNAIDS) 2004)

- Poverty
- Disruption of family and support systems:
  - Conflict
  - Urbanization (rural to urban migration)
  - Children separated from families to seek work
- Deficiencies in the educational system: inaccessible, unaffordable and poor-quality schooling
- Ineffective enforcement of relevant legislation.

What is the relevant legislation?

In most countries this is based on the UN Convention on the Rights of the Child (UNCRC, 1989). This has been a highly influential document in defining rights of all children (defined as under the age of 18) around the world. All but two countries (the US and Somalia) have ratified the Convention and most have incorporated much of the content into national legislature.

The UNCRC has 41 articles, which set standards for the rights of all children to survive, develop, be protected and participate fully in society. Articles include guarantees of:

- Health, education and care
- Protection from violence
- Protection from economic exploitation.

There are also important optional protocols on involvement of children in armed conflict and the sale of children for prostitution and pornography.

Clearly many governments cannot guarantee these rights, partly because of resource constraints, but all signatory countries report to the UN Committee on the Rights of the Child and they need to demonstrate progress at least towards meeting the obligations and standards in UNCRC.

http://www.unicef.org/crc

Full text of the UNCRC

Examples of CDC

There are clearly many CDCs in the UK, but here we are going to focus on the two largest groups from a global perspective: working children, and children who live and work on the street.

Working children

Child labour is defined by the ILO as all economic activities carried out by persons less than 15 regardless of their occupational status, except household work in the parents' or carers' home. An estimated 210 million children under the age of 15 (or 20% of all children in the age group) are involved in some form of economic activity. Around 120 million work full-time while the rest combine work with some form of education. The highest prevalence of child work is in sub-Saharan Africa, where around 40% of all children are primarily involved in work. This compares with around 25% in Asia and 12% in Latin America.

What work do children do?

The major categories of child work are shown in Box 38.7.

Agriculture is clearly by far the most common form of child work, and children in rural areas are twice as likely to be working than children in urban areas. Agricultural work ranges from (usually unpaid) work on family land to plantation work within the formal sector.

Child labour is a necessity for many poor families, who rely on the income or help provided by their children to survive. This fact is acknowledged in the legislative framework for child labour, which is based on the UNCRC. What the legislation now recognizes is that abolition of child labour is not realistic in the foreseeable future, but that policy approaches should instead target work that is harmful to children for early

BOX 38.7 Types of child work	
Agriculture	70%
Domestic work	15%
Manufacturing	8%
Transport	4%
Construction	2%
Mining and quarrying	1%

(Data from 26 countries, ILO 2003)

BOX 38.8 Potential health hazards of child labour

General
- Exhaustion, abuse, loss of educational opportunity*

Agricultural work
- Injuries, pesticides, parasitic diseases, heat

Mining/construction
- Accidents, respiratory illness, musculoskeletal problems

Manufacturing
- Injuries, hearing loss, exposure to toxins/solvents

Domestic service
- Physical/sexual abuse

Street work
- Road traffic accidents, violence, substance abuse

Sex work
- STIs/HIV, violence

* Loss of educational opportunity leads indirectly to poor long-term health, partly through lower earning power, lower socioeconomic status and lower health knowledge. This health disadvantage is now known to extend to the next generation. The education of women is particularly important in improving health outcomes for children.

intervention. Harmful in this context means work that is likely to harm the health, safety or morals of children. Clearly the health of children is crucial to this definition

What are the health effects of child labour?

There is poor evidence of harm to health in many sectors of child labour (partly because of lack of systematic rigorous studies) but we can make certain assumptions (Box 38.8).

http://www.ilo.org/public/english/support/publ/chilwork.pdf

'Children at Work: Health and Safety Risks': a good summary of the potential health hazards

Three final points demonstrate the difficulties in trying to improve conditions for children who have to work:
- Workplace regulations often apply only to employees in the formal sector and most children work in the informal sector.
- Because children are 'not allowed' to work there is often no legislation to protect them from the more hazardous tasks.

BOX 38.9 The two types of street children

Children *of* the streets
- Street is the child's home
- Seek shelter, food, companionship among other street dwellers
- Abandoned, orphaned, runaways
- Relatively small numbers, probably less than 10% of the total

Children *on* the streets
- Have family connections
- Go home (family/extended family/caring adult) to sleep
- Just work on the street

- For the same reason protective clothing and devices are often simply not made in child sizes.

Children who live and work on the street

This is the preferred term for what used to be known as street children (although street children is still used as a shorthand). They are defined as children who live or spend time on the streets, supporting themselves and/or their families through various occupations, and who are inadequately cared for/supervised by caring adults.

The reason that the estimates of their numbers vary hugely (from 10 to 100 million) is partly because of the different classifications used. They are usually divided into two categories: children of the streets and children on the streets. The characteristics of the two groups are shown in Box 38.9.

The largest numbers of street children are in Latin America (an estimated 40 million), followed by Asia with 30 million and Africa with 10 million. Boys outnumber girls by a factor of around 10 to 1.

What jobs do street children do?
- Begging
- Hawking to pedestrians, motorists
- Directing vehicles to parking areas for a tip
- Guarding vehicles for a tip
- Selling drugs
- Petty crime
- Collecting paper/rubbish
- Shoe shining
- Girls: mostly begging and prostitution.

What are the health risks for street children?
- Infectious disease, especially gastrointestinal disorders and skin conditions

BOX 38.10 Street children in the Philippines

- Population c. 87 m
- 2.4 m children on the streets
- 70% go home every night
- 5% completely abandoned
- 25% intermittent home support
- 5.5 m children (aged 5–14) in the labour market
- At least 500 000 girls under 15 in domestic service (ILO 2000)
- 60% exposed to hazardous work: 20% biological, 26% chemical, 51% environmental

- Substance misuse: alcohol, tobacco, cannabis, cocaine and especially solvents
- Mental disorders
- Violence
- Poor nutrition
- Limited access to healthcare
- STIs/HIV
- Pregnancy.

Pregnancy has led to the phenomenon of a second generation on the streets of many cities.

A country example
The Philippines is a good example of a country with large numbers of working and street children (Box 38.10).

 http://www.ilo.org

ILO: International Programme for the Elimination of Child Labour (IPEC)

 http://www.streetchildren.org.uk/

An excellent starting point for information on street children

 http://www.ucw-project.org

The Understanding Children's Work group, a collaboration of the ILO, UNICEF and the World Bank

 http://www.unicef.org

Useful information about all types of CDC; now UNICEF collects specific data on child protection

MODULE SIX

Childhood Disorders II

MODULE SEVEN

Stephen Hodges   Susan Bunn

CHAPTER

39

Gastroenterology and hepatology

LEARNING OUTCOMES

By the end of this chapter you should:

- Know and understand the basic science of bowel function
- Know and understand the common methods for investigating the gastrointestinal tract
- Know and understand the causes and management of common paediatric disorders affecting the bowel
- Know and understand the investigation and management of the common liver disorders.

MODULE SEVEN

Diagnostic investigations

In assessing a child for gastrointestinal conditions a careful and thorough history and examination is crucial (Ch. 5).

The tests undertaken can then be approached systematically. Blood tests may be helpful, but abnormalities are usually non-specific and not diagnostic. A diagnosis will generally be confirmed by a series of relevant tests or targeted therapeutic trials.

An ideal test is sensitive, specific, simple, inexpensive, safe, non-invasive, convenient, acceptable to patients and staff, objective, reliable and amenable to serial measurements to permit the assessment of therapeutic interventions. There are no such tests in paediatric gastroenterology, so a number of tests are often used and those chosen for a specific clinical scenario may differ between centres. General principles and applications are discussed below.

Oesophageal pH monitoring

Oesophageal pH monitoring permits the assessment of the frequency and duration of oesophageal acid exposure and its relationship to symptoms. A pH study monitors intra-oesophageal pH, usually over a period of 24 hours. It can be combined with heart rate and saturation monitoring in a young child to investigate whether respiratory events are associated with gastro-oesophageal reflux (GOR).

A pH study is a safe test, but it is invasive and keeping the probe in place may be difficult in toddlers and uncooperative children. It should therefore only be undertaken if the results will influence management.

The test is performed by the transnasal passage of a microelectrode containing a pH sensor into the lower oesophagus. Its position is usually confirmed radiologically. The child is encouraged to eat, drink and continue as near normal activities as possible during the study. The time of any drinks or meals is recorded so that their effect on the study can be assessed. If the study is being performed to see if other clinical features are associated with GOR (coughing, abnormal movements, crying, pain etc.), then the child or carer is asked to record the time of any of these events during the study. The pH data are recorded on to a portable recording device, from which they are downloaded on to a computer and analysed by software programmes. Usually a graph of intra-oesophageal pH against time is produced, on which meals and 'clinical events' can be shown (Fig. 39.1). The 'reflux index' (the percentage of the study in which intra-oesophageal pH is < 4) estimates the total acid exposure time and is considered the most sensitive and specific measure. A reflux index of up to 12% in the first year of life and up to 6% thereafter is considered normal. An abnormal reflux index is found in 95% of children with oesophagitis but the reflux index does not correlate with the severity of oesophagitis. Additionally, it should be remembered that not all children with significant GOR have oesophagitis. The time taken for acid to be cleared from the oesophagus after a reflux episode can also be assessed by a pH study as a proxy for oesophageal motility.

Limitations of the pH study

It is not a diagnostic test for GOR, as any cause of vomiting can cause an abnormal study. Likewise, a negative test does not exclude GOR, as only acid reflux episodes are detected. Postprandial GOR in particular is missed, as the gastric acid is buffered by foodstuffs and the refluxate tends to have a neutral pH. This can be overcome somewhat by using a dual probe technique (a lower and upper pH probe, the lower probe being placed in the stomach and the upper in the lower oesophagus — hence times can be identified when the intragastric pH is neutral and GOR would not be detected). Some centres also advocate that one feed with a relatively low pH (usually apple juice) is given over the study period so that an increase in postprandial reflux can be identified.

Situations in which a pH study is most helpful

A pH study is useful in determining whether symptoms such as pain, crying and abnormal movements (Sandifer's syndrome) are associated with acid reflux or whether GOR could be contributing to airway complications.

It also has a place in assessing the adequacy of acid suppression in children who remain symptomatic despite being treated with a proton pump inhibitor (PPI).

Radiological contrast studies of the gastrointestinal tract

Radiological contrast studies of the gastrointestinal tract play an important role in assessing a child with gastrointestinal symptoms, but like the pH study they also have their limitations. All involve a significant radiation exposure, and some are invasive and unpleasant for the child. Before requesting a contrast study consideration has to be given as to whether it is the best test available to answer the clinical question posed. Contrast studies are particularly good at assessing for anatomical abnormalities causing symptoms. The commonly used contrast studies and their more usual indications are summarized in Table 39.1.

Hydrogen breath tests

The principle of the H_2 breath test is that any undigested/malabsorbed sugar that reaches a part of the gastrointestinal tract that has organisms within the lumen (most usually the colon but also the small bowel in small bowel overgrowth) is then fermented by the organisms, producing H_2, which is excreted in the breath. The breath H_2 monitor is a small hand-held device into which the older child simply exhales. In a younger child breath can be collected by the use of a face mask. Breath H_2 is plotted against time from carbohydrate ingestion on a graph. The normal small bowel transit time is considered to be approximately 2 hours, such that an increase in breath H_2 at baseline or before 2 hours suggests small bowel fermentation and overgrowth, and after 2 hours colonic fermentation due to sugar maldigestion/malabsorption.

If sugar maldigestion/malabsorption is suspected (for example, lactose), then the candidate sugar is given as an oral bolus after fasting. The study would start with two baseline readings at −30 mins and 0 mins, and then the sugar is administered at time 0. Breath H_2 is measured every 30 minutes for 3 hours. Figure 39.2A shows a normal H_2 breath test in red, where there is no increase in breath H_2, as no significant amount of sugar has reached the colon. The results shown in blue are an abnormal H_2 breath test that suggests sugar malabsorption/maldigestion, as there is an increase in breath H_2 after 2 hours when the malabsorbed/maldigested sugar is fermented by colonic bacteria. Figure 39.2B shows a lactulose H_2 breath test, which is the preferred test for small bowel overgrowth. As lactulose is a non-absorbable sugar, in a normal child the pattern

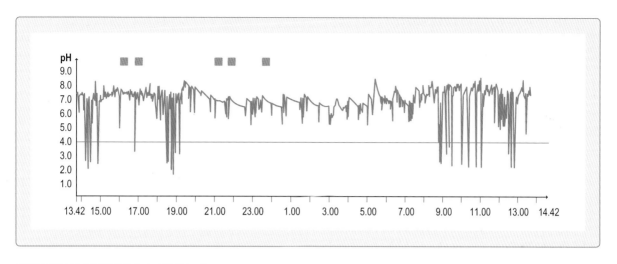

Period table

Item		Total	Upright
Duration of period	(HH:MM)	24:00	24:00
Number of acid refluxes	(#)	31	31
Number of long acid refluxes	(#)	0	0
Longest acid reflux	(min)	1	1
Total time pH below 4.00	(min)	12	12
Fraction time pH below 4.00	(%)	0.8	0.8

▨ Episodes of chest pain
(chest pain not related to
reflux events)

A

Period table

Item		Total
Duration of period	(HH:MM)	23:40
Number of acid refluxes	(#)	392
Number of long acid refluxes	(#)	28
Longest acid reflux	(min)	37
Total time pH below 4.00	(min)	603
Fraction time pH below 4.00	(%)	42.4

B

Fig. 39.1 Results of a pH probe.
(A) Normal pH study in a 12-year-old boy with episodic chest pain. His chest pain is not associated with his (normal) reflux events; (B) pH study in an 8-year-old child with neurodevelopmental delay, showing severe gastro-oesophageal reflux (GOR). She has a reflux index of 42.4% and poor oesophageal clearance of acid, shown by numerous long acid reflux events, the longest being 32 minutes.

Table 39.1 **Radiological contrast studies**

Contrast study	Part of GI tract examined	Indications for use	Conditions identified
Videofluoroscopy	Oropharynx	Concerns regarding aspiration on swallowing Assessment of child's ability to swallow different consistencies of fluid/food safely	Bulbar palsy Pseudo-bulbar palsy
Barium swallow	Oesophagus	Dysphagia To investigate tracheo-oesophageal fistula	Oesophageal pouches/webs/strictures/fistulae
Barium meal	Oesophagus, stomach and duodenum	Recurrent vomiting	Hiatus hernia Gastric outflow obstruction Malrotation (if duodenal–jejunal flexure to right of midline)
Barium meal and follow-through	Oesophagus, stomach, duodenum, jejunum and ileum	To identify presence of small bowel Crohn's disease Partial small bowel obstructive symptoms Note: images are not as good as with small-bowel contrast study	Small bowel Crohn's disease Small bowel strictures due to Crohn's disease or post-surgery
Small-bowel study (requires duodenal intubation)	Duodenum, jejunum and ileum	To identify small bowel Crohn's disease Partial small bowel obstructive symptoms	Small bowel Crohn's disease Small bowel strictures due to Crohn's disease or post-surgery
Contrast enema	Rectum and colon	To reduce intussusception (therapeutic) Very rarely used diagnostically in children	

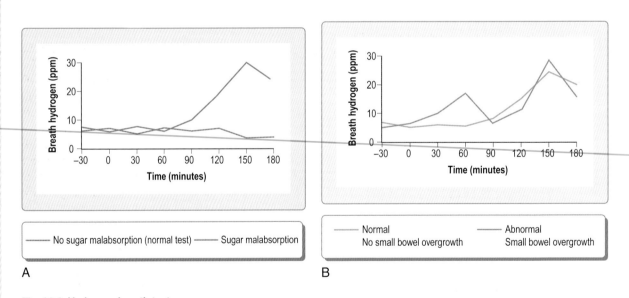

A

B

Fig. 39.2 **Hydrogen breath tests.**
(A) A normal test (red) with no sugar malabsorption, and an abnormal test (blue) when malabsorbed sugar is fermented by colonic bacteria, increasing breath hydrogen; (B) lactulose hydrogen breath test showing a normal test (green) when the non-absorbable sugar is fermented by colonic bacteria, increasing breath hydrogen, and an abnormal test (purple) when small bowel organisms ferment the lactulose, producing an increase in breath hydrogen prior to sugar arriving in the colon (double peak sign).

is as shown in Figure 39.2A; the green line is seen as the non-absorbed lactulose is fermented in the colon. However, in Figure 39.2B the purple line shows an abnormal lactulose hydrogen breath test with an early peak, suggesting that the sugar is being fermented by organisms in the small bowel, and the second peak when the lactulose reaches the colon.

Both false positive and false negative hydrogen breath test results can occur. False positive results are seen with inadequate pretest fasting or recent smoking;

Table 39.2 Serological studies

Antibody	Sensitivity	Specificity
IgA endomysial antibody (IgA EMA)	85–98%	97–100%
IgA tissue transglutaminase antibody (IgA tTG)	90–98%	95–97%
IgA antigliadin antibody (IgA AGA)	80–90%	85–95%
IgG antigliadin antibody (IgG AGA)	75–85%	75–90%

false negative results can be seen after the recent use of antibiotics, in patients with lung disorders or in the approximately 1% of children who are 'non-hydrogen producers'. Oral bacteria may lead to an early hydrogen peak and pretest mouth-washing with an antiseptic is advocated by some units. The H_2 peak occurring from bacterial overgrowth in the distal small intestine may be difficult to discriminate from the normal peak seen when the test sugar reaches the colon. Additionally, rapid delivery of the test sugar to the colon in patients with short bowel syndrome may lead to false positive results.

'Coeliac antibodies'

Four serological studies have been described to aid the diagnosis of coeliac disease (Table 39.2).

Serum IgA endomysial and tissue transglutaminase antibody testing have the highest diagnostic accuracy. The IgA and IgG antigliadin antibody tests have lower diagnostic accuracy, with frequent false positive results, and are therefore no longer recommended for initial diagnostic evaluation or screening. All are less accurate in children under 2 years of age.

The serum antibodies commonly used in testing for coeliac disease are IgA and therefore all have high false negative rates in IgA deficiency. It should be remembered that the coeliac population has a higher rate of IgA deficiency than the non-coeliac population. Thus if coeliac disease is clinically suspected and serum antibodies are checked, IgA deficiency also needs to be excluded. None of the serum antibody tests has 100% sensitivity and specificity and therefore a small bowel biopsy is always needed for a definitive diagnosis. Likewise, when there is a high degree of clinical suspicion a small bowel biopsy needs to be performed, even with negative serological testing.

IgA endomysial antibodies

Endomysial antibodies bind to connective tissue surrounding smooth muscle cells. Serum IgA endomysial antibodies produce a characteristic staining pattern, which is visualized by indirect immunofluorescence. The test result is reported simply as positive or negative, since even low titres of serum IgA endomysial antibodies are specific for coeliac disease. The target antigen has been identified as a tissue transglutaminase.

Anti-tissue transglutaminase antibodies

Enzyme-linked immunosorbent assay (ELISA) tests for IgA anti-tissue transglutaminase antibodies are now widely available and are easier to perform and less costly than the immunofluorescence assay used to detect IgA endomysial antibodies.

IgA EMA, IgA tTG and IgA AGA levels fall with treatment; as a result, these assays can be used as a non-invasive means of monitoring the response and adherence to a gluten-free diet.

Testing for *Helicobacter pylori*

H. pylori can be identified by histological examination or on *Campylobacter*-like organism (CLO) testing of mucosal biopsies collected at upper gastrointestinal endoscopy. However, non-invasive tests have a role in diagnosing *H. pylori* infection and confirming eradication after treatment.

Urea breath testing

H. pylori has the enzyme urease, which converts urea to ammonia and bicarbonate and then carbon dioxide. The presence of this enzyme in the stomach in a child with *H. pylori* infection can be used diagnostically via a stable isotope breath test. In children, urea labelled with C^{13} (non-radioactive) is administered after fasting, usually with fresh orange juice to delay gastric emptying. If *H. pylori* is present the urea is hydrolysed, releasing C^{13}-tagged CO_2, which can be detected in breath samples. Breath is collected and analysed by mass spectrometry. C^{13} is a naturally occurring stable isotope, so it is present in small quantities in the breath, but there is an increase if *H. pylori* infection is present in the stomach. The test is both highly sensitive (> 90%) and specific (> 95%). However, the test becomes less sensitive (has a high rate of false negatives) if used within a month of antibiotic therapy or while the child is taking H_2-blocking agents or PPIs. To prevent false negative results, the child should not have taken antibiotics for at least 4 weeks and antisecretory agents for at least 2 weeks.

H. pylori serology

Laboratory-based serological testing using ELISA to detect IgG or IgA antibodies is inexpensive and widely available. Large studies have found uniformly high

Table 39.3 Common indications for upper gastrointestinal endoscopy and colonoscopy in children

	To diagnose macroscopically or histologically	Therapeutic procedures
Upper GI endoscopy	Reflux oesophagitis Oesophageal/gastric varices Gastritis/gastric ulcer (GU) Duodenitis/duodenal ulcer (DU) *H. pylori* infection Crohn's disease of upper GI tract Enteropathies including coeliac disease (Fig. 39.3)	Dilatation of peptic stricture Sclerotherapy/banding of bleeding varices Bleeding control in bleeding GU/DU Insertion of feeding gastrostomy Passage of nasojejunal tube
Lower GI endoscopy	Polyps Inflammatory bowel disease	Removal of polyps

sensitivity (90–100%) but variable specificity (76–96%). However, the positive and negative predictive values of the test relate to the pretest probability of *H. pylori* in the population being studied. Generally, in children in the UK where the prevalence of *H. pylori* is low, a negative test is helpful to exclude infection, but a positive serological test is more likely to be a false positive. As a result, it is recommended that secondary testing (urea breath test, stool antigen testing, endoscopy) is used to confirm the initial result before initiating treatment. *H. pylori* serology does usually become negative after successful eradication treatment but seroconversion is slow. Serological testing is therefore not useful for follow-up since many patients continue to have antibodies for months or even years after successful eradication therapy.

Stool antigen assay

The presence of *H. pylori* in the stool of infected patients has led to the development of faecal assays. A commercially available enzyme immunoassay is available. The sensitivity and specificity of this test are 94% and 90% respectively when compared to endoscopy and urea breath testing. The stool assay has the same limitations as the urea breath test regarding false negatives after antibiotic use and acid-suppressing drugs.

Confirmation of eradication after treatment

Confirmation of eradication is required after treatment for *H. pylori* and is facilitated by the availability of accurate, relatively inexpensive non-invasive tests. Urea breath testing is the test of choice to confirm eradication of infection. Stool antigen testing is an alternative when urea breath testing is not available, but it is less accurate.

Upper gastrointestinal endoscopy and colonoscopy

These are important tests that are useful both diagnostically and therapeutically. However, they are invasive and in most centres are performed under general anaesthetic. Complications are rare but colonic perforation can occur at colonoscopy. Additionally, colonoscopy requires bowel preparation with laxatives, which most children find unpleasant. Hence, they are only used in selected cases when the symptoms are sufficiently severe, a tissue diagnosis is needed or a therapeutic procedure can be performed.

Common indications for upper gastrointestinal endoscopy and colonoscopy in children are listed in Table 39.3.

Pancreatic function testing

Pancreatic function tests can be either direct or indirect. Direct pancreatic function testing is considered the 'gold standard' but is rarely performed, as it is invasive and requires intubation of the duodenum. Duodenal secretions are aspirated after pancreatic stimulation by intravenous cholecystokinin and secretin or a Lundh test meal (meal composed of standardized nutrients). It allows bicarbonate, amylase, trypsin and lipase to be assayed separately and there are clear normal ranges for comparison.

Several indirect (non-invasive) tests of pancreatic exocrine insufficiency have been developed. Of the available tests, the most commonly used are faecal chymotrypsin and faecal elastase measurements.

Faecal chymotrypsin

Faecal chymotrypsin is easy to measure and levels are stable in stools for several days. Measurement was frequently used in the past as a screening test for pancreatic insufficiency. However, levels are usually low only in advanced pancreatic disease and the sensitivity for pancreatic insufficiency is therefore only 50–60%. Additionally the test cannot be performed when the child is taking pancreatic enzyme replacement therapy.

Faecal pancreatic elastase

Faecal pancreatic elastase estimation is now the most widely used test for pancreatic exocrine insufficiency.

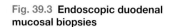
Fig. 39.3 **Endoscopic duodenal mucosal biopsies**

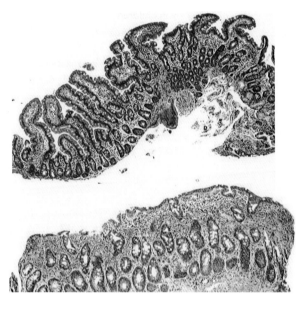

Normal duodenal mucosa with tall, finger-like villi and crypts of normal length

Almost total villous atrophy in a child with coeliac disease with elongation of the crypts, an increase in chronic inflammatory cells and disorganization of the enterocyte layer.

The pancreatic enzyme, elastase 1, is stable during intestinal transit and is measurable as faecal elastase. After 2 weeks of age it has a high sensitivity in the diagnosis of moderate and severe pancreatic insufficiency. The test has a sensitivity and specificity of 93% for pancreatic insufficiency. In addition, its values are independent of pancreatic enzyme replacement therapy and can therefore be used while the child is taking pancreatic enzyme supplements.

Tests of fat malabsorption

If the clinical history suggests significant fat malabsorption (steatorrhoea), then a variety of tests can be employed to identify whether steatorrhoea is present. However, all the tests have limitations and are not universally available.

Currently, the gold standard for diagnosis of steatorrhoea is quantitative estimation of stool fat. The method most commonly used for the measurement of faecal fat is the titrimetric Van de Kamer method. In adults, the test involves a diet containing 100 g of fat for 3–5 days. Stools collected over 72–96 hours are pooled and refrigerated. In children, the collection period is usually 3 days. Children find it difficult to adhere to a strictly regimented diet and therefore a careful dietary record is required to calculate the mean daily fat intake. Steatorrhoea is present if more than 7% of ingested fat is excreted, though infants under 6 months can excrete up to 15% of dietary fat due to the physiological immaturity of the pancreatic and biliary secretions. Despite it being the only quantitative test of fat excretion, 72-hour stool collection is rarely used in children, as it is cumbersome and unpopular with families and laboratory staff. Qualitative (subjective) tests are more commonly used

and faecal Sudan III staining/microscopy and faecal acid steatocrits are the most widely available. Sudan III stain on a spot sample of stool can detect more than 90% of patients with clinically significant steatorrhoea, but it needs to be properly performed and interpreted by an experienced assessor. The acid steatocrit is performed rather like a haematocrit on a spot stool sample and gives the percentage of the stool that is composed of fat. It has a sensitivity of 100%, specificity of 95% and positive predictive value of 90%, as compared to the gold standard 72-hour faecal fat collection.

Enteral and parenteral nutrition

Total or supplementary nutrition can be given via different routes. These routes and their advantages, disadvantages and indications are shown in Table 39.4.

Acute diarrhoea

Diarrhoea is one of the most common causes of morbidity and mortality in children world-wide. World-wide childhood death secondary to diarrhoea declined from an estimated 5 million per year in 1980 to less than 2 million in 1999. The decline is attributed to global improvements in sanitation and the use of oral rehydration therapy (Ch. 38).

Basic science

Gut immunity

The gastrointestinal mucosal immune system protects the mucosal surfaces (400 m^2 surface area in adults)

Table 39.4 Enteral and parenteral routes of nutrition

Route of feed	'Anatomy' of feeding route	Advantages	Disadvantages	Common indications
Oral sip feeds	Drunk by child	No tube	Compliance Needs to like taste	As a supplement when high requirements or poor appetite, e.g. cystic fibrosis, Crohn's disease As therapy in Crohn's disease
Nasogastric	Tube passed via nose to stomach	Easy to place and to remove Can bolus-feed for convenience Can continuously feed	Placement uncomfortable Visible on face Easy to displace or remove accidentally Have to check position before using Blocks easily	Child cannot take full requirements due to problems sucking/swallowing, e.g. cleft palate, neurodisability Child cannot take full requirements due to illness or high requirements, e.g. bronchiolitis, cardiac disease Child needs continuous feeding, e.g. severe GOR, short gut
Nasojejunal	Tube passed via nose to jejunum	Relatively easy to place	Placement uncomfortable Difficult to place and often has to be passed under X-ray screening Position checked by X-ray	Child excessively vomits gastric contents, e.g. severe GOR or gastroduodenal dysmotility Child has pancreatitis (intragastric feeding causes stimulation of pancreas)
Gastrostomy	Tube inserted at endoscopy or surgically into stomach through abdominal wall	Discreet Difficult to pull out accidentally Position does not need to be checked	Needs general anaesthetic for initial insertion Risks of initial surgery Local infections	Child requiring medium- to long-term nutritional support
Jejunostomy	Tube placed surgically into jejunum via abdominal wall	Discreet Difficult to pull out accidentally Position does not need to be checked	Needs general anaesthetic for initial insertion Risks of initial surgery Local infections	Unusual feeding route usually used in child with gastroduodenal dysmotility requiring medium- to long-term nutritional support
Parenteral Peripheral	Intravenous nutrition given via peripheral cannula	Easy to place	Short-term as thrombophlebitis common Have to limit osmolality (and therefore glucose content) of parenteral nutrition Usually inadequate for full nutritional requirements	Child whose gut cannot be used for full nutritional requirements, e.g. post-surgery, during chemotherapy, short gut Short-term nutritional support while awaiting CVL placement
Central	Intravenous nutrition given via central venous line (CVL)	Secure access Can give high glucose concentrations and full nutritional requirements	Needs to be placed under general anaesthetic CVL sepsis a major risk	Child whose gut cannot be used for full nutritional requirements, e.g. post-surgery, during chemotherapy, short gut Can be used long-term

from harmful invasive organisms, but also has to suppress immune responses to food antigens (up to several hundred grams per day, depending on age) and commensal bacteria. Therefore, even under completely physiological conditions, the gastrointestinal tract contains enormous numbers of leucocytes diffusely scattered in the lamina propria and the intraepithelial compartment, or organized in the Peyer's patches and isolated lymphoid follicles of the colon. Combined, they form the gut-associated lymphoid tissue (GALT). In health 40% of lymphocytes in the body are present in the gastrointestinal mucosa and GALT. The majority of them produce dimeric IgA antibodies. At birth, the gut-associated lymphoid tissue possesses the necessary cells with which to serve its function, but having never met foreign antigens, it lacks certain elements found in later life. Full maturity is not achieved for up to 2 years.

Water and electrolyte absorption

In healthy adults the small intestine is presented with approximately 8 litres of fluid each day. This amount includes both ingested liquids and gastrointestinal secretions. By the time the initial 8 litres of fluid reaches the ileocaecal valve, only about 600 ml remains and by the time this reaches the anus, only about 100 ml of fluid

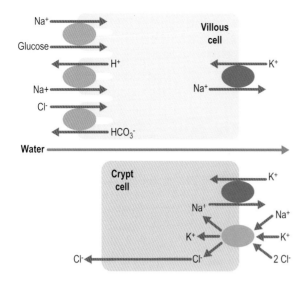

Fig. 39.4 **Main intestinal absorptive/secretory processes for electrolytes and glucose**

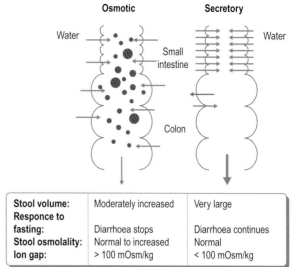

	Osmotic	Secretory
Stool volume:	Moderately increased	Very large
Responce to fasting:	Diarrhoea stops	Diarrhoea continues
Stool osmolality:	Normal to increased	Normal
Ion gap:	> 100 mOsm/kg	< 100 mOsm/kg

Fig. 39.5 **Summary of features of osmotic and secretory diarrhoea**

remains. The efficiency of water absorption in the small and large intestine combined is approximately 99%.

The normal absorption of electrolytes, glucose and water is shown in Figure 39.4.

In the villous cell Na/K adenosine triphosphatase (ATPase) maintains a low intracellular Na concentration, thus allowing the 'downhill' entry of Na, coupled Cl and nutrients. In the crypt cell the low Na concentration drives a carrier in the basolateral membrane coupling the flow of one Na, two Cl and one K from the serosal compartment into the crypt cell. As a result, Cl accumulates above its electrochemical equilibrium and under physiological circumstances leaks into the gastrointestinal lumen across a semipermeable apical membrane. In health the absorptive activity in the villous cell far exceeds the minor secretion from the crypts and the net result is absorption of electrolytes and nutrients. Water absorption then passively follows, mainly through the intercellular tight junctions.

Acute diarrhoea is the abrupt onset of increased fluid content of the stool above the normal value of approximately 10 ml/kg/day. Diarrhoea is the reversal of the normal net absorptive state. This can be due to an osmotic force acting in the lumen to pull water into the gut, as seen in sugar malabsorption (Fig. 39.5). This diarrhoea will stop on fasting. It can also be due to an active secretory state induced in the enterocytes. Secretory diarrhoea continues on fasting. The most common cause of secretory diarrhoea is infection, and different enterotoxins and inflammatory processes affect the transport of electrolytes in different ways. The classic example is cholera enterotoxin-induced diarrhoea, in which there is enhanced anion secretion by the crypt cell and an inhibition of the Na/Cl channels in the apical cell. The consequential increase in electrolytes in the gastrointestinal lumen not only prevents passive water absorption but also reverses water transport, causing water loss into the gastrointestinal tract and profuse watery diarrhoea. The glucose/Na transporter is usually unaffected in infectious secretory diarrhoea, explaining the efficacy of oral rehydration solution.

Infective diarrhoea in the developed world

Approximately 1 in 50 children in developed nations are hospitalized for acute gastroenteritis some time during childhood. More than 95% of this risk occurs in the first 5 years of life.

Viral infections are most common between 6 and 24 months of age, after transplacental antibody is cleared and breastfeeding has stopped and before full acquisition of protective immunity.

Bacterial gastroenteritis is more common in the first few months of life and then again in school-age children. Most bacterial gastroenteritis is due to food-borne pathogens.

Problem-orientated topic:

acute diarrhoea

Karen, an 18-month-old girl, presents with a 2-day history of non-bloody diarrhoea. She is passing more than 8 stools per day. She is pyrexial and vomiting but drinking well and not dehydrated.

Continued overleaf

Q1. What is the likely diagnosis and the most likely pathogen?

Q2. How do the clinical features help with diagnosis?

Q1. What is the likely diagnosis and the most likely pathogen?

The frequency of pathogens isolated in cases of childhood sporadic diarrhoea in developed countries is shown in Table 39.5.

Table 39.5 Frequency of pathogens in acute diarrhoea

Pathogen	Frequency
Viruses	
Rotavirus	25–40%
Calicivirus	1–20%
Astrovirus	4–9%
Adenovirus	2–4%
Norovirus (Norwalk-like virus)	Unknown
Bacteria	
Campylobacter jejuni	6–8%
Salmonella	3–7%
Escherichia coli	3–5%
Shigella	0–3%
Yersinia enterocolitica	1–2%
Clostridium difficile	0–2%
Parasites	
Cryptosporidium	1–3%
Giardia lamblia	1–3%

Q2. How do the clinical features help with diagnosis?

See Table 39.6.

Vomiting and regurgitation

Basic science

Though vomiting can occur due to a wide range of stimuli and causes, regardless of the initiation, the complex vomiting 'reflex' is identical. There are three stages to vomiting:

- *Nausea*: a feeling of wanting to vomit, often associated with autonomic effects including hypersalivation, pallor and sweating. This phase is associated with decreased gastric motility and retrograde propulsion of duodenal contents into the stomach.
- *Retching*: a strong involuntary effort to vomit during which the glottis remains closed and there is contraction of the diaphragm and abdominal muscles.
- *Vomiting*: the expulsion of gastric contents through the mouth after relaxation of the cardia and lower oesophageal sphincter and sustained contraction of the abdominal muscles.

The mechanisms of provocation of vomiting are summarized in Figure 39.6. It should be noted that the presence of an anatomically discreet 'vomiting centre'

Table 39.6 Clinical features of pathogens

Pathogenesis	Predominant site of action	Infective agents	Clinical presentation
Direct cytopathic effect	Proximal small intestine	Rotavirus Adenovirus Calicivirus Norovirus (Norwalk-like virus) Enteropathogenic *E. coli* Giardia	Copious watery diarrhoea, vomiting, mild to severe dehydration; frequent lactose malabsorption; no blood in stools
Enterotoxigenicity	Small intestine	*Vibrio cholerae* Enterotoxigenic *E. coli* (ETEC) Entero-aggregative *E. coli* *Cryptosporidium*	Watery diarrhoea (can be copious in cholera or ETEC); no blood in stools
Invasiveness	Distal ileum and colon	*Salmonella* *Shigella* *Yersinia* *Campylobacter* Entero-invasive *E. coli* *Amoeba*	Dysentery: very frequent stools, cramps, pain, fever and often blood in stools. Variable dehydration. Course may be protracted
Cytotoxicity	Colon	*Clostridium difficile* Enterohaemorrhagic *E. coli* (EHEC) *Shigella*	Dysentery: abdominal cramps, fever, blood in stools. EHEC or *Shigella* may be followed by haemolytic–uraemic syndrome

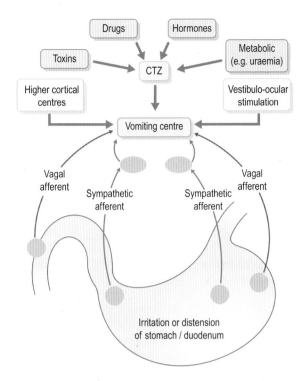

Fig. 39.6 Diagram summarizing the vomiting reflex (CTZ = chemoreceptor trigger zone)

Problem-orientated topic:

regurgitation

Josh, a 4-month-old boy, presents with regurgitation of small volumes of his milk feeds over 20 times per day, particularly in the hour after his feed. He is otherwise well and thriving.

Q1. What is the most likely diagnosis?

Q2. What investigations are indicated?

Q3. What treatment would you consider starting?

Q1. What is the most likely diagnosis?

Gastro-oesophageal reflux (GOR) is the involuntary retrograde flow of gastric contents proximally into the oesophagus. When the gastric contents reach the mouth, this is termed regurgitation. Both are commonly seen in infants. Both regurgitation and GOR are effortless and are not preceded by nausea and retching. The physiology of GOR is summarized in Figure 39.7. Infants and children with GOR have normal resting lower oesophageal sphincter pressures but demonstrate spontaneous relaxation of the lower oesophageal sphincter. It is not clear whether this is a local or centrally mediated process. The drop in the sphincter pressure precedes a drop in intra-oesophageal pH, indicating reflux of gastric contents into the oesophagus (p. 167). The reflux of gastric contents into the distal oesophagus is not caused by an increase in gastric pressure (as in vomiting), as the intragastric pressure remains unchanged.

in the lateral reticular formation of the medulla is now questioned, but there is certainly a central process that functions as a vomiting centre.

The chemoreceptor trigger zone (CTZ) lies outside the blood–brain barrier in the floor of the fourth ventricle. It is stimulated by proemetic agents in the blood or cerebrospinal fluid. Table 39.7 summarizes the effects of antiemetic medication.

Table 39.7 Drugs used to control emesis and their mechanism of action

Drug group	Indication	Mechanism
Antihistamines	Motion sickness and mild chemotherapy-induced vomiting	Labyrinthine suppression via anticholinergic effect H_1-receptor antagonism in vomiting centre
Substituted benzamides e.g. Metoclopramide	Chemotherapy, gastroparesis	D_2-receptor blockade at the CTZ. In high dose has $5\text{-}HT_3$ activity in the gut
$5\text{-}HT_3$ receptor antagonists e.g. Ondansetron	Chemotherapy Postoperative nausea and vomiting	$5\text{-}HT_3$-receptor blockade most important in the gut, but possibly some effect in CTZ and vomiting centre
Benzodiazepines e.g. Lorazepam	Chemotherapy	Central GABA inhibition, producing sedation and anxiolysis
Phenothiazides	Rarely used in children because of extrapyramidal side-effects	D_2-receptor blockade at the CTZ
Butyrophenones e.g. Domperidone	Chemotherapy, gastroparesis, GOR	D_2-receptor blockade at the enteric nervous system

(CTZ = chemoreceptor trigger zone; GABA = gamma-aminobutyric acid; GOR = gastro-oesophageal reflux)

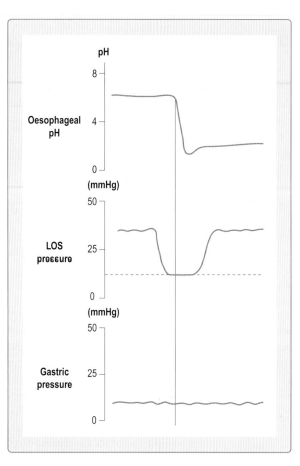

Fig. 39.7 Simultaneous measurements of intra-oesophageal pH, lower oesophageal sphincter (LOS) pressure and intragastric pressure during an episode of gastro-oesophageal reflux

Features of excessive 'physiological' regurgitation in infants

- Natural history: improves with age
- Improves on weaning and on becoming more upright when walking
- Resolution in 80% by 18 months, and in 90–95% by 2 years.

Clinical presentation of gastro-oesophageal reflux disease (GORD) in infants and children is shown in Table 39.8.

Q2. What investigations are indicated?

Many clinicians recommend a therapeutic trial of treatment, rather than investigation. If GOR is clinically suspected and treatment will be implemented, even with a negative test, then the test should not usually be performed. If investigations are indicated, then the investigation chosen depends on the clinical question asked (Table 39.9).

Q3. What treatment would you consider starting?

A general algorithm for treatment is given in Figure 39.8 and a summary of the action of acid-blocking drugs in Box 39.1.

N.B. Cow's milk protein intolerance may mimic GOR and a trial of hypoallergenic formula may be helpful, particularly when there is a strong family history of atopy. Even in families without atopy it is usually recommended before surgical intervention.

Specific management of clinical scenarios

An infant with uncomplicated reflux ('happy puker')

Diagnosis is made on history and examination. No investigations are indicated.

Reassurance without any other specific intervention is usually sufficient. Other treatment options include feed thickeners. Re-evaluation should take place if symptoms worsen or do not improve by the time the child is 18–24 months of age.

Table 39.8 Clinical presentation of gastro-oesophageal reflux disease

	Infants	Children
Excessive regurgitation	Vomiting Growth faltering	Vomiting Growth faltering
Oesophagitis	Irritability with feedings Feeding refusal Arching Haematemesis, anaemia	Heartburn Chest or abdominal pain Dysphagia, odynophagia Haematemesis, anaemia Sandifer's syndrome
Respiratory disorders	Apnoea/stridor Aspiration pneumonia Laryngospasm (apnoea, stridor) Apparent life-threatening events Sudden unexpected death in infancy	Aspiration pneumonia Bronchospasm (asthma) Laryngospasm (apnoea, stridor) Hoarseness

Table 39.9 Regurgitation: investigations based on questions

Question to ask	Test performed
Are there structural abnormalities in the upper GI tract?	Barium meal
Is there a delay in gastric emptying?	Radionucleotide gastric emptying study
Does aspiration occur?	Chest X-ray, videofluoroscopy/barium swallow, bronchoscopy, radionucleotide 'milk scan'
Is oesophagitis present?	Endoscopy and biopsy
Are specific symptoms causally related to GOR?	pH monitoring with event recording
Is a hiatus hernia present?	Barium swallow, endoscopy
Is the quantity of acid GOR abnormal?	pH monitoring
Is there an oesophageal motility disorder?	Barium swallow, oesophageal manometry

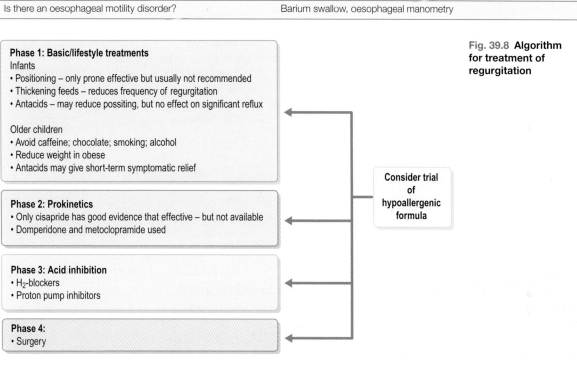

Fig. 39.8 Algorithm for treatment of regurgitation

Phase 1: Basic/lifestyle treatments
Infants
• Positioning – only prone effective but usually not recommended
• Thickening feeds – reduces frequency of regurgitation
• Antacids – may reduce possiting, but no effect on significant reflux

Older children
• Avoid caffeine; chocolate; smoking; alcohol
• Reduce weight in obese
• Antacids may give short-term symptomatic relief

Phase 2: Prokinetics
• Only cisapride has good evidence that effective – but not available
• Domperidone and metoclopramide used

Phase 3: Acid inhibition
• H$_2$-blockers
• Proton pump inhibitors

Phase 4:
• Surgery

Consider trial of hypoallergenic formula

BOX 39.1 Summary of action of acid-blocking drugs

Histamine type 2 receptor antagonists
- Ranitidine, cimetidine
- Inhibit acid secretion by blocking histamine H$_2$-receptors on the parietal cell

Proton pump inhibitors (PPIs)
- Omeprazole, lansoprazole etc.
- Block acid secretion by irreversibly binding to and inhibiting the hydrogen–potassium ATPase pump on the luminal surface of the parietal cell membrane

An infant with recurrent vomiting and poor weight gain

Dietetic assessment is indicated. Poor weight gain despite an adequate intake of calories should prompt evaluation for causes of vomiting and weight loss other than GOR; investigations should include a full blood count, electrolytes, liver function tests, serum ammonia, glucose, urinalysis, urine ketones, reducing substances in the stool and a review of newborn screening tests.

Barium meal is usually required to exclude anatomical abnormalities. An upper endoscopy with biopsy may also be required in selected patients.

If GORD continues to be suspected after the above evaluation, treatment options include:
- Thickening the formula
- Trial of hypoallergenic formula
- Increasing the caloric density of the formula
- Prokinetic therapy, e.g. domperidone (though no evidence in this situation)
- Implementing continuous nasogastric feeding.

An infant with discomfort on feeding

If oesophagitis is suspected, endoscopy with biopsy is the investigation of choice, though a therapeutic trial may be carried out. The best treatment option would be acid inhibition, possibly with feed thickening and/or prokinetic agent.

A child or adolescent with recurrent vomiting or regurgitation

Otherwise healthy children with recurrent vomiting or regurgitation after the age of 2 years usually require evaluation, typically with a barium meal and/or upper endoscopy with biopsy. Treatment should be based upon the findings.

A child or adolescent with heartburn

These patients are usually treated empirically with lifestyle changes accompanied by a 4-week trial of an H_2-blocker or PPI.

Persistent or recurrent symptoms require investigation with an upper endoscopy and biopsy.

Apnoea or apparent life-threatening events

Recurrent vomiting or regurgitation occurs commonly in patients with apparent life-threatening events (ALTE, p. 399). However, an association between reflux and apnoea or bradycardia has not been convincingly demonstrated. In the evaluation of such patients pH monitoring may be useful to link intra-oesophageal acid with events. Infants with ALTE may be more likely to respond to antireflux therapy when:
- Vomiting or oral regurgitation occurs at the time of the ALTE
- Episodes occur while the infant is awake
- ALTE is characterized by obstructive apnoea.

Most infants respond to maximal medical therapy with formula thickening, prokinetic agents and acid suppression. Only a minority require antireflux surgery.

GOR in children with neurodisability

Key points are given in Box 39.2.

Chronic diarrhoea and malabsorption

Basic science

Malabsorption syndromes are characterized by the association of chronic diarrhoea and failure to thrive. The disorders involve inadequate absorption of one or more of the major nutrients and primarily involve the small intestine or the exocrine pancreas.

BOX 39.2 GOR in children with neurodisability

- One-third of children with severe psychomotor retardation have significant GOR
- It is exacerbated in many by the presence of large hiatal hernias and diffuse foregut dysmotility
- Growth faltering and dental erosions are a frequent problem
- All severe sequelae of GOR have a higher incidence in children with neurodisability (recurrent aspiration pneumonia, blood loss from oesophagitis, stricture formation etc.)
- Oesophagitis can respond to H_2-antagonists, but most require 'maximum medical therapy' with high-dose PPIs
- Many of these children will not respond adequately to medical therapy and will require fundoplication
- Fundoplication has a high rate of perioperative and postoperative complications in this group

Causes of malabsorption

- Enteropathy: loss of surface area in small bowel due to inflammation of the mucosa and villi damage
- Defect in a transport mechanism
- Deficiency of an enzyme.

Carbohydrate absorption/ malabsorption

Basic physiology of carbohydrate digestion
(Box 39.3)

Carbohydrates in food comprise starch, sucrose and lactose. Starch molecules (amylase and amylopectin)

BOX 39.3 Basic physiology of carbohydrate digestion

Starch 50–60%
- Digestion by salivary/pancreatic amylase to maltose and maltotriose
- Maltose and maltotriose:
  - ~80% hydrolysed by sucrase–isomaltase → glucose
  - ~20% glucoamylase

Sucrose 30–40%
- Hydrolysis by sucrase–isomaltase → glucose fructose

Lactose 0–20% adults, 40–100% infants
- Hydrolysis by lactase → glucose galactose

and glucose polymers require preliminary intraluminal digestion by amylase, releasing maltose and maltotriose. The final hydrolysis of di- and oligosaccharides occurs at the brush border. Glucose and galactose enter the enterocyte via a sodium-linked carrier (p. 175) and fructose via an energy-independent 'pore'.

Malabsorption of carbohydrate leads to osmotic diarrhoea. The undigested sugar is then fermented in the colon, producing excessive flatus and acidic stools.

Characteristic stools of sugar malabsorption

- Osmotic diarrhoea (stops on fasting)
- Very watery
- Acidic
- Passed with excessive flatus (explosive).

Lactose malabsorption

The most common form of carbohydrate malabsorption is lactase malabsorption. Lactase is found on the brush border in the small bowel. Any mechanism causing damage to the mucosa and villi of the small bowel (enteropathy) will cause secondary lactase deficiency. This can be managed with a lactose-free formula or diet, but resolves spontaneously as the enteropathy resolves.

In all humans the amount of lactase present per area of small bowel reduces towards the middle of the first decade, but in some ethnic groups it falls to a level where symptoms will occur when even a small amount of lactose is ingested. This is termed congenital hypolactasia and is very common. It is simply managed by reducing the ingestion of lactose to that which can be tolerated.

Congenital glucose–galactose malabsorption

This is an extremely rare autosomal recessive condition due to the absence of the sodium, glucose–galactose transporter in the enterocyte. The baby cannot tolerate lactose or glucose polymer-based feeds. Presentation is with life-threatening osmotic diarrhoea. Fructose is the only dietary carbohydrate tolerated and treatment is with a fructose-based formula.

Sucrase–isomaltase deficiency

This is a rare autosomal recessive condition with variable presentation. Watery diarrhoea follows ingestion of sucrose and to a lesser extent starch. It therefore may present at the time of the introduction of solids and

may be confused with toddler diarrhoea. Diagnosis is usually by sucrose hydrogen breath test or a sucrose challenge where explosive watery diarrhoea occurs after ingestion of sucrose, the stools testing positive for sucrose. Treatment is with dietary exclusion of sucrose and to a lesser extent starch.

Protein absorption/malabsorption

Initial digestion of protein is performed by gastric pepsin and pancreatic enzymes. Further hydrolysis of peptides takes place at the brush border of the intestine, where a mixture of peptides and amino acids are absorbed.

Protein-losing enteropathy (Box 39.4)

Loss of serum proteins across the gut mucosa may occur either because of abnormal or inflamed mucosal surface or from abnormal intestinal lymphatics. Methods for documenting enteric loss of protein are available but, in paediatric practice, are rarely used. The serum albumin is low. Alpha$_1$-antitrypsin can be measured in the stool and will be elevated.

Fat absorption/malabsorption

Fat digestion and absorption take place mainly in the duodenum and upper jejunum. The fat content of a normal diet is predominantly insoluble long-chain triglycerides. Digestion begins in the stomach with lipase produced in the gastric fundus. The fat is then emulsified by bile salts in the small intestine. Pancreatic lipase then hydrolyses the triglycerides to monoglycerides and fatty acids. Pancreatic bicarbonate is required to maintain optimum pH for hydrolysis for the next step

---

BOX 39.4 Diseases associated with excessive enteric protein loss

Loss from abnormal/damaged small intestinal mucosa
- Coeliac disease (Fig. 39.3)
- Cow's milk protein enteropathy
- Tropical sprue
- Crohn's disease
- Giardiasis
- Graft versus host disease

Loss from intestinal lymphatics
- Primary intestinal lymphangiectasia
- Secondary intestinal lymphangiectasia: obstructed lymphatics from lymphoma, malrotation or heart disease/failure

Table 39.10 Presentation of coeliac disease

	Classical	Atypical
Stools	Pale, loose, offensive, sometimes watery, 'oat porridge'	Constipated
Weight	Weight loss/failure to thrive	Weight gain/growth failure
Personality	Fretful, clingy, withdrawn	
Anaemia	++	Iron resistant
Abnormal LFTs		Increased alanine/aspartate aminotransferase (ALT/AST)
Skin		Dermatitis herpetiformis
Bone/teeth		Dental hypoplasia Osteoporosis

in fat absorption: the utilization of monoglycerides and fatty acids by bile acids. This consists of their incorporation into aggregates called micelles that are absorbed by the intestinal mucosa cell. The monoglycerides and fatty acids are then re-esterified into triglycerides, which coalesce into chylomicrons. The chylomicrons pass out of the cell and are transported by the lymphatic system into the blood.

Steatorrhoea

Steatorrhoea results from the impaired digestion and absorption of fat due to exocrine pancreatic deficiency, lack of bile salts or damage to the small intestinal mucosa.

Causes of steatorrhoea
- Exocrine pancreatic insufficiency:
  - Cystic fibrosis (p. 252)
  - Shwachman–Diamond syndrome
- Lack of bile salts:
  - Primary: Byler's disease
  - Secondary: obstructive jaundice, ileal resection (due to impaired enterohepatic circulation), small bowel bacterial overgrowth
- Mucosal pathology:
  - Enteropathy (loss of surface area): coeliac disease, cow's milk protein intolerance, giardiasis, tropical sprue, autoimmune enteropathy
  - Co-lipase deficiency
- Failure of chylomicron formation:
  - abetalipoproteinaemia
- Damage to intestinal lymphatics:
  - intestinal lymphangiectasia.

Coeliac disease

This is a disease of proximal small intestine characterized by abnormal small intestine mucosa, associated with a permanent intolerance to gluten (Table 39.10). Removal of gluten from the diet leads to full clinical remission with restoration to normal of small intes-

tinal mucosa. The condition may present at any age and diagnosis is for life.

Coeliac disease is due to T lymphocyte-mediated small intestinal enteropathy induced by gluten in a genetically predisposed individual. There is increased incidence with HLA B8 and DQ. Incidence is 1 in 100–200.

Associations include diabetes mellitus, thyroid disease, autoimmune chronic active hepatitis and IgA deficiency.

Diagnosis
- Screening: page 171.
- Definitive: abnormal small intestinal biopsy with subtotal villous atrophy (Fig. 39.3), crypt hyperplasia and increased inflammatory cells in lamina propria.

When biopsy is abnormal and antibodies are positive, diagnosis is straightforward. If diagnosed at age < 2 years, a gluten-free diet is recommended but a challenge would usually be performed in the second half of the first decade, as there are other conditions that can cause a similar histological appearance. The patient is given either gluten-containing food, or gluten powder whilst continuing on a gluten-free diet. Coeliac disease is confirmed if antibodies become positive and the repeat biopsy shows coeliac disease.

Management
Management involves withdrawal of gluten from the diet (wheat/rye-free) under the supervision of a dietician.

Complications
There is an increased risk of developing small bowel lymphoma and carcinoma of the oesophagus in adult life. Strict compliance with a gluten-free diet reduces risk to that of the normal population.

Shwachman–Diamond syndrome

This rare autosomal recessive cause of pancreatic insufficiency is associated with cyclical neutropenia and other haematological abnormalities. Patients may be developmentally delayed, and have an enlarged liver with abnormal liver function tests. There are associated skeletal abnormalities and patients are at risk of developing haematological malignancies.

Treatment is with pancreatic supplements.

Cow's milk protein intolerance

(Box 39.5)

This is due to an intolerance to cow's milk protein, which is usually transient. The symptoms may be confined to the gastrointestinal tract or there may be other manifestations of atopy: cow's milk protein allergy.

There is a 30–35% cross-sensitivity between cow's milk and soya protein. In children with gastrointestinal manifestations changes in the small intestinal mucosa may vary from normal to patchy to partial to subtotal villous atrophy (Fig. 39.3).

Cow's milk protein colitis

This occurs in children less than 2 years of age, who present with bloody diarrhoea. Often there is a family history of atopy. At sigmoidoscopy there is a colitic appearance and biopsies show an increase in eosinophils in the lamina propria (eosinophilic colitis).

Investigations

There may be an increase in eosinophils in the peripheral blood film. IgE may be elevated. Patients may have a positive radioallergosorbence test (RAST) to cow's milk protein and a positive skin prick to cow's milk. However, cow's milk protein intolerance is often present when all these tests are negative, so a therapeutic trial is indicated when there is sufficient clinical suspicion.

BOX 39.5 Manifestations of cow's milk intolerance

Gastrointestinal manifestations
- Diarrhoea
- Vomiting
- Failure to thrive
- Acute colitis
- Constipation

Non-gastrointestinal manifestations
- Migraine
- Eczema
- Asthma
- Anaphylaxis

Management

Treatment is with a cows' milk protein-free diet, using a casein hydrolysate as a milk substitute. The child should be challenged at the age of 2 years, as most will have outgrown the condition by this age. Whilst anaphylaxis is rare, challenge should usually be carried out in hospital.

Short gut syndrome

This is a problem seen mainly in a small number of surgically treated infants when a large segment of gangrenous small intestine is resected as a result of necrotizing enterocolitis or midgut volvulus. These infants are dependent on parenteral nutrition (PN) following surgery and are prone to fluid and electrolyte disturbance, sepsis from central venous catheters and liver damage (PN cholestasis). They require 40–60 cm of non-dilated upper small intestine, preferably with an intact ileocaecal valve and a colon, to have enough bowel to sustain nutrition without PN in the long term. This length of bowel will not be sufficient initially, as it needs to undergo adaptation to increase its surface area. This process can take up to 1 year.

Acute abdominal pain

Abdominal pain of recent onset should trigger prompt diagnosis and active treatment. While most children with acute abdominal pain have a self-limiting condition, the pain may herald a serious medical or surgical emergency. Primary care aspects are discussed in Chapter 25.

Problem-orientated topic:

acute abdominal pain

A 4-year-old boy, Callum, is admitted to the acute assessment unit with a 24-hour history of right upper quadrant pain that is worse on movement. On examination he has a temperature of 39°C and is grunting. He is tender in the right upper quadrant but has no signs of peritonism. His haemoglobin is 11.6 g/dl, white blood count 23×10^9/l, neutrophils 18×10^9/l, platelets 465×10^9/l, C-reactive protein 135 mg/l and serum amylase 90 IU/l.

Q1. How would you assess this child?
Q2. What is the most likely diagnosis?

History

- Pain:
  - Site, characteristics, exaggerating and relieving factors
  - Young child: unexplained screaming
- Associated symptoms:
  - Diarrhoea, vomiting, urinary, menstrual, rectal bleeding
- Trauma?
- Past medical history

Examination

- General:
  - Temperature, signs of cardiovascular instability, respiratory rate, rash, joints, lymph nodes
- Abdomen:
  - Signs of peritonism, abdominal mass, intestinal obstruction

Investigations

- Blood:
  - Full blood count, urea and electrolytes, liver function tests, amylase
- Urine:
  - Urinalysis for blood, protein and glucose; microscopy and culture
- Radiological:
  - Plain abdominal X-ray, chest X-ray, ultrasound and CT of abdomen

Q1. How would you assess this child?

See Box 39.6.

Q2. What is the most likely diagnosis?

The clinical algorithm shown in Figure 39.9 is helpful in the diagnosis of acute abdominal pain.

Acute appendicitis (Ch. 25)

Initial symptoms are periumbilical pain, nausea, vomiting and anorexia. There may be associated frequency of micturition. Classically the pain then radiates to the right iliac fossa, though with a retrocaecal appendix the pain may be more lateral and in the flank. The patient will have a low-grade temperature and localized peritonism in the right iliac fossa. Once the appendix has perforated, there is a high fever, grunting respiration and generalized signs of peritonitis. The appendix may perforate to form a localized abscess when a mass is palpable in the right iliac fossa. The diagnosis is usually based on the clinical presentation, though an elevated neutrophil white count and C-reactive protein may be helpful in supporting the diagnosis. The diagnosis can be difficult in younger children, who are usually more ill and have generalized peritonitis at presentation as a result of perforation. Treatment is surgical.

Acute pancreatitis

Acute pancreatitis results from autodigestion of the pancreas.

Causes of acute pancreatitis in childhood are:

- Gallstones
- Congenital abnormalities of the pancreas: pancreatic divisum
- Trauma
- Hereditary (autosomal dominant, incomplete penetration)
- Hypercalcaemia
- Hyperlipidaemia.

Clinical features

- *Pain*: upper abdominal, sudden onset, continuous and intense, radiates to back and flank. The severity is related to the degree of peritonism and is caused by liberation of enzymes and haemorrhage.

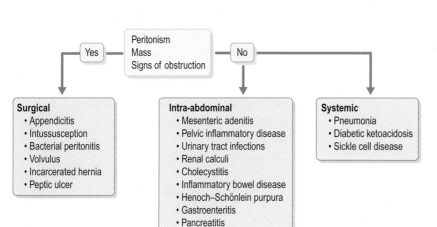

Fig. 39.9 Diagnosis of acute abdominal pain

- *Vomiting*: severe, bilious and may be faeculent as a result of paralytic ileus.
- *Clinical findings*: fever, signs of cardiovascular instability (tachycardia, hypotension), peritonism, ileus; there may be an epigastric mass.

The diagnosis is confirmed by an elevated serum amylase.

Management
- Resuscitation
- Nil by mouth
- Nasogastric aspiration
- Intravenous fluids
- Analgesia: pethidine
- Antibiotics
- Nutritional support: total parenteral nutrition or jejunal feeding.

Once the patient has recovered, the child should be investigated for an underlying cause. If the patient has gallstones, cholecystectomy should be undertaken when the patient is well.

Chronic pancreatitis

Repeated attacks of pancreatitis cause the pancreas to become atrophic and fibrotic. The ducts are obstructed and dilated and cyst-like cavities develop. Exocrine pancreatic insufficiency may occur. In children, this is usually due to hereditary pancreatitis. They either have recurrent bouts of acute pancreatitis or may develop intractable pain. Acute episodes are managed with analgesia and intravenous fluids. Attacks may be prevented with antioxidants and pancreatic supplements.

Pancreatic pleural fistula is a rare complication. The child will develop a pleural effusion that has a high amylase content.

Intussusception

This results from the invagination of one part of the bowel into another (usually the terminal ileum into the caecum). This results in the blood supply to that part of the bowel being severely compromised. It can occur at any time in childhood but the peak incidence is between 3 and 6 months of age following either an upper respiratory infection or gastroenteritis, or coinciding with the introduction of solids when the Peyer's patches become enlarged and act as a lead point. The child has episodes of pain followed by pallor and may pass blood in the stools (redcurrant jelly). A mass is usually palpable though the diagnosis can be confirmed with an ultrasound scan (doughnut sign). Treatment is with either an air or a barium enema.

If this fails or the child has had symptoms for more than 24 hours, a laparotomy plus surgical reduction is indicated. Intussusception may be recurrent.

Volvulus

Volvulus or twisting occurs when a long mobile loop of bowel revolves around its own mesentery. Volvulus of the midgut from malrotation is most common during infancy but may occur at any time in childhood. It may be intermittent or may cause ischaemia and infarction of the gut. The symptoms are abdominal pain and bilious vomiting and there may be associated fullness/abdominal distension. A plain abdominal X-ray may show a double bubble appearance due to air proximal to the obstruction, though there is usually a small amount of distal air. The diagnosis is confirmed with an upper gastrointestinal contrast study, which will demonstrate the ligament of Treitz to be abnormally placed (it should lie to the left of the midline and above the duodenal bulb). Treatment is surgical.

Blood in the stool

(See also Ch. 25.)

> **Problem-orientated topic:**
>
> ### bloody diarrhoea
>
> Ryan, a 2-month-old boy, presents with bloody diarrhoea present for 2 weeks. His mother is well except for poorly controlled asthma. He is formula-fed and thriving.
>
> Q1. What diagnoses would you consider?

Q1. What diagnoses would you consider?

Lower gastrointestinal bleeding (originating distal to the duodenum) is a common problem in paediatrics and, although most causes are self-limiting and benign, serious pathology can present this way. The most likely diagnoses based on history of the bleeding and age of the child are shown in Table 39.11.

Anal fissure

Anal fissure causes bright red blood on the outside of stool, sometimes dripping into the toilet and on the toilet tissue. Usually there is a history of passage of large constipated stool and pain on defaecation.

Table 39.11 **Common causes of blood in the stool**

Description of bleeding per rectum	Likely anatomical source/cause	Most likely diagnoses			
		Birth–1 month	1 month–2 years	2–10 years	10–16 years
Bright red blood coating formed stool	Anus or rectum	Vitamin K deficiency Anal fissure	Anal fissure	Anal fissure Polyp	Polyp Anal fissure Haemorrhoids
Bloody diarrhoea	Colonic/colitis	Food-allergic colitis Vitamin K deficiency Necrotizing enterocolitis Hirschsprung's enterocolitis	Food-allergic colitis Infectious enterocolitis Hirschsprung's enterocolitis Necrotizing enterocolitis	Infectious enterocolitis Inflammatory bowel disease	Infectious enterocolitis Inflammatory bowel disease
Large-volume dark-red blood	'Surgical cause', distal small bowel/ proximal colon	Duplication cyst Volvulus	Meckel's diverticulum Duplication cyst Volvulus	Meckel's diverticulum Angiodysplasia	Angiodysplasia

The fissure is generally posterior and obvious on anal inspection. Treatment is usually by stool-softening agents.

Food allergy

Bloody diarrhoea can be the presenting feature of allergic enterocolitis, most commonly due to cow's milk and/or soy protein. The child is usually less than 3 months old and, though the infant can have associated vomiting and become dehydrated, the bloody stools are often the isolated concern in an otherwise well baby with normal weight gain. The child should be given a hypoallergenic formula, usually a hydrolysate.

Infectious enterocolitis

Bloody stools can occur in infections due to *Salmonella*, *Shigella*, *Campylobacter jejuni*, *Yersinia enterocolitica*, *Escherichia coli* 057 and *Entamoeba histolytica*. Pseudo-membranous colitis due to *Clostridium difficile* should be considered in any child having received broad-spectrum antibiotics. Stool cultures and 'hot' stools for ova, cysts and parasite examination (and *Cl. difficile* toxin, if indicated) are mandatory in any child with bloody diarrhoea.

Meckel's diverticulum

This typically presents before 2 years of age with the painless passage of a large volume of dark red blood in an otherwise healthy child. It is twice as common in boys as girls.

Intussusception

See page 185.

Polyps

Polyps are a relatively common cause of per rectum bleeding in children under 2 years. Bleeding is typically bright red, often on the surface of the stools, small in amount and painless. Ninety percent of childhood polyps are hamartomatous juvenile polyps, which are benign, generally singular and situated in the left colon. They are confirmed and removed at colonoscopy.

Haemorrhoids

Haemorrhoids are rare in infants and children, and if present, are usually due to portal hypertension. They do occur in constipated adolescents, causing bleeding during defaecation with blood on the surface of the stool or the toilet paper or dripping into the toilet bowl. The child may describe something 'coming out' from their anus during defaecation and the pain is typically aching in nature rather than sharp as described with fissures.

Inflammatory bowel disease: Crohn's disease and ulcerative colitis

Crohn's disease is an inflammatory condition affecting any part of the digestive tract and involving the entire thickness of the bowel wall. Isolated ileal disease is less common in children and Crohn's colitis is the commonest distribution. Symptoms include abdominal pain, anorexia, weight loss, poor growth, diarrhoea (which may contain blood and mucus) and fever. Positive physical findings may include anorexia, thickening and fissuring of the lips (oro-facial granulomatosis),

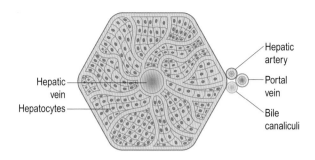

Fig. 39.10 **The anatomy of the liver lobule**

clubbing, abdominal masses, peri-anal fissures and skin tags. Blood tests reveal evidence of chronic inflammation (elevated ESR, CRP and platelet count and hypoalbuminaemia). Definite diagnosis is based an upper GI endoscopy, ileo-colonoscopy and biopsy. Treatments include dietary measures (elemental and polymeric diet), steroids and immunosuppressive agents. Surgery and resection of the affected areas may be needed particularly in severe growth failure or stricturing disease.

Ulcerative colitis is confined to the large bowel. Symptoms include diarrhoea with mucus, rectal bleeding and tenesmus. Diagnosis is based on colonoscopy and biopsy. Treatment is initially with steroids (systemic and local) and 5 aminosalicylic acid. Colectomy +/– ileal pouch is reserved for failure of medical treatment.

Liver disease

Basic science

The liver is divided into the right and left lobe, which are in turn divided into eight segments. Each segment is divided into lobules with a central vein. In the spaces between the lobules are branches of the portal vein, hepatic artery and bile duct canaliculi (Fig. 39.10).

The functions of the liver include formation and secretion of bile, glycogen storage and metabolism, ketone body formation, detoxification of toxins and drugs, and manufacture of plasma proteins and coagulation factors. Whilst biochemical liver function tests reflect the severity of hepatic dysfunction, they rarely provide diagnostic information of individual disease.

Baseline investigations

Bilirubin is nearly always elevated in liver disease; when detected in urine it is always abnormal. It may also be elevated in any condition causing haemolysis. Causes of elevated serum bilirubin are shown in Box 39.7.

Other indices of liver function

(Table 39.12)

Aminotransferases

● Aspartate (AST)
● Alanine (ALT).

These are present in liver, heart and skeletal muscle, and are elevated if there is hepatocyte damage.

Alkaline phosphatase (ALP)

ALP is found in liver, kidney, bone, placenta and intestine. Elevation of this enzyme in liver disease indicates biliary epithelial damage, cirrhosis, rejection or osteopenia secondary to vitamin D deficiency/malabsorption.

Gamma-glutamyl transpeptidases (GGT)

GGT is present in biliary epithelium and hepatocytes, and increased in many forms of liver disease.

Table 39.12 Significance of abnormal investigations in the jaundiced child/child with abnormal liver function tests

Investigation	Significance
Haemoglobin	Low with elevated reticulocytes indicates haemolysis
Bilirubin	Unconjugated increase suggests haemolysis Conjugated increase suggests hepatic or post-hepatic disease
AST/ALT/gamma-glutamyl transferase (GGT)	Elevated with liver damage
Albumin/total proteins	Albumin low in chronic liver disease, total proteins elevated in autoimmune hepatitis
Serology	Identification of virus causing hepatitis
Immunology	Increased IgG, +ve antinuclear antibodies (ANA) (type 1), +ve liver, kidney, microsomal antibodies (LKM) (type 2) in autoimmune chronic active hepatitis
Copper studies	Ceruloplasmin decreased, 24-hour urinary copper pre- and post-penicillamine increased in Wilson's disease

Synthetic function of the liver

- *Albumin*. If decreased, indicates chronic liver disease.
- *Coagulation*. If abnormal, indicates significant hepatic dysfunction, either acute or chronic.
- *Blood glucose*. A finding of fasting hypoglycaemia in absence of other causes suggests poor hepatic function, particularly in acute hepatic failure.

Infectious hepatitis

Causes
- Acute viral:
  - Hepatitis A, B, C (D and E) (Table 39.13)
  - Measles
  - Rubella
  - Erythrovirus 19 (parvovirus B19)
  - Herpes simplex types I and II
  - Varicella zoster
  - Cytomegalovirus
  - Epstein–Barr virus
  - Human herpes virus type 6
  - Yellow fever
- Non-viral:
  - Leptospirosis
  - *Listeria monocytogenes*
  - Toxoplasmosis
  - Hydatid disease.

Hydatid disease

This is caused by *Echinococcus* (tapeworm), whose intermediate host is sheep and dogs. Following ingestion of ova by humans, the embryo develops and penetrates the stomach wall, reaching the liver via the portal vein. Cysts develop in the liver and lungs. Liver cysts are slow-growing, giving asymptomatic hepatomegaly.

Treatment is either by surgical excision, or with mebendazole for 3 months.

Autoimmune liver disease

Autoimmune chronic active hepatitis is a chronic inflammatory disorder affecting the liver, responding to immunosuppression. It may coexist with other autoimmune disorders and the male: female ratio is 1:3. It may present as hepatitis, fulminant liver failure or chronic liver disease (often despite a short history). The diagnosis is confirmed on liver biopsy (interface hepatitis). Investigations typically show raised total proteins and IgG, antinuclear antibody (ANA) and smooth muscle antibody positive (classed as type 1), and liver kidney microsomal (LKM) antibody positive (type 2). Treatment is immunosuppressive, with steroids and azathioprine.

Sclerosing cholangitis is an autoimmune condition predominantly affecting intra- and extrahepatic bile ducts, leading to fibrosis and usually associated with ulcerative colitis. As there are similar autoantibody features to type 1 autoimmune hepatitis, there is probably some overlap between the two conditions.

Wilson's disease

This is a rare autosomal recessive disorder. There is an accumulation of copper in liver, brain (causing behavioural changes and extrapyramidal problems), cornea (Kayser–Fleischer rings) and kidneys (renal tubular problems, vitamin D-resistant rickets). The genetic defect results in decreased synthesis of copper-binding protein ceruloplasmin and defective copper excretion in bile. Children present mostly under 12 years with any form of liver disease or occasionally with haemolytic anaemia.

The diagnosis is based on measurement of serum copper, but this can be unreliable (usually decreased, occasionally normal or increased); decreased ceruloplasmin; increased 24-hour urinary copper after D-penicillamine; and increased liver copper.

Treatment is with penicillamine to chelate and excrete excess copper, and zinc to decrease absorption.

Table 39.13 Clinical features of hepatitis A, B and C

Type	Virus	Incubation period	Transmission	Clinical presentation	Treatment
Hepatitis A	RNA	30 days	Faecal–oral	Acute illness with nausea, abdominal pain, jaundice and hepatomegaly +ve IgM Very rare cause of acute liver failure, rare persistent cholestasis	Supportive, as normally self-limiting illness
Hepatitis B	DNA	30–180 days (mean 100)	Transfusion blood/ blood products Needlestick injury Lateral spread in families Perinatal	May be asymptomatic, classical features of acute hepatitis, fulminant hepatic failure 1–2% +ve serology 30–50% chronic carriage 10% will develop cirrhosis with risk of hepatocellular carcinoma in later life	Interferon and lamivudine may be of benefit Prevention: pregnant women screened for hepatitis B surface antigen (HBsAg) Babies of all HBsAg +ve mothers receive vaccination If mother has hepatitis B e antigen, +ve baby receives immunoglobulin at birth
Hepatitis C	RNA	40–80 days	Transfusion blood/ blood products Vertical transmission 7%	Rarely acute infection 50% will develop chronic liver disease, despite many having normal liver function tests, and progress to cirrhosis with risk of hepatocellular carcinoma in later life	Interferon and ribavirin in combination may be of benefit

Liver transplantation is reserved for acute liver failure and decompensated liver disease.

Acute liver failure

Acute liver failure is rare in childhood and has a high mortality. It is defined as onset of encephalopathy and coagulopathy within 8 weeks of the onset of liver disease. The most common causes are viral hepatitis, undefined metabolic conditions and, in the older child, deliberate overdosage of paracetamol.

The child presents with jaundice, encephalopathy and hypoglycaemia. The signs of encephalopathy may initially be subtle and include drowsiness, night-time wakefulness and periods of irritability and aggression. Initially, the bilirubin may not be elevated but transaminases are very high, coagulation is abnormal and ammonia is elevated.

Principles of management of acute liver failure
- *Hypoglycaemia*: maintain blood glucose > 4 mmol/l with 10% dextrose.
- *Prevent sepsis*: broad-spectrum antibiotics/ antifungals.
- *Coagulopathy*: correct with vitamin K and fresh frozen plasma.
- *Cerebral oedema*: nurse head up, restrict fluid to 60% maintenance, ventilation for encephalopathy.

- *Prevent gastrointestinal bleeding*: H$_2$-blockers/PPIs.
- *Liver protection*: N-acetylcysteine 150 mg/kg/24 hr.
- *Transfer when stabilized*: to supraregional liver transplant unit.

Cirrhosis and portal hypertension

Cirrhosis is a pathological diagnosis that includes the combination of fibrosis and regenerative nodules. It is the end result of many forms of liver disease and causes portal hypertension, ascites, distended veins on the abdominal wall and oesophageal varices.

Complications of portal hypertension
- *Ascites*: results from decreased albumin and sodium retention; treated with diuretics and albumin infusion
- *Hypersplenism*: decreased white cell count and platelet count
- *Oesophageal varices*: may bleed
- *Encephalopathy*: often precipitated by gastrointestinal bleed/sepsis/renal failure.

Management of bleeding oesophageal varices
- *Resuscitation*: blood transfusion, aiming for haemoglobin of 10 g/dl
- *Acid suppression*: H$_2$-blockers/PPIs

- *Lowering portal blood pressure*: octreotide (vasopressin analogue)
- *Endoscopy*: sclerotherapy or banding of varices
- *Resistant bleeding*: liver transplantation/shunt operations.

Extrahepatic portal hypertension/ portal vein thrombosis

Blockage of the portal vein may result from a congenital abnormality of the portal vein, blockage following umbilical venous catheterization, omphalitis and infiltration with tumour. The portal vein is not seen on ultrasound and is replaced by tangled enlarged venous collaterals: cavernous transformation of the portal vein/portal cavernoma. Presentation may be with haemorrhage from oesophageal varices, an enlarged spleen or hypersplenism. If gastrointestinal haemorrhage cannot be controlled endoscopically, blockage can be bypassed by a graft, usually taken from the external jugular vein: mesorex shunt.

Heather Lambert

Urinary system

MODULE SEVEN

LEARNING OUTCOMES

By the end of this chapter you should:

- Know the common presentations of renal disease
- Understand the appropriate choice of investigations
- Know how to assess and manage the dehydrated child
- Understand the investigation and management of urinary tract infection
- Understand the causes and management of hypertension
- Understand the investigation, management and common presenting symptoms of diseases of the urinary tract.

Introduction

The kidneys have a wide range of functions. They are responsible for the control of the volume and electrolyte composition of extracellular fluid by a combination of glomerular filtration and tubular reabsorption. They play a role in maintenance of acid–base status through reabsorption of filtered bicarbonate and regeneration of bicarbonate. The kidney plays a role in the formation of red blood cells through production of erythropoietin; bone biochemistry through generation of 1,25-dihydroxycholecalciferol; and the regulation of blood pressure through the renin–angiotensin system.

Disorders of the urinary tract presenting in primary care are discussed in Chapter 26.

Investigating renal function

Plasma creatinine

Plasma creatinine is the best clinically useful and available guide to renal function. It is easily, quickly and cheaply measured on a small blood sample. Individual measurements are of use in determining whether renal function is within the normal range. Sequential measurements are useful to follow deterioration or improvements of renal function over a short timescale of hours and days or over a long timescale of months and years. Plasma creatinine varies with height, sex and muscle mass.

Concept of fractional excretion

Clearance of any substance that is filtered by the glomerulus and then reabsorbed by the tubule can be compared to the clearance of creatinine, which is filtered and then excreted largely unmodified by the tubule. The fractional excretion is that fraction of substance X that has been filtered at the glomerulus that actually reaches the urine.

$$\text{Fractional excretion (FE) } X\% = \frac{\text{urine } X}{\text{filtered } X} \times 100$$

Fractional excretion of sodium

Normally most of the filtered sodium (Na) is reabsorbed; the majority of this happens in the proximal tubule. When plasma sodium is normal and the patient is not shocked, fractional excretion of sodium can vary physiologically. However, calculating FE Na can give useful clues in pathological states.

The normal renal response to intravascular fluid volume reduction is to excrete urine with low sodium content. The kidney does this via a number of mechanisms, including reduction of glomerular filtration rate (GFR) and aldosterone-stimulated sodium reabsorption, which requires intact tubules.

Calculation of fractional excretion

See Box 40.1.

Table 40.1 shows the clinical picture.

BOX 40.1 Calculation of fractional excretion

Fractional excretion Na %	=	urine Na × 100 filtered Na
Urine Na	=	UNa × V
and filtered Na	=	GFR × P Na
and GFR	=	UCr × V PCr
so **FE Na %**	=	UNa × V × PCr _or_ **U/P sodium × P/U creatinine** PNa × UCr × V

N.B. When calculating, remember to ensure urine and plasma units are the same.

Table 40.1 Clinical picture from equation

Clinical picture	FE Na	Clinical significance
Shock	< 1%	= Tubules functioning = pre-renal failure
	> 1%	= Acute tubular necrosis (AIN)
Hyponatraemia	< 1%	= Salt loss or water overload (appropriate renal response)
	> 1%	= Renal salt wasting
Hypernatraemia	< 1%	= Renal concentration defect
	> 1%	= Salt overload

Table 40.2 Requirements for 24-hour water, sodium and potassium

Age	Preterm	Term	1 year	5 years	12 years
Sodium (mmol/kg)	5	3	2	2	1
Potassium (mmol/kg)	5	3	2	2	1
Water (ml/kg)	200	150	100	75	50
Easy hourly rate (ml/kg/hr)	8	6	4	3	2

Water and electrolyte imbalance

Problems with fluid and electrolyte balance are common in ill children. They can occur in a wide variety of clinical situations and with a wide range of underlying diagnoses. A methodical approach to history-taking and clinical examination is therefore essential and interpretation of biochemical results must always be done in the context of the clinical situation.

Maintenance water, sodium and potassium requirements per 24 hours are shown in Table 40.2.

Dehydration and hypovolaemia

Dehydration represents a deficit between fluid and electrolyte intake and losses. Fluid within the body is normally distributed between the intracellular fluid (ICF) and extracellular fluid (ECF) compartments; the ECF is composed of intravascular and interstitial components. Differential solute composition of ICF and ECF compartments is maintained by cell membrane pump activity and solute size and electrical charge. Fluid movement is regulated by a balance between osmotically active solutes and hydrostatic pressure. It is useful when clinically assessing the fluid volume status of a patient to try to consider which compartment has insufficient or excess volume.

The effects of ECF volume depletion are usually shared between the intravascular and interstitial compartments and are seen as hypovolaemia and dehydration respectively. Assessment can be complex. For example, in a situation like nephrotic syndrome, there may be weight gain and oedema on examination. However, since there is hypoalbuminaemia and albumin is the primary intravascular osmotic component, the intravascular fluid volume may be low but the total ECF volume high. Conversely, in acute renal failure there can be weight gain and oedema in a situation where both the total ECF and the intravascular volume are high. Oedema can therefore occur with high or low intravascular fluid volume.

In a complex situation like intensive care, where there may be multi-organ failure and multiple drug therapies, clinical assessment of fluid status is very difficult and invasive monitoring becomes essential.

Clinical estimation of ECF volume deficit

This is based on symptoms and signs (Boxes 40.2 and 40.3), as well as weight on admission compared with an expected weight.

Often in dehydration, sodium and water have been lost in approximately normal ratio and therefore the deficit should be replaced as normal saline (Box 40.4).

Aim to treat cardiovascular collapse or 'shock' quickly over the first 1–2 hours. Infuse normal saline to restore circulating blood volume and thereafter slow the replacement rate so that total deficit is replaced over 24 hours. In hypernatraemic dehydration, after an acceptable cardiovascular state has been restored, aim to reduce plasma sodium slowly over 24–48 hours

---

BOX 40.2 Symptoms and signs of ECF volume deficit

Mild (3–5% weight loss)
- Thirsty
- Mucous membranes dry
- Decreased skin turgor

Moderate (5–10% weight loss)
- Increased severity of above plus
  - Depressed fontanelle
  - Sunken eyes
  - Tachycardia

Severe (10–15% weight loss)
- Increased severity of above plus
  - Drowsiness, confusion or coma
  - 'Shock'
  - Cool periphery
  - Prolonged capillary refill time
  - Hypotension

BOX 40.3 Practical point: clinical assessment of volume status

Good clinical assessment of volume status comes with experience. A good way of improving those skills is whenever a judgment of reduced ECF is made (for example, when admitting a toddler with dehydration from acute gastroenteritis). Note the percentage assessment deficit and the weight of the child and compare this with the percentage gain in weight of the child once he or she is fully rehydrated (e.g. 48 hours later). This gives an indication, in retrospect, of the accuracy of the initial assessment.

BOX 40.4 Practical point: prescribing rehydration fluids

When prescribing rehydration fluids:
1. Make an assessment of volume deficit and replace this as normal saline (or sometimes human albumin solution in shock)
2. Calculate maintenance fluids and insensible losses
3. Initially estimate and then measure ongoing losses and replace appropriately in volume and content.

   Fluid prescription should consist of 1 + 2 + 3.

---

by altering the sodium concentration of the infusion fluid appropriately and repeatedly monitoring the rate of fall of plasma sodium and the urinary sodium concentration.

Management of fluid and electrolyte disorders depends on measurement of input and output plus *serial*:
- Clinical examination
- Biochemical data on urine and blood
- Weight measurements.

Hyponatraemia

Hyponatraemia is defined as a plasma sodium of less than 130 mmol/l and occurs when there is:
- Sodium loss in excess of water loss
  or
- Water gain in excess of sodium gain.

The total body sodium may be high, low or normal and therefore clinical assessment of ECF volume is essential.

Hypernatraemia

Hypernatraemia is defined as a plasma sodium greater than 150 mmol/l and occurs when there is:

- Water loss in excess of sodium loss

  or

- Sodium gain in excess of water gain.

Again, the total body sodium may be high, low or normal.

In hypernatraemic dehydration the water loss exceeds sodium loss. Because sodium is the principle ECF osmole, the ECF volume is relatively well maintained and signs of dehydration and hypovolaemia are less apparent.

Urinary tract infection

Urinary tract infection (UTI) is an important and common cause of acute illness in children, may be a marker of an underlying urinary tract abnormality and may cause significant long-term morbidity, particularly renal scarring, hypertension and renal impairment, which may not present until adult life (Box 40.5). There is good evidence that UTI in childhood is associated with renal scarring, the risk being highest in the youngest infants. This is the very group in whom diagnosis is often overlooked or delayed because clinical features are frequently non-specific. Thus diagnosis of UTI requires a very high index of suspicion, particularly in the youngest. Accurate diagnosis is essential because of the need for imaging and the risks associated with over- or under-investigation. UTI may be recurrent, about one-third of girls having a further UTI within a year. The recurrence rate in boys is much lower.

BOX 40.5 Clinical features of urinary tract infection

- Affects many children
- May be difficult to diagnose
- May cause acute illness and symptoms
- Is frequently over- or under-diagnosed
- May have long-term sequelae: hypertension, renal scarring, renal failure

---

Problem-orientated topic:

dysuria

Whilst away on holiday, Mary, a 5-year-old girl, complained of soreness and stinging on passing urine for 24 hours. She was taken to see the local doctor, who treated her with a 5-day course of antibiotics. Two weeks after return from holiday the symptoms recur and the girl is taken to see her GP, who telephones you asking for advice.

Q1. Did Mary have a urinary tract infection?

Q2. What is the differential diagnosis of dysuria?

Q3. How would you assess Mary?

Q4. What would be your management?

Q5. Does Mary require further investigation?

Q1. Did Mary have a urinary tract infection?

Clinical features of UTI in childhood are often different to those found in adults and are frequently non-specific. Without a high index of suspicion many UTIs, especially in the very young, will be missed. Classical symptoms of lower UTI (dysuria, frequency and incontinence) and upper UTI (fever, systemic upset, loin pain and renal tenderness) are frequently not seen in paediatric practice. Attempts to distinguish between upper and lower UTI on clinical grounds are unreliable and clinical history is not closely related to findings on imaging. UTI can occasionally produce life-threatening illness, especially in very young infants, who may present severely unwell with shock or septicaemia. Boys and girls are equally affected in infancy but after that the ratio of girls to boys progressively rises. After puberty the incidence of UTI is low in both sexes but rises in females who are sexually active. Renal scarring may occur in association with few or no symptoms.

Preschool children

In general terms, the younger the child, the more diverse and less specific the symptoms and signs. Thus evaluation of any unwell or febrile young child must include examination of urine. Sometimes there is a history of smelly urine or of crying on passing urine. Children may have an altered pattern of micturition and day- or night-time wetting may recur. Non-specific manifestations, such as poor feeding, vomiting, irritability, abdominal pain, failure to thrive, lethargy and restlessness, should always lead to a suspicion of UTI.

Older children

Older children may have more typical signs and symptoms localizing to the urinary tract, including dysuria, frequency, urgency, hesitation and enuresis. Some may have loin pain but absence of loin pain does not exclude upper urinary tract involvement. Generalized symptoms are common and include fever, lethargy, anorexia, abdominal pain, nausea and vomiting.

From the information given by the GP, it is not possible to be sure whether Mary had a UTI.

- Clean catch
- Pads
- Sterile adhesive bags
- Suprapubic aspiration (SPA)
- Potty (washed up)
- Midstream urine (MSU)
- Urethral catheterization

Q2. What is the differential diagnosis of dysuria?

Not all children with dysuria have a UTI. Dysuria may be associated with localized skin conditions, such as candidiasis, vulvitis or excoriation secondary to threadworms or other irritation. Febrile or mildly dehydrated children may complain of pain, stinging or discomfort on passing concentrated or what they term 'strong' urine. Children with quite minor degrees of haematuria — for example, from glomerulonephritis — may present with dysuria.

Q3. How would you assess Mary?

(Boxes 40.7 and 40.8)

Details should be sought of family history of urinary infection, vesico-ureteric reflux (VUR), renal disease or hypertension; antenatal and perinatal history; and drinking, voiding pattern and bowel habits. Examination should include examination of the urine; measurement of blood pressure; abdominal palpation for masses (bladder, kidney); inspection of external genitalia and lower back; and assessment of lower limb sensation and reflexes. When UTI is recurrent, it is particularly important that bladder and bowel habits are evaluated, as UTI may be associated with dysfunctional voiding, bladder instability and constipation.

Making the diagnosis of UTI: urine collection and testing (Boxes 40.6 and 40.8)

Infants with UTI but only non-specific symptoms are frequently under-diagnosed, whereas girls with vulvitis and febrile anorexic children who produce a highly concentrated urine and complain of dysuria are often falsely diagnosed as having a UTI.

Unfortunately, it is common for some children to receive an antibiotic for a presumed UTI without a urine sample being either collected or tested. Once this has happened, it is not possible to reach a certain diagnosis and the decision whether to investigate the child is very difficult.

- Evaluation of any sick child must include examination of urine
- Every young child with unexplained fever should have urine examined
- Clinical features of UTI are often non-specific
- Boys seldom get recurrent UTI in the absence of urinary tract abnormalities

- Accurate diagnosis of UTI is vital to appropriate subsequent management
- Antibiotic treatment should be started as soon as a suitable sample has been collected
- Urine can be collected in any setting by pad or bag, or by clean catch into a bottle or washed potty
- All urine collecting methods may fail or result in contamination
- All methods result in some false positives
- Phase-contrast microscopy is easy to learn and quick to perform
- Microscopy can immediately identify and prevent false positives
- Positive nitrite stick tests diagnose UTI but negative ones do not exclude UTI
- Urine white cell counts do not help make the diagnosis of UTI
- Urine samples that cannot be transported to the laboratory quickly should be refrigerated or inoculated on to a dipslide
- Boric acid bottles should be avoided, as they may produce false negative results

Organisms that cause UTI

About 85% of urine samples from boys and girls with a first UTI grow *Escherichia coli* on culture. *Klebsiella*, *Proteus* and *Streptococcus faecalis* are responsible for most of the rest. Children with abnormal urinary tracts are much more likely to have UTI due to less virulent organisms such as *Pseudomonas* or *Staphylococcus aureus*.

Laboratory culture for bacteria

There may be problems with over-diagnosis if organisms $> 10^5$/ml are used. Using $> 10^8$/ml would reduce false positives but would require special handling by laboratories. Refrigeration is highly effective for minimizing the overgrowth of contaminating organisms during storage and transfer to the laboratory.

Bacterial culture on dipslides

Urine can be cultured at any time and anywhere, and can be posted to the laboratory.

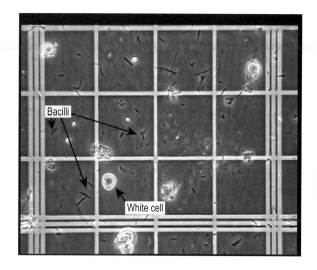

Fig. 40.1 **Phase-contrast microscopy of urine**

BOX 40.9 Treatment of UTI

BOX 40.9 Treatment of UTI

- Treatment goal is prevention of renal injury and symptoms associated with UTI
- Start 'best guess' antibiotic as soon as urine obtained
- Change antibiotic if culture result indicates
- If clinical condition does not improve after 48 hours repeat urine culture and request urgent investigations to exclude urological problems
- Give prophylactic antibiotics until investigations complete
- Clinical experience suggests benefit from increasing fluid intake and treatment of constipation

Phase-contrast microscopy (Fig. 40.1)

Bacteria can be identified very easily in unprepared urine by phase-contrast microscopy. Therefore, phase-contrast microscopy can provide a fast, reliable, efficient and economic near-patient UTI diagnostic service.

When infected urine is examined by phase-contrast microscopy there will typically be tens, hundreds or thousands of identical rods per high-power field, equivalent to bacterial counts of between 10^6 and 10^9/ml. Uninfected urine simply has no organisms to see at all. The urine from a child with a UTI will almost invariably have many rods visible per high-power field, so a completely empty field virtually guarantees an uninfected sample.

Some urine samples will give uncertain results because either just one or two bacteria are seen, or rods and streptococci are present together, or there is amorphous debris, cotton strands etc. present. If these urine samples are cultured, they are likely to give uncertain results several days later. If microscopy is used, a repeat sample can be collected at once.

Identifying bacteria with nitrite stick tests

Most uropathogens produce nitrite as a result of their metabolism. Uninfected urine samples do not contain nitrite, so the specificity is about 100%. A positive test is diagnostic. However, it often takes hours for the bacteria to produce detectable quantities of nitrite and children with UTI tend to void frequently so the test sensitivity is low (53%, range 15–82). If samples test negative for nitrite this must be ignored, as it adds nothing to the diagnostic process.

Urinary white blood cells in UTI

White blood cells in the urine, whether detected by sticks or microscopy, are an unreliable guide to infection. They disappear with time and may be present in febrile children without UTI.

Q4. What would be your management?

(Box 40.9)

Cefalexin, trimethoprim or nitrofurantoin is frequently used but discussion with the local microbiologist should help guide general advice about resistance patterns. Children, particularly infants, who are clinically dehydrated, toxic or unlikely to retain oral fluids, should be given parenteral antibiotics initially. There is no clear evidence about the ideal length of therapy to eradicate acute infection in children.

There is no evidence of benefit from treatment of asymptomatic bacteriuria in girls with normal urinary tracts. They do not therefore require routine screening of urine when well.

Q5. Does Mary require further investigation?

The aims of investigation are to identify children:
- With an underlying renal tract abnormality or predisposition to UTI:
  - Structural abnormality of urinary tract
  - Urinary tract obstruction
  - VUR
  - Abnormal bladder emptying
- Who have already sustained damage to their kidneys
- Who are likely to sustain damage to their kidneys.

Investigation of UTI

- All children should have some investigation after a proven UTI.
- Unnecessary investigations should be avoided.

- VUR is found in up to 30% of children with UTI (see below).
- Babies with antenatal hydronephrosis have increased risk of VUR.
- There is a 20–50-fold increased risk for VUR if there is a family history of VUR.
- There is an association between abnormal urodynamic variables and VUR.
- The relationship between VUR, renal scarring and reflux nephropathy is not clear.
- Renal scarring can occur without VUR.
- Young children and infants warrant intensive investigation.

Which investigations after UTI?
- Ultrasonography (US):
  - No ionizing radiation
  - Good for detecting structural abnormalities
  - In childhood scars are often small and frequently missed on US
- Tc^{99}-dimercaptosuccinic acid (DMSA):
  - Useful for detection of scarring
  - Small dose of ionizing radiation
  - Timing: DMSA scan soon after acute infection may show areas of reduced uptake that are not permanent; therefore delay DMSA scan for 2–5 months post acute UTI
- Micturating cystourethrogram (MCUG) direct contrast study:
  - To show reflux and urethral anatomy
  - Requires insertion of a bladder catheter
  - Ionizing radiation to the gonads
- MCUG direct radioisotope study:
  - Lower radiation dose than contrast MCUG
  - Requires the insertion of a bladder catheter
  - Grading of reflux not possible
  - No anatomical features demonstrated
- Indirect radioisotope study MAG3 (mercaptoacetyltriglycine):
  - No bladder catheter is required but intravenous injection is necessary
  - Lower radiation dose than contrast MCUG
  - Higher false negative rate
  - No anatomical information
- Abdominal X-ray:
  - Useful for localization of stones in selective cases (e.g. *Proteus* infection) or where there is a suggestive history
  - Spinal defects may be identified and constipation demonstrated.

It is important to acknowledge that there is no single test that answers all the essential questions in a child who has had a UTI.

BOX 40.10 Grades of vesico-ureteric reflux

I Into ureter only

II Into ureter, pelvis and calyces with no dilatation

III With mild to moderate dilatation; slight or no blunting of fornices

IV With moderate dilatation of ureter and/or renal pelvis and/or tortuosity of ureter; obliteration of sharp angle of fornices

V Gross dilatation and tortuosity; no papillary impression visible in calyces

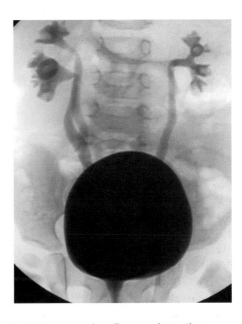

Fig. 40.2 Vesico-ureteric reflux on micturating cystourethrogram (duplex on right side)

Vesico-ureteric reflux (VUR) (Box 40.10 and Fig. 40.2)

VUR is the retrograde flow of urine from the bladder into the upper urinary tract. It is usually congenital. VUR is a major risk factor for progressive renal damage associated with UTI. The incidence of VUR is in the order of 1% in infants and is increased in certain risk groups. There is good evidence that VUR is a genetic disorder.

VUR is thought to predispose to renal damage by facilitating passage of bacteria from the bladder to the upper urinary tract. An immunological and inflammatory reaction is caused by renal infection, leading to renal injury and scarring. Extensive renal scarring causes reduced renal function, reduced renal growth, renal failure, hypertension and increased incidence of pregnancy-related hypertension. Whilst these sequelae may occur in childhood, patients frequently do not present until many years or decades later. Some babies

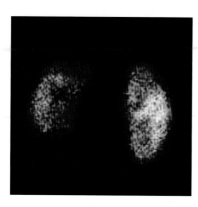

Fig. 40.3 **Unilateral scar seen on DMSA**

born with VUR have associated dysplastic or hypoplastic renal malformations or in utero damage, all of which may impair renal function. Therefore when a child being investigated following a UTI is found to have abnormalities on DMSA scan it may be difficult to distinguish whether this is scarring caused by UTI or a congenital renal abnormality or both (Fig. 40.3).

The risk of scarring following a UTI varies with age, but the precise details of this are not clear. In clinical situations it is often very difficult to know at what age an individual child acquired the scars. Young children appear to be at most risk.

It is thought that children with VUR should be protected from scarring until they outgrow their reflux, rather than up to an arbitrary age.

The child with evidence of scarring diagnosed at any age

When scarring is first detected it is not possible to determine at what age that scar occurred. Thus it is logical to need to know whether there is still VUR present, with the intention of trying to prevent further damage from UTI in those with VUR.

Management of VUR (Boxes 40.11 and 40.12)

Historically, both medical and surgical management strategies for VUR have been introduced without controlled studies documenting long-term benefit.

Resolution of VUR with time

Resolution of VUR over time with medical treatment is related to the grade of VUR and the age of the patient. In general a lower grade of reflux has a better chance of spontaneous resolution. In children with grade I or II reflux there is resolution in about 80–90% after 5 years. Bilateral grade IV and V reflux have the poorest chance, with spontaneous resolution in less than 20% of patients after 5 years.

Medical management

Since it is known that in the vast majority of cases VUR will resolve with time, the aim in medical management of VUR, with prophylactic antibiotics, is to prevent recurrent (or sometimes first) UTI and consequent renal scarring, whilst waiting for resolution of VUR. Breakthrough infections may be problematic and may be due to non-compliance or true bacterial resistance. Trimethoprim, nitrofurantoin or cefalexin is frequently used for prophylaxis.

Surgical management

There are two main forms of surgical treatment of VUR:
- *Endoscopic subureteric injection (STING).* Injection of tissue-augmenting substances is done under general anaesthetic and requires only a short stay (or treatment as a day case) in hospital. The success rate in abolition of VUR varies with the centre,

the material used, the timing of re-evaluation and test used in re-examination. The longevity of the treatment and need for repeat are not fully known.

- *Reimplantation.* Surgical success in curing VUR with reimplantation is high (> 95% overall). This is, however, a major operation requiring a stay of several days in hospital, with the associated risks and costs.

Two large multicentre prospective trials of medical versus surgical treatment for children with severe VUR do not show superiority of either treatment. Breakthrough infection, despite medical treatment or because of non-compliance, remains a commonly used factor for consideration of surgical treatment, as does deterioration of DMSA appearance.

Hypertension

Persistent systemic hypertension is an important risk factor for heart failure, myocardial infarction and stroke in adult life. There is increasing evidence that 'essential' hypertension has its origin in childhood; therefore early detection and treatment is highly desirable. Obesity in childhood is an increasing problem and will be associated with an increasing number at risk of hypertension. The kidney has a very important role in hypertension, both as the 'villain', as in essential hypertension and primary renal disease, and as the 'victim', as demonstrated in the destruction of the kidney in malignant hypertension and the rapid progression of chronic renal insufficiency in the face of poor blood pressure (BP) control.

Accurate measurement is important and there are various methods for measuring BP in children. The mercury or aneroid sphygmomanometer, used with stethoscope or Doppler, is generally considered the gold standard. Automated methods are often used for ease and rapidity, but not all have been validated for use in children and in practice most are not appropriately maintained and calibrated. Therefore BP should always be rechecked by another more reliable method when thought to be abnormal. Twenty-four-hour ambulatory BP monitoring or home BP monitoring may be useful in some situations to monitor borderline cases or monitor therapy. The cuff size used should be no less than two-thirds of the length of the upper arm from antecubital fossa to shoulder and it should also be large enough to encircle the arm. In effect the biggest cuff that will still allow the elbow to bend.

Defining normal blood pressure and hypertension

Definition of normality is difficult. There is a steady increase in blood pressure with age and no significant sex difference. The Second Task Force on Blood Pressure Control in Children has compiled charts of normal ranges for children from birth to 17 years.

 http://ww.nhlbi.nih.gov/guidelines/ hypertension/child_tbl.pdf

Normal ranges by child's height

Since BP is a continuous variable, any definition of hypertension is arbitrary and there are no universally accepted definitions. It is important to exclude errors in measurement. The most common are use of an incorrectly sized cuff, poor technique, use of unvalidated equipment and inappropriate interpretation (failing to use appropriate nomograms for age, height and sex). Reactive rises due to anxiety or pain are common pitfalls. Some conditions cause short-lived rises in blood pressure in otherwise normal children (e.g. hypovolaemia, raised intracranial pressure, drug therapy (e.g. steroids) and iatrogenic intravenous fluid overload). Even when errors have been excluded it is important that BP is measured repeatedly. Children with a systolic BP 15 mmHg or more above the 95th percentile can be considered to be severely hypertensive. For neonates, repeated systolic BP measurements above 90 mmHg at term and above 80 mmHg preterm are hypertensive.

Primary (essential) hypertension is the most common diagnosis in mild hypertension in childhood. Secondary hypertension is usually more severe. The underlying cause is important in determining an acceptable level of BP. For example, in the patient with chronic renal failure or a transplant, BP should ideally be more tightly controlled.

Some specific renal causes of hypertension

Hypertension complicates chronic renal failure and transplantation, most often due to salt and water retention, usually with stimulation of the renin–angiotensin system. By the time children are in end-stage renal failure most will be hypertensive. In patients on dialysis hypertension is usually related to salt and water overload. In transplant patients early hypertension is often related to acute volume expansion and later may be associated with immunosuppressive therapy, rejection or renal artery stenosis.

Renovascular hypertension

This accounts for 5–25% of severe childhood hypertension, usually due to renal artery stenosis with fibromuscular dysplasia. It is often found in relatively young children and is associated with:

- Idiopathic hypercalcaemia
- Marfan's syndrome
- Vasculitis
- Neonatal umbilical arterial catheter
- Abdominal radiation.

A bruit may be found on examination. The definitive investigation is angiography, with or without renal vein renin levels. Treatment may be surgical or medical, depending on whether there is an isolated resectable abnormality or whether there are widespread or small vessel abnormalities.

Reflux nephropathy

This tends to be picked up in children after the age of 5 years. At least 10% of patients with renal scars develop hypertension. Treatment is usually medical but nephrectomy is highly effective where there is unilateral severe scarring.

Other renal causes

- Chronic glomerulonephritis
- Renal damage after haemolytic uraemic syndrome (HUS)
- Autosomal recessive polycystic kidney disease (ARPKD)
- Autosomal dominant polycystic kidney disease (ADPKD).

Important cardiovascular causes

- Coarctation of the aorta
- Renal artery stenosis.

Hypertension may also be a feature of endocrine disease, drug therapy, substance abuse and heavy metal poisoning.

Problem-orientated topic:

hypertension

A family move and register with a new GP. At initial consultation Ruby, a 13-year-old girl, is found to have a systolic blood pressure of 150 mmHg. She is rushed to the paediatric unit where her blood pressure is found to be 160 mmHg systolic.

Q1. How would you assess Ruby?

Q2. What is your management?

Q1. How would you assess Ruby?

Aims
- Identify causes of secondary hypertension; severe hypertension needs aggressive investigation.
- Exclude primary (essential) hypertension.

There is currently no evidence of whether detection and treatment of children with mild hypertension is of any benefit.

History
Many cases in childhood are detected as an incidental finding on examination for another reason. In severe hypertension secondary to renal disease the presentation may be congestive cardiac failure. Hypertension should always be excluded as an explanation for recurrent headache (about one-tenth of children with hypertension will present with neurological symptoms and complications).

The following should be explored:
- Past medical history:
  - UTI
  - Systemic disease
  - Trauma
  - Neonatal intensive care (umbilical catheter)
- Family history
- Growth/weight/puberty
- Medications:
  - Prescription
  - Non-prescription
  - Oral contraceptives
  - Anabolic steroids
  - Diet pills
  - Substance abuse
- Review of systems:
  - Headache
  - Nosebleed
  - Rash.

Physical examination
Assessment of the child with suspected hypertension requires a full cardiac and neurological examination. The abdomen should be examined for possible masses. The following should also be assessed:
- Signs of systemic disease
- Stigmata of syndromes associated with hypertension, e.g. Williams', neurofibromatosis etc.
- Evidence of end-organ damage, e.g. fundi
- Pulses and BP in all four limbs
- Bruits: carotid and renal
- Signs of endocrinopathy.

Investigations
These are done in stages. The initial general stage should include:

- Plasma biochemistry profile
- Full blood count (FBC)
- Peripheral plasma renin and aldosterone levels
- Urinalysis and microscopy
- Urine catecholamine and metabolites
- Chest X-ray (CXR)
- Abdominal ultrasound
- DMSA renal scan
- Electrocardiogram (ECG)
- Echocardiography.

Supplementary investigations to identify a particular diagnosis may include:
- MCUG or voiding isotope scan
- Arteriography
- Selective renal vein renin levels
- Plasma catecholamines
- Isotope scan for phaeochromocytoma
- Other endocrine tests.

Q2. What is your management?

- Treatment of underlying cause
- Weight reduction
- Salt intake reduction
- Lifestyle changes, e.g. exercise.

Medication

In the child with mild hypertension (> 95th percentile) drug therapy is usually not indicated. Appropriate advice on diet, reducing salt intake, avoidance of smoking and regular exercise is usually sufficient, with follow-up measurements of BP.

Severe hypertension as in Ruby's case should be considered a medical emergency and patients should be referred to specialist units. In severe hypertension it is important to reduce BP slowly; precipitous drops are hazardous and may particularly affect vision.

In the longer term the aim should be to maintain the BP at or below the 90th percentile for age, sex and height, or lower if there is continuing renal disease. The choices are:
- Calcium channel blockers
- Angiotensin-converting enzyme (ACE) inhibitors
- Beta-blockers
- Vasodilators.

Glomerular disease

All glomerular diseases are characterized by proteinuria and children may present with a chance finding of proteinuria, with proteinuria associated with other symptoms and signs, or with oedema. However, not all children with proteinuria have glomerular disease. Transient proteinuria is also associated with febrile illnesses, UTI, surgery and trauma. There is also a physiological rise in protein excretion with upright posture and physical exercise. Ideally the first or second urine in the morning after rising should be used to test for proteinuria. Proteinuria in association with oedema, oliguria or hypertension should always be taken seriously and the child must be seen urgently.

Glomerular disease can cause a wide spectrum of clinical pictures:
- Nephrotic syndrome
- Acute glomerulonephritis
- Rapidly progressive glomerulonephritis
- Chronic progressive glomerulonephritis
- Asymptomatic proteinuria/haematuria.

The final diagnosis is often dependent on histology of renal biopsy. The findings may be due to a primary renal disease (most common in childhood) or secondary to a systemic illness (rare in early childhood but increasingly found towards adulthood).

Nephrotic syndrome

Idiopathic nephrotic syndrome in childhood is a disease of unknown aetiology and is characterized by the onset of proteinuria, oedema and hypo-albuminuria, together with hyperlipidaemia. It is more common in boys. Most young children with nephrotic syndrome will have 'minimal change' on renal biopsy. The likelihood of this varies with age of presentation (Fig. 40.4).

The term minimal change is a histological diagnosis and refers to the relative lack of findings on light microscopy of renal biopsy. Most cases of minimal change disease will respond to steroid therapy, and for that reason, children who fit the typical clinical picture should be started on steroids. The long-term prognosis of steroid-sensitive nephrotic syndrome (SSNS) is excellent.

Proteinuria in nephrotic syndrome

Glomerular filtrate is formed by ultrafiltration of plasma across the glomerular capillary wall, which is negatively charged. This wall has three layers: the endothelium, the basement membrane and an outer epithelium consisting of podocytes with interdigitating foot processes. Plasma albumin is negatively charged and there is evidence for a barrier to passage of albumin by electrical charge, as well as a sieve-like size-specific barrier. On renal biopsy in minimal change, whilst there are minimal histological changes on light microscopy, there are changes to the appearance of the foot processes on electron microscopy. It is thought

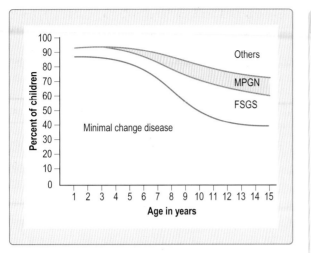

MPGN, membranoproliferative glomerulonephritis;
FSGS, focal and segmental glomerulosclerosis

Fig. 40.4 'Smoothed' representation of the distribution of the major causes of childhood nephrotic syndrome by age.
Based on pooled data from the International Study of Kidney Disease in Childhood and patients investigated at Guy's Hospital, London (n = 566).
Adapted from Postlethwaite RJ (2003) Clinical paediatric nephrology, 2nd edn. Elsevier Science Ltd, with permission.

that loss of negative electrical charge on the basement membrane and epithelium renders the capillary wall permeable to albumin, but the underlying cause remains the subject of extensive research.

Oedema in nephrotic syndrome

Oedema is the central clinical feature in nephrotic syndrome. Its formation is related to changes to the balance of factors affecting the movement of water and small solutes between the intravascular and extravascular compartments.

The Starling equation tells us that oedema can result from an increase in capillary intravascular hydrostatic pressure or from decrease in capillary oncotic pressure. Since plasma protein (mainly albumin) is the main contributor to intravascular oncotic pressure, loss of urinary albumin, causing hypoalbuminaemia, will lead to a shift of fluid from the plasma to the interstitium. This results in contraction of the circulating volume leading to physiological responses (reduction in GFR; activation of the renin–angiotensin–aldosterone system; release of arginine vasopressin (AVP); inhibition of atrial natriuretic peptide (ANP); increased proximal tubular salt and water reabsorption), resulting in salt and water retention.

Problem-orientated topic:

oedema

Trudie, a 4-year-old, has had generalized oedema for 2 days and is found to have proteinurla on stick testing. A diagnosis of nephrotic syndrome is suspected.

Q1. Is this likely to be minimal change disease?
Q2. What complications may be expected?
Q3. What investigations are appropriate at initial presentation?
Q4. What are the indications for consideration of renal biopsy?
Q5. What management is necessary?

Q1. Is this likely to be minimal change disease?

Clinical features suggestive of minimal change disease are:
• Age over 1 year and under 10 years
• Rapid onset of oedema (days rather than months)
• Heavy proteinuria +++/++++ on stick testing.

Q2. What complications may be expected?

Acute complications
• Discomfort or even skin breakdown related to extreme oedema
• Hypoalbuminuria, leading to intravascular hypovolaemia
• Acute renal failure secondary to hypovolaemia
• Hypercoagulability leading to vascular thrombosis (exacerbated by hypovolaemia)
• Infection.

Assessment of hypovolaemia in an oedematous child is difficult. It may be suggested by:
• Cold periphery
• Delayed capillary refill
• Reduced jugular venous pressure (JVP)
• Low sodium (< 20 mmol/l) in urine
• Abdominal pain.

N.B. Abdominal pain in an oedematous child with nephrotic syndrome may be a symptom of hypovolaemia or peritonitis and should be taken seriously.

Chronic complications
• Steroid and other medication side-effects (Box 40.13).

- Change in facial appearance and body shape
- Weight gain
- Poor growth
- Striae
- Acne
- Behavioural changes
- Adrenal suppression
- Infections (especially chickenpox)
- Reduction in bone mineral density
- Proximal myopathy

Q3. What investigations are appropriate at initial presentation?

- Plasma urea, electrolytes, creatinine, albumin, total protein, calcium, phosphate, lipid profile, complement C3 and C4, antistreptolysin O titre (ASOT), antinuclear antibody (ANA), autoantibody screen
- Hepatitis B and varicella serology
- FBC
- Urine: stick test and microscopy; albumin (or protein):creatinine ratio; sodium, osmolality and creatinine.

Q4. What are the indications for consideration of renal biopsy?

Discuss these with the regional centre:
- Age under 1 year or over 10 years
- Gradual onset of oedema
- Macroscopic haematuria
- Hypertension
- Rash or other features of systemic disease
- Low complement C3 or C4
- Failure of response to steroids by 4 weeks.

Q5. What management is necessary?

- *Prednisolone*: current International Study of Kidney Disease in Children (ISKDC) recommendations are 4 weeks of 60 mg/m² followed by 4 weeks of 40 mg/m² on alternate days for initial presentation.
- *Penicillin*: prophylactic to prevent pneumococcal peritonitis.
- *Dietary sodium restriction*: if adequately salt-restricted, the child is unlikely to need fluid restriction.
- *Albumin infusion*: in hypovolaemia.

Assessment of intravascular fluid volume and urine output is essential in the safe treatment of children presenting with acute oedema. Infusion of 20% albumin to restore oncotic pressure and treat hypovolaemia is often appropriate but can be hazardous in children whose GFR is so reduced they are in established renal failure.

Most children with SSNS will have more than one episode and some will go on to frequent relapses. Those having repeated courses of high-dose steroids or requiring long-term continuous steroids (> 0.5 mg/kg/day) or with clinical evidence of steroid toxicity should be considered for second-line therapy using agents such as levamisole, cyclophosphamide or ciclosporin/tacrolimus. Initiation of such treatments is usually done in conjunction or discussion with a tertiary paediatric nephrology centre.

The children who do not have SSNS will turn out to have a variety of different histological findings on renal biopsy and generally have a less satisfactory response to treatments and a worse long-term prognosis. A small number will turn out to have minimal change disease but have a late (4–8-week) response to steroids or, extremely rarely, are steroid-resistant.

Glomerulonephritis

Problem-orientated topic:

haematuria

A 14-year-old boy, Christopher, develops haematuria and is sent by his GP to the paediatric assessment unit. On questioning he admits to some pain on passing urine and also admits this has happened three times in the last year and on each occasion has lasted for a few days before clearing.

Q1. What is the most likely diagnosis? What is the differential diagnosis?

Q2. What investigations would you order?

Q3. How would you decide if Christopher needs referral to a specialist centre?

Q1. What is the most likely diagnosis? What is the differential diagnosis?

Acute glomerulonephritis refers to diseases characterized by the acute onset of haematuria, proteinuria, oedema and often hypertension. There are a wide variety of underlying causes and the prognosis is often related to the underlying diagnosis.

Some children with glomerulonephritis may have a strong nephrotic element to their presentation. Diagnosis is usually histological. In the UK, IgA nephritis is probably more common than post-infectious or post-streptococcal nephritis since the decline in streptococcal infections in recent years.

Q2. What investigations would you order?

- *Blood* FBC: urea, electrolytes, creatinine, albumin, protein, calcium, phosphate, immunoglobulins, complement C3 and C4, ANA, antineutrophil cytoplasmic antibody (ANCA), anti-double-stranded DNA, anti-glomerular basement membrane (GBM) antibodies, autoantibody screen, ASOT, hepatitis B and C status
- *Urine*: sodium, osmolality, creatinine; stix; microscopy for red cell morphology, casts (and to exclude infection); albumin (or protein):creatinine ratio
- *Throat swab*.
- Many children will require renal biopsy

Q3. How would you decide if Christopher needs referral to a specialist centre?

Features suggesting serious pathology include:
- Elevated or rising plasma creatinine
- Oliguria
- Heavy proteinuria
- Persistent proteinuria
- Severe hypertension
- Severe oedema.

Urinary tract stones (Box 40.14)

Urolithiasis is a stone in the urinary tract whereas nephrocalcinosis implies an increase in the calcium content of the kidney.

The incidence and composition of stones vary with geographical region. In the UK incidence is around 2

> **BOX 40.14 Stone formation**
>
> Complex interaction of several factors:
> - Urinary concentration of stone-forming chemicals
> - Urine flow rate
> - Urine pH
> - Balance of promoter and inhibitor factors for crystallization, e.g. citrate, magnesium, pyrophosphate
> - Presence of foreign body
> - Presence of infection
> - Anatomical factors causing urinary stasis.
>   Principles of treatment need to address these factors.

children/million population (cf. 2 adults/thousand population). It is much higher in other parts of the world: for example, the Middle and Far East, North Africa. Factors such as socioeconomic status, climate, race, diet, fluid intake, dehydration and infections may be important. In European children more than half of cases are infective in origin and are frequently related to *Proteus* urine infection. The most common cause of metabolic stones in the West is hypercalciuria.

Clinical features may be non-specific, especially in younger children. About half will have abdominal, flank or back pain. A few will pass a stone and it is vital that such stones are retrieved and analysed chemically. Microscopic haematuria is usually present and renal stones should be part of the differential diagnosis of any child with glomerular haematuria.

Clinical approach
- History and examination, including careful attention to family history, dietary history, growth and blood pressure
- Urinalysis and urine microscopy
- Ultrasound
- Radiology (Ca content determines 'visibility' on abdominal X-ray)
- Plasma biochemistry, including urea and electrolytes, ionized calcium, phosphate, magnesium, bicarbonate, chloride, parathyroid hormone (PTH)
- Urine biochemistry, including calcium, magnesium, oxalate, glycolate, glycerate, urate, cystine:creatinine ratio; urinary pH.

Causes of stone formation
See Box 40.15.

Management
Medical treatment depends on the underlying condition. Avoidance of dehydration is often important and dietary manipulation may be necessary in some conditions.

Surgical treatment may be required and techniques include ureteroscopy, extracorporeal shock-wave lithotripsy, percutaneous nephrolithotomy and open surgery.

Renal tubular disorders

Renal tubular disorders may be congenital or acquired. Since the renal tubule is responsible for the reabsorption of water and electrolytes in the glomerular ultrafiltrate, disorders may lead to profound electrolyte and volume disturbance. Most children with genetic

BOX 40.15 Causes of stone formation

Struvite stones (radio-opaque)
- Associated with urine infections

Calcium stones (radio-opaque)
- Hypercalciuria + normocalcaemia:
  - Idiopathic
  - Distal renal tubular acidosis
  - Furosemide treatment
  - Hyperalimentation
  - Hypophosphataemia
  - Juvenile rheumatoid arthritis
  - Medullary sponge kidney
- Hypercalciuria + hypercalcaemia:
  - Hyperparathyroidism
  - Vitamin D excess
  - Endocrine disorders
- Hypercalciuria associated with low molecular weight proteinuria:
  - Dent's disease

Oxalate stones (radio-opaque)
- Primary hyperoxaluria types 1 and 2
- Enteric hyperoxaluria
- Idiopathic

Uric acid stones (radiolucent)
- Familial
- Over-production
- Hyperuricosuria

Cystine stones (usually radio-opaque)
- Cystinuria

Miscellaneous conditions
- Inflammatory bowel disease
- Cystic fibrosis

tubular disorders present in infancy with non-specific symptoms like failure to thrive or poor feeding.

Bartter's syndrome

The main problem is tubular loss of sodium and chloride and secondarily excess loss of potassium in the distal tubule associated with hyper-reninaemia and hyperaldosteronism. In all forms there is hypokalaemia, hyponatraemia and alkalosis with increased urinary chloride excretion. Inheritance is autosomal recessive.

Fanconi's syndrome

In Fanconi's syndrome there is a generalized failure of proximal tubular reabsorption of sodium, bicarbonate, phosphate, glucose and amino acids, and in addition reabsorptive processes in the distal nephron are overloaded.

Causes
- Genetic:
  - Galactosaemia
  - Mitochondrial disorders
  - Cystinosis
  - Lowe's syndrome
  - Wilson's disease
- Acquired:
  - Drugs:
    Aminoglycosides
    Ifosfamide
  - Renal disorders:
    Recovery phase of acute tubular necrosis
    Early post-renal transplant
    Acute interstitial nephritis
  - Other:
    Heavy metal poisoning
    Multiple myeloma.

Cystinosis

Cystinosis is an autosomal recessive disorder in which there is excess accumulation of intracellular cystine because of a defect of lysosomal cystine transport. This particularly affects proximal tubule cells, leading to Fanconi's syndrome. Progression to renal failure is inevitable, though patients do well after transplantation.

Nephrogenic diabetes insipidus (NDI)

NDI is a disorder in which the kidney fails to respond to the hormone AVP, leading to failure of urinary concentration. The congenital form is most severe and results from genetic defects in the AVP receptor or associated water channels. It is inherited in an X-linked manner and affected boys present in the newborn period with dehydration, poor growth and irritability.

Polycystic renal disease

The use of the term polycystic implies specific diagnoses that should not be confused with the wide spectrum of other cystic kidney diseases that exist. These include glomerulocystic kidney disease, medullary cystic disease and cystic dysplasia. Multicystic dysplastic kidney is the extreme end of the dysplasia spectrum and implies a non-functioning kidney with no connection to the bladder. Cystic kidneys are an important component of a number of syndromes.

Polycystic renal disease is an inherited disorder. In the autosomal recessive form (ARPKD), which is also called infantile polycystic kidney disease, the kidneys are large and are often easily palpated. There may be an antenatal diagnosis and there may be oligohydramnios and pulmonary hypoplasia, so some affected babies do not survive the neonatal period. Progression to renal failure frequently occurs in early childhood. Hepatic fibrosis is invariably present but early on may not be evident clinically or on ultrasound. Management is supportive with aggressive control of hypertension and management of renal failure and eventually renal and/or liver transplant.

Autosomal dominant polycystic kidney disease (ADPKD) may be detected antenatally, in the neonatal period or in early childhood but it is more likely to present in later childhood or in adulthood. Those presenting very early in life are thought to have a more severe outcome and some may progress to end-stage renal failure in childhood. Others may preserve renal function for many decades, though eventual progression into renal failure is a significant likelihood. Control of hypertension is a major factor influencing progression of disease as well as cardiovascular morbidity and mortality. This is an important issue in discussion and decisions about screening asymptomatic family members for the condition.

Urinary tract dilatation

Dilatation of the urinary tract is usually detected on ultrasound. This may be done as a follow-up of anomalies found on antenatal screening or when ultrasound is performed during investigation for urinary tract problems like UTI. Occasionally urinary tract obstruction may present acutely with pain or infection.

Hydronephrosis describes dilatation of the collecting system of the kidney and hydroureter describes dilatation of the ureter, but neither term implies obstruction.

There is no clear definition or test for obstruction, and diagnosis requires clinical and functional assessment as well as imaging.

Causes of a dilated urinary tract
- Obstruction:
  - E.g. stone in ureter
  - Posterior urethral valves
  - Pelvi-ureteric obstruction
  - Neuropathic bladder
- VUR
- Non-obstructed and non-refluxing.

Rarely, reflux and obstruction can occur together in duplex system.

Dilated upper urinary tract presenting in the neonatal period is discussed on p. 392.

Acute renal failure

Acute renal failure (ARF) can result from a wide variety of causes. ARF should be suspected in any patient who is oliguric, though it may be picked up on 'routine' biochemistry of an unwell child.

In childhood, ARF may be seen with a high, normal or low urine output. On plasma biochemistry an increase in urea and creatinine is seen and there is an inability of the kidney to regulate fluid and electrolytes appropriately. ARF may occur in isolation — for example, in intrinsic renal disease like glomerulonephritis — or may coexist or result from other disorders — for example, in multi-organ failure in an intensive care situation.

Causes of ARF
- *Prerenal*: hypovolaemia secondary to gastroenteritis, haemorrhage, burns, septic shock, nephrotic syndrome, cardiac failure
- *Intrarenal*: HUS, acute tubular necrosis (ATN), ischaemia, nephrotoxic agents, acute glomerulonephritis, pyelonephritis, acute interstitial nephritis, cortical or medullary necrosis, bilateral renal artery thrombosis, infiltration by neoplastic disease
- *Postrenal*: bladder outflow obstruction — urethral valves, blocked catheter, bilateral ureteric obstruction, bilateral stones, unilateral obstruction of a single kidney, neuropathic bladder, tumours, trauma (bleeding and clot).

Assessment of volume status is critical to initial treatment strategies. It is important to assess systolic BP together with intravascular volume, either directly with central venous pressure measurements, or indirectly by JVP, core peripheral temperature difference and capillary refill. Urinary urea and electrolytes and creatinine measurements are very useful tools in assessing whether renal failure is prerenal or established intrarenal. In hypovolaemia the urinary sodium and fractional excretion of sodium (Na) are usually low (urine Na < 20 mmol/l, fractional excretion of sodium < 1%) and the urine osmolality may be high.

In the case of suspected intrarenal disease, where there is no clear cause of ATN and no diagnosis of HUS, then a renal biopsy is often required. In the initial stages it is important to establish the diagnosis and identify and manage any life-threatening abnormalities. More complex investigations may take longer to establish the underlying cause, which may be multifactorial. It should be remembered that some children presenting in ARF actually have acute on chronic failure and may have had undiagnosed renal impairment for some time.

Life-threatening emergencies in ARF

- Hyperkalaemia (Box 40.16)
- Shock
- Metabolic acidosis
- Hypertension
- Fluid overload/pulmonary oedema.

Children who are intravascularly hypovolaemic should be given a bolus of 20 ml/kg of 0.9% saline (except when hypovolaemia is due to haemorrhage, when it makes sense to infuse blood, or when nephrotic, when 20% albumin is used). This should be repeated until circulatory volume has been restored, but if a urine output has not been established with good volume status and intravenous furosemide, then fluid restriction related to current urine output should be commenced (Box 40.17).

Indications for renal replacement therapy (RRT)

Indications for institution of RRT (haemo- or peritoneal dialysis or haemofiltration) are complex and there is no set of measurements or biochemical values that indicate RRT should commence. In general the underlying cause, clinical condition, speed of progression of ARF, response to treatments, access availability and setting will influence decisions to start RRT. RRT in children should only be performed in specialist settings, and discussions with specialist centres should take place at an early stage regarding any child whose renal function is deteriorating.

Henoch–Schönlein purpura (HSP)

This condition is discussed in detail on page 269.

Renal involvement is common, with microscopic or macroscopic haematuria or mild proteinuria in over 80% of cases. Generally these features resolve, but if proteinuria persists, nephrotic syndrome may result. Indicators of progressive renal disease are heavy proteinuria, oedema, hypertension and deteriorating renal function. Fewer than 1% of patients develop persistent renal disease and fewer than 0.1% severe renal disease. The principal differential diagnoses of HSP are idiopathic thrombocytopenia and meningococcal disease.

Investigations

- FBC, inflammatory markers, immunoglobulins
- Urine microscopy and dipstick for red blood cells, white blood cells, casts or albumin
- Skin biopsy: rarely needed; will demonstrate a leucocytoclastic vasculitis
- Renal biopsy: similarly, may show IgA mesangial deposition and occasionally IgM, C3 and fibrin.

Haemolytic uraemic syndrome

HUS is the most common cause of ARF in childhood in Europe and North America. Most cases are associated with a diarrhoea prodrome (so-called 'D+ HUS'). HUS without diarrhoea has a large number of rare causes and a worse prognosis. In the UK most D+ HUS cases are associated with infection with verocytotoxin-producing *Escherichia coli*. The natural reservoir is farm animals, though outbreaks have been associated with a wide variety of foodstuffs.

Any age group can be affected but the disease is typically found in preschool children (and the elderly). They frequently have bloody diarrhoea several days to a couple of weeks before presenting with reduced urine output, pallor and malaise. There is microangiopathic haemolytic anaemia, thrombocytopenia and renal failure. The gastrointestinal disease may be severe. Neurological involvement carries a poor prognosis.

Diagnosis is by blood film together with biochemical evidence of renal failure. If HUS is suspected but the initial blood film does not support the diagnosis, a film should be repeatedly examined over the next hours and days.

There is no specific effective treatment though many agents have been tried. Antibiotics should probably be avoided. The mainstay is supportive management with control of fluid and electrolyte disturbance, dialysis and blood transfusion. Most children recover but there is still a significant mortality (reported 2–10%) and up to one-third of survivors have some long-term renal sequelae in the form of ongoing renal impairment, proteinuria or hypertension.

Chronic renal failure

Chronic renal failure (CRF) may present in a wide variety of ways.

Presentation of CRF
- General or non-specific malaise
- Failure to thrive
- Short stature
- Rickets
- Anaemia/pallor
- Hypertension
- Enuresis
- UTI
- Screening: sibling or antenatal
- Acute on chronic renal failure
- Congestive cardiac failure
- Pulmonary oedema.

Because of the wide range of presentations and causes a very detailed history and examination is essential to give clues towards further investigations. The history may help distinguish between ARF, when the child has been previously fit and well, and CRF, when the child may have been non-specifically unwell or have had problems with appetite or growth for many months or even years. There may have been specific urinary symptoms like polyuria, polydipsia, wetting or recurrent UTI.

Major causes of CRF
- Congenital abnormalities
- Hypoplasia/dysplasia
- Reflux nephropathy
- Glomerulonephritis
- Multisystem disease
- Inherited conditions.

Investigations

Often when a finding of impaired renal function is confirmed on initial blood biochemistry results, it is not possible to determine how much renal recovery is possible. Therefore repeated biochemistry over days, weeks and months is important in determining both the chronicity of the condition and the actual level of renal function, once other factors like infection or hypertension are corrected.

Findings of non-haemolytic anaemia, small or dysplastic kidneys on ultrasound, X-ray evidence of rickets and end-organ damage from hypertension point towards chronic rather than acute renal failure.

Investigations in CRF may include:
- Urine microscopy and urinalysis
- Urine albumin:creatinine ratio
- Urine biochemistry, urea and electrolytes, creatinine, osmolality, calcium, phosphate, oxalate, cystine

- Blood biochemistry including liver function tests, bone biochemistry, bicarbonate, intact PTH, ferritin, lipid profile
- Renal tract ultrasound
- CXR
- Wrist X-ray
- Echocardiography
- MCUG
- Isotope scans, DMSA, MAG3
- Immunology bloods complement C3 and C4, ANCA, ANA, anti-GBM antibodies, autoantibodies, anti-double-stranded DNA antibodies
- Renal biopsy
- White cell cystine.

Management

The first aim of management is to treat any underlying disorder and associated conditions, then to preserve and improve renal function to prevent a decline into end-stage renal failure for as long as possible. Meticulous attention needs to be paid to maintaining nutrition and growth; controlling BP; treating fluid, electrolyte and acid–base imbalance; controlling renal osteodystrophy; and treating anaemia.

Indications for RRT

The indications for RRT are complex and dependent on a holistic view of the child, not specific biochemical values. In general RRT is started when the child becomes symptomatic from renal failure, with tiredness, anorexia and vomiting, or when blood biochemistry approaches hazardous levels despite therapy and dietary restrictions.

End-stage renal failure and transplantation

Renal failure is a continuum from mild renal impairment through preterminal renal failure to the end stage. End-stage renal failure is when the need for RRT is imminent. The ultimate aim of therapy is renal transplantation because it places far less restriction on normal life and is associated with lower morbidity and mortality. Dialysis is generally considered as a therapy used before or between transplantation, except for those few individuals who are currently unable to be transplanted when dialysis is used as long-term therapy over many years and even decades. Transplantation before dialysis is common when the child is to receive a living donor kidney. Some children are not suitable for pre-emptive transplantation.

The choice of dialysis modality is individual to the child and family. Haemodialysis for children is based in a few specialist centres and therefore travel to and from the centre for a 3–5-hour session three times a week may be an issue. Fluid restriction is normally more severe when on haemodialysis, but the family is relieved of some stresses and responsibilities and the child retains some independence. Home peritoneal dialysis is usually done by machine overnight. This enables normal school attendance. There is a huge burden on the care-givers and the child is very dependent on them on a regular basis. Sudden fluid and electrolyte shifts are avoided. Fluid and dietary restrictions are minimized. It is particularly suited to younger patients. Peritoneal dialysis is often the first choice of dialysis modality.

Successful renal transplantation offers the nearest to a normal lifestyle and is the preferred form of treatment for end-stage renal failure. Living donor kidneys have better graft survival figures than cadaveric. Immunosuppression medication needs to continue indefinitely and non-compliance with medication is a significant cause of graft failure in teenagers and young adults.

Frank Casey   Brian Grant

Cardiovascular system

LEARNING OUTCOMES

By the end of this chapter you should:

- Know the factors distinguishing an innocent and pathological murmur
- Be able to assess and manage the child in heart failure
- Be able to recognize the typical ECG appearance of the common arrhythmias and know the basic management of each
- Be able to recognize the historical and clinical features in the child with chest pain of cardiac origin
- Know the clinical features of the common cardiac conditions presenting in childhood
- Be able to recognize chest X-ray abnormalities associated with cardiac disease.

Assessment

Congenital heart disease (CHD) is the most commonly occurring severe congenital abnormality. The prevalence is 0.8–0.9 per 1000 live births. For those with major CHD early and accurate diagnosis can be vitally important to morbidity and mortality. The presentation can vary from the asymptomatic child presenting with a murmur to the child who presents acutely unwell with cyanosis or heart failure.

History and physical examination

History

Key symptoms in the history to elicit when assessing a child for possible heart disease are as follows.

Infants
- Feeding difficulties: breathlessness, sweating or tiring with feeds
- Failure to thrive
- Episodes of central cyanosis.

The older child
- Breathlessness and fatigue with exertion
- Palpitations
- Chest pain
- Dizziness or syncope on exertion.

Physical examination
- An initial assessment of growth parameters is important since failure to thrive is a common presentation of CHD in infancy.

BOX 41.1 Assessment of heart murmurs

I Intensity: grade 1–6

II Timing — systolic, diastolic or continuous:
- Systolic murmurs are classified as ejection systolic, pansystolic or late systolic
- Diastolic murmurs should be classified as early or mid-diastolic

III Character: e.g. harsh, musical, vibratory, blowing

IV Area of maximal intensity

V Radiation: back, axilla, neck

- Is there central cyanosis? Assess the lips, tongue, mucous membranes and nail beds.
- Is the child in heart failure? The classical signs are tachycardia, tachypnoea and hepatomegaly.
- Check the pulses in all four limbs. Are they of normal, increased or decreased volume? Palpation of the femoral pulses is one of the most important points in the examination.
- Check the blood pressure in the right arm and also a leg blood pressure.
- Palpate the precordium: note the presence of any heaves or thrills, locate the apex beat.
- Finally auscultate the heart:
  - Assess the heart sounds. Is their intensity normal?
  - Is there normal splitting of the second heart sound?
  - Are there any additional heart sounds or clicks?

Any murmur should be evaluated according to the parameters in Box 41.1.

The specific clinical findings found in the more common congenital heart problems are described in later sections dealing with each in turn. Some lesions occur more commonly in association with certain syndromes (Table 41.1).

The electrocardiogram (ECG)

The ECG remains an important basic investigation in the assessment of any child suspected of having CHD. Consideration of the age of the patient is important in the interpretation of any ECG change. It is very difficult to remember normal values for all the ECG parameters at various ages, but the important ones are summarized in Box 41.2.

Congestive cardiac failure

Basic science

The cardiac output is governed by the equation:

Table 41.1 Congenital heart disease and syndromes

Syndrome	Associated defects
Down's (trisomy 21)	Atrioventricular septal defect Ventricular septal defect Tetralogy of Fallot Atrial septal defect Patent ductus arteriosus
Edwards' (trisomy 18)	Ventricular septal defect Atrial septal defect Double outlet right ventricle
Patau's (trisomy 13)	Ventricular septal defect Atrial septal defect
Turner's (XO)	Coarctation of aorta Aortic stenosis
Klinefelter's (XXY)	Tetralogy of Fallot Ventricular septal defect Atrial septal defect Patent ductus arteriosus
22q11	Interrupted aortic arch Truncus arteriosus Tetralogy of Fallot Pulmonary atresia
Noonan's	Pulmonary stenosis Atrial septal defect Hypertrophic cardiomyopathy
Marfan's	Aortic root dilatation Dissecting aortic aneurysm Mitral valve prolapse and mitral regurgitation
Williams'	Supravalvular aortic stenosis Pulmonary artery stenosis
Cri-du-chat	Ventricular septal defect Atrial septal defect Patent ductus arteriosus

Cardiac output (l/min) = stroke volume (l) × heart rate (bpm)

The stroke volume is governed primarily by the preload, the myocardial contractility and the afterload (Table 41.2). In simple terms, the preload of a ventricle is the degree to which it is stretched prior to contraction, and the afterload is the vascular resistance against which it ejects.

The Frank–Starling law states that the energy of contraction is proportional to the initial length of the cardiac muscle fibre. There is therefore a close relationship between the ventricular end-diastolic volume and the stroke volume (Fig. 41.1).

Problem-orientated topic:

lethargy and breathlessness

Peter, an 8-week-old baby boy, presents to the accident and emergency department

Continued overleaf

with a history of decreased feeding over the previous week. His parents report that they feel he is more lethargic this morning. Initial assessment reveals a respiratory rate of 60 breaths per minute, subcostal recession and intercostal indrawing. Oxygen saturations in room air are 94% and heart rate is 160 beats per minute. Capillary refill time is 3 seconds. The precordium is active and a harsh pansystolic murmur is audible. The liver is enlarged 3 cm below the right costal margin. Peripheral pulses are normal in volume.

Q1. What is your differential diagnosis?

Q2. What investigations are you going to request?

Q3. What is your initial management plan?

BOX 41.2 A logical approach to reading the ECG

Must include analysis of the following parameters:

1. *Rhythm*. Is there sinus rhythm? In sinus rhythm a p wave should precede each QRS axis and the p wave axis should be normal, as indicated by the presence of an upright p wave in leads 2, 3 and aVF.

2. *Heart rate*. Is it within the normal range for age?

3. *P wave*. Axis and magnitude. Is there atrial enlargement? A p wave in any lead that is peaked and > 3 mm in magnitude is suggestive of right atrial enlargement. A bifid p wave in lead 2 is the traditional sign of left atrial enlargement but this can occasionally be observed in normal children.

4. *PR interval*. Is it shorter or longer than normal?

5. *QRS frontal axis*. In the newborn period the normal QRS axis is rightward; as the child grows, it becomes leftward, such that at age 1–3 years the 50th percentile is 60° and it remains at that level during the rest of childhood.

6. *QRS duration*. Is it prolonged?

7. *QT interval*. The important figure is the QTc, which is the QT interval corrected for heart rate. The upper limit of normal is 440 msec.

8. *T wave axis*. In the first few days of life the T wave is upright in lead V_1 but, in most cases, by days 5–7 the T wave axis has changed, so that the T wave becomes negative in this lead. Persistence of an upright T wave beyond 1 week of age is indicative of right ventricular hypertrophy. In the normal heart the T waves usually remain inverted until later childhood, when they again become upright.

BOX 41.2 A logical approach to reading the ECG (cont'd)

9. *Magnitude of R and S waves*. Is there evidence of hypertrophy of the right or left ventricle? In addition to an upright T wave the presence of a Q wave in V_1 is also an indicator of right ventricular hypertrophy. A frontal QRS axis of less than 30° is suggestive of left ventricular hypertrophy (LVH). In the newborn infant LVH is indicated by an SV_1 of > 19 mm or an RV_1 of > 11 mm.

Table 41.2 Factors influencing stroke volume

Factor	Affected by
Preload	Length of diastole Venous return Atrial systole Myocardial compliance
Myocardial contractility	Sympathetic nervous system Metabolic abnormalities Electrolyte imbalance Inotropic drugs Intrinsic myocardial dysfunction
Afterload	Aortic resistance Peripheral vascular resistance Haematocrit (blood viscosity) Vasodilator drugs

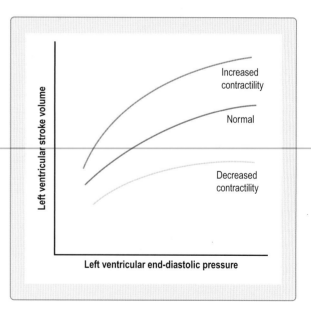

Fig. 41.1 The relationship between left ventricular end-diastolic volume and stroke volume.
As left ventricular end-diastolic pressure increases, stroke volume increases up to a critical point.

Q1. What is your differential diagnosis?

Peter's history and examination findings suggest that he has congestive cardiac failure (Box 41.3). He displays the

BOX 41.3 Clinical presentation of heart failure in infants

Symptoms

- Breathlessness
- Poor feeding
- Sweating (especially with feeds)
- Restlessness
- Lethargy
- Poor weight gain

Signs

- Pallor
- Poor peripheral perfusion
- Tachypnoea
- Increased work of breathing
- Tachycardia
- Gallop rhythm (4th heart sound)
- Hepatomegaly
- Ventricular heave
- Murmur (due to underlying cause)

BOX 41.4 Aetiology of heart failure

Volume overload

- Left-to-right shunt: e.g. ventricular septal defect, atrioventricular septal defect, patent ductus arteriosus, atrial septal defect
- Valvular regurgitation: e.g. aortic regurgitation, mitral regurgitation
- Complex congenital cardiac lesions: e.g. univentricular heart
- Arteriovenous malformation: e.g. vein of Galen, haemangioma

Pressure overload

- Left heart obstructive lesions: e.g. severe aortic stenosis, coarctation of aorta, hypoplastic left heart syndrome
- Acute hypertension: e.g. haemolytic uraemic syndrome, acute glomerulonephritis
- Right heart obstructive lesions: severe pulmonary stenosis

Cardiac arrhythmias

- Congenital complete heart block
- Supraventricular tachycardia
- Ventricular tachycardia

Ventricular dysfunction

- Myocarditis
- Cardiomyopathy: dilated, hypertrophic, restrictive
- Sepsis
- Pericardial effusion/cardiac tamponade
- Ischaemia: e.g. anomalous left coronary artery, birth asphyxia

typical triad of tachypnoea, tachycardia and hepatomegaly associated with heart failure. Heart failure occurs when the cardiac output can no longer meet the circulatory and metabolic needs of the body.

In Peter's case the most likely diagnosis is a congenital cardiac lesion causing a significant left-to-right shunt, such as a large ventricular septal defect (VSD).

The most common causes of heart failure in childhood are summarized in Box 41.4.

Q2. What investigations are you going to request?

- *Chest X-ray* (CXR): will usually show cardiomegaly and plethoric lung fields as a result of increased pulmonary blood flow or pulmonary venous congestion (Fig. 41.2).
- *ECG*: may demonstrate evidence of chamber enlargement.
- *Echocardiogram*: enables identification of the underlying cardiac lesion and provides information regarding ventricular function.

Q3. What is your initial management plan?

The initial management goal is to stabilize the patient by maximizing oxygen delivery to the tissues. This can be achieved by a combination of preload reduction, optimization of myocardial contractility and afterload reduction (Box 41.5).

Box 41.5 summarizes management. Continual reassessment is important in the management of the child with

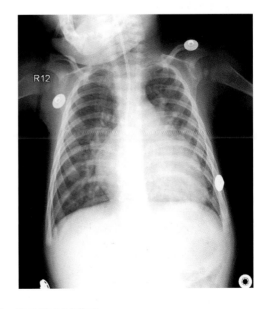

Fig. 41.2 Heart failure.
Chest X-ray showing cardiomegaly and pulmonary oedema due to a large ventricular septal defect.

BOX 41.5 Medical management of heart failure

Oxygen
- Judicious use if duct-dependent lesion suspected

Diuretics
- Result in preload reduction by inhibiting sodium and water reabsorption in the renal tubules
- Oral or i.v. furosemide (loop diuretic) often used in conjunction with a potassium-sparing diuretic (e.g. spironolactone or amiloride)

Inotropes
- Improve myocardial contractility
- Oral or i.v. digoxin: inhibits Na^+–K^+ adenosine triphosphatase in myocardium, which in turn increases intracellular Ca^{2+}. Patient is usually given loading doses followed by twice daily maintenance dose
- Beta-adrenergic agonists: i.v. infusion dopamine and/or dobutamine

Angiotensin-converting enzyme (ACE) inhibitors
- Result in afterload reduction by decreasing peripheral vascular resistance (inhibit conversion of angiotensin I to angiotensin II)
- May also produce venodilatation (and therefore preload reduction) and interfere with aldosterone production
- Oral captopril: commenced at low dose and built up in increments. Monitor for hypotension with dose increase, renal dysfunction and serum potassium

heart failure. Further measures, such as ventilation and management in the intensive care setting, may be appropriate.

It is important to exclude concomitant aggravating factors, such as anaemia, and treat accordingly. Nutrition is also an important consideration and should be optimized with the addition of high-calorie supplements to feeds if necessary. Following medical stabilization, surgical or cardiac catheter intervention may be required to repair or palliate the underlying cardiac lesion.

Pathophysiology of left-to-right shunts

A congenital cardiac lesion that causes a left-to-right shunt essentially places a volume load on the heart. This results from a communication between the systemic and pulmonary circulations, which allows shunting of fully oxygenated blood back to the lungs. If we consider a VSD, there are two main factors that determine the magnitude of the left-to-right shunt and therefore the degree of volume loading:

- The size of the defect
- The pulmonary vascular resistance (PVR).

For a small VSD the degree of shunting is restricted by the size of the lesion. For a large VSD, the defect size could allow unrestrictive shunting, the degree of which is determined by the PVR. With a high PVR, such as occurs in the first weeks of life, there is minimal shunting and few symptoms. When the PVR falls at around 6–8 weeks of life, the magnitude of the left-to-right shunt increases and the symptoms of heart failure increase accordingly. It should be noted that it is the left heart that is volume-loaded in this scenario.

Ventricular septal defect

A VSD is a developmental defect in the interventricular septum, resulting in communication between the two ventricles. It is the most prevalent form of congenital heart defect, accounting for 30% of CHD. A VSD may occur as an isolated defect, or it may be a component of such anomalies as tetralogy of Fallot, coarctation of the aorta, transposition of the great arteries or complete atrioventricular septal defect. Broadly, VSDs may be classified as perimembranous, muscular or subarterial defects.

Clinical features
Symptoms and signs associated with an isolated VSD largely relate to the degree of left-to-right shunt. In those with a moderate to large VSD, at around 6–8 weeks of age when the PVR has fallen significantly, symptoms and signs of congestive cardiac failure become apparent. It should be noted that this change may occur earlier in preterm infants. An infant or child with a small VSD may well have normal growth and be free of symptoms, with suspicion raised by the presence of a murmur during routine examination.

Examination may reveal an active precordium, with a right ventricular heave and possibly a systolic thrill present at the left lower sternal border. Typically there is a pansystolic murmur that is harsh in character and loudest in this area. In the presence of a large left-to-right shunt there may be a mid-diastolic murmur over the apex from increased flow across the mitral valve.

Investigations
CXR may demonstrate cardiomegaly and increased pulmonary vascular markings, with the degree being directly related to the size of shunt. ECG may demonstrate evidence

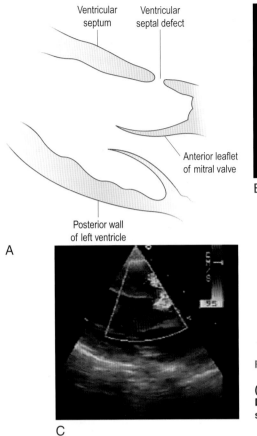

Ventricular septum   Ventricular septal defect

Anterior leaflet of mitral valve

Posterior wall of left ventricle

A

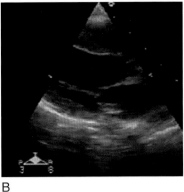

B

C

Fig. 41.3 **Ventricular septal defect. (A) Diagram showing locations; (B) echocardiogram; (C) Colour Doppler study showing left to right shunting.**

of chamber enlargement, typically of the left heart. Two-dimensional echocardiography allows diagnosis of the position and size of the VSD (Fig. 41.3). Colour and continuous wave Doppler interrogation allows assessment of the direction and magnitude of the flow across the defect.

Management

Initial management is directed towards medical treatment of symptomatic congestive cardiac failure and optimization of calorific intake. Early surgical closure of VSD is indicated when congestive cardiac failure/failure to thrive is unresponsive to medical therapy. Other indications include a Qp:Qs (ratio of pulmonary and systemic blood flow) greater than 2:1, when there is evidence of increasing PVR, and when closure will prevent the progression of associated aortic incompetence.

Pulmonary artery banding may be necessary in the infant with multiple VSDs or in the presence of associated anomalies. Transcatheter device closure of VSD may be possible in selected cases.

Children with a small VSD are usually asymptomatic and most do not require any active treatment. The defects tend to become smaller with time and the majority undergo spontaneous closure.

Complete atrioventricular septal defect

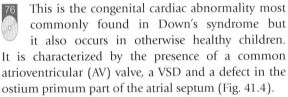

This is the congenital cardiac abnormality most commonly found in Down's syndrome but it also occurs in otherwise healthy children. It is characterized by the presence of a common atrioventricular (AV) valve, a VSD and a defect in the ostium primum part of the atrial septum (Fig. 41.4).

As a result of the excessive pulmonary flow patients usually present with severe heart failure, failure to thrive and feeding difficulties. Early management involves medical anti-failure therapy with diuretics and angiotensin-converting enzyme (ACE) inhibitors in conjunction with maximizing calorie intake with the aid of nasogastric feeding. Since there is a significant risk of developing pulmonary vascular disease, especially in those with Down's syndrome, early surgical repair is required. Surgical correction now has an operative mortality of approximately 5%. The most common problem post-surgery is residual left AV valve (mitral) regurgitation.

Left heart obstructive lesions

Where there is obstruction to normal blood flow there is an increased pressure load on the heart. In mild or

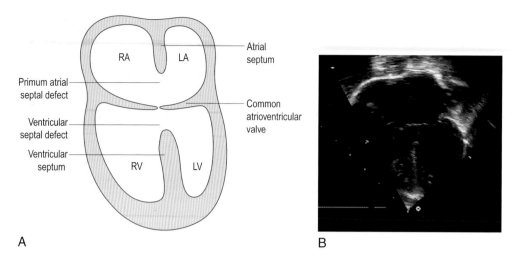

Fig. 41.4 Atrioventricular septal defect.
(A) Diagram showing location (RA = right atrium; LA = left atrium; RV = right ventricle; LV = left ventricle); (B) echocardiogram.

moderate aortic stenosis there is compensatory left ventricular hypertrophy (LVH) and the cardiac output may be maintained with minimal symptoms of heart failure. However, with severe coarctation of aorta, critical aortic stenosis or hypoplastic left heart syndrome, infants can present within hours of birth with acute circulatory collapse.

Coarctation of aorta

This is the most common left heart obstructive lesion presenting with heart failure in childhood. Coarctation of the aorta is a narrowing that can occur at any point along the course of the aorta. It most frequently occurs in the thoracic aorta in the region of insertion of the ductus arteriosus. Coarctation accounts for 6–8% of live births with CHD and occurs more commonly in males, with a preponderance of 1.5–2:1. Coarctation may occur in isolation or it may be associated with other anomalies, with bicuspid aortic valve and VSD being the most common associations (see Table 41.3 below). An increased incidence of 15–20% occurs in Turner's syndrome.

Pathophysiology

It is hypothesized that coarctation results from decreased antegrade blood flow across the aortic valve in fetal life, as a result of an associated cardiac anomaly. Discrete coarctation most commonly occurs between the origin of the left subclavian artery and the insertion of the ductus arteriosus, and takes the form of an isthmal waist with the ductus open (Fig. 41.5). In the majority of cases, there is an extension of ductal tissue into this waist, such that when the ductal tissue constricts, the isthmal narrowing increases. Therefore, with ductal closure in neonatal life, there may be an

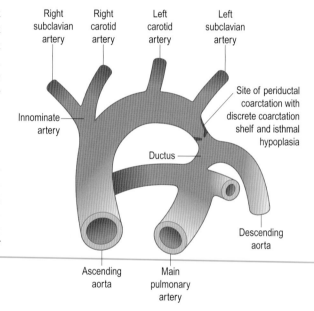

Fig. 41.5 Coarctation at site of ductus arteriosus remnant

acute increase in afterload on the left ventricle and the infant may rapidly decompensate. Where the increase in afterload is more gradual, compensatory ventricular hypertrophy results. Low blood pressure beyond the coarctation equates to decreased renal perfusion. This results in activation of the renin–angiotensin system in an attempt to improve renal perfusion pressure, causing hypertension proximal to the coarctation.

Presentation of coarctation

Clinical presentation can be largely considered as early (neonatal) or late presentation. The key features of early and late presentation are summarized in Table 41.3.

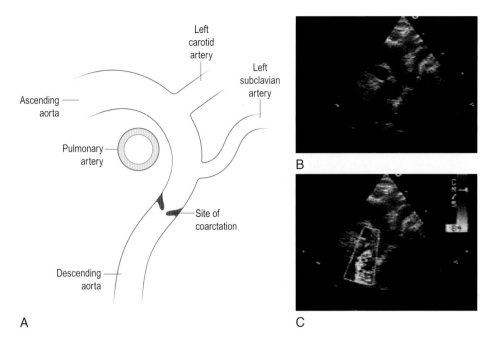

Fig. 41.6 Severe periductal coarctation of the aorta.
(A) Diagram showing locations; (B) echocardiogram; (C) colour Doppler study.

Table 41.3 Possible presenting features of coarctation of the aorta

	Early presentation	Late presentation
Symptoms	Poor feeding Dyspnoea Lethargy	Usually asymptomatic Headaches Epistaxis Calf claudication
Signs	Tachypnoea Increased work of breathing Tachycardia Prolonged capillary refill Active precordium Gallop rhythm Systolic murmur Absent/diminished femoral pulses Hepatomegaly	Upper limb hypertension Diminished/absent femoral pulses Radiofemoral delay Left ventricular impulse Systolic murmur Continuous murmur (collaterals)

Investigations

In infants, a CXR frequently demonstrates cardiomegaly and pulmonary oedema (Fig. 41.2). In older children, the heart size may be normal, but more commonly there is cardiomegaly due to LVH. A pathognomonic sign, which may be seen on the chest radiograph of older children, is rib notching. This is rarely seen before 5 years of age and is due to enlargement of the intercostal arteries, with pressure erosion of the inferior border of the posterior ribs.

ECG in the neonate may reveal right ventricular hypertrophy due to increased in utero afterload but may be normal. Later, changes due to LVH with left ventricular strain may occur.

Diagnosis of coarctation in infancy is now almost always confirmed by echocardiography (Fig. 41.6). It allows evaluation of the aortic arch from the suprasternal notch view and assessment of the severity of coarctation. Using colour Doppler, a turbulent jet may be seen through the coarctation, and interrogation with continuous wave Doppler may demonstrate an increased velocity with typical 'sawtooth' pattern.

In neonatal presentation, echocardiography is useful to assess the size of the ductus arteriosus and response to prostaglandin therapy. It also allows delineation of intracardiac anatomy to look for possible associated anomalies.

In most cases of coarctation, particularly in the infant, clinical examination and echocardiography alone provide sufficient information to formulate a management plan. Cardiac catheterization is only necessary when echocardiographic findings are inconclusive. More commonly, it may be used in older children to provide further structural and haemodynamic information prior to catheter intervention in the form of balloon angioplasty. Magnetic resonance imaging (MRI) and computed tomogram (CT) angiography may be useful modalities in older patients or in post-operative patients.

Management

In neonatal presentation of coarctation, initial management focuses on medical stabilization prior to elective surgical repair. Ductal patency is maintained by administration of an intravenous infusion of pro-staglandin E1. This allows possible partial reduction in the severity of coarctation and improves lower body perfusion, albeit with systemic venous blood. In children presenting beyond 2 weeks of age pro-staglandin is unlikely to be effective. In the critically ill infant with coarctation and left ventricular failure ventilatory and inotropic support is often necessary to stabilize the child prior to surgery. It should be noted that drug pharmacokinetics may be altered due to renal hypoperfusion.

It is generally accepted that, for native coarctation in infancy, surgical repair is the best option. Surgical repair can take three forms:

- Resection of coarctation and end-to-end anastomosis
- Left subclavian flap repair
- Patch aortoplasty.

The particular technique employed depends on a number of factors, including location of the coarctation, aortic arch anatomy, associated problems such as transverse arch hypoplasia, and age and size at presentation.

In late presentation, the treatment of upper extremity hypertension, usually with β-blocker therapy, takes priority initially. Beyond 1 year of age, cardiac catheterization and balloon angioplasty of native coarctation may be considered as an alternative to surgical treatment.

Prognosis

For most children with coarctation the prognosis is good. About 10% of those requiring a procedure in infancy will require further treatment later in life.

The child with an asymptomatic murmur

(See also Ch. 23.)

Problem-orientated topic:

asymptomatic murmur

Gemma, a 4-year-old girl, attends her GP with an upper respiratory infection. She is a previously healthy girl with no cardiovascular symptoms. An incidental finding on examination is that she has a grade 3/6 ejection systolic murmur loudest at the lower left sternal edge. Both heart sounds are normal and on palpation the precordium is quiet. Pulses are normal in volume in all four limbs. Blood pressure in the right arm is 92/63 mmHg.

Q1. What is the differential diagnosis?

Q2. What features help differentiate between an innocent and a pathological murmur?

Q3. What are the relevant investigations?

Q4. When is a referral to a paediatric cardiologist indicated?

Q5. What advice would you give to the parents of a child with an innocent murmur?

Q1. What is the differential diagnosis?

The differential diagnosis is between an innocent or functional murmur and asymptomatic CHD.

Q2. What features help differentiate between an innocent and a pathological murmur?

Innocent murmurs are extremely common and the key features associated with them are summarized in Box 41.6.

In the attempt to differentiate those with CHD from those with innocent murmurs key features in history-taking are birth history, feeding patterns, growth, breathing difficulties and cyanosis.

Clinical assessment of the child with a murmur requires a full cardiovascular examination. This includes assessment of colour, heart and respiratory rates, and palpation of the precordium for heaves or thrills. Palpation of pulses in all four limbs and measurement of blood pressure is essential to rule out coarctation of aorta. On auscultation attention should first be focused on the heart sounds and then on the murmur. The murmur should be defined under the headings in Box 41.1 (p. 211).

Features suggesting that a murmur may be patho-logical are summarized in Box 41.7.

Very important congenital heart conditions such as aortic stenosis and hypertrophic cardiomyopathy may be asymptomatic in childhood and present as a

---

BOX 41.6 Clinical characteristics of an innocent murmur

- No symptoms
- Normal heart sounds
- No added sounds
- No thrills/heaves
- Intensity grade 3 or less
- Musical or vibratory quality
- Intensity changes with posture

murmur. Recognition of such conditions is, however, vitally important since both are known causes of sudden death in young people, particularly during exertion. The common conditions presenting as an asymptomatic murmur are summarized in Box 41.8. Each of these conditions is described in more detail under the relevant headings in this chapter.

Innocent murmurs

By far the most commonly occurring innocent murmur is the Stills murmur, often first detected at the routine preschool examination. The classical Stills murmur is ejection systolic, has a musical or vibratory quality, and diminishes in intensity when the child sits upright. It is usually loudest at the lower left sternal edge. Venous hums are also very common in the preschool and school-age groups. A venous hum is a continuous noise, heard when the child is sitting upright. The murmur is created by blood returning through the great veins to the heart and it can be made to disappear by laying the child flat or applying gentle pressure over the great veins in the neck.

The pulmonary flow murmur is heard over the base of the heart and is more common in adolescents, particularly girls. It is distinguished from valvular pulmonary stenosis by the absence of an ejection click. It also alters with posture and may decrease in intensity or disappear with a Valsalva manoeuvre. Finally it is common in young healthy children to be able to hear a bruit over the carotid arteries in the neck. These murmurs are caused by the flow from aorta into the head and neck vessels, and in contrast to the murmur of aortic stenosis, the carotid bruit is louder over the neck than over the precordium.

Q3. What are the relevant investigations?

In many cases it is clear after clinical examination that the murmur is highly likely to be innocent. In practice most paediatricians assessing a child with a heart murmur will request an ECG and CXR. The ECG may be helpful in identifying an abnormal axis or evidence of atrial or ventricular enlargement (Table 41.1).

The main parameters to be assessed on the CXR are:
- Shape of the cardiac silhouette
- The cardiothoracic ratio: below 55% is considered to be normal
- Pulmonary vascularity: normal/increased/ decreased.

It should be noted that a normal ECG and CXR does not preclude the presence of a congenital cardiac abnormality.

The gold standard investigation for the evaluation of cardiac structure and function in children is echocardiography.

Q4. When is a referral to a paediatric cardiologist indicated?

If there is uncertainty after clinical examination that the murmur is innocent or there is any abnormality on the ECG or CXR, then referral to a paediatric cardiologist is indicated so that a definitive diagnosis can be obtained. Children with a family history of inheritable cardiac conditions such as hypertrophic obstructive cardiomyopathy (HOCM) should also be referred.

In many cases an experienced paediatric cardiologist will be able to confirm on clinical examination that the murmur is innocent. In the remainder echocardiography is necessary either to rule out or confirm pathology. It is crucial that someone skilled in paediatric echocardiography performs this investigation.

Q5. What advice would you give to the parents of a child with an innocent murmur?

For those children with an innocent murmur it is extremely important that a very clear message is given to the parents that their child's heart is normal. It should be made clear that the child should have no restrictions with regard to physical activity and that antibiotic prophylaxis for dental treatment is not necessary. The best way to reinforce the message that there are no ongoing concerns is to discharge the child from further follow-up.

Pathological lesions presenting as a murmur in childhood

Atrial septal defect (ASD)

The majority of children with an isolated secundum ASD will not present until school age. They may be found to have a murmur on routine examination or may have symptoms of dyspnoea or fatigue on exertion. These symptoms become more prominent as the child gets older. Some may have been more prone to respiratory infections and misdiagnosed as asthmatic. Increasingly infants having echocardiography for other reasons are found to have small ASDs and the long-term significance of these is unclear.

Clinical features

If there is a significant left-to-right shunt through the ASD there is usually a palpable left parasternal impulse. The classical finding is fixed splitting of the second heart sound due to delayed emptying of the dilated right ventricle. An ejection systolic murmur is audible in the pulmonary area due to the increased flow across the pulmonary valve. In those with a large ASD a mid-diastolic murmur due to increased flow across the tricuspid valve may be heard.

Investigations

CXR will indicate cardiomegaly, with a prominent main pulmonary artery and increased pulmonary vascularity.

The ECG will usually show sinus rhythm with evidence of right atrial enlargement in about 50% of cases. In the majority there will be an 'RSR' (incomplete right bundle branch block) pattern due to the right ventricular diastolic volume overload.

The diagnosis is confirmed by echocardiography. This allows measurement of the size and location of the defect, and assessment of the degree of right atrial and right ventricular enlargement. The addition of colour Doppler imaging quantifies the direction and magnitude of shunting and also helps with excluding any associated anomaly of pulmonary venous drainage.

Management

For significant ASDs closure is indicated to prevent long-term complications. Closure is commonly performed around the age of 4–5 years but can be carried out earlier if there is evidence of heart failure. In the modern era the choice is between surgical and device closure at cardiac catheterization. Small to moderate secundum ASDs can often be closed by interventional catheter techniques, avoiding the need for surgery. Large secundum ASDs, sinus venosus ASDs and defects in the primum area of the atrial septum require surgical closure.

Both surgical and device closure have a very low mortality and patients with secundum ASD have an excellent long-term prognosis if corrected in childhood.

Sinus venosus ASD

This type of defect accounts for 5–10% of all ASDs. The defect usually lies posterior to the fossa ovalis and the superior vena cava overrides its upper margin. It is commonly associated with anomalous connection of the right upper pulmonary veins to either the right atrium or the superior vena cava.

Ostium primum ASD (partial ASD)

In this condition the defect lies antero-inferiorly to the fossa ovalis and is always associated with an abnormal mitral valve with a variable degree of mitral regurgitation. The degree of left-to-right shunting may be large and patients may present with heart failure in infancy, particularly if there is significant mitral regurgitation. Correction requires patch closure of the primum defect and, in most cases, repair of the 'cleft' in the anterior septal leaflet of the mitral valve also.

Pulmonary stenosis

Pulmonary valvular stenosis may occur as an isolated abnormality or as part of more complex abnormalities such as tetralogy of Fallot. Patients with Noonan's syndrome commonly have a dysplastic stenotic pulmonary valve.

Clinical features

Those with mild or moderate pulmonary valve stenosis (PS) are often asymptomatic and the diagnosis is only made after a murmur has been detected on routine examination. At the other end of the spectrum those with critical PS may present with cyanosis in the neonatal period.

In children with PS palpation of the precordium may reveal a right ventricular systolic impulse and a palpable thrill. On auscultation the characteristic finding is an ejection click audible over the pulmonary area. There is also an ejection systolic murmur loudest over the upper left sternal border but radiating widely, particularly through to the back. In infants with critical PS and heart failure a second pansystolic murmur of tricuspid regurgitation is often audible.

Investigations

In mild or moderate PS the ECG may be normal. In severe PS there will be evidence of right ventricular hypertrophy. The most striking feature on CXR is prominent pulmonary artery conus caused by post-stenotic dilatation in the main pulmonary artery. In infants with critical PS there is generally very marked cardiomegaly with mainly right atrial enlargement secondary to tricuspid regurgitation. The diagnosis is easily made by echocardiography. The pulmonary valve leaflets appear thickened and doming with poor mobility, and the pulmonary valve annulus is often small. In those with critical PS the right ventricle will appear very hypertrophied with a small cavity and there will be tricuspid regurgitation with right atrial dilatation. Colour Doppler will demonstrate turbulent flow across the valve with increased velocity, and continuous wave Doppler allows accurate measurement of the peak systolic gradient across the valve.

Management

In infants and older children the preferred mode of treatment is now balloon pulmonary valvuloplasty performed at cardiac catheterization. In this group a Doppler gradient across the pulmonary valve of 60 mmHg or greater is often used as the cutoff point for intervention. The dysplastic pulmonary valve in patients with Noonan's syndrome is usually also associated with a narrowed valve annulus and is less likely to have a good result from valvuloplasty.

In neonates with critical pulmonary stenosis, where pulmonary blood flow is ductus-dependent, initial management is to maintain patency of the ductus using a prostaglandin infusion. To relieve the obstruction the choice is between surgical pulmonary valvotomy and balloon pulmonary valvuloplasty. If there is hypoplasia of the right ventricle with a small main pulmonary artery it may be necessary to augment pulmonary blood flow with a Blalock–Taussig shunt.

For the vast majority of patients with PS the long-term prognosis is excellent. Some may need pulmonary valve replacement in adult life because of pulmonary regurgitation.

Small ventricular septal defect (VSD)

The typical finding in a small VSD is a blowing pansystolic murmur, usually loudest at the lower left sternal edge. There may be an associated thrill. The patient will be asymptomatic and will not require any treatment but antibiotic prophylaxis against infective endocarditis is important.

Patent ductus arteriosus (PDA)

PDA is the most common congenital heart lesion found in the newborn period, accounting for about 10% of all CHD in babies born at term. In the majority of newborns there is complete functional closure of the ductus within 72 hours of birth.

The most common clinical situation in which persistent patency of the ductus is important is in the ventilator-dependent premature infant with lung disease of prematurity. This is discussed in detail on page 356. In the older child the presentation may be with failure to thrive, with breathlessness on exertion or with the incidental finding of a murmur.

Clinical features

The severity of symptoms is related to the magnitude of left-to-right shunting from aorta to pulmonary artery. A large PDA will in most cases lead to symptoms of breathlessness and often an increased tendency to respiratory infection. There may be gradual onset of heart failure due to volume overload of the left heart.

In the presence of a significant PDA the peripheral pulses will be increased in volume and may be bounding. The child may be tachycardic and tachypnoeic at rest with the precordium active. In the newborn period the murmur is usually ejection systolic, and with a moderate to large PDA there may be multiple ejection clicks. In the infant or older child the classical continuous machinery murmur is easily audible. Very rarely with a large ductus, if the pulmonary vascular resistance remains high, the continuous murmur may never appear. This group are at risk of developing early irreversible pulmonary vascular disease.

Investigations

CXR will show cardiomegaly and increased pulmonary flow. Echocardiography will readily identify whether the ductus is patent and also establish its size. Colour Doppler will indicate the direction of shunting, which in the absence of pulmonary hypertension should be left-to-right (Fig. 41.7). Dilatation of the left atrium and left ventricle is an indicator of significant left-to-right shunting.

Management

Management of PDA in the premature ventilator-dependent infant is dealt with elsewhere (p. 356). In older children, when ductal patency has been established, the commonly accepted management is to proceed to closure. With a moderate to large PDA the indication for closure is to prevent the risk of developing pulmonary vascular disease. The indication for closure of the small PDA is the prevention of infective endocarditis. If the PDA is very large surgical ligation remains the treatment of choice. Surgical closure is performed through a left thoracotomy incision. For small to moderate PDA device occlusion at cardiac catheterization is usually possible. Both treatment options have a low morbidity

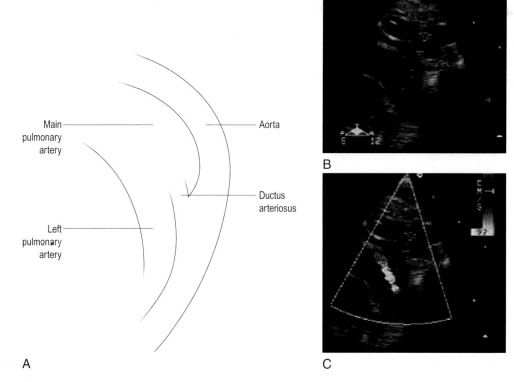

Main pulmonary artery

Aorta

Ductus arteriosus

Left pulmonary artery

A

B

C

Fig. 41.7 Patent ductus arteriosus (PDA).
(a) Moderate PDA; (b) echocardiogram; (c) Doppler study.

and mortality. Occlusion devices may be in the form of coils or 'plugs'.

Aortic stenosis

Aortic stenosis accounts for about 5% of CHD diagnosed in childhood. The stenosis is most commonly valvular but subvalvular obstruction and more rarely supravalvular obstruction can occur. In valvular aortic stenosis the valve is often bicuspid with thickened leaflets and commissural fusion. Subvalvular obstruction is caused in most cases by a discrete fibromuscular ring. Supravalvular aortic stenosis is more common in children with Williams' syndrome.

Clinical features

Children are often asymptomatic, even in the presence of severe stenosis. When symptoms do occur there may be a history of fatigue and/or chest pain with exertion. The first presentation may be with an episode of collapse during exercise, and aortic stenosis is a recognized cause of sudden death in young people.

With moderate to severe aortic stenosis there may be a palpable left ventricular heave and a thrill. The thrill is easily palpable in the suprasternal notch as well as over the aortic area. In valvular aortic stenosis an ejection click is audible. The murmur is harsh and, although loudest in the aortic area, radiates widely down to the apex and up into the neck. If there is mixed aortic valve disease with aortic regurgitation a diastolic murmur will also be audible. In severe aortic stenosis all pulses will be of reduced volume and blood pressure measurement will reveal a reduced pulse pressure.

Investigations

In severe aortic stenosis the ECG will usually show evidence of left ventricular hypertrophy but correlation between ECG change and the valve gradient is not good. The appearance of a left ventricular 'strain' pattern with ST depression and T wave inversion in the left precordial leads is an important indicator of the need for intervention to relieve the obstruction.

The diagnosis is easily confirmed by two-dimensional echocardiography. Imaging will clarify the level of obstruction (subvalvular, valvular or supravalvular) and its mechanism. The degree of left ventricular hypertrophy can be determined from wall thickness measurements and an ejection or shortening fraction calculated as a measure of left ventricular function. Colour Doppler also helps to clarify the level of the obstruction and quantify any associated aortic regurgitation. Continuous wave Doppler measurement estimates the transvalvular gradient.

Management

All patients, even those with mild obstruction, require endocarditis prophylaxis. Those with moderate or severe stenosis should not participate in competitive sport.

In the ill neonate with severe aortic stenosis the treatment of choice is still surgical aortic valvotomy. In the older child balloon aortic valvuloplasty performed at cardiac catheterization can be an effective and less invasive means of relieving the stenosis. The decision to intervene with surgery or valvuloplasty in childhood aortic stenosis can be difficult and intervention may be necessary in the asymptomatic child. In children a Doppler gradient of greater than 70 mmHg or a mean gradient of greater than 35 mmHg is often used as a level above which intervention needs to be considered. The ECG changes of ST depression or T wave inversion are further evidence of the need for treatment. Subvalvular aortic stenosis is potentially a much more dangerous lesion because of its dynamic nature, and in this condition surgery is indicated for even moderate degrees of obstruction.

Prognosis

Children with aortic stenosis require life-long follow-up. Since the valve is intrinsically abnormal a significant percentage of those who require surgery or valvuloplasty in childhood will go on to require further treatment. As the patient gets older aortic regurgitation may be the dominant problem, and valve replacement with a prosthetic valve is required in approximately 35% within 15–20 years of the original procedure. Those with a prosthetic valve require long-term anticoagulation.

Cyanotic heart disease

This usually presents in the neonatal period and is discussed in Chapter 47.

Chest pain in childhood

(See also Ch. 23.)

Problem-orientated topic:

chest pain

A 12-year-old boy, Danny, has complained intermittently of chest pain over the past 4 months. He describes a left-sided pain occurring mainly with exercise but sometimes also at rest. Each episode lasts less than 5 minutes.

Q1. What points in the history help distinguish cardiac from non-cardiac chest pain?

Q2. What should you look for on clinical examination?

Q3. What is the differential diagnosis?

Q4. What investigations are appropriate?

Q1. What points in the history help distinguish cardiac from non-cardiac chest pain?

It is important to identify factors that bring on the pain:

- Is it related to exercise?
- What are the location, intensity and duration?
- Does it get worse with deep inspiration?
- Does it stop the child from doing any activity when it comes on?
- Is there any association with breathlessness, palpitations or dizziness?
- Is the pain associated with eating?
- Has there been any chest trauma?

It is also important to elucidate:

- Any history of wheezing, since exercise-induced asthma is a relatively frequent cause of chest pain in childhood
- A good social and family history, possible psychogenic factors influencing the child's symptoms, particularly recent stresses at school or at home.

Brief, infrequently occurring chest pain occurring over months or years in an otherwise well child is unlikely to have a serious aetiology. On the other hand, pain that is constant or frequently occurs with exercise and interferes with the child's activities needs to be taken more seriously. Cardiac pain due to ischaemia is often crushing in nature and associated with sweating, nausea, dyspnoea or syncope.

Q2. What should you look for on clinical examination?

As for any illness with an unknown aetiology, a complete physical examination should be performed. This should include a detailed cardiovascular examination, including measurement of blood pressure. On examination palpation for any signs of tenderness, particularly over the costochondral junctions, may reveal the diagnosis of costochondritis. In those with a musculoskeletal cause the pain may be increased in certain positions or activities and often is made worse by deep inspirations.

An active precordium, abnormal pulses or presence of a murmur will point towards a cardiac cause of the

BOX 41.9 Causes of chest pain in childhood

- Idiopathic
- Musculoskeletal
- Pulmonary
- Psychological
- Gastrointestinal
- Cardiac

BOX 41.10 Cardiac causes of chest pain in childhood

- Left ventricular outflow tract obstruction: aortic valve stenosis, subaortic stenosis, hypertrophic obstructive cardiomyopathy
- Coronary artery stenosis: post-Kawasaki disease or Takayasu arteritis
- Anomalous origin of coronary arteries
- Tachyarrhythmias
- Inflammatory: myocarditis, pericarditis, rheumatic carditis, dissecting aortic aneurysm (Marfan's syndrome)
- Mitral valve prolapse
- Coronary vasospasm

pain that needs to be further investigated. Auscultation of the lungs may reveal evidence of infection or bronchospasm. Abdominal examination may reveal epigastric tenderness, suggesting a gastrointestinal cause.

Q3. What is the differential diagnosis?

The most common causes of chest pain in childhood are summarized in Box 41.9.

In the majority of children who complain of chest pain the cause will be non-cardiac. It does, however, provoke a lot of parental anxiety, particularly in young people who are participating in sport. It may not be possible to identify a clear cause and many cases are idiopathic, but in such cases both patient and parents need to be reassured that there is no cause for concern. Those in whom the cause is idiopathic will often describe sharp pain of very short duration occurring either at rest or during exercise. The cardiac causes of chest pain are summarized in Box 41.10.

Q4. What investigations are appropriate?

If the history is not suggestive of serious pathology and a thorough physical examination is normal, then further investigation is usually not indicated. In the remainder the investigations are guided by particular causes of

concern from the history or clinical examination. For those with a possible cardiac aetiology ECG and echocardiography are mandatory. If possible an ECG should be obtained during an episode. The most useful investigation for those old enough to cooperate is a treadmill exercise test during which there is ECG and blood pressure measurement. A normal exercise test provides reassurance in many cases and in the remainder may more clearly help with the differential diagnosis between musculoskeletal and cardiac pain if the symptoms are reproduced during the test.

Arrhythmias

Problem-orientated topic:

palpitations

Sarah, a 12-year-old girl, presents to the accident and emergency department with a history of her 'heart beating strongly and very fast'. This feeling started while she was watching television and has continued for over an hour. She states that this has never happened before. She appears nervous but well. Colour is pink and there is no evidence of respiratory distress. Pulse is very fast and difficult to count. Capillary refill time is less than 2 seconds. Her rhythm strip is shown in Figure 41.8.

Q1. What does the rhythm strip demonstrate and what is the most likely diagnosis?

Q2. How are you going to manage this patient?

Q3. What are the long-term treatment options?

Q1. What does the rhythm strip demonstrate and what is the most likely diagnosis?

The rhythm strip demonstrates a narrow complex tachycardia with a rate of 240 beats per minute. The most likely diagnosis is of a supraventricular tachycardia (SVT) or, more specifically, an atrioventricular re-entry tachycardia. It can sometimes be difficult to differentiate sinus tachycardia from SVT, particularly at a heart rate around 200 bpm. In such cases, a 12-lead ECG should be performed. Box 41.11 sets out factors that help make this distinction.

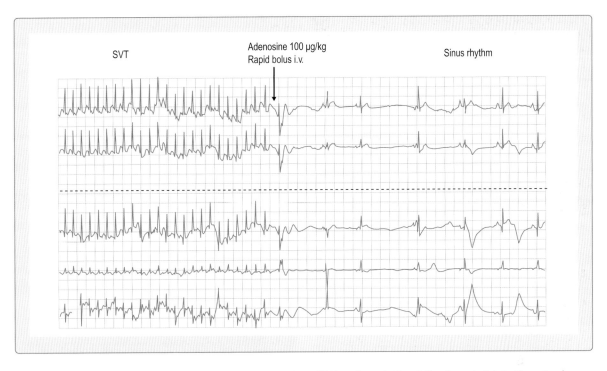

Fig. 41.8. Sarah's rhythm strip demonstrating conversion from SVT to sinus rhythm following administration of intravenous adenosine (arrow head)

BOX 41.11 Factors distinguishing sinus tachycardia from supraventricular tachycardia

Sinus tachycardia

- May have history of preceding systemic illness
- Heart rate rarely exceeds 200 bpm
- P waves upright in leads II, III and aVF (may be difficult to identify at fast rates)
- Beat-to-beat variability can be seen
- Heart rate gradually slows with treatment (e.g. fluid resuscitation)

Supraventricular tachycardia

- Previously well with no preceding systemic upset
- May report sudden onset
- May have had similar previous episodes, which terminated abruptly
- Heart rate generally above 220 bpm (may be lower if on treatment)
- P waves may be absent: negative in leads II, III and aVF if present
- No beat-to-beat variability in SVT
- Rate abruptly changes following intervention

Q2. How are you going to manage this patient?

After assessment of airway, breathing and circulation, it is clear that Sarah is not in shock. It is reasonable to attempt manoeuvres, which result in vagal stimulation and may terminate the arrhythmia (e.g. Valsalva manoeuvre, one-sided carotid sinus massage). In a neonate or infant application of an ice pack to the face is an appropriate vagal manoeuvre but this should not be performed in older children.

It is important that Sarah is put on a heart monitor from which the rhythm is archived and retrievable, or which is printing during such interventions, so that any change in rhythm can be analysed and documented.

If vagal manoeuvres fail, the treatment of choice is intravenous adenosine, at an initial dose of 50 µg/kg, which should be administered rapidly through a large-bore cannula in a large proximal vein and flushed through with normal saline (Fig. 41.8). Adenosine has a short half-life of a few seconds and works by blocking the AV node. Sarah should be warned before administration that she will feel unpleasant for a short time following the injection. Again, continuous ECG monitoring should be in place. Further doses of adenosine at 100 µg/kg and then 250 µg/kg should be administered if the arrhythmia is not terminated.

If Sarah remains in SVT following adenosine, it is important that she is discussed with a paediatric cardiologist, who may suggest synchronous DC cardioversion under sedation/anaesthesia, or other drugs (such as propranolol, flecainide, amiodarone or digoxin).

 http://www.aplsonline.com

Sarah should have an echocardiogram to look for evidence of any CHD, although the majority of children presenting with SVT will have a structurally normal heart.

Q3. What are the long-term treatment options?

Sarah should commence regular prophylaxis to prevent further episodes of SVT. This is usually in the form of a β-blocking drug. Some patients who have infrequent, self-terminating episodes of SVT may choose not to be on regular medication.

In recurrent or resistant SVT, identification of the accessory pathway by electrophysiological mapping in the cardiac catheter laboratory, along with its ablation, may be considered.

Supraventricular tachycardia (SVT)

SVT is the most common arrhythmia seen in children (Fig. 41.8). It commonly results from the presence of an accessory pathway between the atria and the ventricles, with normal electrical conduction across the AV node and retrograde conduction across the abnormal pathway. The best-known example of this phenomenon is Wolff–Parkinson–White syndrome. During sinus rhythm, antegrade conduction across the pathway may be possible and results in ventricular pre-excitation, with classical ECG findings of a delta wave and short PR interval.

About half of all cases of SVT in childhood present in infancy, with presentation ranging from a history of irritability or poor feeding, to presenting in extremis with heart failure. Older children tend to present earlier as they can vocalize symptoms and rarely present in heart failure.

Problem-orientated topic:

syncope

Simon, a 10-year-old boy, is referred to outpatients with a history of syncope. This occurred most recently after playing football with his friends, when he fainted, lost consciousness briefly and complained of 'feeling funny' for a short time afterwards. Further questioning reveals that this has occurred on several other occasions, and he is awaiting an outpatient EEG for investigation of possible seizures. His cardiovascular examination is unremarkable. His 12-lead ECG is shown in Figure 41.9.

Q1. What abnormality does the ECG demonstrate?

Q2. What may have caused Simon's episodes of syncope?

Q3. What is your further management?

Q1. What abnormality does the ECG demonstrate?

The QT interval appears prolonged, and when corrected for heart rate ($QTc = QT/\sqrt{R-R}$ interval) is 0.5 seconds. The causes of a prolonged QT interval are listed in Box 41.12.

The most likely cause in this scenario is congenital long QT syndrome. This condition is inherited and results from a mutation in the genes controlling the sodium and potassium channels in the myocardial cell wall.

BOX 41.12 Causes of an abnormal QT interval

Shortened QT interval
- Hypoxia
- Hypercalcaemia
- Digoxin
- Short QT syndrome

Prolonged QT interval
- Congenital long QT syndrome
- Hypocalcaemia
- Hypothermia
- Head injury
- Amiodarone
- Sotalol
- Tricyclic antidepressants

Q2. What may have caused Simon's episodes of syncope?

The syncope could have resulted from episodes of arrhythmia, in particular ventricular tachycardia. Episodes of collapse in children with long QT syndrome are typically precipitated by activities or events that produce an increase in catecholamine levels.

Q3. What is your further management?

Given Simon's history he should be commenced on a β-blocking agent, such as propranolol. A 24-hour ambulatory ECG recording should be arranged and analysed. Genetic screening should be arranged for Simon, as an increasing number of genetic mutations are being identified, which help confirm the diagnosis and guide treatment. First-degree relatives should

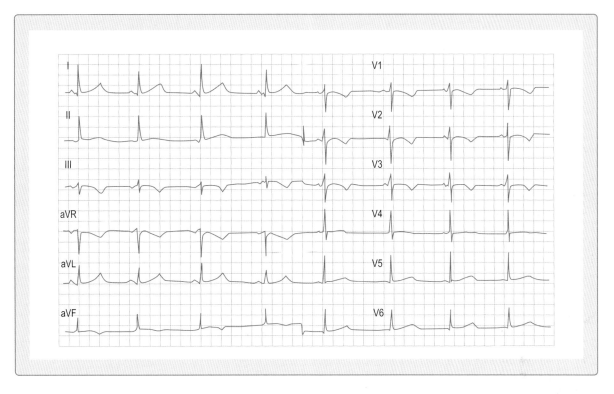

Fig. 41.9 Simon's ECG strip

receive ECG and genetic screening. Avoidance of competitive sport and swimming should be advised.

Ventricular tachycardia (VT)

VT is defined as a series of three or more premature ventricular contractions. It typically has a rate of over 120 beats per minute and the QRS morphology is wide (Fig. 41.10).

VT is relatively uncommon in childhood. In the management of a child with VT it is important to consider possible underlying causes (Box 41.13).

This is potentially a very dangerous arrhythmia because of the possibility of its degenerating into ventricular fibrillation. If the patient is not clinically shocked then intravenous administration of amiodarone in a dose of 5 mg/kg given over 30 minutes is an appropriate initial treatment. In the clinically shocked patient DC

BOX 41.13 Causes of ventricular tachycardia

- Congenital heart disease
- Previous cardiac surgery
- Congenital long QT syndrome
- Drugs (e.g. tricyclic antidepressants, cisapride, erythromycin)
- Electrolyte imbalance (e.g. hyperkalaemia)

---

cardioversion under sedation or anaesthesia should be undertaken. For treatment algorithms refer to APLS guidelines.

Inflammations and infections

Infective endocarditis

Infectious endocarditis is rare in childhood but remains a potential cause of serious morbidity and mortality. The vast majority of those affected will have underlying structural heart disease as a result of either congenital or rheumatic heart disease. With increasing survival following surgery for CHD the population potentially at risk is increasing. The lesions most commonly complicated by endocarditis are VSDs, aortic stenosis or incompetence, tetralogy of Fallot and PDA. An increasing group is those with artificial conduits or prosthetic valves. Endocarditis can occur in those with structurally normal hearts: for example, those with indwelling central venous lines or intravenous drug users.

In most series streptococci (*Strep. viridans* more than enterococci) are the most common causative organism, with staphylococci (*Staph. aureus* and *Staph. epidermidis*) being the second largest group. In the paediatric age group 80% of cases are due to these two organism groups.

The clinical features of the illness depend on the virulence of the organism and host resistance. The most useful clinical features are summarized in Box 41.14.

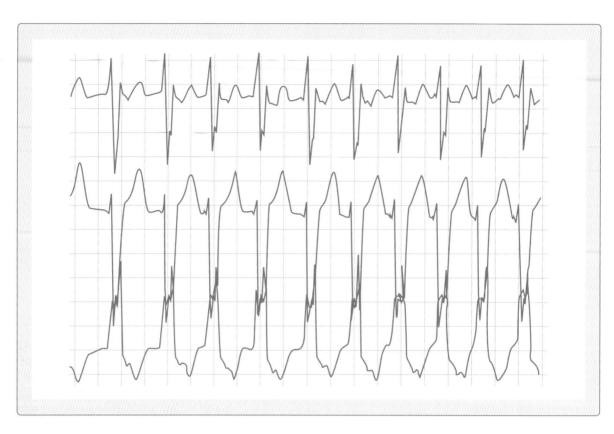

Fig. 41.10 **Ventricular tachycardia.**

- Fever
- Heart murmur (N.B. new or changing murmur)
- General malaise (myalgia, arthralgia)
- Heart failure
- Splenomegaly
- Microscopic haematuria
- Petechiae
- Embolic phenomena: neurological or pulmonary
- Osler nodes, Janeway lesions, splinter haemorrhages

Isolation of the infecting organism from blood culture is crucially important in making the diagnosis and guiding appropriate antimicrobial therapy. Two or three blood cultures over a 24-hour period are usually adequate. Diagnostic difficulty can arise in patients partially treated with antibiotics prior to a diagnosis of endocarditis being considered. *Candida* infection should be considered in those with negative blood cultures.

In most cases transthoracic echocardiography will demonstrate the vegetations attached to affected valves and will also help quantify any associated valve regurgitation (Fig. 41.11). Transoesophageal echocardiography may be necessary where the transthoracic images are inadequate.

Management

Treatment is required for a minimum of 4 weeks and is usually continued for 6.

For *Strep. viridans* a combination of penicillin and gentamicin given intravenously is effective. For *Strep. faecalis* a combination of amoxicillin and gentamicin is used. Flucloxacillin and gentamicin is the first-choice therapy for staphylococcal infection. *Candida* infection is difficult to treat and may require a combination of amphotericin and flucytosine. It may prove impossible to eradicate infection on a prosthetic valve, patch, homograft or pacemaker with antimicrobial therapy alone and surgical exploration may be necessary.

Prophylaxis

Bacteraemia can occur in relation to dental or surgical procedures. It has been estimated that extraction of an abscessed tooth produces bacteraemia in up to 80% of cases. Streptococci form part of the normal flora of the

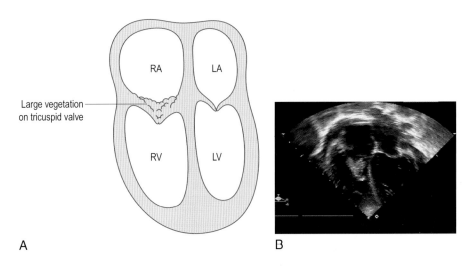

Fig. 41.11 Infective endocarditis.
(A) Diagram of infective endocarditis and large vegetations on the tricuspid valve (RA = right atrium; LA = left atrium; RV = right ventricle; LV = left ventricle); (B) echocardiogram.

mouth and are the usual cause of endocarditis following dental procedures. The most important prophylactic measure is good oral hygiene. In addition to extraction antibiotic prophylaxis is also indicated for scaling, major root fillings and orthodontic procedures. Prophylaxis should be given less than 1 hour prior to the procedure. Other procedures for which prophylaxis is indicated include:

- Tonsillectomy and adenoidectomy
- Appendicectomy
- Bronchoscopy
- Endotracheal intubation
- Urethral catheterization.

Rheumatic fever

Rheumatic fever is the most common cause of acquired heart disease in children and young adults world-wide. It is an inflammatory disease involving the joints and heart, and less frequently the central nervous system, skin and subcutaneous tissues. It arises as a complication of group A streptococcal infection. There is a 2–3-week latent period between the upper respiratory tract infection and the onset of rheumatic fever. The peak incidence is in children aged 5–15 years and there may be a genetic influence as family clustering occurs. The incidence is strikingly higher in people living in overcrowded conditions. Current theories suggest that the inflammatory process is mediated by an immunological reaction precipitated by the streptococcal infection.

Pathology
In the early stages there is an acute inflammatory exudative reaction. This lasts 2–3 weeks and involves the myocardium, valves and pericardium. This is followed by a proliferative phase, during which Aschoff bodies form. This pathognomonic lesion consists of a perivascular infiltrate of large cells with polymorphous nuclei and basophilic cytoplasm arranged in a rosette around an avascular centre of fibrinoid. Subsequently fibrotic scarring occurs in the region of the Aschoff bodies.

Rheumatic carditis
Mitral valve involvement is the most common, with aortic valve involvement second. The tricuspid valve is infrequently involved and the pulmonary valve only very rarely. Valve lesions begin as small verrucae composed of fibrin and blood cells along the borders of the valves. Particularly with the mitral valve, this may progress to some loss of valve tissue and shortening and thickening of the chordae tendinae. With persistent inflammation fibrosis and calcification occur. Chronic mitral regurgitation leads to left atrial dilatation, which may in turn lead to atrial fibrillation. There is also the risk of endocarditis.

Clinical features
The diagnostic criteria of Duckett Jones, drawn up in 1944 (Box 41.15), are still used to guide the diagnosis of rheumatic fever. The presence of two major criteria or one major plus two minor criteria indicates a high probability of acute rheumatic fever, if supported by evidence of recent group A streptococcal infection.

Supporting evidence of streptococcal infection includes:

- Increased antistreptolysin O titre (ASOT)
- Positive throat culture for group A streptococcus
- Recent scarlet fever.

BOX 41.15 Jones criteria for guidance in the diagnosis of rheumatic fever

Major manifestations
- Carditis
- Polyarthritis
- Chorea
- Erythema marginatum
- Subcutaneous nodules
- Leucocytosis

Minor manifestations
- Clinical:
  - Fever
  - Arthralgia
  - Previous rheumatic fever or rheumatic heart disease
- Laboratory:
  - Acute phase reactants: elevated erythrocyte sedimentation rate (ESR) and/or C-reactive protein (CRP)
  - Prolonged PR interval

Joint symptoms are the most common feature, occurring in 75%. Typically there is a migratory polyarthritis. The joint symptoms disappear in 3–4 weeks. Carditis occurs in 40–50% of initial attacks. Tachycardia disproportionate to fever is a typical finding. The most distinctive sign of rheumatic carditis is a new distinctive murmur. This is most commonly the blowing pansystolic apical murmur of mitral regurgitation. With aortic valve involvement the early diastolic murmur of aortic regurgitation may be heard. Other signs of carditis are finding a pericardial rub or evidence of congestive cardiac failure. Sydenham's chorea occurs in about 15% of patients. Subcutaneous nodules are found in 5–10% and erythema marginatum in less than 5%.

Laboratory findings

ESR and CRP are elevated. Around 80% will have an elevated ASOT. Values of > 300 are abnormal. A moderate normochromic normocytic anaemia is common.

The ECG will demonstrate a prolonged PR interval in one-third of patients. Flattened T waves occur with myocarditis and elevated ST segments are found in pericarditis.

Management

- Eradicate streptococcal infection with oral or intramuscular penicillin.
- Bed rest is recommended for the period of carditis.
- Prescribe salicylates, initially aspirin 75–100 mg/kg/day.
- Give prednisolone (2 mg/kg/day) if there is evidence of carditis. This dose is continued for

2–3 weeks, followed by gradual withdrawal over a further 2–3 weeks. As the steroid is withdrawn, salicylate is introduced to prevent clinical rebound. Salicylate should be continued for at least 4–6 weeks.
- Give diuretics in heart failure.
- Digoxin can be used with careful monitoring of levels.

Prognosis

Cardiac involvement is the major factor determining morbidity in acute rheumatic fever. Around 75% of patients with congestive heart failure during the initial attack will have evidence of chronic valvular disease after 10 years. The 10-year mortality rate is approximately 4%.

Prevention

Prophylaxis needs to be continued through childhood and adolescence. Lifetime prophylaxis is recommended in patients with rheumatic valvular disease. Oral penicillin may cause the emergence of resistant alpha-streptococci in the oral cavity.

Myocarditis

Myocarditis is an inflammatory disorder of the myocardium, causing necrosis of myocytes. It is most commonly caused by a viral infection, such as Coxsackie B or adenovirus. Other infective agents have been implicated, including meningococcus, *Mycoplasma*, *Diphtheria*, *Toxoplasma*, and rickettsiae. Rarely, myocarditis may be caused by drugs, toxins or autoimmune disease. An autoimmune response to the initial viral insult may play a part in disease progression and this may have a genetic basis. Myocarditis can occur at any age, including the newborn period. As many cases are subclinical, incidence is difficult to determine.

Clinical features

Presentation varies widely from acute collapse to a subclinical picture. History may reveal a recent respiratory or gastrointestinal infection. There may be symptoms and signs of congestive cardiac failure (Box 41.3). Older children may complain of chest pain (from myocardial ischaemia or concurrent pericarditis) or palpitations.

Investigations

CXR may reveal cardiomegaly and pulmonary oedema. ECG abnormalities include resting tachycardia, low-voltage QRS, ST segment changes, Q waves and arrhythmia, including atrioventricular conduction disturbances. Two-dimensional echocardiography demonstrates a dilated and poorly contracting left ventricle, with reduced ejection fraction. Mitral regurgitation due to a dilated mitral valve annulus may be demonstrated and a pericardial effusion may be present. ESR, CRP and cardiac enzyme levels are usually elevated. Evidence of an infective agent should be sought, including blood culture, acute and convalescent viral serology, and throat swab and faeces for viral culture.

Management

Management is largely supportive, with some patients requiring intensive care, including intubation, ventilation, inotropic support, afterload reducing agents and prompt treatment of arrhythmia. There is no specific treatment for the disease process, with the use of steroid and immunosuppressive therapy remaining controversial. Many children will recover completely but some may progress to chronic dilated cardiomyopathy. Heart transplantation may be necessary.

Cardiomyopathy

Cardiomyopathy is a disease of the myocardium. Cardiomyopathies may be primary, but increasingly secondary causes are being identified.

Cardiomyopathies are broadly divided into the following categories:

- *Dilated cardiomyopathy.* The most common cardiomyopathy in childhood; characterized by ventricular dilatation and reduced systolic ventricular function.
- *Hypertrophic cardiomyopathy.* Characterized by asymmetric septal hypertrophy leading to left ventricular outflow tract obstruction in the more severe cases.
- *Restrictive cardiomyopathy.* Rare in childhood; characterized by abnormal diastolic ventricular function and atrial dilatation.

Pulmonary hypertension

Pulmonary hypertension is defined as a pulmonary artery systolic pressure greater than 30 mmHg or a pulmonary artery mean pressure greater than 20 mmHg.

Primary pulmonary hypertension (PPH)

PPH is a rare disorder of unknown aetiology. Incidence in the general population is 1–2 per million, with onset in childhood rare. While there is a female preponderance in adulthood (1.7:1), prior to puberty incidence is equal between genders. The majority of cases are sporadic but familial forms may account for 10%. For a diagnosis of PPH to be made, other causes of pulmonary hypertension must be excluded

> **BOX 41.16 Diagnostic classification of pulmonary hypertension (World Health Organization 1998)**
>
> - Pulmonary arterial hypertension:
>   Primary pulmonary hypertension:
>   - Pulmonary hypertension associated with:
>   Collagen vascular diseases
>   Portal hypertension
>   Congenital systemic to pulmonary shunts
>   Drugs/toxins
>   HIV infection
>   Persistent pulmonary hypertension of newborn (PPHN)
> - Pulmonary venous hypertension
> - Pulmonary hypertension associated with disorders of respiratory system and/or hypoxaemia
> - Pulmonary hypertension due to chronic thrombosis and/or embolic disease
> - Pulmonary hypertension due to disorders affecting pulmonary vasculature

(Box 41.16). PPH is caused by precapillary obstruction of the pulmonary vascular bed, as a result of intimal and medial proliferation in the arteriolar wall.

Secondary pulmonary hypertension

Secondary pulmonary hypertension is more common in childhood and is largely a consequence of pulmonary or cardiac disorders. Chronic hypoxaemia may occur in the setting of severe asthma, cystic fibrosis, interstitial lung disease or obstructive sleep apnoea. This causes pulmonary vasoconstriction through a variety of mechanisms (Fig. 41.12). Cardiac conditions may result in pulmonary hypertension because of volume and/or pressure overload on the pulmonary vasculature. This can occur from any left-to-right shunt, such as a VSD. Where pulmonary vasculature changes are severe and pulmonary arterial pressures are supra systemic, reversal of the shunt from right to left may occur. This is termed Eisenmenger's syndrome. Left heart problems, such as mitral stenosis, aortic stenosis, cor triatrium or left ventricular dysfunction, may result in left atrial hypertension and hence pulmonary venous hypertension. This results in pulmonary arterial hypertension, with intimal proliferation of pulmonary vessel walls occurring over time. Pulmonary veno-occlusive disease is a rare cause of pulmonary hypertension. Obliteration of the pulmonary vascular bed, such as can occur in connective tissue disorders or chronic pulmonary emboli, can result in progressive pulmonary hypertension.

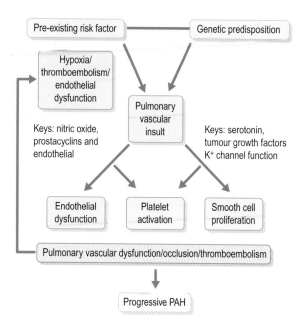

Fig. 41.12 Causes of pulmonary vasoconstriction.
(PAH = pulmonary artery hypertension)

BOX 41.17 Symptoms and signs of secondary pulmonary hypertension

Symptoms
- Fatigue
- Exertional dyspnoea
- Syncope
- Chest pain
- Headaches

Signs
- Right ventricular heave
- Loud P2 (may be palpable)
- Pansystolic murmur (tricuspid regurgitation)
- Hepatomegaly
- Peripheral oedema
- Elevated jugular venous pulse (older children)

Clinical features

In cases of secondary pulmonary hypertension, presenting features will be dominated by the underlying primary disease (Box 41.17).

Investigations

ECG demonstrates evidence of right axis deviation and right ventricular hypertrophy. CXR may demonstrate cardiomegaly, with prominent main and branch

Table 41.4 Medical management of pulmonary hypertension

Treatment	Effect
Oxygen	May provide symptomatic improvement
Calcium channel blockers	E.g. nifedipine. Systemic and pulmonary vasodilator. Prescribed in 'responders' (i.e. demonstrating acute reversibility of pulmonary vascular resistance in the catheter laboratory in response to a pulmonary vasodilator, such as inhaled nitric oxide)
Prostacyclin analogues	Epoprostenol: potent pulmonary vasodilator and inhibitor of platelet aggregation. Given by continuous i.v. infusion via a central line. May cause systemic hypotension. Nebulized iloprost is an alternative but due to short half-life requires regular administration. Oral (beraprost) and subcutaneous (treprostinil) analogues available
Inhaled nitric oxide	Potent and selective pulmonary vasodilator requiring continuous inhalation. May be given in the intensive care setting
Sildenafil	Oral phosphodiesterase-5 inhibitor. Results in increased cyclic guanosine monophosphate (GMP) levels and therefore an increase in endogenous endothelial nitric oxide production
Bosentan	Oral dual endothelin receptor antagonist. Competitively binds to endothelin-1 receptors ET$_A$ and ET$_B$. Reduces smooth muscle cell proliferation

pulmonary arteries and paucity ('pruning') of the peripheral pulmonary vascular markings. Echocardiogram shows a hypertrophied right ventricle with reduced function. Pulmonary arterial pressure may be indirectly assessed by Doppler interrogation of any regurgitant jets. It may also identify a CHD as a cause of secondary pulmonary hypertension. Cardiac catheterization may be considered for direct measurement of pulmonary arterial pressures, to look for secondary causes and to assess for reversibility of pulmonary hypertension, which can aid treatment options. Other investigations to look for secondary causes may be necessary.

Management and prognosis

In cases of secondary pulmonary hypertension, management is largely targeted at the underlying cause. Medical treatment options are summarized in Table 41.4. Blade septostomy may improve prognosis. In end-stage disease, lung or heart–lung transplant should be considered. If PPH is untreated, most children will die within 1 year of diagnosis.

Michael D. Shields   B.S. O'Connor

CHAPTER

42

Respiratory paediatrics

LEARNING OUTCOMES

By the end of this chapter you should:

- Be able to identify the different respiratory noises and know their causes and significance
- Understand the role of pulmonary function testing and radiological imaging in investigating respiratory disorders
- Know how to diagnose the common and important respiratory disorders of childhood
- Know how to assess the severity of the common respiratory conditions
- Be able to outline a management plan for the common respiratory conditions
- Understand the important underlying problems that are associated with poor control of chronic respiratory disorders such as asthma and cystic fibrosis.

Approach to respiratory disease

Disorders of the respiratory system make up a substantial part of a general paediatrician's workload. Acute respiratory tract infections are frequent in childhood and range from the trivial to the serious and the life-threatening. Infections may be limited to the upper respiratory tract (e.g. head cold, pharyngitis/tonsillitis, otitis media and croup) or may also involve the lower respiratory tract (e.g. bronchiolitis, pneumonia, tuberculosis). Common chronic disorders include asthma and cystic fibrosis.

Typical signs of respiratory disease may be subtle or absent in the young child.

History (see also Ch. 5)

It is important to establish at an early stage what the parent/child's primary concern is. The main reasons for parents seeking medical attention are:
- Cough
- Noisy breathing
- Recurrent chest infections
- Shortness of breath.

It is important to determine the onset, duration and severity of that problem, the particular triggers or relievers of the symptoms, and the impact on the child's life.

In children who present with some form of noisy breathing, accurately identifying what the noise is and its timing in the respiratory cycle is helpful in arriving

MODULE SEVEN

at a diagnosis and in particular establishing the location of the problem. If the noise is not currently present, make sure you understand what the parent is describing. You may have to try and make the noise yourself.

Following this, specific questions within the conventional history will shed further light on the problem.

Examination

Examination may need to be repeated several times, especially during an evolving illness where signs may initially be absent or very subtle.

While attention is paid to the respiratory examination, it is important to determine whether there are features suggestive of an underlying chronic disease (Table 42.1). General features to look for include:

- Failure to thrive: plot height and weight against percentile
- Scoliosis
- Ear, nose and throat: signs of allergic rhinitis, allergic salute
- Signs of atopic eczema.

Noisy breathing

Can you define and describe the following noises? Do you understand how each noise is produced?

- Snoring
- Stridor

Table 42.1 Signs to consider in respiratory disease

Examination	Clinical features to consider
Inspection	Finger clubbing (Fig. 41.1): suggestive of suppurative lung diseases Cyanosis Chest deformity: possible chronic condition (Figs 42.2 and 42.3) Effort of breathing/signs of respiratory distress
Palpation	Chest expansion reduced Hepatomegaly
Percussion	Reduced percussion note (may be omitted in the smaller child)
Auscultation	Breath sounds Crepitations Wheeze Cardiac murmurs
Sputum inspection	Volume Colour
Growth chart	Weight and height plotted

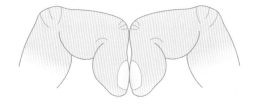

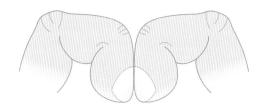

Fig. 42.1 Clubbing (loss of angle at the nail bed)

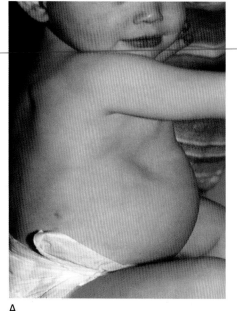

A

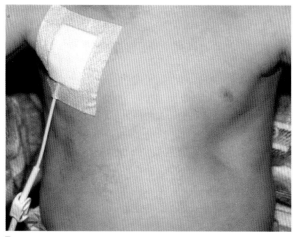

B

Fig. 42.2 A toddler who had a long history of breathlessness and indrawing.
(A) Side view; (B) front view. Note the valley that has been created where the diaphragm is attached to the ribs anteriorly and how the ribs distal to this then point outwards (marked Harrison's sulci).

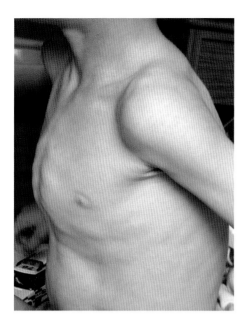

Fig. 42.3 Over-inflated 'barrel-shaped' chest

- Congestion/rattly breathing
- Grunting
- Wheezing
- Cough.

See Box 42.1 for a description of the common respiratory noises.

Shortness of breath

When parents report that a young child experiences 'shortness of breath' this is likely to be based on their opinion of the child's appearance. This is probably correct when the child is overtly wheezing and has recession:

- Obese children report and appear to have 'shortness of breath' that is most likely due to deconditioning. In these children it can be difficult to exclude asthma.
- Parents of children with a spasmodic cough or children who are having difficulty expectorating phlegm often report that the child has 'shortness of breath'.
- 'Tightness in the chest' will cause the sensation of 'shortness of breath' and is a feature of asthma, even if audible wheezing is not heard.
- The lungs may be stiff, e.g. pneumonia.

Rarer causes of 'shortness of breath' include:

- Pulmonary hypertension
- Interstitial lung diseases.

In both these conditions the shortness of breath may be manifest initially with exercise, when the child becomes hypoxic.

Investigations

Lung function testing (Box 42.2)

It is important not to forget that blood gas analysis (pH, $PaCO_2$, PaO_2) and O_2 saturation monitoring are important measures of lung function.

More complicated lung function tests will involve the measurement of lung volumes via body box plethysmography and determination of gas transfer (transfer factor) to detect gas transfer abnormalities across the alveoli to capillaries in the pulmonary circulation.

Chest imaging

Radiological imaging of the chest is an integral part of the diagnosis and follow-up of many respiratory diseases.

Plain chest X-ray

The plain chest X-ray is usually the initial study in the diagnostic work-up. Some general patterns occur but with overlap (Table 42.2). Always ask if the defect is localized or generalized (symmetrical versus asymmetrical).

Ultrasound scan (USS)

USS is especially useful for studying pleural disease, as air in the lung prevents penetration of the ultrasound beam; for example, in a child with a unilateral 'white lung' it might not be clear how large an effusion is relative to underlying intraparenchymal consolidation. Pleural effusions can be measured and the presence of loculations and debris determined. USS is also useful for observing diaphragmatic function.

Computed tomography (CT)

CT can give high-quality detailed images of the intrathoracic structures. The radiation dose needs to be kept to a minimum.

Bronchoscopy

Bronchoscopy can be via either a rigid or a flexible bronchoscope. This allows direct observation and access to the airways.

Rigid bronchoscopes allow good ventilation through the bronchoscope during the procedure and are best for removal of foreign bodies and larger tissue biopsies.

Flexible bronchoscopy requires the child to breathe around the solid bronchoscope. It is best for visualization of more difficult areas and allows samples to be obtained from different areas of the lung (bronchoalveolar lavage (BAL), brushings, mucosal biopsy).

Indications include:

BOX 42.1 Description of the common respiratory noises

Snoring
- Rough inspiratory vibratory noise due to airflow obstruction in the hypopharyngeal region
- Occurs during sleep when muscle tone lax

Stridor

- Harsh crowing sound that is predominantly inspiratory due to airflow obstruction of the larynx or upper trachea
- The intrathoracic airways tend to collapse in inspiration and stridor is predominantly inspiratory
- An expiratory component suggests either a lower tracheal obstruction or a more severe fixed obstruction

Congested or 'rattly' breathing

- Mucus is allowed to lie in the hypopharynx, trachea and large bronchi and the child 'breathes through' these secretions
- Parents say that they can feel the infant's chest to be 'rattly' and have the impression that a good cough would clear the problem
- Sounds are produced from the upper and larger airways of infants with mucus hypersecretion
- Causes:
    Transient mucus hypersecretion, e.g. with viral upper respiratory tract infection
    - Persistent mucus hypersecretion, e.g. with early asthma or cystic fibrosis

Grunting

- An end-expiratory noise that occurs when an infant breathes out against a partially closed glottis
- Produces an end-expiratory break and thus provides a positive end-expiratory pressure that prevents the bronchioles and alveoli from collapsing

Wheezing
- A musical high-pitched noise heard audibly or by auscultation
- Can be described to parents as a 'whistling noise in the chest when your child breathes out'
- Produced by intrathoracic airway narrowing causing turbulent airflow and therefore wheezing is predominantly expiratory

Cough

- The sudden forceful expulsion of air with the aim of:
    - Generating high-velocity airflow to expel material from the airway
    - In certain situations, squeezing the lung parenchyma and moving material (mucus/pus) further up the airway so that it can be expelled with further coughing

---

BOX 42.2 Use of lung function tests

Diagnostic
- To determine if and to what extent a child has an obstructive or restrictive lung disorder
- Single measure may confirm diagnosis but is rarely diagnostic
- Serial measurements are more useful

Measuring morbidity
- Baseline values
- Disease progression

Monitoring response
- Short-term response, e.g. bronchodilator responsiveness
- Long-term response, e.g. cystic fibrosis therapy

- Visualizing anatomy, e.g. stridor, fixed wheeze
- Obtaining BAL samples for microbiology or cytology
- Biopsy
- Therapeutic removal of mucus plugs and foreign bodies.

Pulmonary function testing (PFT)

Physiology of PFT

In normal breathing inspiration is an active process that begins with the contraction of the diaphragm, the intercostal muscles functioning to fix the chest wall. If greater work of breathing is required the accessory

Table 42.2 Patterns in chest imaging

Pattern	Pathology

Hyperinflation
  Depressed diaphragms
  Narrow cardiothymic shadow/elongated heart
  Horizontal spread ribs
  Separation of vessels
	Symmetrical
	  Hyperinflation alone or associated with generalized and irregular opacities/areas of collapse
	  Causes: bronchiolitis, asthma, aspiration, cystic fibrosis or other chronic suppurative lung disease, neonatal chronic lung disease
	Asymmetrical (Fig. 42.4)
	  Foreign body
	  Partial airways obstruction (unilateral 'ball valve' effect)
	  Localized lobar collapse
	  Hypoplastic lung with compensatory emphysema
	  Congenital lobar emphysema

Air space disease	Consolidation
	  Fluid, pus or blood is in the alveolar spaces
	  Characterized by fluffy opacities that have irregular margins and coalesce
	  Air bronchograms are produced by the contrast between the adjacent airspace disease with alveolar consolidation with a patent airway standing out in contrast
	  Distribution: lobar (Fig. 42.5), often with sharply defined margins along a fissure (suggest lobar pneumonia), or generalized and patchy (suggests bronchopneumonia, Fig. 42.6)
	Pulmonary oedema
	  Look for fluid in fissures and interlobular septa
	  'Bat's wing' distribution extending from hilum
	Collapse
	  Produces a similar density as consolidation but without air bronchograms
	  Look for displacement of horizontal fissure
	  If large may show compensatory hyperinflation
	  ± Mediastinal shift (Fig. 42.7)
	Bronchiectasis
	  Thickened dilated bronchial walls
	  Cross-sectional appearance: ring shadows or white round shadows if plugged
	  Longitudinal appearance: 'tram lines' (Fig. 42.8)

Pleural disease	Pleural fluid accumulates below the diaphragmatic surface of the lung causing:
	  In upright position:
	    Blunting of the lateral costophrenic angle
	    Meniscus formation; increases superiorly (Fig. 42.9)
	    Lung compression or mediastinal shift
	  In supine position:
	    Fluid gravitates posteriorly
	    If large the whole lung will be white
	    ± Associated mediastinal shift

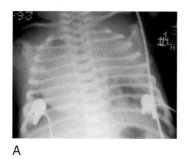

A

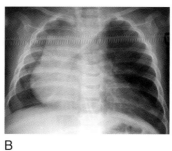

B

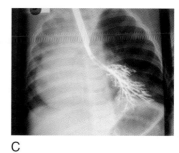

C

Fig. 42.4 Patterns in chest imaging.
(A) Unilateral hyperinflation: chest X-rays of a neonate with respiratory distress. **(B)** Once the delayed clearance of lung fluid had occurred the left upper lobe became massively over-inflated, herniating to the right and compressing the left lower lobe. Reduced air entry was heard on the left side. **(C)** A bronchogram confirmed no ventilation or perfusion to the left upper lobe. This child had a congenital left upper lobar emphysema, which was acting as a space-occupying lesion and therefore was removed.

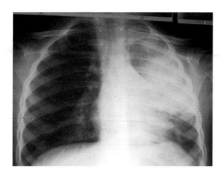

Fig. 42.5 Dense lobar consolidation in the left upper lobe

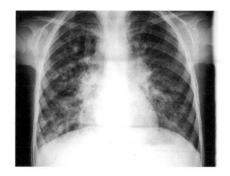

Fig. 42.6 Bronchopneumonia.
Bilateral fluffy shadows that are more confluent near the heart border. There is perihilar lymphadenopathy. This child had a late presentation of cystic fibrosis.

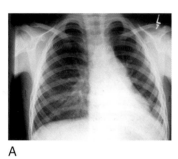

A

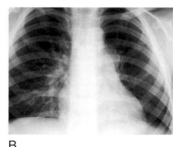

B

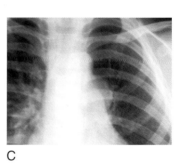

C

Fig. 42.7 Three chest X-rays from a boy whose wheezing and cough were being treated unsuccessfully with asthma therapy.
(A) There is left lower lobe collapse. Note the sharp line running behind the heart to the left costophrenic angle, and the absence of a visible left diaphragm. (B) After physiotherapy the left lower lobe has almost completely re-expanded (the left diaphragm is becoming visible) and the bronchogenic cyst at the left hilar region can be better visualized. (C) Focuses on the left hilar region; a bronchogenic cyst was compressing the left lower lobe bronchus. This patient did not need any asthma therapy after the cyst was removed surgically.

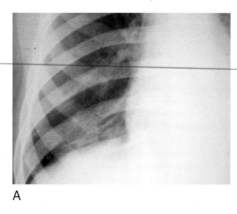

A

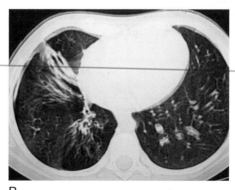

B

Fig. 42.8 Localized bronchiectasis (tramlines) in the right mid-zone.
(A) Chest X-ray; (B) high-resolution CT confirming localization of disease. A retained inhaled foreign body should be ruled out in localized bronchiectasis.

muscles (which are normally inactive during quiet respiration) are recruited. These include the scalene and sternocleidomastoid muscles. However, the diaphragm is the most important muscle used in inspiration.

Exhalation is usually a passive process. When the lungs are stretched, e.g. full of air after a maximal inspiration, the elastic recoil pressure of the lung outplays the natural tendency of the chest wall to expand.

The child is asked to inspire to total lung capacity (TLC) and then to do a maximal forced expiration

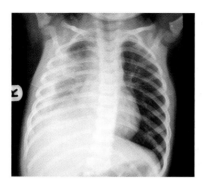

Fig. 42.9 Chest X-ray of an infant with a right-sided pleural effusion

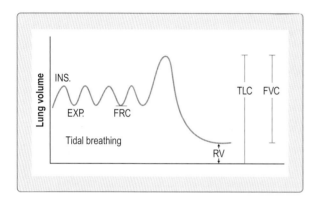

Fig. 42.10 Lung volume analysis.
The left-hand aspect shows the volume (y axis) against time (x axis) of a child during normal tidal breathing. Remember inspiration is active and expiration is passive. The passive end-expiratory 'resting point' or trough occurs when the forces of elastic recoil of the lung balance the chest wall expansive forces and no airflow is occurring. This point is referred to as the functional residual capacity. (RV = residual volume; TLC = total lung capacity; FVC = forced vital capacity)

manoeuvre to residual volume (RV). A visual incentive may be used to encourage the child to keep blowing out maximally until airflow has ceased. The forced vital capacity (FVC) is the volume of air shifted with this manoeuvre. From the FVC plot we can measure the volume exhaled at given time points. Most frequently used is the volume exhaled at 1 second or forced expiratory volume in 1 second (FEV_1) (Fig. 42.10).

Figure 42.11 shows a flow–volume (F–V) curve. Flow is volume moved (inspired or expired) per unit of time (seconds).

During forced expiration the rate of airflow rises rapidly to a maximum. As the lung volume decreases, the intrathoracic airways narrow and the expiratory airflow progressively falls until no further airflow is occurring.

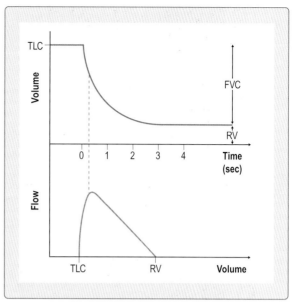

Fig. 42.11 Flow–volume curve.
The flow–volume (F–V) curve is derived from the same forced expiratory manoeuvre used to show the volume–time curve, with volume on the upper y axis versus time (x axis), and flow on the lower y axis versus volume (x-axis).

'Normal' is usually taken to be greater than the 2.5 percentile, i.e. 97.5% of healthy well children will be above this value after adjustment is made for age, height, gender and race.

Peak expiratory flow rate (PEFR)

The child gives a short sharp blow into a mini-handheld PEFR meter.

Advantages

- Cheap and easily available.
- Can be used at home to monitor airway calibre that varies over time. The normal diurnal variation (airways narrower in the morning and wider in the afternoon) is increased in asthmatics. The finding of exaggerated diurnal variability ('shark's teeth' pattern, Fig. 42.12) that improves with trial of asthma treatment is helpful diagnostically.

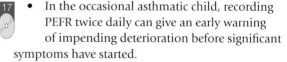

- In the occasional asthmatic child, recording PEFR twice daily can give an early warning of impending deterioration before significant symptoms have started.

When using PEFR monitoring it is important to find out the maximum PEFR for the child. This may require a short course of intense anti-asthma therapy. Serial monitoring compares day-to-day values against the child's 'personal best' recording.

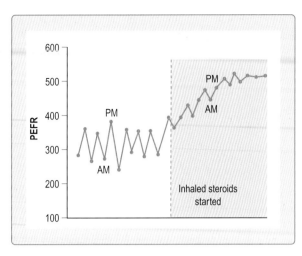

Fig. 42.12 Peak expiratory flow rate (PEFR) showing 'shark's teeth' pattern

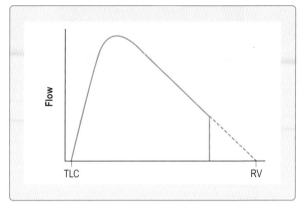

Fig. 42.13 The F–V loop from a 'short blow', where the flow can be seen abruptly dropping to the zero line.

Unless the child has blown for longer than 1 second the FEV_1 and the FVC will be almost equal and all that can be claimed is that the FEV_1 is at least that which was recorded. Clearly the FVC and mid-flow measurements will be inaccurate.

Disadvantages

- Some asthmatic children learn to 'check blast' into the PEFR meter in order to achieve high results. This illustrates that PEFR is measuring large airways calibre and that reduction in PEFR is a relatively late indicator of airways obstruction.
- Some children/parents invent the results that are recorded on diary cards.
- Overall, chronic asthma management using PEFR measurement action plans has not been shown to be superior to symptom-based plans.

Spirometry

Children over 5 or 6 years can generally perform spirometry, including F–V curves, FEV_1 and FVC manoeuvres.

When performing spirometry, first check if the spirogram is technically adequate. Common technical problems in children performing F–V loops include:

- Failure to blow to flow cessation, i.e. a short blow (Fig. 42.13).
- Double blow, when the child does a second blow into spirometer.
- The child who takes a submaximal inspiration and does not blow from TLC. This can be difficult to spot on the F–V loop, as the curves with and without a good inspiration will look similar.
- Younger children who take several attempts to optimize their technique but often start to tire after a further 2–3 attempts, with a deterioration in performance.
- The process can make some children cough.

Bronchodilator responsiveness (BDR)

Finding out if there is BDR is helpful confirmatory evidence that a child is likely to benefit from bronchodilators and is a feature of asthma (p. 248).

Problem-orientated topic:

respiratory function testing

Andrew is an 8 year old. His paediatrician is not sure whether his respiratory symptoms indicate asthma. He tries to get Andrew to blow into his new spirometer, which has a visual incentive. His FEV_1 is below normal at 63% predicted for his height (134 cm) and age (8 years).

Andrew is given salbutamol (100 µg/puff, six puffs) via a small-volume holding chamber and 25 minutes later Andrew performs another spirometry manoeuvre (Table 42.3).

Before interpretation check that both F–V loops (Fig. 42.14) are technically satisfactory and that Andrew has blown out until there is no further flow.

Q1. Do these tests suggest that Andrew's test is technically satisfactory?

Q2. How do you interpret the findings on these loops?

Table 42.3 Andrew's spirometry results

	Before (% predicted)	After (% predicted)
FEV$_1$	1.10 (63%)	1.51 (86%)
FVC	2.00 (96%)	2.11 (101%)

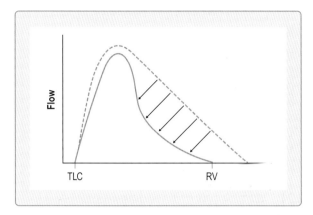

Fig. 42.14 Andrew's F–V loops

Q1. Do these tests suggest that Andrew's test is technically satisfactory?

Andrew has blown out to flow limitation as the FV loop reaches baseline without a sudden drop. Looking at the two F–V loops, the dashed post-bronchodilator trace shows much less sagging (concavity), suggesting better flow at low lung volumes.

Q2. How do you interpret the findings on these loops?

There has been a significant increase in both FEV$_1$ and FVC, suggesting BDR. Generally an increase of > 10–15% in FEV$_1$ or FVC is taken as indicating BDR.

Tests of bronchial hyper-reactivity (BHR)

Often children attending clinics with a history in keeping with asthma have normal lung function and the question arises: does the patient have 'twitchy airways' or BHR? To answer this, bronchoprovocation tests are used. The typical challenge agents used are methacholine, histamine and adenosine. The concentration at which the FEV$_1$ falls by 20% is recorded. The lower the dose or concentration, the greater the BHR. The asthmatic typically responds to challenge at a lower than normal dose.

Exercise can also be used as the 'challenge'. This is mostly carried out on a treadmill but can be done using free running. Patients with asthma often have an exaggerated drop in lung function after exercise. FEV$_1$ should be measured before and 15 mins after cessation of exercise. A drop in FEV$_1$ > 15% suggests a positive test.

Stridor

> **Problem-orientated topic:**
>
> **acute stridor (part I)**
>
> Ben is a 14-month-old baby who presents at 1 a.m. He has a 1-day history of a runny nose and had developed a barking cough the previous evening. He is brought to the accident and emergency department because he is making an inspiratory crowing noise and has difficulty breathing.
>
> He is assessed as having a loud inspiratory stridor when upset, which decreases in intensity but is still present at rest. His saturations are 95% in room air, with a respiratory rate of 40 breaths per minute, with some subcostal recession. He has good air entry on auscultation, with a heart rate of 90 beats per minute.
>
> Q1. What is the differential diagnosis?
> Q2. What is your assessment of the severity of Ben's condition?
> Q3. What is your initial management plan?

Q1. What is the differential diagnosis?

The most likely diagnosis of acute stridor in a toddler is laryngotracheobronchitis (croup) (Box 42.3).

Q2. What is your assessment of the severity of Ben's condition? (Box 42.4 and Table 42.4)

Overall Ben is active and has good air entry and no signs of hypoxaemia, suggesting that the airways obstruction is currently not severe. However, he has stridor at rest associated with some increased working of breathing (indrawing), indicating that the airways obstruction is not mild. He has mild to moderately severe airways obstruction.

- Laryngotracheobronchitis (croup)
- Epiglottitis
- Bacterial tracheitis
- Foreign body
- Angioedema

Timing?
- The most prominent phase of the respiratory noise should be inspiratory
- Expiratory stridor indicates more severe or intrathoracic airways obstruction

Work of breathing?
- Increased respiratory rate
- Sternal (supra- and sub-)recession

How effective is the breathing?
- Chest expansion
- Breath sounds for air entry

Is there adequate oxygenation?
- Is heart rate increased?
- Pallor, cyanosis
- O_2 saturation
- Activity levels

Q3. What is your initial management plan?

You decide Ben's condition is severe enough to give budesonide via nebulizer. You assess him 30 mins after treatment and feel that he no longer has stridor at rest. You therefore allow him to be discharged home.

Problem-orientated topic:

acute stridor (part II)

Unfortunately, Ben reattends 2 days later, with similar symptoms. The stridor is loud with an expiratory component. His respiratory rate is 60 breaths per minute, with subcostal and intercostal retraction. His saturations are 90% on room air, heart rate is 120 bpm, capillary refill time is > 3 seconds and temperature 38°C.

Q1. What is your plan/diagnosis?

Q1. What is your plan/diagnosis?

Ben has had an acute deterioration and is unwell. He needs an immediate supply of oxygen and assessment of airway, breathing and circulation (ABC).

The differential diagnosis is between severe croup, epiglottitis and bacterial tracheitis. Ways of differentiating between these diagnoses are shown in Table 42.5.

He needs admission and further assessment by paediatric intensive care. The anaesthetist decides to intubate Ben to secure the airway. Purulent exudates are noted during intubation, confirming the diagnosis of bacterial tracheitis. Following intubation, swab cultures via endotracheal tube and blood cultures are taken to confirm the organism.

Intravenous antibiotics are given to cover *Staphylococcus aureus* and *Haemophilus*.

Laryngotracheobronchitis ('croup')

(See also Ch. 23.)

Croup is an acute clinical syndrome that usually starts with a runny nose, followed by a barking cough and hoarse voice. Acute stridor often starts in the early

Table 42.4 Assessment and evaluation of croup

Croup	Assessment	Treatment
Mild	Active, well child, barking cough, stridor with agitation, minimal signs of increased work of breathing	Nil
Moderate	Stridor at rest, some signs of increased work of breathing	Oral dexamethasone and/or nebulized budesonide
Severe	Stridor at rest with expiratory component, marked increased work of breathing (indrawing), increased respiratory and heart rate, agitation and pallor. As airways obstruction becomes very serious, the stridor becomes quieter but sounds 'tighter', agitation eventually turning into exhaustion	Oxygen to maintain O_2 saturation > 92% Nebulized adrenaline (epinephrine) may buy time, followed by oral or nebulized steroid Intubation and ventilation may be required

Table 42.5 Croup, epiglottitis and tracheitis: differential diagnosis

Typical features	Croup	Epiglottitis	Bacterial tracheitis
Prodrome	URTI	Nil/mild URTI	URTI
Age	6 mths–3 yrs	1–8 yrs	6 mths–8 yrs
Onset	Slow (1–2 days)	Rapid (2–8 hr)	Variable
Barking cough	Yes	No	Yes
Hoarseness	Yes	No	Yes
Loud stridor	Yes	No, usually soft	Yes
Drooling	No	Yes	No
Dysphagia	No	Yes	No
'Toxic appearance'	No	Yes	Yes
Ability to lie flat	Yes	No	Yes
Microbiology	Viral: Parainfluenza 1,3 RSV	*Haemophilus influenzae* B	*Staph. aureus* *Haemophilus influenzae*

(URTI = upper respiratory tract infection; RSV = respiratory syncytial virus)

hours of the morning. Children are usually between 6 months and 5 years.

Peak incidence is in autumn, often with a second peak in spring. Parainfluenza virus accounts for 75% of cases (especially type 1,3), with other respiratory viruses (respiratory syncytial virus (RSV), influenza, metapneumovirus, adenovirus) causing the remainder.

The illness resolves within 3 days but occasionally symptoms persist. Less than 5% of children need to be hospitalized and very few require intubation and ventilation.

Acute spasmodic croup

This does not have signs of a preceding head cold; children are afebrile and awake suddenly with acute stridor during the night. Recurrences typically occur on the subsequent 2–3 nights. This syndrome occurs in children of the same age as in infectious croup, during the same seasons, and similar viruses can be isolated. Some would therefore say that they are not different conditions. However, children with recurrent spasmodic croup often have a strong atopic or asthmatic family background.

Bacterial tracheitis

The infection causes purulent secretions and mucosal necrosis. The child has a croupy cough but also looks toxic, febrile and ill. Some regard it as a bacterial superinfection after viral croup. Since routine immunization against *Haemophilus influenzae* was introduced, bacterial tracheitis is probably now more common than epiglottitis.

Epiglottitis

This presents with fever and a toxic look, which comes on over 4–6 hours. Patients have a quieter muffled stridor and often sit up, extending their neck slightly to maintain maximal airway patency. They do not like swallowing and therefore saliva pools in the mouth and drooling occurs. The epiglottis is inflamed and 'cherry red' with swollen arythenoids. Children with epiglottitis do not like being disturbed. Management is shown in Box 42.5.

Problem-orientated topic:

persistent stridor

Anna, a 2-month-old baby, has had persistent noisy breathing (which the GP believes to be stridor) from the first week of life. The stridor was initially intermittent and only occurred with crying or when she was lying supine, but has now become persistent and more severe. Anna has some indrawing at rest, the stridor is both inspiratory and expiratory and you note that she sleeps with her neck extended. Her weight has dropped to the second centile.

Q1. What are the causes of persistent stridor in an infant?

Q2. Why is Anna not thriving?

Q3. What investigations are indicated?

Do not

- Examine the throat
- Lay the child flat
- Order a lateral X-ray of the neck
- Upset the child by trying to gain intravenous access or place an oxygen mask

Do

- Call the airway team (ENT and consultant anaesthetist)
- Stay with the child
- Allow the child to sit on mother's knee
- Measure O_2 saturation if possible
- Give O_2 therapy if absolutely needed and only if well tolerated

Q1. What are the causes of persistent stridor in an infant?

- Laryngomalacia
- Subglottic stenosis (congenital or acquired: usually preterm baby who was intubated)
- Subglottic web
- Subglottic haemangioma
- Vascular ring
- Tracheal stenosis
- Vocal cord paralysis.

Q2. Why is Anna not thriving?

Anna has signs of significant airways obstruction (inspiratory and expiratory stridor, holds neck extended). The poor weight gain is likely to be due to energy expended with the extra work required for breathing. In addition, some children with congenital laryngomalacia (the most common cause of chronic stridor in an infant) have swallowing difficulties and gastro-oesophageal reflux, making it difficult to get adequate calories into the child.

Q3. What investigations are indicated?

Bronchoscopy and upper airways laryngoscopy confirm the diagnosis. These should be performed in all who have significant stridor and especially those with stridor that progressively becomes more severe. They need to have a progressive lesion (such as an expanding haemangioma) ruled out.

Laryngomalacia

The stridor results from collapse of the supraglottic structures inwards during inspiration. Typically, stridor begins during the first 2 weeks of life and becomes more obvious by 2–6 months. It increases with activity, with lying supine or with respiratory tract infections. Over time (by 2 years) the stridor will usually disappear. The diagnosis is confirmed by flexible laryngoscopy/bronchoscopy.

Expectant observation and parental reassurance are required for the majority. Stridor can be associated with gastro-oesophageal and laryngopharyngeal reflux, which may need to be treated. Laryngomalacia will become more severe with a concomitant viral respiratory tract infection but with progressive stridor an expanding lesion (such as an expanding haemangioma) needs to be ruled out. For those with very severe obstruction, often associated with failure to thrive, cyanosis or apparent life-threatening events (ALTEs), endoscopic supraglottoplasty can be used to avoid tracheotomy.

Other causes of stridor

Subglottic stenosis

This may be congenital but is more often acquired. Always suspect subglottic stenosis in a preterm baby that was intubated for a considerable time. If severe, repeated dilations or a tracheostomy may be required.

Haemangioma

Subglottic haemangiomas often enlarge in the first few months of life and are therefore associated with progressive development of increasingly severe stridor. Improvement occurs over the next few years.

Vocal cord paralysis

Bilateral recurrent laryngeal nerve palsy is associated with bilateral adducted vocal cords, causing stridor that can be severe. It may occur in infants with spina bifida and the Arnold–Chiari malformation. Acute onset of stridor in such an infant with a ventriculo-peritoneal shunt would suggest possible shunt malfunction.

Vascular compressions

These include vascular rings, such as the double aortic arch (Fig. 42.15), or aberrant origins of the subclavian arteries causing the subclavian artery to cross anterior to the trachea, resulting in some degree of pulsatile anterior compression of the trachea.

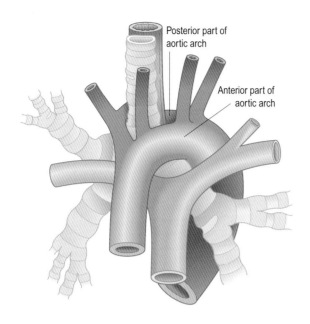

Fig. 42.15 Double aortic arch.
The ascending aorta divides into two, with the posterior part passing behind and trapping the trachea and oesophagus before rejoining the descending aorta. There may therefore be swallowing difficulties and a barium swallow will show a fixed posterior indentation. The anatomy can be better defined using echocardiography but usually angiography (contrast or MRI) is required.

Posterior part of aortic arch

Anterior part of aortic arch

Problem-orientated topic:

snoring and obstructive sleep apnoea (OSA)

George, an 8-year-old boy with Down's syndrome, has been noted by his teachers to have become unduly sleepy in his class. His parents describe loud snoring associated with rib recession after he has gone to sleep and they get very worried when the snoring stops and he appears to have stopped breathing. He is very restless at night.

Q1. What is the differential diagnosis of George's problem?

Q2. What are the risk factors for obstructive sleep apnoea?

Q3. What is the physiological sequence of an episode of OSA?

Q4. What are the long-term risks involved?

Q5. What investigations would you order?

Q6. What are the principles of management?

Q1. What is the differential diagnosis of George's problem?

Obstructive sleep apnoea syndrome (OSAS)

OSAS occurs when a child who snores experiences periods of complete obstruction, initially associated with increased respiratory efforts but followed by apnoea. These episodes can be associated with significant hypoxia and hypercarbia.

Primary snoring

Many children snore, which is due to partial obstruction of the nasal airways or pharynx.

Central apnoea/hypoventilation

This is defined as an elevated $PaCO_2$ due to a decreased central nervous system ventilatory drive. It is usually associated with hypoxaemia. Children fail to breathe normally, despite having normal airways, lungs, respiratory muscles and chest wall:

- *Congenital hypoventilation syndrome.* In this rare disorder children have intact voluntary control of breathing and are well when awake. They lack automatic breathing control and therefore hypoventilate when asleep. To remain alive these children need nocturnal ventilatory support at night.
- *Secondary central hypoventilation*:
  - Conditions associated with raised intracranial pressure (e.g. brain tumour in the hypothalamic region)
  - Rare neurological conditions, some with hypothalamic and endocrine dysfunction.

N.B. Children with Prader–Willi syndrome may have both OSAS (due to associated obesity) and central hypoventilation. It is also important not to blame OSAS for daytime somnolence when the cause is inadequate sleep. Increasingly we observe children who watch television or play computer or video games in their bedrooms into the early hours and become sleep-deprived.

Q2. What are the risk factors for obstructive sleep apnoea?

- Small airway relative to large tongue or adenotonsillar hypertrophy
- Relatively hypotonia, as in Down's syndrome
- Pierre Robin syndrome
- Obesity, e.g. Prader–Willi syndrome.

Q3. What is the physiological sequence of an episode of OSA?

- *Loud snoring.* This is due to upper airways obstruction.
- *Complete obstruction.* Snoring stops attempts to breathe against complete obstruction.
- *Apnoea.* Stops breathing completely
- *Arousal.* PaO_2 falls and $PaCO_2$ rises, stimulating an arousal response and improved muscle tone with re-establishment of breathing.

Q4. What are the long-term risks involved?

- Poor-quality sleep and feeling unrefreshed in morning
- Sleepy by day:
  - Reduced school performance
  - Deterioration in behaviour
- Pulmonary hypertension if prolonged hypoxaemia.

Q5. What investigations would you order?

- Full clinical and ENT examination
- Overnight continuous recording of:
  - O_2 saturation
  - Respiratory movements
  - Airflow at nose/mouth
  - Heart rate.

In some studies this was regarded as adequate for OSAS screening, but other studies have suggested a high false negative rate compared with full polysomnography. A video of the snoring obstructed breathing and subsequent apnoea is helpful.

In polysomnography, electroencephalography, sleeping staging, end-tidal CO_2, electro-oculograms, submental electromyography, and thoracic and abdominal movements are additionally measured.

Q6. What are the principles of management?

- Adenotonsillectomy
- Trial of nasal corticosteroids
- Nasal continuous positive airway pressure (CPAP)
- Uvulopalatopharyngoplasty
- Rarely, tracheotomy
- Weight loss for obese children.

Wheeze

Problem-orientated topic:

wheeze and lethargy

Over Christmas, 3-month-old Conor attends the accident and emergency department after 3 days of being generally unwell at home. His mother is anxious, as he has been breathing noisily for a few days but has now become sleepy and will not take his feeds. He has otherwise been a well child.

Conor is assessed to be lethargic but maintaining his colour; his respiratory rate is 80 breaths per minute, and he has a hyperexpanded chest and intercostal recession. There is an audible wheeze but predominantly widespread crepitations on auscultation.

Q1. What is the likely clinical diagnosis of Conor's illness?
Q2. What is your initial management?
Q3. What are the risk factors for more severe acute disease and can this disorder be prevented in high-risk infants?

Q1. What is the likely clinical diagnosis of Conor's illness?

Wheezing needs to be clearly defined, as parents may not have the same idea as you of what wheeze is. Specific details recorded from the history include timing and duration of wheeze episodes, precipitants such as dust, pollen, recent viral infection and seasonality, and other associated symptoms such as cough or shortness of breath.

Causes of wheezing in infants and preschool children

- Acute bronchiolitis (the most likely cause in Conor)
- Post-bronchiolitis recurrent wheezing
- Asthma:
  - True atopic asthma
  - Recurrent viral-induced wheeze
- Bronchopulmonary dysplasia
- Recurrent pulmonary aspiration
- Congenital bronchial stenosis, vascular rings, bronchogenic cysts
- Tracheobronchomalacia
- Inhaled foreign body
- Conditions causing chronic supportive lung disease, e.g. cystic fibrosis
- Primary ciliary dyskinesia
- Immune deficiencies.

Q2. What is your initial management?

- ABC
- Assessment of breathing
- Further evaluation of history.

Subsequent management is largely supportive (Box 24.6).

Q3. What are the risk factors for more severe acute disease and can this disorder be prevented in high-risk infants?

Risk factors

- Prematurity, especially if there is neonatal chronic lung disease, congenital heart disease, immune deficiency and cystic fibrosis.

Prevention

- High-risk babies can be given a monoclonal antibody (palivizumab) to RSV to try to prevent hospital admission.
- In hospital prevention measures to stop cross-infection are important but unproven. Sensible measures include cohort segregation of cases, strict hand washing, and the wearing of face masks and gowns.

Acute bronchiolitis

This is discussed in Chapter 23.

BOX 42.6 Management of acute bronchiolitis

Humidified oxygen
- Aim for O_2 saturation > 92%

Maintenance of clear airway
- Gentle nasopharyngeal suction

Hydration
- May require nasogastric or i.v. fluids
- Take care not to overload the circulation, as bronchiolitis may be associated with inappropriate antidiuretic hormone (ADH) secretion and hyponatraemia

Apnoea
- Infants under 6 weeks may have seemingly milder disease but this may still be complicated by apnoeic episodes
- Prematurity or cardiac disease increases risk of severe disease
- May require paediatric intensive care unit (PICU) and ventilation

Nebulizer therapy
- Nebulized adrenaline (epinephrine) may benefit a few children
- May be considered but discontinue if no response
- Overall no specific treatment, including adrenaline, bronchodilators and corticosteroids, has been shown conclusively to be beneficial

Asthma

Problem-orientated topic:

asthma

Aidan is a 4-year-old boy who has been referred by his GP. He has suffered frequent wheezing episodes in winter associated with head colds. Aidan also experiences day-to-day symptoms of cough and is breathless with exercise. Last month he was up all night wheezing after having a 'pillow fight' with his sister.

Aidan's mother has asthma and hay fever and his older sister had frequent wheezing episodes in infancy in addition to eczema. Aidan has mild eczema.

Aidan is diagnosed as having asthma and started on regular inhaled corticosteroids with salbutamol for relief medication.

Continued overleaf

Q1. What are the typical patterns of asthma in young children?

Q2. What issues need reviewing when a child does not seem to respond to anti-asthma therapy?

Q3. What are the principles of pharmacological management of chronic asthma?

Q1. What are the typical patterns of asthma in young children?

See Box 42.7. Note the flow chart in the British Thoracic Society/Scottish Intercollegiate Guidelines Network (BTS/SIGN) Guidelines for Asthma Management (see URL below).

Aidan is seen at the asthma clinic several months later. Mum reports that he still has day-to-day exercise wheezing and breathlessness and is up at night with cough on 2–3 nights per week. Mum feels the salbutamol gives him good relief but is not sure of the preventive 'steroid' inhaler (beclomethasone 100 µg twice daily).

BOX 42.7 Asthma patterns

Episodic viral-associated wheezing
- Episodes are more frequent in winter months
- Almost always associated with head colds
- Usually completely asymptomatic between episodes
- Evidence suggests that, for the majority of these children, the response to regular anti-inflammatory therapy is poor

Classic atopic asthma
- May have an atopic background (allergies or eczema)
- Positive family history of atopy and asthma
- Day-to-day symptoms triggered with exercise or occurring at night when no head cold
- Should respond well to regular anti-inflammatory asthma therapy

Cough variant asthma (CVA)
- Nocturnal and/or exercise-induced cough when free from head colds
- Wheezing may just simply never have been heard
- A personal or family history of other atopic disorders is a helpful supporting finding
- Child responds rapidly to anti-asthma medication
- Symptoms relapse when therapy withdrawn

BOX 42.8 Review of management

Non-compliance
- Lack of knowledge that inhaled corticosteroids need to be taken regularly even when well
- Forgetting/chaotic family lifestyle
- Hidden health beliefs, e.g. fear of dependency on inhalers or fear of side-effects

Poor inhaler technique
- Check at each visit
- Remember a fighting crying child is unlikely to receive much medication administered via a spacer and face mask. Crying is predominantly expiratory. The face mask should have a seal against the child's face
- Choose a suitable age-appropriate inhaler device

Ongoing trigger factors
- Aero-allergens
- Environmental tobacco smoke

Concomitant disease
- Allergic rhinosinusitis
- Gastro-oesophageal reflux

Is asthma the correct diagnosis?
- Before stepping-up medication review whether the diagnosis of asthma is correct

Q2. What issues need review when a child does not seem to respond to anti-asthma therapy?

See Box 42.8.

Q3. What are the principles of pharmacological management of chronic asthma?

- Control symptoms
- Prevent exacerbations
- Achieve best possible pulmonary function
- Minimize side-effects.

Asthma management should follow a stepwise approach. Start at the step most appropriate to initial severity to achieve early control and maintain control by stepping treatment up and down according to symptoms.

 http://www.sign.ac.uk/guidelines/published/#Respiratory

BTS/SIGN Guidelines for Asthma Management: full text version p. 8, Fig. 2 for flow chart for diagnosis of asthma in children, specific link to figure given

acute exacerbation of asthma (part I)

A year later, Aidan is brought to accident and emergency by ambulance. He has had an upper respiratory tract infection for 2 days and has become increasingly wheezy and short of breath. His parents gave him some salbutamol using his inhaler and spacer device, but it only produced a slight and short-lived improvement.

In accident and emergency he is pale, cyanosed, agitated and in marked respiratory distress and only gasps out single words at a time. His heart rate is 160/min and respiratory rate 60/min.

Q1. What immediate actions are needed in the accident and emergency department?

Q2. What are the features of severe and life-threatening asthma?

Q3. What tests are indicated if there is no improvement or if Aidan deteriorates?

Q1. What immediate actions are needed in the accident and emergency department?

Assessment of ABC is mandatory.

Airway

Aidan's upper airway appears patent; he can speak single words and is breathing, and there is audible expiratory wheeze.

Breathing

- Check respiratory rate.
- Assess work of breathing: marked indrawing (suprasternal, subcostal recession) and only able to speak in single words.
- Assess efficacy of breathing: pallor, cyanosis and agitation along with tachycardia suggest that Aidan is hypoxic.

You have identified a problem with breathing. Therefore:

- Check O_2 saturation with pulsed oximetry.
- Give O_2: enough to bring O_2 saturation > 92% and preferably > 94%.

Circulation

- Heart rate
- Capillary refill time
- Blood pressure.

Pulsus paradoxus occurs in acute severe asthma but is not always present.

Q2. What are the features of severe and life-threatening asthma?

According to guidelines Aidan has had a severe exacerbation of asthma. He is therefore given nebulized β_2-agonist combined with ipratropium bromide (3 nebulizations of each in the first hour), along with supplemental oxygen and prednisolone orally.

N.B. If a patient is unable to take steroid orally, then an i.v. line should be inserted and steroids given systemically.

 http://www.sign.ac.uk/guidelines/fulltext/63/annex5.html

This refers to flow chart for the assessment of severity of acute asthma

Q3. What tests are indicated if there is no improvement or if Aidan deteriorates?

See Box 42.9.

When frequent bronchodilator therapy has not produced the desired response, additional therapy includes:

- I.v. aminophylline
- I.v. salbutamol
- I.v. magnesium.

A paediatric intensive care anaesthetist should also assess Aidan.

BOX 42.9 Investigations in severe asthma

Arterial blood gases

- A normal $PaCO_2$ in a child with very severe asthma is an ominous sign since in mild/moderately acute asthma the hyperventilation is associated with a low $PaCO_2$
- An elevated $PaCO_2$ is associated with exhaustion (Fig. 42.16)

Chest X-ray

- Performing a CXR is *not* usually a priority but should be done if a pneumothorax is suspected

PEFR or FEV$_1$

- This is an objective measure of airflow obstruction in children with acute asthma but it is difficult to teach a child or perform the test correctly during an acute severe attack

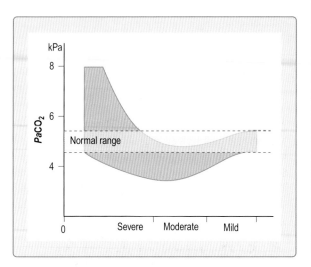

Fig. 42.16 In an asthmatic child with marked breathlessness the finding of a normal $PaCO_2$ should *not* be reassuring but taken as an indication of severe airways obstruction

---

Problem-orientated topic:

acute exacerbation of asthma (part I)

Aidan starts to respond to treatment and avoids intensive care. After several days he is back on his regular inhaled therapy and ready for home.

Q1. Before Aidan is discharged home what should be checked?

Q1. Before Aidan is discharged home what should be checked?

See Box 42.10.

Cough

Problem-orientated topic:

chronic cough (part I)

Lucy is an 8-year-old who gives a 6-month history of a progressive cough. In the past she has had a problem dry cough, which lasted several weeks after each head cold. A tentative diagnosis of asthma has been made and stepping up anti-asthma therapy

---

along with oral antibiotics gas seemed to coincide with eventual improvement of each coughing episode. She has been hospitalized for acute pneumonia on several occasions to be given intravenous antibiotics. Her present cough is described as productive of purulent phlegm.

Q1. What are the causes of a chronic productive (moist or wet) cough and what are the key investigations for each cause?

Q2. What treatment will you start Lucy on?

All advice, verbal and written, should be documented in the patient's hospital notes.

Advice on reducing asthma triggers at home
- Environmental tobacco smoke exposure
- Anti-house dust mite measures
- Consideration given to removing pets

Advice on when to take medications
- Understanding importance of taking preventive anti-inflammatory therapy regularly

Advice on how to take medications
- 'Inhaler technique': it is not adequate to show a child/parent how to use an inhaler. Technique should be checked and shown to be satisfactory

Action plan for 'acute asthma attack'
- Recognizing severity and treatment of an exacerbation

Q1. What are the causes of a chronic productive (moist or wet) cough and what are the key investigations for each cause?

See Table 42.6.

Lucy has a moist/wet or productive cough suggesting a condition causing a chronic endobronchial infection, and serious underlying conditions need to be excluded. It is important to obtain sputum for culture and order a CXR; high-resolution CT is likely to indicate cylindrical bronchiectasis.

Figure 42.17 shows her CXR and CT scan. This appearance followed an acute pneumonia with residual crackles heard in the left lung on follow-up. No foreign body was detected at bronchoscopy.

Table 42.6 Causes of cough

Causes of productive cough	Investigations
Cystic fibrosis (CF)	Sweat test, CF gene phenotyping
Primary immune deficiency	IgGs, IgG subclasses, functional antibody response to tetanus, pneumococcus or *Haemophilus influenzae* vaccination
Primary ciliary dyskinesia	Saccharine test and nasal nitric oxide can be used as screening tests. Epithelial brushing for electron microscopy or cilial beat frequency should be obtained from nasal or bronchial mucosa when free from infection
Retained foreign body	History of sudden onset of symptoms, localized disease on CXR/high-resolution CT. Diagnostic and therapeutic test is rigid bronchoscopy
Recurrent aspiration	Observation of feeding, videofluoroscopy, barium swallow, milk scan and 24-hr pH studies

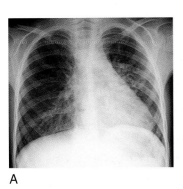

A

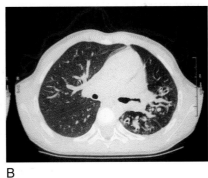

B

Fig. 42.17 Lucy's investigations. (A) Chest X-ray. The left mid-zone and lower lobe show cylindrical bronchiectasis. Ring shadows can be seen. (B) CT scan.

Q2. How will you treat Lucy?

Short term
- Antibiotics and intensive physiotherapy to clear infection.

Long term
- Advise regular chest physiotherapy with postural drainage.
- Aim to control infections:
  - Sputum culture should be routinely monitored.
  - Antibiotics, oral or intravenous, are dictated by sputum culture and sensitivities.
  - Give an annual influenza vaccination.

Bronchiectasis

This is irreversible abnormal dilatation of the bronchial tree and represents a common end stage of a number of different processes.

Mechanisms
- Chronic endobronchial infections: progressive bronchial wall damage and dilatation
- Obstruction of the airway.

Causes
- Widespread disease:
  - Cystic fibrosis
  - Immune deficiencies
  - Primary ciliary dyskinesia
  - Recurrent pulmonary aspiration.
- Localized disease:
  - Retained inhaled foreign body
  - Infection in a congenital lung malformation
  - Local airways compression, e.g. tuberculosis, enlarged lymph node and active infection.

Clinical features
- Cough and copious purulent sputum
- Poor growth
- Crackles with or without wheeze, especially during infections
- Finger clubbing
- Severe extensive disease: dyspnoea, hypoxaemia.

Investigations
- Pulmonary function tests:
  - Obstructive/restrictive or mixed pattern
- CXR:
  - Bronchial wall thickening
  - Tramlining: parallel shadows of thickened dilated bronchial walls
  - Ring shadows: cross-sectional view of thickened dilated bronchial wall
- High-resolution CT:
  - Better than CXR for gauging the extent of disease and determining whether it is localized.

Management

- Order chest physiotherapy for postural drainage.
- Aim to control infections.
- Sputum culture should be routinely monitored.
- Antibiotics, oral or intravenous, are dictated by sputum culture and sensitivities.
- Give annual influenza vaccination.
- Order local surgery for local severe disease.
- Advise a transplant for end-stage disease.

Problem-orientated topic:

chronic cough (part II)

Earlier in life Lucy was given a tentative diagnosis of asthma based on prolonged coughing following head colds. At this stage her GP considered that Lucy was otherwise well. She was growing along the 25th centile.

Q1. What are the other causes of problem coughing in an otherwise previously healthy child?

BOX 42.11 Causes of problem coughing in an otherwise healthy child

Specific infections causing cough

- Pertussis and pertussis-like syndromes, parapertussis, *Chlamydia/Mycoplasma* and viral infections
- Recurrent viral bronchitis and prolonged postviral cough
- Children with these conditions seem to have heightened 'cough receptor sensitivity' and the coughing is typically very troublesome and irritating for the child

Isolated cough with no other respiratory symptoms

- Cough variant asthma: atopic background, reversible airflow obstruction (history of recurrent wheezing, objective bronchodilator responsiveness or fall in FEV_1 after challenge)
- Clear-cut response to anti-asthma therapy with relapse when therapy withdrawn
- Postnasal drip
- Gastro-oesophageal reflux (rarely)
- Psychogenic cough: usually a dry habit cough or a bizarre honking cough that does not irritate the child (but does irritate parents and teachers). These coughs abate when the child is asleep or distracted

Q1. What are the other causes of problem coughing in an otherwise previously healthy child?

See Box 42.11. Other rare causes of chronic cough are interstitial lung diseases, such as the pulmonary fibrosis that can occur with connective tissue diseases.

Key points regarding cough are summarized in Box 42.12.

BOX 42.12 Key points: cough

- Parental reporting of cough frequency and severity does not correlate well with objective cough audiotapes, especially at night
- Parental and doctor characterization of cough as wet (moist with phlegm production) versus dry is generally correct and this classification is important
- Children < 5 years do not cough up phlegm/sputum but rather swallow it
- Cough receptors are concentrated in the larynx and upper tracheobronchial tree and coughing is a natural protective mechanism
- Many children with persistent isolated, postviral or recurrent viral coughing have heightened 'cough receptor sensitivity'
- Cough is a symptom not a disorder and treatment therefore should be targeted at the cause
- Short-term symptomatic relief of coughing associated with an URTI has *not* been proven to be effective

Cystic fibrosis (CF)

Problem-orientated topic:

cystic fibrosis (part I)

Emma is the second child of non-consangineous parents. She was born after an uncomplicated pregnancy by normal delivery at term +5. Birth weight was 3.1 kg. She has an older brother who is 2 years old and well. There is no significant family history.

She was discharged well at 48 hours. Mum felt Emma was a hungry baby compared to her older brother but was generally pleased with her progress. She had her routine heel prick blood test carried out on day 5 of life.

About a week later mum is called to say that the blood spot test for cystic fibrosis was high. She phones her GP for some advice.

Q1. What advice would you give her?

Q1. What advice would you give her?

CF screening tests for raised immunoreactive trypsinogen (IRT) in the dried blood spot. If the test is positive or borderline a second test will be performed to confirm. If the second test is positive the child will be referred for a sweat test (Box 42.13).

Proposed nationwide neonatal screening throughout the UK with a blood spot sample for IRT taken at 5 days will proceed to DNA analysis where a very high IRT is found (> 99.5th centile) on the first test. A second IRT is indicated if only one CF mutation is found on subsequent DNA analysis.

BOX 42.13 The quantitative pilocarpine ionotrophoresis sweat test

- Remains the gold standard for confirming the diagnosis of CF
- Must be done in a specialized laboratory used to dealing with this test to decrease inaccuracies
- A minimum of 100 mg of sweat must be collected

Positive test	Na⁺ > 60 mmol/l
Borderline test	Na⁺ 40–60 mmol/l
Negative test	Na⁺ < 40 mmol/l

Positive test $Na^+ > 60$ mmol/l
Borderline test Na^+ 40–60 mmol/l
Negative test $Na^+ < 40$ mmol/l

 http://www.ich.ucl.ac.uk/newborn/cf/consultation.htm

This link is information on the screening for cystic fibrosis.

Problem-orientated topic:

cystic fibrosis (part II)

Emma is subsequently sent for a sweat test. Her results are: sweat volume 153 μl, chloride 116 mmol/l and sodium 119 mmol/l.

Following her sweat test Emma and her parents are admitted to the ward for initial assessment and to meet the CF team. Emma is then seen at clinic. Retrospectively, mum feels that Emma probably has not put much weight on since she was born. She notes that the baby has always been a bit chesty but just thought that she had caught her brother's head cold. Mum is upset about the results but does not know much about CF and is concerned that her baby will die very young.

Q1. What information and advice will you give this family?

Q2. What further investigations might be necessary?

Q3. What is your initial management plan?

Q1. What information and advice will you give this family?

Specific information regarding CF is tailored to the parents' needs at the time. Some wish to receive all the information at once, while others prefer to digest it more slowly. It is important that they are given written information, with the ability to come back with questions as required.

Some units have their own parent sheets, while others distribute the information pack from the Cystic Fibrosis Trust. An overview is given in Box 42.14.

 http://www.cftrust.org.uk

This links to Cystic Fibrosis Trust.

BOX 42.14 Key points: cystic fibrosis

Presentation
- Classic presentation of recurrent chest infections, bulky, greasy, difficult-to-flush stools and malnutrition
- Spectrum of disease can be very wide, however, from classic CF presenting in early years to relatively asymptomatic patients who present later: e.g. adult males diagnosed on molecular genetic testing when seeking infertility treatment

Incidence
- 7500 people in UK
- 1/25 people in UK are carriers; 1/2500 infants have CF

Life expectancy
- Current mean life expectancy is 31 years, compared with 5 years in 1960

Pathophysiology
- Impairment of cystic fibrosis transmembrane regulator (CFTR) function causes reduced fluid production and enhanced sodium resorption through the epithelial Na⁺ channels (EnaC) and basolateral Na/ATPase pumps of the airways epithelium. This results in increased fluid absorption, leading to decreased airway surface liquid and impaired ciliary clearance

Genetics
- Autosomal recessive disorder, defect on chromosome 7
- Now over 1000 different mutations of CFTR responsible for CF
- Most common mutation is ΔF508; others include G551d, R117H, 621 +1 (G > T), G542X

- Mutations have been classified depending on the action that the mutation has on the production and/or transport of CFTR to the apical membrane of the cell

Q2. What further investigations might be necessary?

See Box 42.15.

A full history and examination of the child is needed, in particular growth parameters (weight, height, head circumference).

BOX 42.15 Baseline investigations in cystic fibrosis

- Sputum/cough swab:
  - Microbiology
- Chest X-ray
- Blood investigations:
  - DNA for genotyping
  - Full blood count
  - Urea and electrolytes
  - Liver function tests
  - Coagulation screen
  - Immunoglobulins
  - Vitamin A, D and E levels
- Faecal elastase:
  - ?Pancreatic insufficiency

Q3. What is your initial management plan?

See Box 42.16. From the time of diagnosis CF needs a multidisciplinary approach to care. The family will require support from all health professionals, and will also need to be reviewed by a social worker to help with application for benefits and allowances. Most children will also be seen in their homes after diagnosis by a specialist CF nurse to maintain support and education.

Problem-orientated topic:

deterioration in a child with CF

Emma was started on the standard CF regimen, with support and education for the family from social worker and CF community nurse.

Over the next few months Emma remains well. She gains weight and is developing well. Her parents are coming to terms with her diagnosis and treatment but still find it difficult at times. Unfortunately Emma develops a cough so her mum brings her to clinic for some advice. She has a fruity cough and crepitations are heard on auscultation.

BOX 42.16 Specific medical management of cystic fibrosis

Respiratory management

- 90% morbidity in CF is a result of chronic pulmonary sepsis and its complications
- Much of therapy is aimed at prevention of lung damage and early treatment of infection to minimize lung damage secondary to inflammation

Prevention of infection

- Prophylactic oral flucloxacillin against *Staphylococcus aureus* infection
- All regular immunizations
- Additional vaccine such as pneumovax and influenza; consider palivizumab for RSV protection
- Good infection control policy to prevent cross-infection

Physiotherapy

- Learnt at an early stage
- Multiple techniques that are adapted to patient age and severity of disease
- Reduces airways obstruction by improving clearance of secretions

- Decreases severity of infection by clearance of infected material
- Maintains respiratory function and exercise tolerance

Nutritional/gastrointestinal

- Direct link between pulmonary health and the patient's nutritional status
- Increased energy requirements due to increased demand and increased losses:
  - High-energy diet
- Malabsorption of fat:
  - > 90% patients require exocrine pancreatic supplements, e.g. Creon
    Vitamin A, D and E supplements
- Close monitoring of weight, particularly in the younger child, to ensure growth and development:
  - Intervention with oral calorie supplements and use of enteral feeding via nasogastric tube or gastrostomy may be required in some patients

Her weight has also dropped slightly since her last visit. She has a CXR and sputum is sent for culture and sensitivities. Emma's chest X-ray shows a right lower lobe consolidation.

She is commenced on oral antibiotic initially and is reviewed 1 week later. She is still unwell and her recent sputum has grown *Pseudomonas aeruginosa* for the first time.

Q1. What respiratory pathogens are found in the CF lung?

Q2. What is your respiratory management?

Q3. What other treatment may aid resolution of the right upper lobe consolidation?

Q1. What respiratory pathogens are found in the CF lung?

- *Staphylococcus aureus*
- *Haemophilus influenzae*
- *Pseudomonas aeruginosa*
- *Burkholderia cepacia*
- *Stenotrophomonas maltophilia.*

Q2. What is your respiratory management plan?

See Box 42.17.

Emma's right lower lobe collapse/consolidation was slow to improve, so Emma had a bronchoscopy and bronchial washout.

BOX 42.17 Management of cystic fibrosis exacerbations

Acute exacerbations

- Oral antibiotics for 10–14 days, based on most recently colonized organisms

1st isolate *Pseudomonas*

- Aggressive treatment of 1st isolate can lead to eradication of *Pseudomonas* and delay the onset of chronic infection (3 months' oral ciproxin + 3 months' inhaled colomycin)

Chronic *Pseudomonas*

- Reduce bacterial load and minimize lung damage
- Regular elective i.v. antibiotics and/or regular nebulized colomycin ± tobramycin

Q3. What other treatment may aid resolution of the right upper lobe consolidation?

Mucolytics such as Dnase (dornase alfa) or hypertonic saline may aid breakdown of the mucus plugging, allowing physiotherapy to clear it more easily. Both reduce sputum viscosity and therefore improve its clearance.

Problem-orientated topic:

CF and acute cough

Helen is 14 years old and was diagnosed with cystic fibrosis by routine neonatal screening. She is homozygous for the DF508 gene and has been chronically colonized with *Pseudomonas aeruginosa* since she was 9 years old. She is generally well but usually requires intravenous antibiotics 1–2 times a year. Her mother phones for an urgent appointment, as she is concerned that Helen is coughing and more tired than usual.

Helen arrives at clinic and is annoyed at her mum for bringing her. She does not want to miss more school as she has exams next month. She claims she feels well but her mother argues that Helen is coughing more, especially at night, and would be more productive with physiotherapy. She also says Helen comes home from school very tired and has to lie down to rest. Her weight has dropped just over 1 kg since her last visit 6 weeks ago.

Q1. What areas would you cover during this consultation?

Q2. What is your management plan?

Q3. What other diagnoses would you consider?

Q1. What areas would cover during this consultation?

History
- School work
- Exercise tolerance
- Compliance

Table 42.7 Differential diagnosis of acute cough in cystic fibrosis

Diagnosis	Investigations
CF-related diabetes	Glucose tolerance test (GTT)
Allergic bronchopulmonary aspergillosis (ABPA)	ABPA work-up: Full blood count (eosinophilia) Skin prick test *Aspergillus* antigen Serum IgE Specific *Aspergillus* IgE/IgG Sputum for *Aspergillus*
Atypical infections	Sputum for atypical mycobacteria

- Nutrition/appetite
- Cough/amount of sputum production.

Investigations

- Lung function tests
- Sputum for culture.

Helen's previously stable lung function with FEV_1 around 95% predicted has dropped to 83% predicted. On assessment the physiotherapist feels the girl's chest was more productive than usual and has sent a good sputum sample to the laboratory, dirty-green in colour.

Q2. What is your management plan?

You send Helen home with course of oral ciproxin to commence immediately and arrange for her to reattend next week for review. At this second appointment her chest is a lot worse, with FEV_1 now 70% predicted, and her weight has dropped a further 0.5 kg. You arrange for Helen to be admitted for intravenous antibiotics.

Helen's sputum grew mucoid *Pseudomonas* at the last clinic and her antibiotics were chosen from best sensitivities. However, after 7 days on antibiotics her FEV_1 is still only 75% predicted.

Q3. What other diagnoses would you consider?

See Table 42.7.
Helen's GTT result was:
- Baseline glucose: 4.2 mmol/l
- Blood glucose 2 hours after glucose challenge: 15 mmol/l.

The diagnosis is CF-related diabetes. This and other complications of CF are shown in Table 42.8.

Lung infections

Problem-orientated topic:

lower respiratory tract infection

Owen, a 2-month-old boy, has been lethargic and not interested in feeding for 24 hours

Table 42.8 Complications of cystic fibrosis

Complication	Presentation/diagnosis	Treatment
Constipation/distal intestinal obstruction syndrome (DIOS)	Meconium ileus equivalent	Osmotic laxatives, hydration Gastrograffin orally
CF-related diabetes	Exclude in all patients with poor weight gain ± unexplained poor lung function Distinct from types 1 and 2 diabetes mellitus Polyuria and polydipsa are rare presentation Oral glucose tolerance test is gold standard for diagnosis	Involve diabetic team Dietician Insulin regimen tailored to individual lifestyle and eating patterns No evidence of benefit of oral hypoglycaemics
Liver	Abnormal bile flow and inspissated secretions. Leads to focal biliary cirrhosis Screened by annual liver function tests and ultrasound	Ursodeoxycholic acid Taurine: monitor response 6-monthly
Arthropathy	Up to 10% of children with CF Age 13–20 years Episodic pain and swelling of large joints Ciproxin-induced arthropathy separate problem	Spontaneous resolution Non-steroidal benefit Remember renal toxicity with non-steroidal inflammatory drugs and aminoglycosides
Osteoporosis	10–20% of adolescents/adults Low vitamin D and K levels Use of inhaled and oral steroids Poor exercise Diagnosed via dual-energy X-ray absorptiometry (DEXA) scan	Increased calcium intake Vitamin bisphosphonates
Other respiratory complications	Pneumothorax Haemoptysis Allergic bronchopulmonary aspergillosis	

Table 42.9 Investigations in respiratory tract infection

Investigation	Bacterial	Viral
Chest X-ray (specificity is poor for predicting viral versus bacterial disease but can be useful)	Lobar pneumonia Inflammation localized to one or more lobes that are completely consolidated Generally indicates bacterial infection Pneumatoceles suggest *Staph. aureus* or anaerobic infection	Bronchopneumonia Inflammation of the lung, centred around the bronchioles, mucopurulent secretions block or obstruct small airways Patchy infiltrates of adjacent lobules Generally indicates viral infection
Sputum/nasal pharyngeal aspirate	Microbe identification Cultures Sensitivity of organism to guide antibiotic treatment	Rapid antigen diagnostic tests (immunofluorescence for RSV, polymerase chain reaction (PCR) for many respiratory viruses)
White cell count	Bacterial infections typically elevated, e.g. 15 000–40 000/mm³, with granulocyte predominance	Viral infections typically normal or mildly elevated and usually < 20 000/mm³ with lymphocyte predominance
Blood cultures	Blood cultures are rarely positive (10–30% cases) but are worth obtaining in sick children	
Serology	Requires paired samples (acute and convalescent), looking for a fourfold rise in specific antibody titres Cold agglutinins are positive in 50% of *Mycoplasma* cases but this test is not specific	
Inflammatory markers	Erythrocyte sedimentation rate (ESR) and C-reactive protein (CRP) levels tend to be higher in bacterial infections but neither test is specific enough to rule out a bacterial cause	

and has had a 'runny nose'. On examination, he is pale, febrile (temperature 39°C) and limp, and has rapid shallow breathing (respiratory rate 80/min) with minimal nasal flaring and retractions. He has grunting respirations. His heart rate is 180/min.

Q1. What is the likely diagnosis?
Q2. What is your assessment?
Q3. What investigations should be done?
Q4. What are the principles of management?

Q1. What is the likely diagnosis?

Acute pneumonia is an inflammation of the lung parenchyma. It usually presents with fever (children often have had a preceding URTI), tachypnoea, cough, grunting respiration, nasal flaring and recession. Crackles typically are auscultated and in older children there may be reduced intensity of breath sounds.

The most common cause of pneumonia in children is viral. Bacterial infection occurs in approximately 10–30%.

Q2. What is your assessment?

- Owen is very sick. Therefore use the ABC approach, including assessment of capillary refill time.
- He has an infection: elevated temperature and lethargy after an URTI ('runny nose').

- His work of breathing is increased but there is no respiratory noise that points to an airways obstruction.
- The grunting respirations and tachypnoea suggest pneumonia. (N.B. Sometimes infants in shock can have grunty respirations with tachypnoea.)
- His work of breathing is likely to be inadequate; tachycardia, pallor and lethargy suggest hypoxia. However, these findings may be contributed to by the fever and sepsis.

Q3. What investigations should be done?

See Table 42.9.

Q4. What are the principles of management?

Mildly ill
- Oral antibiotic (e.g. amoxicillin) at home
- In an older child consider a macrolide antibiotic to cover *Mycoplasma*.

Hospitalized child
- O₂ therapy
- Maintenance of hydration
- Intravenous antibiotics, e.g. cefuroxime.

 http://www.brit-thoracic.org.uk/iqs/bts_guidelines_pneumonia_html

BTS 2002 Guidelines for the Management of Community Acquired Pneumonia in Childhood. Thorax 57: suppl 1

Table 42.10 **Common organisms causing pneumonia**

Age	Bacteria	Viruses	Others
Neonate	Group B streptococcus *Staphylococcus aureus* *Staph. epidermidis* *Escherichia coli*	CMV Herpes virus Enterovirus	*Mycoplasma hominis* *Ureaplasma urealyticum*
1–4 months	*Staph. aureus* *Haemophilus influenzae* *Strep. pneumoniae*	RSV Influenza Parainfluenza CMV	*Chlamydia trachomatis* *U. urealyticum*
< 5 years	*Strep. pneumoniae* *Staph. aureus* *H. influenzae* Group A streptococci	RSV Adenovirus Influenza	
> 5 years	*S. pneumoniae* *H. influenzae*	Influenza	*Mycoplasma pneumoniae* *Chlamydia pneumoniae* *Legionella pneumoniae*
Special cases Immunocompromised patients	In addition to those listed above: *Pneumocystis carinii* Enteric Gram negatives	CMV RSV Parainfluenza Influenza	Fungi *Aspergillus* *Histoplasma* Mycobacteria
Cystic fibrosis	*Staph. aureus* *Pseudomonas aeruginosa* *Burkholderia cepacia* *Stenotrophomonas maltophilia*		*Aspergillus*

(CMV = cytomegalovirus; RSV = respiratory syncytial virus)

Problem-orientated topic:

deteriorating pneumonia

Ben is a 6-year-old boy who attended his GP's practice with a short history of fever, dry cough and mild tachypnoea. His GP prescribed oral amoxicillin and referred him to the local accident and emergency department for a CXR. This showed a small area of dense consolidation in the left lower zone.

Three days later Ben reattends accident and emergency looking much sicker. He is febrile and toxic-looking, and has increased tachypnoea (respiratory rate 65/min) and grunty respirations. He appears to have developed a scoliosis and is avoiding movement of the left side of his chest due to pain. His trachea and apex beat are displaced to the right and there is reduced intensity of breath sounds and stony dullness to percussion on the left.

Q1. What are the common organisms causing pneumonia?

Q2. What complication of pneumonia is likely to have occurred in Ben?

Q1. What are the common organisms causing pneumonia?

See Table 42.10. Remember, respiratory viruses are probably more common than bacteria as causes of pneumonia and include RSV, parainfluenza, influenza A and B, and adenovirus. Always consider *Tuberculosis* as a possible organism.

Q2. What complication of pneumonia is likely to have occurred in Ben?

He has developed a parapneumonic pleural effusion or an empyema. The features that suggest this complication are:

- Continuing fever and increasing 'toxicity' despite 3 days of oral antibiotic
- Mediastinal shift to left (deviation of trachea and apex beat)
- Stony dullness and reduced breath sounds on the right.

Ben's X-ray shows pleural fluid. Ultrasound scan is now important to determine the location and extent of this pleural fluid and whether it is loculated.

Principles of management of pleural fluid/ empyema

- Pleural drainage
- Intravenous antibiotics.

BOX 42.18 Differential diagnosis of recurrent pneumonia

Genetic disorders
- Cystic fibrosis
- Sickle cell disease

Immune disorders/deficiencies
- Bruton agammaglobulinaemia
- IgG subclass deficiencies
- Severe combined immunodeficiency disease (SCID)
- AIDS

Leucocyte disorders
- Chronic granulomatous disease
- Hyperimmunoglobulin E syndrome
- Leucocyte adhesion defect

Ciliary disorders
- Immotile cilia syndrome
- Kartagener's syndrome

Anatomical disorders
- Sequestration
- Bronchial cyst
- Lobar emphysema
- Oesophageal reflux
- Recurrent aspiration
- Foreign body
- Transoesophageal fistula
- Bronchiectasis

 http://www.brit-thoracic.org.uk/iqs/bts_guidelines_pleurainfchild_html

BTS 2005 Pleural Infection in Children Guideline. Thorax 60: suppl 1

Recurrent lung infections

When a child presents with recurrent lung infections (Box 42.18) ascertain the following.

Have there been frequent upper respiratory viral infections?

This becomes especially noticeable if the child becomes febrile or lethargic, has a chesty cough and is given antibiotics with each head cold. Some children with early asthma give this history, i.e. viral triggered cough and wheeze episodes.

Is there a serious underlying cause?

Local abnormality associated with recurrent local infections
- Retained inhaled foreign body
- Sequestered lobe (an area of lung tissue that is not connected to the normal airways and has its own arterial blood supply, often from the descending aorta)
- Bronchial cyst.

Disorder eventually leading to chronic suppurative lung disease
Look for signs of chronic respiratory disease (finger clubbing, chest over-inflation) or chronic infection elsewhere (chronic ear infections with discharge).

Further reading

Lakhanpaul M, Atkinson M, Stephenson T 2004 Community-acquired pneumonia in children: a clinical update. Archives of Disease in Childhood, Education and Practice Edition 89: ep29–ep34

Rossi UG, Owens CM 2005 The radiology of chronic lung disease in children. Archives of Disease in Childhood 90:601–607

Smyth R 2005 Diagnosis and management of cystic fibrosis. Archives of Disease in Childhood, Education and Practice Edition 90: ep1–ep6

43

Blood and reticulo-endothelial disorders

LEARNING OUTCOMES

By the end of this chapter you should:

● Know the basic scientific principles of blood clotting
● Know the common causes of disease in children who present with anaemia, bruising, thrombocytopenia or pancytopenia
● Know the risks of blood transfusion
● Know the causes and risks of asplenism.

Introduction

The practice of haematology encompasses a close relationship between the clinical assessment and management of patients and the appropriate use of the laboratory. The haematology multidisciplinary team includes not only medical, nursing and allied professions but also the laboratory scientists in the haematology department. The fun of the topic is that, despite the advances in basic science, an individual haematologist can see the patient, undertake diagnostic procedures, interpret the results themselves and inform the patient of the diagnosis, often within a few hours of their presentation. The aims of this chapter are to introduce a rational approach to addressing common presentations of haematological disorders in order to formulate diagnostic algorithms and therefore appropriate use of laboratory facilities. It will also introduce basic principles of management.

A general principle in all paediatric haematology is the need to refer to age-specific normal ranges.

Anaemia

Problem-orientated topic:

pallor

Amir, a 3-year-old boy whose family originate from Pakistan, presents to his GP with a cough. The GP notices pallor and checks a full blood count (FBC). The results indicate haemoglobin of 7.5 g/dl (normal range 11.5–13.5), mean corpuscular volume (MCV) of 64 fl (75–87), platelet count 550×10^9/l (150–450) and white cell count 4.5×10^9/l (5–17).

Q1.   What are the potential causes of this anaemia?
Q2.   What critical features would you elicit in the history?
Q3.   What investigations would you request?
Q4.   What management would you instigate?

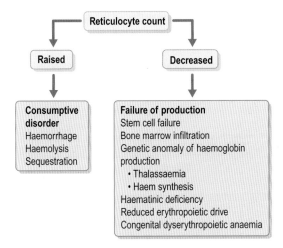

Fig. 43.1 Diagnostic algorithm of anaemia based on the reticulocyte count

Q1. What are the potential causes of this anaemia?

There are multiple causes of childhood anaemia. A rational approach to the diagnosis of any cytopenia involves the consideration of causes of a reduced rate of production and increased rate of either consumption or sequestration. The marker of the rate of red cell production is the reticulocyte, a red cell that retains ribonucleic acid permitting identification using special stains. Increased reticulocyte numbers infer an increased rate of bone marrow red cell production and vice versa. A diagnostic algorithm of anaemia using the reticulocyte count is outlined in Figure 43.1. The alternative pragmatic approach is use of the red cell size, represented by the mean corpuscular volume (MCV; Fig. 43.2). At birth, severe anaemia requiring treatment generally reflects haemorrhage (fetomaternal transfusion, placental abrup-

tion or twin-to-twin); however, haemolysis, secondary to either enzymopathies or fetomaternal incompatibility and α-thalassaemia, may present during the neonatal period.

The most frequent cause of childhood anaemia is iron deficiency, which in turn is most commonly caused by inadequate dietary intake. However, the diagnosis is most commonly seen in the UK in those ethnic populations in whom the incidence of thalassaemia is greatest, this being the principle alternative diagnosis. The most urgent need is to exclude ongoing haemorrhage that may be life-threatening, such as with a Meckel's diverticulum or pulmonary haemosiderosis. Chronically inadequate iron intake or thalassaemia trait does not constitute a medical emergency.

Q2. What critical features would you elicit in the history?

- Is the child failing to thrive?
- Dietetic assessment of iron intake
- Evidence of blood loss:
  - Gastrointestinal tract (parasitic infestation, Meckel's diverticulum, peptic ulceration)
  - Menstruation
  - Urinary (including paroxysmal nocturnal haemoglobinuria)
  - Pulmonary haemosiderosis
- Evidence of malabsorption/enteritis/bowel resection
- Ethnic origin:
  - Mediterranean, Middle East, Indian subcontinent, South-East Asia
- Family history of anaemia, coagulation disorders, consanguinity
- Drug intake associated with high gastric pH.

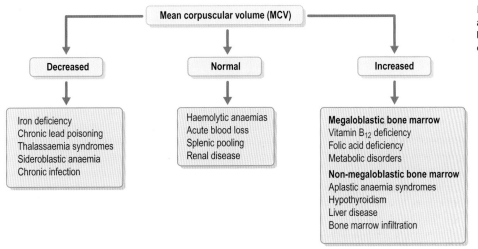

Fig. 43.2 Diagnostic algorithm of anaemia based on the mean corpuscular volume

Clinical signs
- Anaemia, jaundice
- Angular cheilosis (ulceration of angle of lips), smooth shiny appearance of tongue, koilonychia (spoon-shaped nails rare in childhood)
- Signs of malabsorption:
  - Failure to thrive, clubbing, abdominal distension
- Signs of gastrointestinal blood loss:
  - Telengiectasia, oral ulceration
- Facial appearance:
  - Frontal or parietal bossing.

Q3. What investigations would you request?

- Blood film and red cell indices:
  - Iron deficiency leads to hypochromia, microcytosis, anisocytosis (increased range of red cell sizes) and poikilocytosis (variation of shapes), including pencil cells and target cells.
  - Mixed iron/folate/B_{12} deficiency will produce a dimorphic population of red cells, one with a high MCV, one with a low MCV. The mean MCV may be misleadingly normal.
- Reticulocyte count: reduced in iron deficiency
- Frequent elevation of platelet count
- Measures of iron deficiency:
  - Serum ferritin: reduced in iron deficiency but elevated in inflammatory conditions, therefore may be falsely normal.
  - Zinc protoporphyrin: elevated in iron deficiency, also affected by inflammation
  - Percentage hypochromic red cells: increased in iron deficiency.
- Thalassaemia screen:
  - Elevation of HbA_2, is diagnostic of β-thalassaemia.
  - May be reduced into normal range by coexistent iron deficiency.
  - Rare forms of β-thalassaemia are associated with normal levels of HbA_2.
  - No confirmatory test for α-thalassaemia other than polymerase chain reaction (PCR)-based mutation screening.
- Therapeutic trial of iron replacement:
  - Laboratory investigations may identify iron deficiency but may not be able to exclude the coexistence of thalassaemia trait, notably α-thalassaemia trait. Prolonged iron replacement may lead to excess iron loading in children who have a diagnosis of thalassaemia trait, but a short therapeutic trial of iron for 3–6 months with close monitoring of haemoglobin is a reasonable diagnostic and therapeutic approach.
- Bone marrow for assessment of marrow iron stores and exclusion of congenital sideroblastic anaemia.

Q4. What management would you instigate?

- Give dietetic advice.
- Give oral iron supplementation for at least 6 months:
  - Predicted response is 1 g/dl increment after each week of initial replacement
  - If inadequate, consider:
    Poor compliance (stool colour is dark when iron is being taken orally)
    Alternative/additional diagnosis
    Blood loss/malabsorption.
- Stop supplementation after 6 months.
- If there is further progressive anaemia, investigate for blood loss including gastrointestinal tract imaging.

Does chronic iron deficiency matter?
The effects of anaemia are well recognized as leading to weakness, fatigue, palpitations and lightheadedness. Less common effects of iron deficiency are the epithelial changes seen in the mouth and pica, the consumption of non-nutritive substances including soil and clay. Chronic iron deficiency can also impair growth and intellectual development. Studies of the effect of iron replacement on cognitive development have yielded disparate results.

Thalassaemia

Thalassaemia is a recessively inherited anaemia caused by abnormal imbalanced production of the globin chains within the haemoglobin molecule. It predominantly affects populations centred on the Mediterranean, the Middle East, the Indian subcontinent and South-East Asia. However, all ethnic groups may be affected. The thalassaemia syndromes are caused by underlying gene defects that are generally deletions of varying length. The nature of the deletion correlates with the resultant clinical phenotype. They all result in microcytic red cells and hypochromic anaemia of variable severity. The clinical phenotype is variable; thalassaemia major is a fatal disease if not managed with regular blood transfusions, thalassaemia intermedia is characterized by anaemia that may not require intervention, and thalassaemia trait is an asymptomatic carrier state.

BOX 43.1 Alpha-thalassaemia phenotype	
Four-gene deletion	Haemoglobin Bart's hydrops fetalis
Three-gene deletion	HbH disease: anaemia (Hb 7–11 g/dl), splenomegaly, occasional transfusion dependence
Two-gene deletion	Thalassaemia trait: borderline anaemia, low mean corpuscular volume (MCV) and mean cell haemoglobin (MCH)
One-gene deletion	Silent carrier: low MCV, MCH

Alpha-thalassaemia

Alpha-thalassaemia results in reduced production of α-chains, the resulting excess of β-chains causing red cell instability and haemolysis. The haemoglobin molecules present at birth contain α-chains, so that α-thalassaemia syndromes are present at delivery. Each individual has four α-genes; the clinical phenotype correlates with the number of gene deletions (Box 43.1).

Beta-thalassaemia

Beta-thalassaemia results in reduced production of β-chains, the resulting excess of α-chains causing red cell instability and haemolysis. Beta-thalassaemia syndromes only present at the age of 6 months, at the time of the major haemoglobin switch from HbF to HbA. Beta-thalassaemia major presents with a severe anaemia and a compensatory increase in the rate of erythropoiesis. Children present with failure to thrive, splenomegaly and expansion of the bone marrow space, resulting in skeletal anomalies including osteoporosis. Children not transfused die within the first few years of life. Diagnosis is based on quantitation of the different classes of haemoglobin.

Thalassaemia trait

The most common presentation of this disorder is thalassaemia trait or a silent carrier status, characterized by a mild microcytic anaemia often mistaken for and coexisting with iron deficiency. Beta-thalassaemia trait is identified by the presence of an elevated concentration of HbA_2; however, there is no simple test for α-thalassaemia, which is generally a diagnosis of exclusion. Thalassaemia trait has no clinical consequences for the individual; however, it is important to provide counselling that iron replacement is only indicated if

iron deficiency has been confirmed. Genetic counselling is also important, given the recessive inheritance.

Initial treatment consists of red cell transfusion. This has a dual role: first, to abolish the symptoms and sequelae of anaemia, and second, to suppress endogenous erythropoiesis, so preventing bone marrow expansion and the skeletal and splenic consequences. The options for longer-term management are continuation of a hypertransfusion programme or allogeneic stem cell transplantation from a tissue type-matched sibling donor. Frequent red cell transfusions are complicated by tissue iron loading, which can result in multi-organ toxicity affecting the heart, liver, pancreas and endocrine organs. Prevention of such toxicity necessitates a chelation regimen currently involving subcutaneous infusions of desferrioxamine. Alternative oral iron chelators will hopefully soon be available.

Transfusion of blood products

Blood products may be donated as whole blood, which undergoes subsequent processing into individual components, or cell separator techniques can be utilized to collect specific cellular components or plasma from donors. The transfusion of blood products should be guided by haematological investigations and not done on the basis of non-substantiated clinical need. Individual components, either alone or in combination, should be used rather than whole blood. Cellular components include red cells, platelets and occasionally white cells. Plasma components include fresh frozen plasma, cryoprecipitate and cryosupernatant. The indications for use of these products can be found elsewhere. The transfusion of blood products constitutes one of the most dangerous aspects of patient care (Box 43.2). General principles of transfusion include avoidance, if at all possible, documentation of the indication for use in the clinical notes and the limitation of donor exposure. Scrupulous attention must be paid to the administrative aspects of requesting blood products for patients since most transfusion errors are consequent on documentation errors.

 http://www.bcshguidelines.com

Transfusion guidelines for neonates and older children

Sickle cell disease

Sickling disorders are those in which red cells adopt a shape change in environments of low oxygen concentration to become a crescent or boat shape similar to the shape of the blade on a sickle. This shape results in red cells becoming lodged in small capillaries, leading to

BOX 43.2 Adverse effects of transfusion*

Immediate

- Febrile transfusion reaction:
  - White cell antibodies
  - Plasma protein antibodies
- Haemolytic transfusion reaction:
  - ABO-incompatible blood
- Bacterial infection
- Volume overload
- Air embolism
- Transfusion-associated lung injury (TRALI)

Delayed

- Haemolytic transfusion reaction:
  - Red cell antigens other than ABO
- Post-transfusion purpura
- Pathogen transmission (viruses, possibly variant Creutzfeldt–Jakob disease (vCJD))
- Graft versus host disease
- Transfusion haemosiderosis

* Most transfusion errors are consequent on administrative mistakes

Table 43.1 Causes of haemolysis

	Intrinsic to red cell	Extrinsic to red cell
Congenital	Haemoglobin defects: Haemoglobinopathy Thalassaemia Red cell enzyme defects: Glucose-6-phosphate dehydrogenase Pyruvate kinase Red cell membrane defects: Hereditary spherocytosis Hereditary elliptocytosis	Nil
Acquired	Paroxysmal nocturnal haemoglobinuria (increased red cell lysis by complement)	Immune: Autoimmune: Cold Warm Alloimmune: HDN Transfusion reaction Drug-mediated Red cell fragmentation: Microangiopathic: TTP HUS DIC Cardiac valve grafts Infections: Malaria Clostridium Meningococcus Burns

(HDN = haemolytic disease of the newborn; TTP = thrombotic thrombocytopenic purpura; HUS = haemolytic uraemic syndrome; DIC = disseminated intravascular coagulation)

obstruction to blood flow, tissue ischaemia and further sickling. The most frequent disorders characterized by sickling are homozygous HbSS, compound heterozygous HbSC and coinheritance of HbS and β-thalassaemia trait. Sickle cell disease is seen most commonly in black Africans, Americans and Afro-Caribbeans but is also seen in the Mediterranean, Middle East and parts of India. The abnormal haemoglobin molecules result from structural abnormalities of the globin chains resultant on gene mutations. Diagnosis is based on electrophoresis of haemoglobin, in which structural variants move at different speeds along an electrical gradient. Newer techniques are suitable for population screening programmes.

Sickle cell disease constitutes a chronic haemolytic anaemia complicated by acute crises. Vaso-occlusive events cause painful crises most frequently in bones, lungs and the spleen. A crisis involving the brain may result in a stroke. In young children dactylitis (infarcts of the small bones of the hand) may lead to digits of variable length. Sequestration crises represent sickling within organs and the pooling of blood with severe exacerbation of anaemia.

A severe chest syndrome is the most common cause of death; hepatic or splenic sequestration may require urgent blood transfusion. Other crises include aplastic crises and priapism. Splenic infarction consequent on sickling leads to an increased risk of overwhelming sepsis from encapsulated microorganisms. To protect against

this, patients are immunized against encapsulated organisms and receive life-long penicillin prophylaxis. The universal neonatal haemoglobinopathy screening programme is centred around an early diagnosis of sickle cell disease and early introduction of prophylactic penicillin. Other complications of sickle cell disease include proliferative retinopathy, avascular necrosis of the hips and ulcers of the lower limbs.

 http://www.bcshguidelines.com

Guidelines for the management of the acute painful crisis in sickle cell disease

Haemolytic anaemia

Haemolysis describes the destruction of circulating red cells at a pathologically increased rate. The potential causes of haemolysis are either intrinsic to the red cell or extrinsic (Table 43.1). The cardinal clinical features of haemolysis include anaemia, jaundice, gallstones and splenomegaly. Investigations reveal a raised level of bilirubin (predominantly unconjugated), reduced concentration of serum haptoglobin and increased urinary urobilinogen. There may be red cell morphological changes, including spherocytes. Intravascular haemolysis is also characterized by haemoglobinaemia and haemosiderinuria. A healthy bone marrow will respond by a compensatory increased rate of red cell production, evidenced by a raised reticulocyte count. Clinically there will be pallor and jaundice. There may be associated splenomegaly reflecting the principal site of red cell destruction.

Principles of management are supplementation of folic acid, avoidance of precipitants of acute crises and occasionally red cell transfusion, splenectomy and cholecystectomy. Specific disease states will require specific treatment.

Spherocytosis

The normal shape of a red cell is a biconcave disc; spherocytes are abnormal spherically shaped red cells. They are formed either as a consequence of immune-mediated red cell destruction or as an inherited defect of red cell membrane. The binding of immunoglobulin antibodies to the red cell membrane may result in an increased rate of haemolysis. Macrophages in the reticulo-endothelial system bind the Fc fragment of the immunoglobulin molecule and remove small areas of the membrane. As the area of available membrane is reduced, the red cell adopts the shape in which the maximum volume is enclosed by the minimum surface area. This shape is a sphere. The alternative mechanism leading to an increased number of spherocytes is the inheritance of a defect of spectrin, the main structural protein of the red cell membrane, which causes the red cell to adopt a spherical shape. The spherical shape itself leads to premature red cell breakdown. This inherited condition is known as hereditary spherocytosis and is inherited in an autosomal dominant fashion. It is characterized by a low-grade jaundice and moderate splenomegaly. Gallstones are common. Viral infections may precipitate an acute haemolytic crisis or an aplastic crisis in which the rate of erythropoiesis is reduced. Folate deficiency may also lead to a failure of erythropoiesis. Chronic haemolysis may lead to a failure to thrive with an increase in school non-attendance.

Management consists of appropriate counselling, supplementation of folic acid, and occasional red cell transfusions in the event of significant anaemia, especially in the neonatal period and following an aplastic crisis. The disease may be moderated by splenectomy, which may be indicated in patients with brisk haemolysis and gallstones.

 http://www.bcshguidelines.com

Guidelines for the diagnosis and management of hereditary spherocytosis

Coagulation disorders

Basic science

A rational approach to diagnosis requires some understanding of the normal process of coagulation, which for ease can be considered to consist of primary and secondary haemostasis. A breach of the endothelial lining of the blood vessel will lead to the release of von Willebrand factor. This large multimeric molecule binds to circulating platelets via specific membrane receptors and draws the platelets to the breach in the blood vessel wall, creating a structure of cells across the blood vessel defect akin to a dam of pebbles across a stream. The creation of this dam constitutes primary haemostasis. Secondary haemostasis is the process of sealing the gaps between the platelets. The process of coagulation involves the sequential activation of enzymes to produce a crucial enzyme known as thrombin. Thrombin leads to the cleavage of fibrinogen to form fibrin, which is the cement that binds the platelets together. Ten enzymes are crucial to this process and deficiencies of eight are associated with a clinically significant increased risk of haemorrhage. The balance of haemostasis is ensured by the parallel control system of natural anticoagulants in the blood, principally antithrombin, protein C and protein S. Inherited deficiencies of the anticoagulants lead to an increased risk of thrombosis, a condition known as thrombophilia. Finally, recannulation of thrombosed blood vessels is undertaken by a process called fibrinolysis, the active enzyme being plasmin.

A rational approach to a child with excess bleeding or bruising

It is important to approach a child who presents with symptoms of excess haemorrhage in a systematic fashion (Fig. 43.3). It is necessary to determine whether the symptoms represent a congenital or acquired condition and to consider each part of the haemostatic system in the analysis of the cause.

There are distinct patterns of bleeding in defects of primary and secondary haemostasis. Defects of primary haemostasis lead to bruising and petechiae as well as mucosal haemorrhage, including epistaxis, oral haemorrhage, gastrointestinal haemorrhage and increased

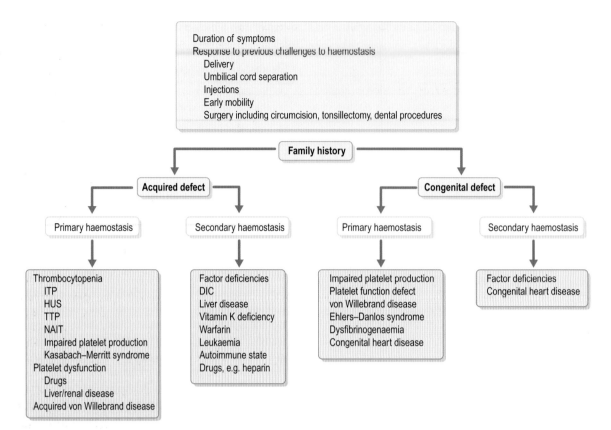

Fig. 43.3 Diagnostic algorithm for a patient with increased bleeding tendency
  (ITP = idiopathic thrombocytopenic purpura; HUS = haemolytic uraemic syndrome; TTP = thrombotic thrombocytopenic purpura; NAIT = neonatal alloimmune thrombocytopenia; DIC = disseminated intravascular coagulation)

menstrual losses. Defects of secondary haemostasis cause deep-sited bleeding in joints, muscles, internal organs and the central nervous system. Some disorders may lead to both types of bleeding, including type III von Willebrand disease.

Aspects of the history in delineating specific congenital defects include prolonged umbilical stump bleeding associated with factor XIII deficiency or fibrinogen deficiency and the association of factor XI deficiency with Ashkenazi Jewish descent. A thorough family history is essential in defining autosomal dominant, recessive and X-linked pedigrees. Assessment of acquired causes includes evidence of current organ dysfunction, recent viral infections and the ingestion of drugs. Examination should elicit current signs, including petechiae, bruising, oral haemorrhage, arthropathy and fundal bleeds, signs of concurrent illness, dysmorphism and signs of increased skin and joint laxity.

A rational algorithm for investigation is essential but beyond the scope of this chapter. Important tests include the following:

Defects of primary haemostasis

- Full blood count (FBC)
- Platelet morphology
- Prothrombin time (PT)
- Activated partial thromboplastin time (APTT)
- Fibrinogen
- Von Willebrand screen
- Assessment of platelet function:
    - Platelet aggregometry
    - Platelet nucleotide analysis
    - Platelet surface glycoprotein expression.

Defects of secondary haemostasis

- FBC
- PT
- APTT
- Fibrinogen
- Assays of specific coagulation factors: sequence of analysis will follow pattern of PT/APTT abnormalities

- Factor XIII assay
- α_2-antiplasmin assay.

Idiopathic thrombocytopenic purpura

Problem-orientated topic:

spontaneous bruising

Jane, a previously healthy 13-year-old girl, presents with a month-long history of fatigue and a week of spontaneous bruising and heavy menstrual loss. Examination is unremarkable other than bruises and petechiae. An FBC reveals haemoglobin of 10.1 g/dl (12–16), MCV of 78 fl (78–95), platelet count $13 \times 10^9/l$ (150–450) and white cell count $4.5 \times 10^9/l$ (4.5–13), of which neutrophils are $3.1 \times 10^9/l$ and lymphocytes $0.9 \times 10^9/l$.

Q1. What do you consider Jane's most probable diagnoses?

Q2. What investigations would you request?

Q3. What treatment would you offer?

Q1. What do you consider Jane's most probable diagnoses?

Childhood idiopathic thrombocytopenic purpura (ITP) has an incidence of between 4.0 and 5.3 per 100 000. The typical presentation is a rapid onset of bruising and petechiae in an otherwise well child. This reflects an impairment of primary haemostasis. There is frequently an association with a previous viral infection or immunization in a younger child; this is less frequent in an older child, in whom association with other autoimmune diseases is more frequent. Additional signs or symptoms should raise the possibility of an alternative diagnosis, such as acute leukaemia, evolving marrow aplasia or thrombocytopenia in association with disorders such as systemic lupus erythematosus (SLE) or the antiphospholipid syndrome.

Q2. What investigations would you request?

Diagnosis is one of exclusion of other disorders and can in general be made by careful clinical assessment, an FBC and review of the blood film by an experienced morphologist. The most feared misdiagnosis is that of acute lymphoblastic leukaemia (p. 418), which has an annual incidence similar to that of ITP. This fear has encouraged the early assessment of bone marrow morphology; however, current advice is to delay such an invasive investigation until a time at which the course of ITP in an individual patient is atypical or prolonged or prior to the use of corticosteroids.

Patients with chronic ITP should be investigated to exclude other immune dysregulation disorders, such as autoimmune disorders like SLE, immune deficiency states and the rare condition, autoimmune lymphoproliferative syndrome.

Q3. What treatment would you offer?

The natural history in 80% cases of ITP is spontaneous resolution within 6–8 weeks. Patients have chronic ITP if disease duration exceeds 6 months. Intracranial haemorrhage occurs with a frequency of approximately 0.1–0.5% and is most frequent in children with chronic disease. The initial management of newly presenting children is reassurance, observation and provision of routes of rapid access to advice or support. Management should be guided by the patient's clinical condition and not solely the platelet count. In the event of significant haemorrhage in excess of petechiae and bruising, treatment options to elevate the platelet count include the use of corticosteroids, intravenous immunoglobulin and anti-D immunoglobulin (in patients who are red cell rhesus-D positive). Transfusion of platelets should only be considered in the event of life-threatening haemorrhage since they will be consumed as rapidly as endogenously produced platelets. None of the above measures will alter the underlying natural course of the disorder. The management of chronic ITP is highly specialized and should be performed in a regional centre. Treatment options include chronic immunosuppression and splenectomy.

 http://www.bcshguidelines.com

Guidelines for the investigation and management of ITP in adults and children and in pregnancy

Henoch–Schönlein purpura

The diagnosis of Henoch–Schönlein purpura (HSP) relies on the recognition of a group of clinical signs, namely:
- A characteristic rash
- Arthralgia
- Periarticular oedema
- Abdominal pain
- Glomerulonephritis.

The peak incidence is between the ages of 3 and 10 years; boys are affected more frequently than girls. HSP is often preceded by a history of an upper respiratory tract infection; hence the incidence is greatest during winter. The clinical features may appear simultaneously over a short time period or there may be a gradual onset over weeks or months. Low-grade fever and fatigue occur in excess of half of affected children.

Clinical features

- *Rash*. This begins as pinkish maculopapules that initially blanch on pressure and progress to purpura. The purpura may be palpable and evolve from red to purple to rusty brown before fading. The rash can appear in crops over 3–10 days and may be episodic, occurring at intervals that vary from a few days to 4 months. The rash may recur rarely several years after the initial presentation. The classic localization of the rash is a symmetrical distribution on the buttocks, extensor surfaces of the arms and legs and the ankles. The trunk is spared unless lesions are induced by trauma. There may be local angioedema, especially in dependent areas such as below the waist and over the buttocks (or the back and scalp of an infant). Oedema may also occur in areas of tissue distensability, such as the eyelids, lips, scrotum or the dorsal surfaces of the hands and feet.
- *Arthritis*. This is present in excess of two-thirds of children, affecting predominantly the knees and ankles. There may be effusions that resolve after a few days without residual deformity or joint damage.
- *Abdominal symptoms*. Inflammation of the vascular supply to the gut may lead to intermittent colicky abdominal pain. Diarrhoea is well recognized and there may be passage of blood rectally and haematemesis. The symptoms may mimic an abdominal emergency. Intussusception may occur, which can be complicated by complete obstruction or infarction with bowel perforation.
- *Renal involvement*. Renal involvement is common; microscopic or macroscopic haematuria or mild proteinuria is present in more than 80% of cases (p. 203).
- *Other complications*. These include hepatosplenomegaly, lymphadenopathy and rarely testicular torsion. Central nervous system involvement may precipitate fits, paralysis or a coma. Other rare complications include rheumatoid-like nodules, cardiac and eye involvement, mononeuropathies, pancreatitis and pulmonary and intramuscular haemorrhage.

Differential diagnosis

The principle differential diagnoses of HSP are ITP and meningococcal disease. Patients with ITP will have thrombocytopenia. Meningococcal disease may be difficult to exclude initially but a more benign clinical course and negative microbiology will exclude it. HSP may occur in association with other systemic disorders such as autoimmune disorders, vasculitides, familial Mediterranean fever or inflammatory bowel disease. Similar but distinct presentations occur with polyarteritis nodosa, meningococcal disease, purpura fulminans, Kawasaki disease and systemic onset juvenile rheumatoid arthritis.

Investigations

There may be an elevated platelet and white cell number and an elevated erythrocyte sedimentation rate (ESR). Immune complexes are often present and levels of IgA and IgM may be increased. Renal involvement is demonstrated by red blood cells, white blood cells, casts or albumin in the urine. A skin biopsy demonstrates a leucocytoclastic vasculitis, and renal biopsy may show IgA mesangial deposition and occasionally IgM, C3 and fibrin.

Management

This is generally supportive, with adequate analgesia and hydration. Management of an acute abdominal crisis may require surgical or radiological reduction of an intussusception. However, steroids may have a role in improving both gastrointestinal and central nervous system complications. Management of renal complications may include the use of immunosuppressive drugs and require long-term follow-up.

Haemophilia

Haemophilia describes an increased tendency to bleed consequent on a failure of secondary haemostasis. Deficiencies of coagulation factors I, II, V, VII, VIII, IX, X, XI and XIII can result in an increased bleeding diathesis. The most frequent deficiencies are those of factor VIII (1:5000–10 000 males) and factor IX (1:35 000–50 000 males), known respectively as haemophilia A and B. Haemophilia A and B are inherited in an X-linked fashion. The severity of the clinical phenotype is correlated with the plasma concentration of the deficient factor (Table 43.2). Untreated severe haemophilia A or B is characterized by chronic arthropathy consequent on repeated haemarthroses (joint bleeds). However, life-threatening haemorrhage can follow minor surgery in patients in whom haemophilia has not been considered, whether that is mild, moderate or severe. The results of diagnostic tests are described in Table 43.3.

Table 43.2 Classification of haemophilia A and B

Plasma concentration of coagulation factor (IU/dl)	Severity of haemophilia	Clinical symptoms
< 1	Severe	Spontaneous bleeding into joints, muscles or other internal organs
1–5	Moderate	Bleeding episodes following minor trauma
5–50	Mild	Bleeding episodes following significant trauma
50–150	Normal individual	Nil

The initial presentation with haemophilia will depend on the challenges to haemostasis sustained by the individual patient and the severity of the disease. Severe haemophilia is associated with a risk of intracranial haemorrhage following delivery. It may cause excess bruising in a toddler raising concerns of non-accidental injury, a haemarthrosis in a 1-year-old boy or excess bleeding following minor surgery such as dental extraction many years later.

Haemophilia care encompasses education, avoidance of drugs that impair haemostasis and activities associated with a high risk of trauma. The expectations of modern care are a normal life expectancy and joint integrity and a life of normal activities undertaken with caution. Treatment for an individual minor bleed involves local measures and antifibrinolytic agents but for significant bleeds elevation of the level of the deficient factor is required. This is achieved by infusion of vials of the relevant factor concentrate via the intravenous route in a dose that is proportional to the weight of the individual. For patients with mild haemophilia A, administration of DDAVP desmopressin may elevate the levels of von Willebrand factor and factor VIII to therapeutic levels. DDAVP is ineffectual in haemophilia B and should be used with caution in children under the age of 2 years.

Haemophilia treatment has progressed from treatment of an established bleed, so-called on-demand therapy, to prophylactic administration of concentrate to prevent bleeds. The most significant complication of haemophilia treatment has been the transmission of plasma bone infections including HIV and hepatitis B and C. This risk has now been virtually eliminated by the use of recombinant products, infection screening and viral inactivation. The remaining complication of coagulation factor replacement is inhibitor development, alloantibodies that bind to and destroy the exogenously administered coagulation factor. Genetic counselling is essential in any inherited disorder and carrier identification of female members of the family can be offered in the majority of cases. However, 30% of new patients with haemophilia A or B have no previous family history since they represent new mutations.

Von Willebrand disease

This is the most common inherited bleeding disorder, which according to some series affects 1:100 of the population. It is characterized by a deficiency of von Willebrand factor (vWf). The clinical features reflect the roles of vWf: namely in the adherence of platelets to the endothelium, in primary haemostasis, and in protecting circulating factor VIII, a role in secondary haemostasis. The deficiency of vWf may be quantitative (type 1, mild; type 3, severe) or qualitative (type 2, in which the function of the molecule is impaired).

The symptoms of type 1 disease are typical of the features of failure of primary haemostasis. The symptoms of type 3 disease combine those of primary haemostatic defects with deep-seated haemorrhage more commonly associated with defects of secondary haemostasis. Type 2 von Willebrand disease usually presents with symptoms similar to those of type 1 disease but a particular disorder, type 2b von Willebrand disease, is associated with thrombocytopenia. The symptoms of types 1 and 2 von Willebrand disease are relatively mild. Treatment consists of conservative measures and DDAVP desmopressin infusions when normal haemostasis is required. Type 3 and some subtypes of type 2 require infusion of intact vWf in the form of specific factor VIII concentrates. The clinical phenotype of von Willebrand disease is influenced by multiple genetic influences but type 1 disease follows an autosomal dominant inheritance. Type 3 disease results from the coinheritance of two vWf genetic defects which may present as type 1 disease in the parents; it is effectively inherited as an autosomal recessive disorder.

Table 43.3 Investigation of haemophilia, von Willebrand disease and vitamin K deficiency

Investigation	Haemophilia A	von Willebrand disease	Vitamin K deficiency
Prothrombin time	Normal	Normal	Prolonged
Activated partial thromboplastin time	Prolonged	Prolonged/normal	Prolonged
Factor VIII	Reduced	Reduced/normal	Normal
vW factor antigen	Normal	Reduced	Normal
Platelet aggregation	Normal	Reduced with ristocetin	Normal

Table 43.4 Classification of haemorrhagic disease of the newborn

	Early	Classical	Late
Age of onset	Days 1 or 2 Rarely up to day 5	Days 2–7 Rarely up to 1 month	2–12 weeks

Risk factors	Maternal ingestion of drugs during pregnancy
	Anticonvulsants
	Coumarin anticoagulants
	Anti-tuberculosis treatment
		Failure to administer vitamin K at birth	Failure to administer vitamin K at birth
			Breastfeeding
			Impaired vitamin K absorption:
			  Liver disease
			  GI malabsorption

Features	May not be prevented by vitamin K at birth	Haemorrhage may be intracranial, gastrointestinal or in other internal organ	Haemorrhage may be intracranial, gastrointestinal or in other internal organ

Vitamin K-deficient bleeding

Four of the coagulation factors — namely, factors II, VII, IX, X — and two of the anticoagulant factors, proteins C and S, require vitamin K to modify the precursor molecules and render them fully functional. Vitamin K is necessary for the post-translational gamma-carboxylation of these molecules. The principal effect of vitamin K deficiency is an increased risk of bleeding, as is seen in haemorrhagic disease of the newborn (HDN, p. 370), following the use of coumarin anticoagulants such as warfarin, and in certain malnourished children. However, if warfarin anticoagulation is initiated without concurrent heparin, the initial deficiency of protein C can lead to the thrombotic complication, purpura fulminans.

There is considerable evidence that the newborn infant is deficient in vitamin K; however, only a minority of neonates have clotting abnormalities at birth as a consequence. Vitamin K deficiency is intensified in the first few days of life unless the baby receives an exogenous source of vitamin K either by specific injection or as a dose by mouth or by inclusion in cow's milk or formula feeds. Breast milk contains little vitamin K.

The differentiation of haemorrhagic disease of the newborn (HDN) from other bleeding disorders is shown in Table 43.4.

A deficiency of the vitamin K-dependent coagulation factors will prolong the PT and APTT. Further evidence of vitamin K deficiency can be obtained from increased levels of proteins produced in the absence of vitamin K (PIVKA). The prevention of HDN by administration of vitamin K at birth is well established. This established efficacy justifies its use despite the previously suggested risks of haemolysis and leukaemia. Emergency treatment of vitamin K deficiency consists of intravenous administration of vitamin K. If life-threatening bleeding is recognized, immediate replacement of the deficient factors will be required, ideally with a coagulation factor concentrate of factors II, VII, IX and X. If no such concentrate is available fresh frozen plasma may be used, although the concentration of coagulation factors is insufficient for complete reversal of the haemorrhagic state.

Asplenism

The spleen serves as an efficient filter of red blood cells as they pass through large pools of blood, where they encounter macrophages and other immune effector cells. During their passage through this organ abnormal red cells may be removed by virtue of their senescence, abnormal membrane caused by binding of immunoglobulin, abnormal membrane structure, haemoglobin or cytoplasmic enzymes. The spleen also plays an important role in the immune system, allowing antigen-presenting cells to be exposed to circulating antigens and allowing macrophages to remove blood-borne bacteria, especially encapsulated organisms. The absence of the spleen will result in an increased risk of overwhelming bacterial sepsis, especially secondary to *Streptococcus pneumoniae*, *Haemophilus influenzae* type b and *Neisseria meningitidis*. The patient is also at risk of increased levels of parasitic infection with *Plasmodium* and *Babesia*.

Impaired splenic function can be seen on examination of the peripheral blood film. Red cells with abnormal morphology may circulate and red cell inclusions, including Howell–Jolly bodies (nuclear fragments), are frequently seen. There is an associated elevated platelet and white cell count (predominantly a monocytosis and lymphocytosis) in the peripheral blood.

Causes of a hyposplenic state are listed below. The clinical importance is the protection against overwhelming post-splenectomy sepsis with appropriate immunizations and penicillin prophylaxis.

Causes of asplenia
- Neonatal period, especially in premature infants
- Congenital absence or hypoplasia (associated with situs invertus and cardiac anomalies)
- Congenital polysplenism

- Surgical splenectomy
- Splenic infarction (sickling disorders and splenic torsion)
- Splenic atrophy (associated with coeliac disease, dermatitis herpetiformis, ulcerative colitis, Crohn's disease, tropical sprue, autoimmune disorders including SLE, graft versus host disease and splenic irradiation
- Splenic infiltration with malignancy or sarcoidosis.

Causes of splenomegaly
- Haematological:
  - Chronic myeloid leukaemia
  - Juvenile myelomonocytic leukaemia
  - Acute leukaemia
  - Lymphoma
  - Thalassaemia major or intermedia
  - Sickle cell anaemia (before infarction in HbSS)
  - Haemolytic anaemia
  - Megaloblastic anaemia
- Portal hypertension
- Storage diseases:
  - Gaucher's
  - Niemann–Pick
  - Histiocytosis X
- Systemic diseases:
  - Sarcoidosis
  - Collagen vascular disease, SLE, juvenile idiopathic arthritis
- Acute infections:
  - Bacterial: septicaemia, bacterial endocarditis, typhoid
  - Viral: infectious mononucleosis, cytomegalovirus and others
  - Protozoal: malaria, leishmaniasis, toxoplasmosis
- Chronic infections:
  - Tuberculosis, brucellosis
  - Tropical: malaria, leishmaniasis, schistosomiasis.

Causes of hepatomegaly
- Infection:
  - Congenital, hepatitis A, B and C, infectious mononucleosis, septicaemia, malaria
- Inflammation:
  - Hepatitis secondary to toxins, autoimmune disorders

- Infiltration:
  - Primary tumours:
    Hepatoblastoma
    Hepatocellular carcinoma
  - Secondary tumours:
    Leukaemia
    Lymphoma
    Haemophagocytic lymphohistiocytosis
- Liver disease:
  - Neonatal liver disease
  - Chronic liver disease
  - Autosomal dominant polycystic liver/kidney disease
  - Alpha$_1$-antitrypsin deficiency
- Storage disorders:
  - Lipid, e.g. Gaucher's, Niemann–Pick
  - Mucopolysaccharidoses, e.g. Hurler's syndrome
  - Glycogen
- Haematological:
  - Sickle cell anaemia, thalassaemia
  - Leukaemia, lymphoma
- Cardiovascular:
  - Right heart failure, tricuspid regurgitation.

Bone marrow failure

Marrow failure presents with a reduced number of circulating peripheral blood cell numbers. The pathology frequently affects one cell line before the others so that a single cytopenia may be the initial presentation. The symptoms will depend on the nature of the cytopenia with pallor, fatigue and reduced exercise tolerance reflecting anaemia, atypical bacterial infections reflecting neutropenia, and bleeding and bruising reflecting thrombocytopenia. Bone marrow failure may reflect abnormalities of the stem cell, either deficiency (aplasia) or abnormal maturation (dysplasia); absence of the raw materials for haemopoiesis, including iron, vitamin B$_{12}$ and folic acid, and hypopituitarism; and infiltration of the bone marrow by abnormal cells such as leukaemia or neuroblastoma or bone as in osteopetrosis (Table 43.5).

Table 43.5 Causes of pancytopenia

Disease category	Specific disorders	Associated features

Marrow aplasia	Congenital:
	  Fanconi anaemia
	  Dyskeratosis congenita
	  Shwachman–Diamond syndrome
	  Reticular dysgenesis
	  Amegakaryocytic thrombocytopenia
	Acquired:
	  Idiopathic
	  Drugs:
	    Predictable
	    Idiosyncratic
	  Viruses
		Congenital disorders are associated with somatic anomalies
		Fanconi anaemia: short stature, hyperpigmentation, abnormal radii and thumbs, renal anomalies
		Dyskeratosis congenita: dystrophic nails, leucoplakia of mucous membranes
		Shwachman–Diamond syndrome: exocrine pancreatic insufficiency

Myelodyoplasia	Stem cell disorder characterized by atypical cellular maturation and morphology	Rarely seen in childhood Frequent associated cytogenetic abnormalities

Haematinic deficiency	Megaloblastic anaemia:
	  Vitamin B_{12} deficiency
	  Folic acid deficiency
	Predominant feature is macrocytic anaemia with atypical peripheral blood morphology
	Leucopenia and thrombocytopenia in B_{12} deficiency
	Hypercellular marrow
	Atypical marrow morphology
		Vitamin B_{12} deficiency:
		  Causes: inadequate dietary intake or malabsorption, including pernicious anaemia
		  Associated neuropathy
		Folic acid deficiency:
		  Causes: inadequate dietary intake or malabsorption, increased use as in haemolysis and pregnancy

Bone marrow infiltrate	Malignant:
	  Leukaemia
	  Metastatic solid tumours including:
	    Neuroblastoma
	    Rhabdomyosarcoma
	Other:
	  Osteopetrosis
	  Haemophagocytosis
	  Myelofibrosis
	  Storage disorders
		Clinical features dependent on primary disorder
		Leucoerythroblastic peripheral blood film with evidence of immature cellular forms circulating in peripheral blood

Further reading

British Committee for Standards in Haematology: General Haematology Task Force 2003 Guidelines for the investigation and management of idiopathic thrombocytopenic purpura in adults, children and in pregnancy. British Journal of Haematology 120(4):574

British Committee for Standards in Haematology: General Haematology Task Force 2003 Guidelines for the management of the acute painful crisis in sickle cell disease. British Journal of Haematology 120(5):744

Nathan DG, Orkin SH, Look AT et al. 2003 Nathan and Oski's Haematology of infancy and childhood, 6th edn. WB Saunders, Philadelphia

Zipurski, A 1999 Review: prevention of vitamin K deficiency bleeding in newborns. British Journal of Haematology 104:430–437

Julia Clark   Noura Al-Aufi   Huda Al-Hussamy   Sachin Mannikar

Immunology and infectious disease

LEARNING OUTCOMES

By the end of this chapter you should:
- Know the body's basic immune mechanisms
- Understand some basic principles of immunology
- Know the principles of allergy
- Know how to investigate and manage recurrent infection
- Understand the prevention and management of HIV/AIDS
- Understand the investigation of fever with rash
- Understand the investigation and management of prolonged fever
- Know how to investigate a child with suspected tuberculosis
- Understand the management of meningitis and septicaemia
- Understand the investigation and management of allergy.

MODULE SEVEN

Basic science

The immune system relies on the interaction of many different parts. Different pathogens stimulate and are controlled by different arms of this system, yet at the same time all components depend on each other, working as a team. The body has both innate and adaptive responses to pathogens (Box 44.1) and the component parts are discussed here. Different defence mechanisms are provoked by different pathogens (Table 44.1).

Phagocytes

Phagocytes are 'eating cells'. They include neutrophils (or polymorphonuclear cells) and the mononuclear phagocyte system (monocytes in blood, macrophages in tissues). Neutrophils are critical for immunity to bacteria and fungi. Phagocytosis of extracellular pathogens is followed by their destruction by superoxides, proteases etc. within the neutrophil phagosomes. Macrophages also phagocytose and are important in T-cell activation, taking up and presenting antigens to T cells.

Antibodies (from B cells)

Immunoglobulins are γ-globulins of differing size that play important roles in humoral and cellular defence mechanisms; they are present in varying amounts through childhood. They participate in complement-dependent and independent opsonization, bactericidal activity, virus and toxin neutralization, and the forma-

273

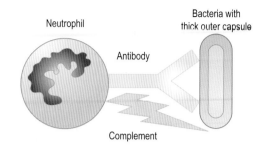

Fig. 44.1 **Antibodies and complement**

Immunology and infectious disease

BOX 44.1 Innate and adaptive responses

Innate (natural Immunity)
First line; no memory
- Phagoctyes
- Natural killer (NK) cells
- Dendritic cells
- Mast cells
- Cytokines
- Complement
- Acute phase proteins (C-reactive protein, CRP)

Adaptive
Second line; specific; memory
- T cells
- B cells
- Antibodies
- Cytokines

Humoral
- B cells, producing antibody

Cellular
- NK cells
- T cells
- CD4 (T-helper)
- CD8 (T-cytotoxic)

Table 44.1 **Defence mechanisms by pathogen**

	Pathogen	Mechanism
Intracellular pathogens	Viruses	T cells
	Salmonella	Natural killer (NK) cells
	Mycobacteria	Macrophages
	Listeria	
	Fungi	
Extracellular pathogens	Polysaccharide bacteria	Neutrophils
		Complement
		Antibodies

tion of immune complexes. IgM is produced early in infection, then interaction with CD4 cells by the binding of CD40 ligand to CD40 on B cells produces immunoglobulin class switching to IgA, IgG or IgE.

Complement

Complement attracts neutrophils to pathogens, helps attach pathogen to phagocyte (opsonization), enhances degranulation of mast cells (hence inflammation), and aids killing by cell lysis.

Antibodies and complement are particularly important for immunity to bacteria with thick carbohydrate capsules (e.g. *Streptococcus pneumoniae*, *Haemophilus influenzae*, *Neisseria meningitidis*). This is because the thick capsule prevents direct phagocytosis of the bacteria. Antibodies and complement act as a link (e.g. opsonin) between the bacteria and the neutrophil (Fig. 44.1).

T cells

T lymphocytes are the key orchestrators of the immune system (Fig. 44.2). They interact directly with cells via major histocompatibility complex (MHC) molecules

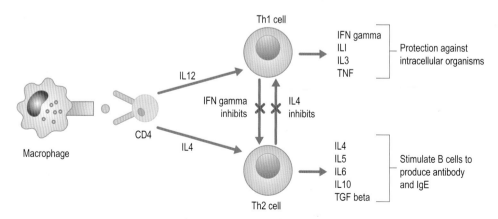

Fig. 44.2 **Th1/Th2 responses**
(IL = interleukin; IFN = interferon; TNF = tumour necrosis factor; TGF-β = transforming growth factor-β)

on the surface of cell targets. CD4 cells help control intracellular pathogens and help B-cell responses; CD8 cells kill infected cells. CD4 cells produce different cytokine responses depending on the stimulus. Th1 responses are proinflammatory, producing interferon-gamma (IFN-γ), tumour necrosis factor-alpha (TNF-α) and interleukin 2 (IL-2); they activate and recruit macrophages and help CD8 responses, hence intracellular killing.

Th2 responses produce IL-4, 5 and 6 and promote B-cell proliferation and differentiation to IgA, IgE and IgG2, as well as eosinophil recruitment. These are important in improving defence of mucosal surfaces, eradication of parasites and polysaccharide antigen responses.

Natural killer (NK) cells

These kill 'self-cells' infected with a virus.

Recurrent infection

Problem-orientated topic:

recurrent infections

Jason, a 10-month-old boy, presents acutely unwell with a short history of cough and fever. He has a respiratory rate of 60 breaths per minute, is using accessory muscles showing marked subcostal recession, and has an SaO₂ of 94% in air. He is thin and has some oral thrush. His chest X-ray (Fig. 44.3) shows bilateral interstitial shadowing.

Mum says Jason has been in hospital on two or three occasions before and has had antibiotics, but has never really been back to normal. The history is vague and this is clearly a large chaotic family that includes three other older children who are well. Hospital notes show Jason was admitted at the age of 7 months with an acute parotid abscess that responded rapidly to intravenous antibiotics, and again at 9 months with a left lower lobe pneumonia; this required oxygen and again responded to antibiotics, but it took about 5 days for his fever to settle and to start to improve. The boy seems to have gained little weight since then.

Q1. What is the differential diagnosis of Jason's problem?

Q2. What, if any, underlying disorders will you want to look for? How will you seek them?

Q3. What other family and social history would be useful?

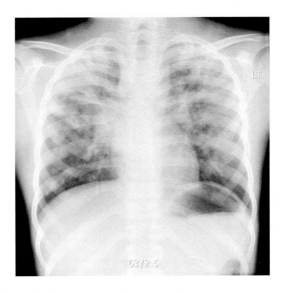

Fig. 44.3 **Bilateral interstitial shadowing**

Q1. What is the differential diagnosis of Jason's problem?

In thinking of underlying causes of recurrent infection, the type of infection is important. Viral and fungal infections suggest problems with T-cell function, whereas bacterial infections may indicate humoral, neutrophil or complement defects. This boy has had two previous invasive bacterial infections, but now has candida and a pneumonitic chest X-ray picture, suggestive in this context of virus or *Pneumocystis carinii (jirovecii)* pneumonia (PCP). You would thus be thinking mainly of T-cell defects, though antibody and neutrophil problems could have been considered after the first two apparently bacterial infections (see Table 44.2 below).

Q2. What, if any, underlying disorders will you want to look for? How will you seek them?

See Table 44.2.

Table 44.2 Immune deficiencies

Type	Disease	Family history	Features
T-cell defect (always ask about consanguinity)	HIV (see text)	Maternal infection almost certain — antenatal screening completed?	
	Severe combined immune deficiency	Previous miscarriages or early infant deaths	Initial low lymphocyte counts — < 2.5 Absent T- and B-cell function Infections in first few months of life with viral, bacterial or fungal pathogens Death if untreated by bone marrow transplantation
	CD40 ligand deficiency (Hyper-IgM)	X-linked — previous infants or maternal male relatives	B cells produce IgM but unable to switch to IgG, IgA Neutropenia
	Di George syndrome	Microdeletion at chromosome 22q11.2	Congenital heart defect (tetralogy of Fallot), immunodeficiency (T-cell disorder) and hypocalcaemia Dysmorphic face, palatal abnormalities, autoimmune phenomena, renal anomalies, neuropsychiatric disorders and short stature
	Wiskott–Aldrich syndrome	X-linked: previous infants or maternal male relatives	Recurrent infection due to combined immunodeficiency, eczema, thrombocytopenia with small platelet volume Autoimmune haemolytic anaemia and malignancy increase with age
	Ataxia telangiectasia	Most cases are sporadic	Developmental delay, cerebellar ataxia, oculomotor apraxia, choreoathetosis, dystonias, progressive spinal muscular atrophy, progressive neurological deterioration T-cell lymphopenia/dysfunction/secondary poor antibody responses
	Common variable immune deficiency (CVID)	Some are AR, AD, XLR	Combined T- and B-cell deficiency Low serum level of IgG, IgA and possibly IgM Recurrent pyogenic infections of upper and lower respiratory tracts, persistent diarrhoea (*Giardia lamblia*) High incidence of autoimmune disorders Common genetic basis for CVID and selective IgA deficiency High risk of malignancy (lymphoma and GI carcinomas)
B cell defects	Selective IgA deficiency	Most cases occur sporadically but AR, AD or multifactorial pattern may oocur Family history of CVID	Serum IgA low, other Ig levels normal The most common type of primary immune deficiency Usually asymptomatic but might be associated with recurrent sinopulmonary infections, allergy, GI disease, neurological disease, autoimmunity and malignancy
	X-linked agammaglobulinaemia (XLA, Bruton's disease) See text	X-linked disease, family history of affected boys Maternal asymptomatic carrier New mutations common	Very low or absent IgG, IgM, IgA and IgE Recurrent otitis media, pneumonia and sinusitis before the age of 1 year with extracellular encapsulated bacteria, recurrent attacks of diarrhoea (*Giardia, Campylobacter*), chronic pulmonary disease, paucity of lymph nodes
Neutrophil defects	Severe congenital neutropenia (including Kostmann syndrome)	?AD form	Recurrent mouth ulcers and pyogenic infections (sinopulmonary and abscesses)
	Chronic granulomatous disease (see text)	X-linked form (similar problems in maternal male cousins) AR Mother may have symptoms of SLE	Symptoms suggestive of inflammatory bowel disease Previous abscesses, recurrent bacterial infections, fungal infections Clinical features indicative of cystic fibrosis (CF) but sweat test and CF mutation screen normal
	Shwachman–Diamond syndrome	AR	Neutropenia, pancreatic insufficiency, anaemia Recurrent bacterial infections, symptoms of malabsorption Short stature

(AR = autosomal recessive; AD = autosomal dominant; XLR = X-linked recessive; SLE = systemic lupus erythematosus)

Q3. What other family and social history would be useful?

See Table 44.2.

Human immunodeficiency virus (HIV)

HIV is an enveloped RNA virus. There are two types: HIV-1 and HIV-2. HIV-1 is the most prevalent and therefore the most important. Up to 40% of the population are HIV-positive in some African countries, and about 800 children were infected in the UK in 2005. (See p. 154 for HIV in developing countries.)

Transmission (Box 44.2)

- Vertical: main route in children. Average risk of transmission is around 25%. Risk increases with:
  - Higher maternal HIV viral load
  - The presence of maternal sexually transmitted infections (STIs) or chorioamnionitis
  - Prolonged rupture of membranes
  - Prematurity
  - Breastfeeding
  - Risk of blood-to-blood contact, such as vaginal delivery or interventions (e.g. fetal scalp electrodes)
- Blood-to-blood: intravenous drug use, infected transfusions or contaminated injections
- Sexual contact: infected semen, vaginal secretions, oral sex (rarely).

Principles of prevention of mother-to-child transmission (MTCT) of HIV

- Provide good maternal antenatal care.
- Low maternal viral load: start maternal highly active antiretroviral therapy (HAART) in pregnancy, aiming for viral load < 50.
- Treat maternal STIs.
- Give intravenous AZT (zidovudine) to the mother just before and during delivery.
- Prescribe oral AZT for the baby for the first 4–6 weeks of life.

- Perform elective caesarean section (although vaginal delivery may be considered by some where all other risk factors are very good, i.e. viral load < 50, mother well).
- Avoid prolonged rupture of membranes.
- Bottle-feed the baby.

Diagnosis of HIV in an infant born to an HIV-positive mother

HIV antibody (IgG) is placentally transferred and so does not indicate neonatal infection, reflecting maternal status only.

HIV proviral DNA polymerase chain reaction (PCR) detects viral DNA and is a specific and sensitive marker of infection. However, at birth PCR is less sensitive, as infection may have only just been acquired and the viral load is very low. By 3 months sensitivity is > 99%. HIV infection is unlikely when there has been any of:

- Two negative PCRs, one after 3 months
- Two negative antibody tests if < 12 months
- One negative antibody test after 18 months.

Presentation

HIV infects and affects CD4 cells as well as macrophages and neuronal and glial cells, and steadily decreases CD4 counts. Hence opportunistic infections that require T-cell help for control are the hallmark of progressive infection, with falling CD4 counts. Clinical presentations of HIV disease in children are shown in Box 44.3. HIV itself can cause encephalopathy and failure to thrive (FTT). Untreated, about one-fifth of children progress rapidly to severe infection and death in the first few years of life; others progress more slowly and a few do not present with clinical features until their early teens.

BOX 44.3 Clinical presentations of paediatric HIV disease

- *Pneumocystis carinii* (*jirovecii*) pneumonia (PCP)
- *Candida* oesophagitis
- Cytomegalovirus (CMV)
- Atypical mycobacteria
- Cryptosporidiosis
- Toxoplasmosis
- Cryptococcal meningitis
- Recurrent bacterial infections
- Parotitis/parotid swelling
- HIV encephalopathy
- Neoplasms
- Wasting/failure to thrive (FTT)
- Lymphocytic interstitial pneumonitis (LIP)

Acquired immune deficiency syndrome (AIDS) is essentially HIV disease rather than infection. CD4 counts have decreased such that illness as either opportunistic infection or effects of HIV itself is found. Hence the CD4 count, as well as the amount of virus in the blood (HIV viral load), is important in disease progression. However, CD4 counts vary by age, with a peak for infants under 1 year; they have less variation when expressed as a percentage of total T-cell count.

The US Centers for Disease Control (CDC) have produced a classification for symptoms/signs and immune suppression using CD4 counts and percentages. Clinical categories range from N (non-symptomatic) to A (mildly symptomatic), B (moderately symptomatic) and C (severely symptomatic). Immune categories are simply no immunosuppression (CD4 > 25%), mild immunosuppression (15–25%) and severe immunosuppression (< 15%)

 http://www.aidsmap.com/en/docs/289A9ABC-1D62-467E-924E-6B9D79789327.asp

Revised classification system for HIV infection in children less than 13 years of age

 www.ctu.mrc.ac.uk/penta/ http://www.ctu.mrc.ac.uk/penta/hppmcs/calcProb.htm

A risk calculator for disease progression and death

Management

Treatment depends on combinations of at least two, and preferably three, elements of antiretroviral therapy (HAART). The aim is to decrease viral replication to an undetectable level and hence to increase CD4 count.

Combinations are chosen from three main categories: nucleoside transcriptase inhibitors, non-nucleoside transcriptase inhibitors and protease inhibitors.

Treatment decisions are made on viral load, CD4 percentage (count in older children and adults), and disease category as defined by CDC.

 www.AIDSinfo.nih.gov http://www.bhiva.org/chiva/

For information on HIV infection

Primary T cell defects

Children with primary immunodeficiencies of T lymphocytes may present with unusual or severe viral infections, unusual autoinflammatory disorders (which, although often triggered by infections, particularly viruses, frequently result from bystander damage of neural tissue) and also an increased propensity to primary lymphoma/lymphoproliferative disease (LPD). With LPD there is often an increased susceptibility to lymphotrophic herpes virus infections (e.g. Epstein–Barr virus, EBV).

Chronic granulomatous disorder (CGD)

This is a rare inherited immunodeficiency disorder of defective phagocytes. Incidence is about 1 in a million, with the male:female ratio being 4:1. About 80% are X-linked recessive; the rest are autosomal recessive.

Basic science

The underlying defect lies within phagocytes (neutrophils, monocytes, eosinophils and macrophages), which lack microbiocidal reactive oxidant superoxide anion, which is important for killing bacteria and fungi. This results in recurrent life-threatening bacterial and fungal infections and granuloma formation. Granulomas are a result of exuberant anomalous chronic inflammatory response to frequent infections; hence the name of the condition. Infections are commonly caused by catalase-producing microorganisms like *Staphylococcus*, *Serratia*, *Aspergillus*, *Burkholderia* and *Nocardia*.

Clinical features

Presentation is usually with unusual infections by 2 years of age (suppurative lymphadenitis, osteomyelitis, pneumonia, recurrent soft tissue infections, brain abscess, sepsis and hepatosplenomegaly with or without a liver abscess).

Granulomas can be symptomatic if they are causing gastrointestinal or genitourinary obstruction. Gastrointestinal symptoms are often prominent and inflammatory bowel disease with diarrhoea and FTT can be the sole presentation.

Maternal carriers may have features of autoimmune disease, including SLE.

Prenatal diagnosis for siblings of affected individuals could be achieved by DNA analysis, obtained by either chorionic villus biopsy or fetal blood sampling.

Diagnosis and significance

Diagnosis is based on observation of a pattern of recurrent atypical infections and tests to demonstrate the defective oxidative function in neutrophils:

1. *Nitro-blue tetrazolium (NBT) reduction.* This is used as a screening test and demonstrates oxidase activity of leucocytes during phagocytosis.
2. *Dihydroflavonol-4-reductase (DHR) reduction.* This is a flow cytometry test and shows fluorescent rhodamine in the presence of oxidative burst.

    These two tests also help in detecting carriers for CGD.
3. *Genetic tests.* Direct genetic tests can detect mutations and help find the nature of the genetic inheritance (XLR vs. AR).

Management

Early diagnosis, aggressive and prompt treatment of infection with prolonged high doses of antibiotics, aggressive search for an infectious agent, and antimicrobial and antifungal prophylaxis together with IFN-γ form the cornerstone of management. Haematopoietic stem cell transplant, from a human leucocyte antigen (HLA)-matched donor, is curative.

Prognosis

Overall prognosis has improved over the last 2 decades. Mortality rates are highest in childhood because of infections. However, most patients now live up to 20–25 years, with a mortality rate of 2–5% each year.

X-linked agammaglobulinaemia (XLA, Bruton's disease)

Basic science

B cells fail to develop from B-cell precursors; hence immunoglobulin is not produced. A defective gene (*btk*) on the X chromosome codes for tyrosine kinase, which is essential for B-cell maturation.

Presentation

As maternal antibody (> 6 months) wanes, bacterial infections become common. Recurrent respiratory and ear infections are typical, with meningitis, bone and joint infections often seen, as are FTT and chronic diarrhoea. Chronic lung infection may lead to bronchiectasis. Interestingly, enteroviral infection may cause a chronic meningo-encephalitis. There is sometimes an association with growth hormone deficiency.

Management

Treatment is with immunoglobulin: either intravenous or subcutaneous. Immunoglobulin levels should be maintained well within the normal range, and prompt and prolonged antibiotic treatment should be given for infections.

Live oral polio vaccine should not be given, as virus may fail to clear.

Fever and rash

Causative organisms

Viruses

Viruses are very small (10–400 nm), have a simple acellular organization consisting of one or more molecules of DNA or RNA enclosed in a coat of protein, and are obligate intracellular parasites (Box 44.4). The genome (DNA or RNA) codes for the few proteins necessary for replication.

BOX 44.4 Virus classification	
The DNA viruses	
Herpesviridae family	Varicella zoster virus (VZV), Herpes simplex virus (HSV), Human herpes virus 6 (HHV 6), Cytomegalovirus (CMV), Epstein–Barr virus (EBV)
Adenoviridae	Adenovirus
Poxviridae	Molluscum
Parvoviridae	Erythrovirus 19 (parvovirus B19)
Hepadnaviridae	Hepatitis B virus (HBV)
The RNA viruses	
Astroviridae	Astrovirus
Caliciviridae	Small round structured virus (SRSV), norovirus (Norwalk virus)
Picornaviruses	Poliovirus, Coxsackie A and B, rhinovirus, hepatitis A virus (HAV), echovirus
Paramyxoviridae	Measles virus, mumps virus, respiratory syncytial virus (RSV), parainfluenza virus
Orthomyxoviridae	Influenza virus
Retroviridae	Retrovirus, human immunodeficiency virus (HIV)
Filoviridae	Ebola virus
Reoviridae	Rotavirus
Flaviviridae	Dengue virus, hepatitis C virus (HCV), Japanese encephalitis (JE) virus

Bacteria

Staphylococci

- Staphylococci live on the skin and mucous membranes (nose) of humans.
- *Staphylococcus aureus* is an important pathogen but can be a skin commensal, as can *Staph. epidermidis*.
- *Staph. aureus* is a Gram-positive β-haemolytic facultative coagulase- and catalase-positive coccus. It may occur singly or be grouped in pairs, short chains or grape-like clusters.

Diseases caused by staphylococci include:
- *Skin infections*: abscess, impetigo, cellulitis
- *Invasive infections*: septicaemia, osteomyelitis, pyelonephritis

- *Toxin-mediated infections*: food poisoning, toxic shock, staphylococcal scalded skin syndrome.

Streptococci

- Streptococci that cause human disease are usually facultative anaerobes, are Gram-positive cocci, either spherical or ovoid in shape, and tend to form chains with each other.
- They are classified into subtypes based on sugar chains expressed on their outer shell (Lancefield group) and their behaviour when grown in the laboratory (α- or β-haemolysis).
- Most streptococci important in rashes or skin infections belong to the Lancefield groups A (*Streptococcus pyogenes*), C and G, and are β-haemolytic.
- *Strep. pneumoniae* (pneumococci) are important bacteria in sepsis, pneumonia and meningitis but rarely cause skin rashes. Pneumococci are α-haemolytic and do not belong to the Lancefield groups.
- Group B streptococci (also known as *Strep. agalactiae*) are important pathogens in the neonate.

Superantigens

Superantigens are proteins (toxins) that bind non-specifically to T-cell receptors (TCR) and MCH class II molecules on antigen-presenting cells (APCs), bypassing the normal peptide groove and hence activating large numbers of T-lymphocytes. Between 5% and 30% of the entire T-cell population may be activated (Fig. 44.4).

Superantigens lead to a massive release of cytokines, especially TNF-α, IL-1 and IL-6. These cytokines are responsible for a capillary leak syndrome and account for many of the clinical signs of toxic shock syndrome (TSS).

Problem-orientated topic:

fever and rash

Rhys, a 4-year-old boy, is seen in the accident and emergency department. He has been unwell for the preceding 4 days, being pyrexial with headaches, aches and swollen glands, and is sleepy and tired most of the time. He has lost some weight and missed nursery school. An antibiotic (amoxicillin) was prescribed by his GP yesterday and a fine rash developed afterwards. On examination there is an erythematous non-itchy maculopapular rash all over his body, his temperature is 39°C and large swollen bilateral posterior cervical lymph nodes are palpable, as is a 3 cm spleen.

Q1. What are the most likely diagnoses?

Q1. What are the most likely diagnoses?

Clearly there are many causes of fever and rash in childhood to be considered when confronted with a history as outlined above. Viruses are most common, but some bacteria such as *Strep. pyogenes* (group A streptococcus), *Staph. aureus* or *Mycoplasma* cause erythematous rashes, as do inflammatory processes such as Kawasaki disease.

Rhys's symptoms could be due to:
- Infection
- Inflammation: Kawasaki disease (p. 286), juvenile idiopathic arthritis (p. 283)
- Autoimmune disorders (p. 283)
- Malignancy (Ch. 51)
- Drugs: especially antibiotics (Ch. 10).

Infective causes are summarized in Tables 44.3 and 44.4. Remember measles and rubella too, though both are now rare in the UK. Rarer causes include meningococcal sepsis, Lyme disease (common in the New Forest and Scotland) and leptospirosis.

Infectious mononucleosis (glandular fever; Epstein–Barr virus, EBV)

Incubation period is 30–50 days. Respiratory transmission is through saliva, coughing and sneezing.

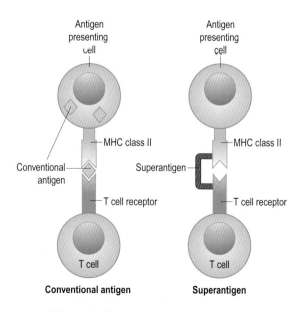

Fig. 44.4 Mechanism of superantigen T-cell stimulation (MHC = major histocompatibility complex)

Table 44.3 Other viral causes of fever and rash

Disease	Virus	Clinical features
Adenovirus	Adenovirus	Different serotypes cause either GI (40, 41) or respiratory disease Fever, purulent conjunctivitis, erythematous rash, respiratory symptoms Associated with bronchiolitis obliterans
Cytomegalovirus (CMV)	CMV	Can cause glandular fever-like illness
Erythema infectiosum (slapped cheek/Fifth disease)	Erythrovirus 19 (parvovirus B19)	Fever, sore throat, GI symptoms, lymphadenopathy, bright erythematous macular rash on face (slapped cheek), lacy reticular rash spreading to rest of the body Complications include arthropathy and marrow aplasia
Roseola infantum (exanthema subitum/Sixth disease)	Human herpes virus 6 (or 7)	Infants, young children High fever for 3–6 days; fever drops and child is better then small red/pink flat raised lesions appear on trunk then extremities Associated with febrile convulsions
Herpangina	Coxsackie virus (A1–10, 16, 22), enterovirus	Fever with small vesicles or ulcers on the posterior oropharynx, cervical lymphadenopathy, anorexia and sometimes macular, papular or vesicular rash
Hand, foot and mouth disease	Coxsackie virus (A16), enterovirus	Fever, blisters to the mouth, tongue, hands and feet Resolves spontaneously, rarely severe
Gingivostomatitis	Herpes simplex virus	

Table 44.4 Other non-viral infective causes of fever and rash

Disease	Pathogen	Clinical features
Scarlet fever	Group A streptococcus (*Strep. pyogenes*)	Throat infection with streptococci producing exotoxin Tonsillitis with an erythematous fine punctate rash, which characteristically has a sandpaper texture, initially on the trunk but spreading rapidly Other features are glossal inflammation with prominent papillae, a strawberry tongue and circumoral pallor, with rash sparing the skin around the mouth There is often desquamation of the fingers and toes on resolution
Staphylococcal scalded skin syndrome	*Staph. aureus*	Caused by exotoxins in young children, particularly neonates and immunocompromised individuals Initially fever, irritability and widespread redness of skin; within 24–48 hr fluid-filled blisters form Rash spreads all over the body and the top layer of skin peels off in sheets, leaving exposed moist red and tender area (Nikolsky's sign) Fluid and pain management essential

Clinical features

These include fever, fatigue, 'flu-like symptoms, sore throat, swollen tonsils, enlarged lymph nodes (cervical, epitrochlear), palatal petechiae, maculopapular rash, eyelid oedema and hepatosplenomegaly. A florid erythematous macular rash is often seen after ampicillin/amoxicillin has been given.

Complications

Complications include chronic fatigue, 0.1–0.5% splenic rupture, hepatitis, jaundice, anaemia, meningo-encephalitis and Guillain–Barré syndrome.

Diagnosis

Diagnosis is by Monospot and Paul–Bunnell reaction (detects heterophile antibody, not sensitive), EBV IgM (or early antigen IgG) antibody titre, EBV PCR and viral culture from throat swab.

Management

Treatment is non-specific and is based on supportive medical care, e.g. analgesia. Steroids and aciclovir are of limited use. Treatment may be surgical in case of organ rupture.

Chickenpox (varicella)

See Ch. 23.

Toxic shock syndrome (TSS)

This is a 'superantigen' disease with fever, hypotension, rash, vomiting and multi-organ failure from toxin-producing *Staph. aureus* or *Strep. pyogenes*. Delay in recognizing the early signs of TSS is associated with increased morbidity and mortality, which may be as high as 15%.

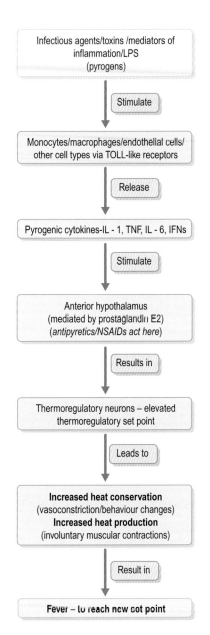

Fig. 44.5 **Pathophysiology of fever**
(LPS = lipopolysaccharide; IL = interleukin; TNF = tumour necrosis factor; IFN = interferon; NSAIDs = non-steroidal anti-inflammatory drugs)

http://www.emedicine.com/MED/topic2292.htm

Information and case definitions for TSS

Prolonged fever: pyrexia of unknown origin

Basic science of fever (Fig. 44.5)

- Fever is 'a state of elevated core temperature, which is often, but not necessarily, part of the defensive responses of multicellular organisms (host) to the invasion of live (microorganisms) or inanimate matter recognized as pathogenic or alien by its host'.

- Thermoregulation is controlled by a centre within the hypothalamus. Normal body temperature is around 37°C but varies with age, time of day (increasing in the late afternoon) and activity.

- Core temperature is best measured rectally; oral measurement is an alternative. Axillary and tympanic measurement are other possibilities but temperature here may be variable and is usually 0.5–1°C lower than rectal temperature.

- High temperature may inhibit viral replication and virulence, and enhance phagocytosis, interferon production and leucocyte migration.

Problem-orientated topic:

prolonged fever

An 11-year-old boy, Patrice, presents to the casualty department with a 10-week history of intermittent fever, night sweats, lethargy, muscle aches and pains, anorexia and possibly some weight loss, though this is not obvious. He has had no cough and is not breathless but feels he does get out of breath playing football.

He is an asylum seeker recently arrived from the Congo and is one of six children ranging from 2 to 16 years old. Mum is a single parent, is pregnant again (now 30 weeks) and thus has had a recent HIV test, which is negative; the rest of the family are well. Patrice was immunized as a baby and has a BCG scar.

On examination his height is on the 25th centile for age and his weight is on the 9th centile. He is pale, is not jaundiced or clubbed, has cervical lymphadenopathy but none elsewhere, has a temperature of 38°C but does not look unwell. He has some scattered crepitations over all lung fields, and a liver edge and spleen tip can be felt.

Q1. What differential diagnoses can you think of?

Q2. How will you investigate these?

Table 44.5 Investigations and their significance in prolonged fever

History/examination	Possible diagnoses	Investigations
Travel abroad	Tuberculosis	Mantoux test; ≥ 10 mm induration
	Typhoid	Stool culture, blood culture
	Legionella infection	Urinary antigen, serology
	Brucellosis	Serology
	Viral haemorrhagic fever	Viral detection, serology
Mosquito bites abroad	Malaria	Thick and thin blood films
	Arbovirus infection: yellow fever, dengue	Viral detection, serology
Animal exposure	Toxoplasmosis	Serology
	Leptospirosis	Urinary antigen, serology
	Q fever (*Coxiella*)	Serology
	Cat scratch disease	Serology (*Bartonella henselae*)
Conjunctivitis	Kawasaki disease	Serology to exclude other diagnoses
	Measles	Measles IgM
	Adenovirus infection	Serology (blood PCR)
Rigors, high swinging fever	Septicaemia	Blood culture and PCR
	Malaria	Thick and thin blood films
	Brucellosis	Serology
	Abscess	Pus aspiration; microscopy and culture
GI symptoms	*Giardia, Salmonella, Campylobacter* infection	Stool culture
	Inflammatory bowel disease	Barium enema, white cell scan
	Appendicitis, abscess	Ultrasound scan
Sore throat	Glandular fever	Serology (EBV IgM)
	CMV	Serology
	Tonsillitis	Throat swab (ASOT)
Lymphadenopathy	Glandular fever, CMV	Serology
	Tonsillitis	Throat swab (ASOT)
	Cat scratch disease	Serology (*Bartonella henselae*)
	Mycobacterial infection	Mantoux, IFN-γ blood test, tissue TB culture
	Toxoplasmosis, toxocariasis	Serology
	Hodgkin's disease	Tissue histology
	Malignancy	Blood film, bone marrow, tissue histology
Respiratory	Pneumonia	CXR
	TB	CXR, Mantoux, IFN-γ blood test
ESR > 100	TB	CXR, Mantoux, IFN-γ blood test, autoantibodies
	Kawasaki	Blood film, bone marrow, tissue histology
	Autoimmune (JIA)	
	Malignancy	

(PCR = polymerase chain reaction; EBV = Epstein–Barr virus; CMV = cytomegalovirus; ASOT = antistreptolysin titre; IFN = interferon; TB = tuberculosis; ESR= erythrocyte sedimentation rate; CXR = chest X-ray; JIA = juvenile idiopathic arthritis)

Q1. What differential diagnoses can you think of?

- History is vital: fever pattern, when started, travel, immunization status (Table 44.5)
- Family history: genetic background (periodic fevers)
- Symptoms: pain to localize infection (bones, GI, respiratory)
- Signs: foci of infection
- If in doubt: admit patient to document fevers and pattern
- Do not start antibiotics until the patient is assessed.

Fever without focus and prolonged fever is often referred to as 'pyrexia (or fever) of unknown origin' (PUO). This is usually defined as fever over 38°C for more than 3 weeks with no cause identified even after 1 week's hospital assessment.

A fever continuing for more than 3 weeks is unusual in children. Causes are:
- Infective
- Malignant
- Autoimmune (Fig. 33.2)
- Factitious
- Undiagnosed.

Q2. How will you investigate these?

See Table 44.5.

Tuberculosis

Basic science

- TB is caused by *Mycobacterium tuberculosis* (MTB) and rarely by *M. bovis*.
- MTB is usually inhaled and so first lodges and begins to multiply in the lungs (known as the Ghon or primary focus).
- Bacilli are then carried to regional lymph nodes, where non-specific immunity controls infection and prevents dissemination. After a period of 4–8 weeks, cell-mediated immunity either:
  - Eradicates the infection
  - *Or* walls it off to an asymptomatic focus (latent TB infection)
  - *Or* fails to control it and mycobacteria replicate to produce TB disease.
- The primary focus and the infected regional lymph node together make the primary complex.
- During the formation of this primary complex and for some months later, bacilli may escape intermittently into the blood stream and may lodge anywhere in the body, but particularly in the central nervous system, bones or kidneys.
- If circumstances favour the organism rather than the host — for example, in a young child or if nutrition is poor — then haematogenous disease occurs either as a localized lesion or multiple lesions (miliary disease).

Transmission

- TB is spread by airborne particles that contain *M. tuberculosis*.
- These particles are expelled when a person with infectious TB coughs or sneezes.
- Higher infectivity is associated with cavitatory disease, laryngeal TB and frequent cough.
- Children rarely form cavities and have poor tussive force; they are therefore rarely infectious.
- Close contact is the most important risk factor for acquiring infection.
- Persons with latent TB infection but no disease are not infectious.

Natural history of TB infection (Fig. 44.6)

Primary infection before 2 years of age may progress to serious disease (including miliary or disseminated) within the first 12 months without significant prior symptoms. Primary infection between 2 and 10 years of age generally produces significant symptoms but rarely progresses to serious disease. Primary infection after 10 years of age often produces adult-type disease.

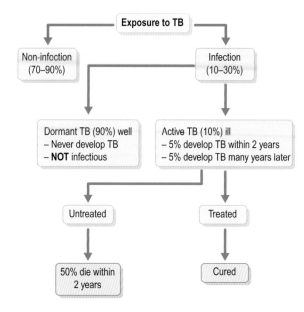

Fig. 44.6 **The natural history of tuberculosis infection**

Clinical features of TB

- May be non-specific, especially in young children
- Fever
- FTT or weight loss
- Lethargy
- Poor feeding
- Cough
- Night sweats
- Lymphadenopathy
- Pleural effusion
- Hepatosplenomegaly
- History of headache, vomiting and drowsiness lasting several weeks
- Erythema nodosum
- Phlyctenular conjunctivitis
- Choroidal tubercles.

Diagnosis of TB in children

TB should be suspected when two of the following are present and is likely when three are present:

- Positive Mantoux test (Box 44.5)
- Clinical findings compatible with TB
- History of contact with TB
- Suggestive CXR
- Positive histological findings from a tissue biopsy.

Positive culture of MTB from secretions or tissue biopsy on its own confirms the diagnosis.

BOX 44.5 Skill: Mantoux test

Perform and read an intradermal Mantoux test.

 This is described on the MasterCourse website.

Table 44.6 Investigations and their significance in tuberculosis

Investigation	Significance
Mantoux	Skin test identifies tuberculin sensitivity Positive in TB, BCG and non-tuberculous mycobacterial infection Infection with TB usually taken as ≥ 6 mm without BCG, ≥ 15 mm with prior BCG using 2TU Mantoux (Danish SSI)
IFN-γ stimulation test (Quantiferon Gold or T SPOT TB)	Identifies an immune response to MTB (independent of BCG status), hence prior infection with MTB Does not distinguish latent infection from TB disease
CXR	Identifies focal lesions and mediastinal lymphadenopathy
Sputum, induced sputum, BAL	Respiratory specimens suitable for identification and culture of mycobacteria
Gastric aspirate	Early morning aspiration of gastric contents may identify swallowed acid-fast bacilli 30% yield
TB smear	The older Ziehl–Neelsen stain is now being superseded by auramine stains in TB reference labs, giving higher sensitivity for smear-positive diagnoses
TB culture	Developments have also progressed in TB culture with rapid liquid culture and gene probes decreasing time to positive culture result from 6 weeks to 2–3 weeks
PCR	The sensitivity of PCR for detecting *M. tuberculosis* in CSF of patients with TBM is reported in recent studies as between 33% and 93%
Contact tracing	If no known TB contact, then screening close contacts may be helpful diagnostically, as finding active pulmonary TB suggests the diagnosis in the child
ESR, CRP	Often elevated, but non-specific markers of inflammation

(BCG = Bacille Calmette–Guérin; MTB = *Mycobacterium tuberculosis*; IFN = interferon; BAL = bronchoalveolar lavage; PCR = polymerase chain reaction; ESR = erythrocyte sedimentation rate; CRP = C-reactive protein)

Investigations

See Table 44.6.

Management

See Box 44.6.

 http://www.nice.org.uk/page.aspx?o=CG033N ICEguideline

Guideline on tuberculosis

BOX 44.6 Principles of management of tuberculosis

- NICE guidelines (2005) suggest quadruple therapy:
  - Isoniazid
  - Rifampicin
  - Pyrazinamide
  - Ethambutol
  for adults and children as standard *unless* they are Caucasian, with no travel or high-risk behaviour, in which case initial therapy is triple (minus ethambutol)
- 6 months of treatment includes 2 months of triple or quadruple and 4 months of isoniazid only. TB meningitis requires 12 months in total
- Treatment must be taken regularly; if there is doubt about compliance, it can be directly observed (DOT)
- Contact tracing is central to the control of TB
- Prevention: BCG vaccination for neonates at high risk of TB

Malaria

There are four species of the protozoan parasite *Plasmodium: falciparum, vivax, ovale* and *malariae*:

- Human reservoir, transmitted by the bite of the female *Anopheles* mosquito
- Imported to UK after travel to tropics or subtropics
- *P. falciparum* more likely in travellers from Africa, *P. vivax* in those from South Asia
- First symptoms usually 10 days to 4 weeks after transmission.

The life cycle of the parasite in the human phase is shown in Figure 44.7.

Clinical features

- Fever
- Influenza-like symptoms: headache, myalgia, rigors, cough, diarrhoea, vomiting
- Splenomegaly, thrombocytopenia, anaemia, jaundice, but these may be absent
- Decreased conscious level
- Seizures
- Shock.

Diagnosis and investigations

- Microscopy of thick and thin blood films: three films 12 hours apart
- Rapid diagnostic tests: dipsticks for malaria antigen
- Full blood count

Fig. 44.7 **Human stages of the malaria parasite**

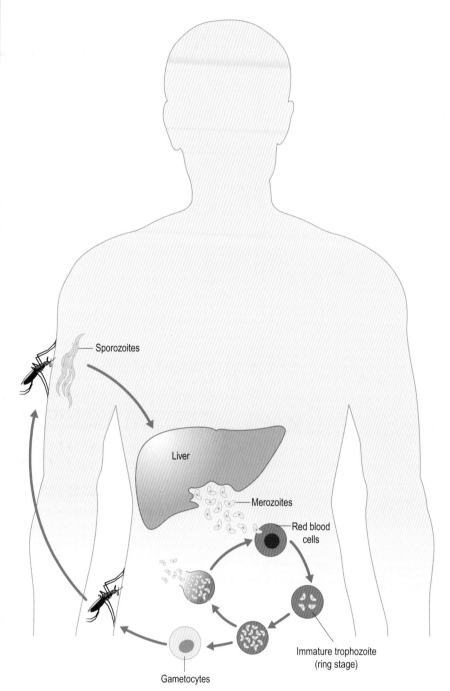

- Sporozoites
- Liver
- Merozoites
- Red blood cells
- Immature trophozoite (ring stage)
- Gametocytes

- Urea and electrolytes
- Liver function tests
- Blood glucose.

Management
- Depends on type and severity.
- Check glucose-6-phosphate dehydrogenase (G6PD) status.
- *P. vivax, ovale, malariae*:
  - Oral chloroquine for 3 days then oral primaquine for 14–21 days.
- *P. falciparum*:

  - Oral proguanil with atovaquone (Malarone)/ mefloquine/artemether with lumefantrine
  - Oral or intravenous quinine.

Prevention is better than cure. Advise prophylaxis and avoidance of mosquito bites (cover up with clothes, use impregnated mosquito nets) when travel is planned to endemic areas.

Kawasaki disease

This is an acute, self-limiting vasculitis occurring predominantly in infants and young children.

Aetiology

- Infectious agent (young age, winter seasonality, epidemicity) but still no specific organism identified
- Superantigen-mediated (vβ4 and vβ8 family expansion)
- Immune perturbation: marked cytokine cascade and endothelial cell activation.

Clinical features

There is a sudden-onset high spiking fever, with malaise and irritability (Box 44.7).

KD is also associated with other non-specific features, such as arthritis, nausea, vomiting, diarrhoea, abdominal pain, extreme irritability, aseptic meningitis and urethritis.

Coronary artery aneurysms are the most serious complication, with possible long-term morbidity and mortality.

Investigations

See Box 44.8.

Management

- Aspirin 80–100 mg/kg/day in four divided doses
- IVIg infusion 2 g/kg in a single infusion
- Aspirin reduced to 3–5 mg/kg/day after fever settled for > 48 hours and continued until absence of coronary abnormalities by 6–8 weeks after the onset is confirmed.

Severe infection

Septicaemia

Structural components of microorganisms such as lipopolysaccharide (LPS, endotoxin) in Gram-negative bacteria and the cell wall fragments (teichoic acid) of Gram-positive bacteria or the exotoxins synthesized by them have been shown to be potent activators of a wide range of cells. These include monocytes/macrophages, neutrophils and endothelial cells. These cells release proinflammatory mediators that activate complement and coagulation, hence producing endothelial damage and capillary leak.

Inflammation is essential for host defence. Unfortunately excessive inflammatory reactions, as occur in septic shock, are detrimental. This is illustrated in Figure 44.8.

Meningitis

Meningitis is an inflammation of the meninges, the membranes that cover the brain and spinal cord. This inflammation is usually caused by bacteria, viruses or fungi (Table 44.7).

Access to the CNS is gained by:
- The blood stream (the most common mode of spread)
- A retrograde neuronal pathway (some viruses)
- Direct contiguous spread, e.g. sinusitis, otitis media, congenital malformations, trauma.

Bacteria are frequent nasopharyngeal colonizers of young children and this is a prerequisite for invasion. Host factors such as local secretory immunity (IgA), integument lesions (picked nose!) and intercurrent viral infections, as well as microbial 'virulence' where certain strains attach to mucosa more strongly, all contribute to bacterial invasion. Once in the blood stream bacteria disseminate and may attach to cerebral endothelium or

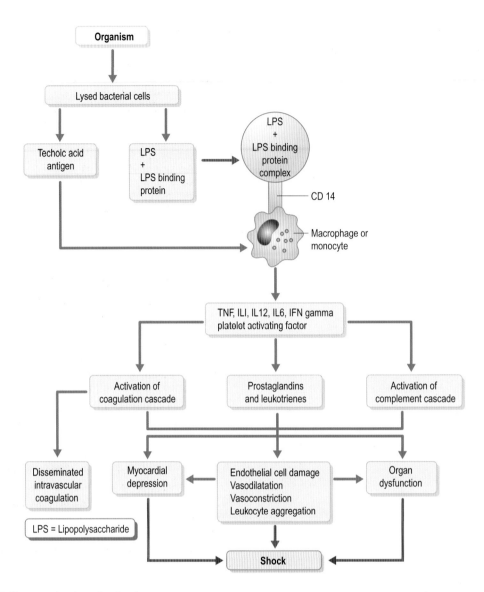

Fig. 44.8 Pathogenesis of septic shock
(LPS = lipopolysaccharide)

choroid plexus. The systemic inflammatory response includes IL-1 and TNF secretion, stimulating vascular endothelial cells and breaking down the tight junctions within the blood–brain barrier (BBB), making this permeable to larger molecules such as white cells, IgG and organisms. Once breached, white cells, inflammatory cells, organisms within the CSF and resident microglia continue the cytokine cascade with platelet activating factor (PAF), complement, prostaglandin and leuco-trienes. This continues to make the BBB permeable and increases vasculitis, oedema, CSF outflow and intracranial pressure.

This systemic inflammatory response accounts for many of the clinical symptoms and signs, and acute and long-term neurological morbidity and mortality.

Actual neuronal injury and death are also primarily due to an immunological response.

Brain oedema contributes to high intracranial pressure; consequently low cerebral blood flow occurs, resulting in anaerobic metabolism and low CSF glucose, which also stems from decreased glucose transport into the spinal fluid.

Aseptic meningitis

Aseptic meningitis is a non-pyogenic cellular response, which may be caused by many different aetiological agents. The most common cause are viruses such as enteroviruses, CMV, EBV, VZV, HSV 1 and 2, HHV6, mumps and measles.

Table 44.7 Characteristics of the three most common bacterial agents

Bacterial agent	Description
Streptococcus pneumoniae	Gram-positive coccus, common colonizer of the human nasopharynx (20–40% of healthy children) The most common overall cause of invasive bacterial sepsis, meningitis and pneumonia Conjugate vaccine covering seven serotypes effective in young children
Neisseria meningitidis	Gram-negative diplococcus, carried in the nasopharynx of otherwise healthy individuals Groups A, B, C, W135 and Y most frequently pathogenic, with B and C most common in the UK Polysaccharide vaccine available for A, C, W135, Y, and a conjugate C vaccine for young children is now in the primary immunization schedule People with deficiencies in terminal complement components are at risk of recurrent infection
Haemophilus influenzae type B	Small Gram-negative coccobacillus, normal flora in the upper respiratory tract Before the introduction of the HiB vaccine it was the most common cause of invasive bacterial disease, meningitis and epiglottitis in children under 5 years. Since HiB vaccine introduced, carriage rates have decreased

Problem-orientated topic:

acute fever, no focus

Shamin, a 9-month-old girl, presents to casualty with a history of fever, vomiting and loose stools over the last 3 days. She had a brief convulsion just before arrival at the hospital in the form of a generalized clonic seizure with uprolling of the eyes, which settled spontaneously. Mum feels that the child has not been herself for the last few days and seems irritable most of the time.

On examination Shamin is febrile at 39°C, drowsy and irritable but had appropriate reactions on being handled, is mildly dehydrated and has cool peripheries. Her throat is slightly inflamed.

Q1. What are the most important differential diagnoses?

Q2. What examination findings and observations would you like to establish immediately?

Q3. Management will depend on cause. What is the management of these conditions?

Q1. What are the most important differential diagnoses?

This little girl appears acutely unwell with a fever but no obvious source of infection is described. Clearly you will be most concerned about bacterial infection causing septic shock and meningitis. However, a young child requires careful assessment then investigation for an initially unapparent focus.

Q2. What examination findings and observations would you like to establish immediately?

Look for a focus:

- Ears: otitis media, mastoiditis
- Throat: tonsillitis, epiglottitis, glandular fever, quinsy
- Mouth: hand, foot, mouth (Coxsackie), gingivostomatitis (herpes simplex), membrane (diphtheria)
- Skin: impetigo, cellulitis, abscess
- Chest: bronchiolitis, upper respiratory tract infection, pneumonia, influenza
- Abdomen: appendicitis, perforation, abscess
- Bone or joint: osteomyelitis, septic arthritis
- Blood: septicaemia, toxic shock, acute viraemia
- Renal: urinary tract infection, pyelonephritis
- Gastrointestinal tract: gastroenteritis, viral or bacterial
- Central nervous system: meningitis, encephalitis, brain abscess.

Clinical features

- Fever, headache, neck stiffness, photophobia, nausea, vomiting and signs of cerebral dysfunction (e.g. lethargy, confusion, coma)
- Cranial nerves palsies, focal neurological signs, seizures and papilloedema.

Symptoms depend on the age of the patient; younger children may not have meningism (Box 44.9).

Investigations in acute fever with no apparent focus
See Table 44.8.

Investigations in suspected meningitis
Brain computed tomography (CT) or magnetic resonance imagining (MRI) is indicated if there are focal

BOX 44.9 Detecting signs of meningeal irritation

Kernig sign

- In a supine patient, flex the hip to 90° while the knee is flexed at 90°. An attempt to extend the knee further produces pain in the hamstrings and resistance to further extension

Brudzinski sign

- Passively flex the neck while the patient is in a supine position with extremities extended. This manoeuvre produces flexion of the hips in patients with meningeal irritation

Neck stiffness

- Resistance to passive neck flexion

BOX 44.10 Findings and their significance in septicaemia and septic shock

Fever	Increasing
Tachycardia	severity
Tachypnoea	
Cool peripheries (toe: core temperature > 3°C)	Decreasing intravascular volume
Prolonged capillary refill (> 3 seconds)	Acidosis
Poor urine output	Electrolyte and glucose loss
Irritability, restlessness, confusion	Disseminated intravascular coagulation
Deteriorating conscious level	Multi-organ failure
Hypoxia	
Hypotension (late sign)	

neurological signs, signs of raised intracranial pressure (ICP) or prolonged fever. These are helpful in the detection of CNS complications of bacterial meningitis, such as hydrocephalus, cerebral infarct, brain abscess, subdural empyema and venous sinus thrombosis.

Diagnosis is only definitively made by lumbar puncture (Ch. 12). Findings are interpreted in Table 44.9.

Q3. Management will depend on cause. What is the management of these conditions?

General management

- Airway.
- Breathing.

- Circulation: fluid resuscitation where there are signs of capillary leak and decreased intravascular volume (sepsis; Box 44.10).
- Dexamethasone: improves neurological outcome when given before or with first dose of antibiotics in *H. influenzae* B and *Strep. pneumoniae* meningitis. Neurological outcome in meningococcal meningitis is generally good and the benefit of dexamethasone is not proven. Its use in meningococcal meningitis is therefore still debated; some experts recommend it, some do not.
- Antibiotics (Table 44.10).

Table 44.8 Investigations and their significance in acute fever with no apparent focus

Investigation	Significance
Urine dipstick/microscopy	Nitrites, leucocytes; white cells, organisms seen — urinary tract infection
CXR	Consolidation, collapse, effusion — lower respiratory tract infection
Neutrophil count	Raised in bacterial infection, low in severe sepsis
Lymphocyte count	Raised or 'atypical' in viral infection
Platelet count	Raised in longstanding inflammation, low in severe sepsis
CRP	Raised suggests bacterial infection or adenovirus
ESR	Raised suggests bacterial infection or inflammation
Blood culture	Bacteria or fungi grown from blood
PCR	Detection of bacterial or viral genomic material in blood indicates infection (*Strep. pneumoniae*, *N. meningitidis*, herpes simplex virus, enterovirus)
Immunofluorescence of nasopharyngeal secretions (or sputum)	Detection of respiratory tract viruses, e.g. respiratory syncytial virus, influenza A and B, adenovirus, indicates infection
Culture of nasopharyngeal secretions (or sputum)	Detection of bacteria or fungi — may be infection or commensal
Serology	Detection of IgM or four-fold rise in IgG on paired samples suggests infection
Lumbar puncture	Glucose, protein, cells, organisms seen or cultured — meningitis

Table 44.9 Lumbar puncture and its significance

Condition	Leucocytes (mm³)	Protein (g/l)	Glucose (mmol/l)	Comments
Normal	< 5 ≥ 75% lymphocytes	0.2–0.45	> 5 (or 75% serum glucose)	
Acute bacterial meningitis	100–10 000 or more; usually 300–2000 PMNs predominate	1–5	Decreased, usually < 4 (or < 66% serum glucose)	Organisms may be seen on Gram stain and recovered by culture Latex agglutination of CSF may be positive
Partially treated bacterial meningitis	5–10 000 PMNs usual but mononuclear cells may predominate if pretreated for extended period of time	1–5	Normal or decreased	Organisms may be seen on Gram stain Latex agglutination of CSF may be positive Pretreatment may render CSF sterile
Viral meningitis or meningo-encephalitis	Rarely > 1000 cells PMNs early but mononuclear cells predominate through most of the course	0.5–2.0	Generally normal; may be decreased to < 4 in some viral diseases, particularly mumps (15–20% of cases)	Herpes simplex virus (HSV) encephalitis is suggested by focal seizures or by focal findings on CT, MRI or EEG HSV and enteroviruses may be detected by PCR of CSF
Brain abscess	5–200 CSF lymphocytes may predominate If abscess ruptures into ventricle, PMNs predominate and cell count may reach > 100 000	0.75–5	Normal unless abscess ruptures into ventricular system	No organisms on smear or culture unless abscess ruptures into ventricular system

(PMNs = polymorphonuclear leucocytes)

Table 44.10 Antibiotics and suggested duration of therapy for acute bacterial meningitis

Patient	Medication	Organism	Days of treatment
Neonate	Cefotaxime/ceftriaxone + Amoxicillin ± Gentamicin	Group B streptococcus (GBS) Escherichia coli Listeria monocytogenes	14 21 21
Infant (1–3 months)	Cefotaxime/ceftriaxone ± Amoxicillin	GBS E. coli Strep. pneumoniae H. influenzae B N. meningitidis	14 21 10–14 7–10 7
Child	Cefotaxime/ceftriaxone ± Dexamethasone	Strep. pneumoniae H. influenzae B N. meningitidis	10–14 7–10 7
Resistant pneumococcus possible	Cefotaxime/ceftriaxone + Vancomycin/rifampicin		10–14
HSV suspected	Aciclovir		21

Chemoprophylaxis

Prevention of secondary cases by eradication of nasal carriage is effective for infections with HiB and *N. meningitidis*. Rifampicin is offered to the index case and:

- All close contacts with *N. meningitidis*: rifampicin 10 mg/kg/day × 2 days or a single injection of ceftriaxone
- Only those contacts under 5 years for HiB: rifampicin 20 mg/kg/day × 4 days.

Complications

- Extent depends on the infecting pathogen. HiB and *Strep. pneumoniae* have poorer neurological outcome than does *N. meningitidis*.
- Early complications include seizures, the development of venous sinus thrombosis, subdural empyema and brain abscess, obstructive hydrocephalus, cerebral infarction and brain parenchymal damage, cranial nerve palsies.
- Later complications include visual and hearing impairment (p. 71) and motor deficits; cerebral palsy, learning disabilities, mental retardation, cortical blindness, continued seizures.

 http://www.inmed.co.uk/resources/resourcepack.htm/

Meningitis Trust

www.meningitis.org

Go to health professionals then doctors in training

Herpes simplex virus (HSV) encephalitis

HSV is the most common treatable cause of encephalitis in the UK, causing direct inflammation of brain tissue.

Presentations of HSV infection

- Neonatal: skin, eye, mouth; encephalitis; disseminated
- Acute encephalitis
- Mild/subacute encephalitis
- Psychiatric syndromes
- Brainstem encephalitis
- Aseptic meningitis
- Benign recurrent meningitis
- Myelitis.

Diagnosis

- Clinical presentation
- CT: diffuse oedema initially, atrophy, parenchymal calcification or cystic encephalomalacia
- MRI: frontobasal and temporal lesions can be seen as hypointense lesions on T1 weighted images and hyperintense on T2 early in disease
- EEG: periodic high-voltage spike/wave activity and slow wave complexes
- CSF: white cell count 5–500, protein < 0.5, HSV PCR (for 1 and 2)
- HSV IgG, IgA, IgM (CSF and blood)
- Viral culture.

Management

Treatment is with aciclovir:
- 0–3 months 20 mg/kg/dose t.d.s.
- 3 m–12 yr: 50 mg/m^2 every 8 hours
  There is no evidence for the use of steroids.

Tonsillitis (see also p. 75)

Fever, sore throat, cervical lymphadenopathy and enlarged inflamed tonsils often with exudates may be caused by:
- Adenovirus
- Enterovirus
- EBV
- Group A streptococcus (GAS) (*Strep. pyogenes*)
- *Corynebacterium diphtheriae*.

Clinical examination cannot distinguish viral from bacterial causes. In primary care most sore throats are self-limiting and do not need antibiotics or throat swabs. Paracetamol or ibuprofen provides symptomatic relief. Those with severe symptoms and signs do improve more quickly with antibiotics, as do those with proven GAS infection. Penicillin V, amoxicillin (or erythromycin) for 10 days is suggested.

Complications of bacterial (GAS) tonsillitis include:
- Cervical abscess
- Scarlet fever: pharyngitis, erythematous 'sandpaper' rash, strawberry tongue
- Rheumatic fever: following tonsillitis.

Influenza

- Caused by an RNA virus. Influenza A and B circulate within the UK. The antigenic structure changes slightly each year; hence new vaccines are produced each year.
- Respiratory pathogen: fever, headache, aches and pains, coryza, sore throat, cough.
- Can cause myositis, pneumonia or sepsis, especially in infants.
- Secondary bacterial infection common: otitis media, pneumonia.
- Diagnosis by immunofluorescence of nasopharyngeal secretions, virus culture or serology.
- Zanamivir and oseltamivir decrease severity and duration of symptoms from influenza A or B by 1 day. Oseltamivir is 60–90% effective in preventing illness from influenza when used prophylactically.

Allergy

Basic science

Atopy

Atopy nowadays describes a hereditary predisposition to produce IgE antibody against common environmental allergens in a type 1 hypersensitivity reaction (Fig. 44.9). In sensitized individuals contact with allergen may result in respiratory, cardiovascular, mucocutaneous and gastrointestinal manifestations, and when severe can be life-threatening (anaphylaxis).

Anaphylactoid reactions are identical to anaphylaxis other than not being IgE-mediated, e.g. reactions to radio contrast media, non-steroidal anti-inflammatory drugs (NSAIDs) etc.

Immunological responses to allergens

Central to an allergic response is T-cell differentiation (Th2) to cells that produce appropriate stimulatory

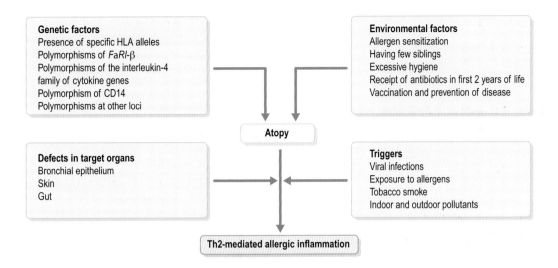

Fig. 44.9 Factors influencing the development of atopy
(HLA = human leucocyte antigen)

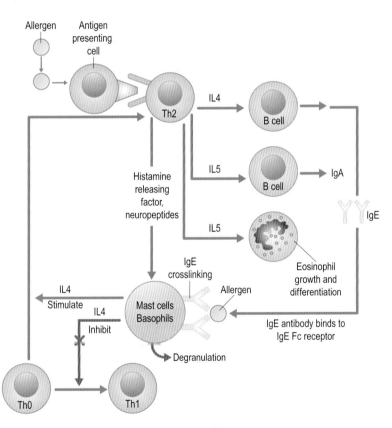

Allergen Antigen presenting cell

MODULE SEVEN

Fig. 44.10 **Immunological response to allergens**
(IL = interleukin)

cytokines (IL-4) and promote class switching of antigen-specific B cells for the production of IgE.

When an allergen is encountered by an antigen-presenting cell (APC), it is taken up and carried from the periphery to T cells in the local lymph node. Depending on the amount of antigen, interaction of T cell with APC, relative production of IL-4, IL-12, IFN-γ and the presence of CpG (cytidine-phosphate-guanosine) repeats in the microbial DNA, differentiation to Th1 or Th2 occurs. Allergen is then presented to this Th2 cell via an allergen-specific B cell and this is stimulated to produce IgE antibody (Fig. 44.10).

These IgE-specific antibodies bind to IgE receptors on the surface of mast cells. On re-exposure to the same allergen, it will bind to two adjacent IgE molecules on the mast cell and basophils (cross-linking), leading to its degranulation and the release of pharmacological mediators inducing vasodilatation and inflammation (Fig. 44.11).

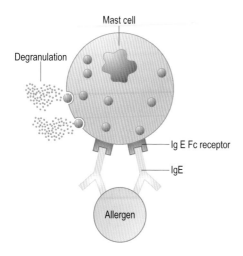

Mast cell

Degranulation

Ig E Fc receptor

IgE

Allergen

Fig. 44.11 **Type 1 hypersensitivity**

Cells and mediators

Mast cells

Mast cells are found mainly in the epithelial tissue of the respiratory and gastrointestinal tract, and of skin. They include preformed substances stored in granules of mast cells and basophils (histamine, tryptase, heparin, chymase and cytokines), or newly synthesized mediators, like derivatives of arachidonic acid metabolism (prostaglandins and leucotrienes). These are released on stimulation. They precipitate:

- Smooth muscle contraction
- Vasodilatation
- Increased vascular permeability
- Mucus hypersecretion.

Histamine is considered to be the prime mediator of anaphylactic shock through its binding to receptors.

Eosinophils

Eosinophilia is usually present in atopy. Granules contain proteins mediating:

- Damage to epithelial cells
- Degranulation of basophil and mast cells
- Airway hyper-responsiveness
- Blocking of muscarinic receptors, increasing acetylcholine and resulting in airway hyper-reaction.

Effects of mast cell mediators

See Table 44.11.

Late phase response

On exposure to allergens atopic people develop immediate hypersensitivity, which may, depending on the amount of allergen, be followed by a late phase reaction after 6–9 hours.

Table 44.11 **Mast cell mediators**

Physiological effect	Clinical presentation	Potential complication
Capillary leak	Urticaria Angioedema Cutaneous Laryngeal Hypotension	Respiratory arrest Shock
Mucosal oedema	Laryngeal oedema Asthma Rhinitis	Respiratory arrest Respiratory arrest
Smooth muscle contraction	Asthma Abdominal pain	Respiratory arrest

Table 44.12 **Immunological response**

Immediate type	Delayed type
Skin wheal and flare within minutes	Within hours
Nose sneezing, running nose	Sustained blockage
Chest wheezing	Further wheezing

Eosinophils and neutrophils accumulate, then CD4 and basophils infiltrate. Depending on the target organ involved, a late phase reaction can be provoked by a mast cell or T cell. If skin is involved mast cells provoke both immediate and late phases, while when lungs are involved T cells are responsible (Table 44.12).

Allergic rhinitis

Clinical features include sneezing, nasal congestion, stuffiness, rhinorrhoea, cough, itching of the nose, eyes and throat, sinus pressure and epistaxis. Rhinitis is induced by specific allergy, often pollen (seasonal rhinitis; hay fever), animals or house dust mite.

Symptoms and signs include large pale turbinates, nasal polyps, allergic salute, eosinophils in nasal smear, blood eosinophilia, raised IgE, and a positive blood IgE or skin prick test to allergen.

Management includes avoidance of allergens if known, oral and nasal antihistamines, nasal steroids, cromoglicate and oral steroids. Immunotherapy can be useful in severe pollen hay fever and may be offered in specialist allergy centres.

Problem-orientated topic:

atopy

John is a 6-year-old boy who has been referred by his GP to the children's outpatient clinic with a history of recurrent episodes of 'nettle rash', which seem to appear after some meals and settle with antihistamine.

On reviewing his medical records it is noticed that he was admitted last year because of an acute attack of respiratory distress associated with difficulty breathing and cough but no rash. His chest examination on that admission revealed rhonchi bilaterally and diminished breath sounds; the CXR showed hyperinflation but no evidence of infection. He was treated with bronchodilators, oxygen and short-course steroids and made a good recovery.

He had eczema as a baby, but this has improved over the last few years and now he is troubled only with patches on flexor areas of his limbs.

Q1. How would you assess the cause of the rash?

Q2. What family and social history might be relevant?

Q3. What treatment could you offer?

Q4. How will you advise John and his parents about how to manage his diet?

Q1. How would you assess the cause of the rash?

Urticaria is a cutaneous vascular reaction characterized by sudden but transient appearance of erythematous wheals, often itchy. These usually disappear in 20 minutes to 3 hours but may continue for up to 48 hours. They are often described as nettle rash. Recurrent episodes for > 6 weeks indicate 'chronic urticaria' and may be associated with angioedema: local soft tissue swelling, most often of the face, eyelids, hands or feet.

Urticaria is caused by extravasation of plasma into the dermis, while angioedema is subcutaneous oedema resulting in deep swelling. Immunologically, it may be IgE-mediated (drugs/food/insect venom) but can also be non-IgE-mediated (infection, physical) (Table 44.13).

Q2. What family and social history might be relevant?

Children with IgE-mediated diseases are 'atopic'. There is often a family history of atopy. If one parent is atopic, the risk to the child is roughly 25%; if both parents are atopic, the risk rises to 50%. Atopic diseases include atopic dermatitis, asthma, hay fever and allergic rhinitis, urticaria and food allergies.

Table 44.13 Urticaria

Type	Precipitant
Infectious	Follows infection; streptococci, Epstein–Barr virus, hepatitis A, B and C, enteroviruses, adenoviruses
Sting bites	Bee, wasp, scorpion, spider
Drugs and food	Peanuts, nuts, milk, eggs, wheat, fish Antibiotics
Physical	Cold, heat, pressure, sunlight or vibration
Papular	In contact with fleas or mites; usually toddlers; resolves in 6–12 months
Secondary to underlying systemic disease	Connective tissue, autoimmune, thyroid or coeliac disease
Idiopathic	Unknown precipitant; frequent

Q3. What treatment could you offer?

- Establishing the precipitant, if possible
- Avoidance of the allergens where possible
- Antihistamine as required for acute treatment or regularly for prevention (second generation long-acting); may use higher doses
- Steroids: local or systemic depending on the severity of the disease
- Chronic urticaria: combination of H_1-blockers with H_2-blockers or leucotriene antagonists may help.

Q4. How will you advise John and his parents about how to manage his diet?

Food allergy

The terms shown in Box 44.11 need to be considered and understood.

Adverse reactions to food consist of any abnormal reaction resulting from eating or swallowing even a tiny amount of a particular food (Fig. 44.12).

The major food allergens are water-soluble glyco-proteins, are generally resistant to proteolysis and are heat-stable (Box 44.12 and Table 44.14). Sensitization to food allergens occurs in the gastrointestinal tract, or in the respiratory tract with inhalant allergens.

Food allergy is a world-wide problem and like other atopic disorders it appears to be on the increase. It remains a leading cause of anaphylaxis treated in emergency departments and the public has become increasingly aware of the problem. Around 6% of infants and children experience food allergy reaction in the first 3 years of life, and 33% of children with moderate to severe atopic disorders have IgE-mediated food allergy.

Most infants and young children outgrow milk (90%) and egg (75%) allergy by 2–4 years. Around

BOX 44.11 Food allergy: terminology

Food intolerance

- Non-allergic food hypersensitivities include any physiological response such as metabolic disorders, e.g. lactose intolerance, coeliac disease, dietary protein enterocolitis

Food allergy

- Adverse immunological response usually due to IgE, occasionally non-IgE-mediated immune mechanisms

Toxic

- Toxic or pharmacological contaminants inherent in a food

Food aversion

- Where patients are convinced that they are allergic to food but when challenged with food no reactions appear

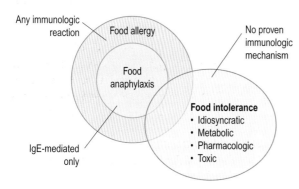

Fig. 44.12 **Adverse food reactions**

20% of young children with a peanut allergy within the first 5 years of life may outgrow this; however, older children tend to be allergic for life.

Occasionally there may be cross-reactions:

- Peanuts: soybeans, green beans and peas
- Wheat: rye
- Cow's milk: soya, goat's milk
- Kiwi fruit: avocado, banana, raw potato, chestnut, latex
- Pollen: hazelnuts, green apples, peaches and almonds.

Clinical features of food allergies

See Table 44.15.

Diagnosis

History is most important and should cover:

- Food suspected to have provoked the reaction
- Quantity of the food ingested
- Length of time between ingestion and development of symptoms

BOX 44.12 Major food allergens

In children

- Milk
- Egg
- Peanut
- Tree nut
- Fish
- Soya
- Wheat

In adults

- Peanut
- Tree nut
- Fish
- Shellfish

Table 44.14 **Food allergens**

Food	Prevalence	Allergen
Milk	2.5–7.5%	Bos d3, Bos d5
Egg	1.3%	Gal d1, Gal d2, Gal d3
Peanut	0.8%	Arah1, Arah 2, Arah 3
Fish	0.1%	Gad c1
Tree nut	0.2%	

BOX 44.13 Skill: allergen skin prick tests

- Are highly reproducible and are often utilized to screen patients with suspected IgE-mediated food allergies
- A food allergen eliciting a wheal at least 3 mm greater than the negative control is considered positive. Anything else is considered negative
- A negative skin test confirms the absence of an IgE-mediated reaction (overall negative predictive accuracy is > 95%)
- A positive skin prick test to food indicates the possibility that the patient has symptomatic reactivity to that specific food (overall the positive predictive accuracy is less than 50%)

- Description of the symptoms provoked
- Similar symptoms developed on other occasions when the food was eaten
- Other factors, e.g. exercise
- Length of time since the last reaction.

Investigations should include:

- Skin prick test (Box 44.13)
- Allergen-specific IgE
- Food elimination
- Food challenge.

Management of food allergy

- Food allergen avoidance: advice from dietitian
- Medication:
  - Antihistamine
  - Adrenaline (epinephrine) autoinjector (Epipen or Anapen) *with training*
  - For reactions involving respiratory involvement: α-agonist effect causes peripheral vasodilatation, while β-agonist effect causes bronchodilatation
  - Oral corticosteroid
- Optimization of asthma control
- Management plan outlining indications for above
- 'Medic Alert' identification
- School support and education
- Psychological support.

Anaphylaxis

Anaphylaxis is a severe life-threatening allergic reaction. Symptoms can include urticaria, swelling (especially of the lips and face), difficulty breathing (because of either swelling in the throat or an asthmatic reaction), vomiting, diarrhoea, cramping, and in anaphylactic shock, a fall in blood pressure, circulatory collapse and death.

Causes

See Box 44.14.

BOX 44.14 Common causes of anaphylaxis

- Foods: peanuts, tree nuts (almond, brazil nut, hazelnut), milk, egg, fish, shellfish, pulses, kiwi fruit
- Bee and wasp stings
- Drugs: antibiotics (especially penicillin IV), anaesthetic agents, aspirin, NSAIDs
- Latex rubber

BOX 44.15 Conditions that may mimic anaphylaxis

- Vasovagal syncope
- Cardiogenic and hypovolaemic shock
- Status asthmaticus
- Seizure disorder
- Systemic mastocytosis
- Hereditary or acquired angioedema
- Panic attacks
- Drug overdose
- 'Red man syndrome' following vancomycin infusion

Investigations

Diagnosis of anaphylaxis in acute settings is based on a brief directed history of presenting symptoms and evaluation to focus on manifestations that are likely to be life-threatening. History should include questions regarding common causative factors (Box 44.14) and past history of atopy and anaphylaxis, and ruling out conditions that may mimic anaphylaxis (Box 44.15).

The only immediate test that is useful at the time of reaction is mast cell tryptase. It is only raised transiently; therefore blood should be taken when it peaks at about an hour after the onset of reaction.

Principles of management

1. Anaphylaxis is a clinical diagnosis; diagnose the presence or likely presence rapidly.
2. Place the patient in a recumbent position and elevate the lower extremities.
3. Assess and maintain the airway. An oropharyngeal airway device may be needed to keep the airways patent.
4. Assess and support breathing with provision of 100% oxygen. A nebulized β_2-agonist agent, like salbutamol, may be needed to treat bronchospasm.

Table 44.15 **Clinical features of food allergies**

Type	IgE-mediated	Cell-mediated	Mixed IgE-mediated
Gastrointestinal	Oral allergy syndrome, GI anaphylaxis	Food protein-induced enterocolitis (cow's milk protein intolerance), proctocolitis, enteropathy syndrome, coeliac disease	Allergic eosinophilic oesophagitis, allergic eosinophilic gastroenteritis
Cutaneous	Urticaria, angioedema, morbilliform rashes, flushing	Contact dermatitis, dermatitis	
Respiratory	Acute rhinoconjunctivitis, bronchospasm		
Generalized	Anaphylactic shock		

5. Assess circulation (heart rate, capillary refill and blood pressure). Fluids — 20 ml/kg of normal saline (0.9% saline), 5% human albumin solution or Ringer's lactate solution — may be used as fluid resuscitation to treat hypotension.

6. *Adrenaline (epinephrine) is the most important drug for anaphylaxis* and should be given intramuscularly if airway compromise or circulatory collapse is suspected. Dose: 0.01 ml/kg of 1:1000 aqueous solution, to a maximum of 0.3–0.5 ml (subcutaneous or intramuscularly only). If necessary, repeat every 15 minutes, up to two doses.

7. Give 0.2 mg/kg of intravenous chlorphenamine once the emergency measures described above have been instigated.

8. Administer 4 mg/kg of hydrocortisone or approximately 250 mg intravenously to reduce the risk of protracted or recurring anaphylaxis. Further doses could be repeated 6-hourly.

9. In refractory cases not responding to adrenaline because a β-adrenergic blocker is complicating management, glucagon, 1 mg intravenously as a bolus, may be useful. A continuous infusion of glucagon, 1–5 mg/hour, may be given if required.

10. Severe cases may need transfer to the intensive care unit, while less severe cases may need a period of observation before discharge.

11. All children with anaphylactic reactions should be referred to a paediatrician for an outpatient clinic assessment, education, further investigations and follow-up.

An important aspect of treatment is prevention of further events, which includes education of the patient regarding strategies for allergen avoidance and being aware of cross-reacting allergens, particularly nuts and drugs.

Adrenaline (epinephrine) autoinjector pen training for the patient, parent and school is also important for success of future treatment.

Patients prone to anaphylaxis should also receive information on wearing 'Medic Alert' bracelets.

 http://www.resus.org.uk/pages/anafig2.pdf

Anaphylaxis, guidance for first responders

Further reading

Maitland K et al 2005 Management of severe malaria in children: proposed guidelines for the United Kingdom. British Medical Journal 331:337–343

For use of adrenaline see Drug and Therapeutics Bulletin 2003; 41(3):21–24

Edited by Michael Hall

The child in hospital

MODULE

EIGHT

Michael J. Marsh, Jason Barling

Care of the critically ill child

LEARNING OUTCOMES

By the end of this chapter you should:

- Understand the basis of physiological control of the circulation and organ perfusion
- Understand circulatory responses to insults
- Understand the factors influencing blood pressure and cardiac output
- Understand the causes and management of the acute respiratory distress syndrome.

You should also:

- Know how to recognize a severely ill child
- Know the principles of cardiopulmonary management and be able to perform this effectively
- Know the causes and management of coma
- Know the causes and management of shock.
- Have attended a life support course such as Advanced Paediatric Life Support (APLS), Paediatric Advanced Life Support (PALS) etc.

MODULE EIGHT

Basic science

Control of the circulation

The circulation is vital for providing tissues with the nutrients they need and for taking away their waste products so that they may function optimally. In order to understand the control of the circulation it is first important to remind ourselves of some fundamental basic facts about its physical characteristics.

The flow of blood (Q) in the circulation is dependent on two factors:

- Pressure difference (ΔP)
- Resistance (R).

They are related by Ohm's Law:

Q = ΔP/R

From this it is clear that a pressure drop across a blood vessel is required for forward flow and that the lower the resistance, the higher the flow.

The most important determining factor in vessel resistance is the radius (r) of that vessel. This is described by Poiseuille's Law:

Q = πΔPr⁴/8ηl

Simplified, this expresses the fact that blood flow is proportional to the radius of the vessel to the power of 4. When we look at the vasculature we see that the arterioles have a very muscular wall that enables them to change diameter and they therefore provide a very powerful method of controlling blood flow.

In order to assess circulation the measurement of arterial pressure is crucial, as it is this pressure gradient to a negligible venous pressure that enables forward flow and tissue perfusion. The elastic nature of arteries reduces the pressure changes that would occur between systole and diastole and enables continuous flow. The pressure difference between systole and diastole is known as the pulse pressure. The blood pressure changes from the aortic root to the arterioles and therefore the concept of a single measurement that represents the driving force of the arterial tree is known as the mean pressure. This is not simply the average of the systolic and diastolic pressures but can be approximated by the formula:

Mean pressure = diastolic pressure + ⅓ pulse pressure

The characteristic of veins is that they are normally partially collapsed and are therefore able to distend (compliance) and act as a store for up to 60% of the circulating volume. This can be very useful when there is acute loss of blood but can be a disadvantage when the right side of the heart is not working effectively. Because of their low resistance they require very little pressure difference to enable venous return. They also make use of non-cardiac pumps such as skeletal muscle and the negative intrathoracic pressure effect of respiration to improve venous return and subsequently cardiac output.

Local control of blood flow by tissues

Tissues control their own circulation in order to achieve metabolic demands. The mechanism behind this can be divided into acute and chronic types.

Acute

- *Vasodilator theory*. When tissue metabolism increases, blood, oxygen and nutrient supply reduces. A vasodilator substance (lactic acid, CO_2, K^+, adenosine) is released by tissues, causing dilatation of the arterioles.
- *Oxygen demand theory*. Tissue is very sensitive to oxygen supply and when levels decrease it is thought that precapillary sphincters relax and encourage blood supply.
- *Autoregulation*. Tissues respond to a sudden change in blood pressure to enable continuous blood flow. This may be partly explained by the above-mentioned metabolic theories. It may also be explained by the response of the vessel to sudden stretch, which is to contract and, in the absence of stretch, to relax (myogenic theory).

Chronic

The body adapts to long-term changes in circulation by altering tissue vascularity, so that if metabolic demand increases in a particular tissue, so does the vascularity. Many angiogenic factors have been found to enable this, such as endothelial cell growth factor and fibroblast growth factor.

Neural control of blood flow in tissues

The sympathetic part of the autonomic nervous system plays a powerful role in the acute regulation of the circulation. This is done through specific fibres that innervate the heart and blood vessels. The sympathetic fibres secrete noradrenaline (norepinephrine), which causes vasoconstriction of both arterioles and veins as well as increasing heart rate and contractility.

The parasympathetic fibres play less of a role through fibres that innervate blood vessels of the head and body viscera and the heart. These fibres secrete acetylcholine, which causes vasodilatation and reduction in heart rate.

Blood pressure regulation

Acute

We have seen how the body goes to extraordinary lengths to maintain blood pressure in order to provide tissues with the nutrients they require. There have to be feedback mechanisms to enable coordination of these systems. The most acute of these are the baroreceptors. Located in the carotid sinus and aortic arch, they respond to stretch and send impulses to the vasomotor centre in the brainstem, which controls autonomic stimulation. They provide excellent acute control but reset themselves to the new blood pressure if it is sustained for more than 1–2 days. As well as these baroreceptors, there are chemoreceptors that exist in the carotid body and aortic arch, which respond to oxygen lack, CO_2 and acid excess. They also stimulate the vasomotor response to increase arterial pressure. The vasomotor centre itself is an intensely powerful controller of blood pressure and the strongest response is seen when it is subjected to ischaemia (i.e. cerebral ischaemia) itself. The stimulus is so strong that other organs and tissues in the body are potentially sacrificed. It may also be influenced by higher centres in the brain, as is seen in the rise in temperature that leads to vasodilatation.

Intermediate

Three mechanisms exist for intermediate control:

- *Transcapillary volume shift*. As blood pressure rises, fluid moves into the extracellular space and vice versa. The extracellular space thus provides a fluid reserve for the vascular system.
- *Vascular stress relaxation*. As the veins are stretched they expand slowly, absorbing any change in pressure over 10–60 minutes. Thus when the pressure falls the veins are able to return the pressure to normal over a similar time frame.
- *Renin–angiotensin system*. This is the more familiar method by which the kidneys start to regulate blood pressure. The juxtaglomerular cells of the kidney secrete an enzyme, renin, in response to a fall in blood pressure. Renin then converts angiotensinogen to angiotensin I in the plasma. Angiotensin I is converted to angiotensin II in the lung; this is a powerful vasoconstrictor and directly causes the kidney to retain salt and water. Angiotensin II also stimulates the adrenals to secrete aldosterone, causing more salt and water retention.

Long-term

The kidney regulates the fluid balance in the body, responding to changes in blood pressure by varying urine output. This mechanism is mediated by two hormones:

- *Aldosterone*. This hormone is secreted in the adrenal cortex in response to angiotensin II and III, leading to salt and water retention. Aldosterone takes 2–3 hours to be stimulated and almost a week to reach peak effect.
- *Antidiuretic hormone (ADH)*. Secreted in the hypothalamus in response to reduced atrial stretch receptor response, this hormone then acts on the kidney to promote water reabsorption. In high concentrations it also causes strong vasoconstriction; hence its other name of vasopressin. The atrial stretch receptor is now

known to produce a hormone called atrial natriuretic peptide, which promotes salt and water excretion and counteracts the effects of aldosterone and ADH.

Cardiac output

An understanding of the concept of cardiac output is essential to understanding the control of the circulation, for it is the cardiac output that ensures a sustainable blood pressure and therefore tissue perfusion. It can be described in different ways:

Cardiac output = heart rate × stroke volume
Cardiac output = arterial pressure/total peripheral resistance

Different methods also exist to measure it. The Fick method uses the principle that by looking at the oxygen consumption (O_2/min) of a particular organ and then measuring the venous (O_2ven) and arterial (O_2art) oxygen concentrations, one can estimate the cardiac output (CO):

$$CO = \frac{O_2/min}{O_2art - O_2ven}$$

The heart needs to be able to respond to the changing demands of the body, whether they are physiological or pathological. Control of cardiac output can be divided into intracardiac and extracardiac mechanisms.

Intracardiac mechanisms

These rely on the physical properties of the cardiac muscle. When this muscle is stretched, it responds with a more forceful contraction up until a certain point. This relationship is well described by the Frank–Starling curve. It plays particular importance in ensuring that the left and right ventricles perform equally and fluid does not accumulate in the lungs.

Extracardiac mechanisms

These rely on the autonomic nervous system, as already described. The sympathetic system increases rate and contractility, thus increasing output, and the parasympathetic reduces the heart rate.

It is quickly apparent that the body has many ways of controlling the circulation, which on initial inspection seem quite complex. However, by applying basic principles, one can see that they are all working towards the same goal, that of tissue perfusion. In the approach to the care of the critically ill child it is therefore important that there is an appreciation of the circulatory status and methods by which it may be supported.

Recognition and management of the seriously ill child

All paediatric senior house officers should have attended APLS, PALS or a similar course.

In this section an introduction will be given describing the importance of a structured approach to the seriously ill child. The outcome of cardiac arrest in children is poor; therefore, in order to reduce both morbidity and mortality, it is essential that early recognition is achieved and appropriate action taken. The primary assessment systematically looks at respiratory, cardiovascular and neurological status and addresses problems as they are found. A secondary assessment is then performed, looking at each system in turn and instituting emergency treatment.

Primary assessment

- A (Airway):
  - Look for chest movement
  - Listen for additional sounds, e.g. wheeze, stridor etc.
  - Feel for breath
- B (Breathing):
  - Effort, e.g. rate, accessory muscles
  - Efficacy, e.g. oxygen saturations
  - Effect, e.g. heart rate, skin colour, conscious level (*N.B. Severe respiratory distress may present with little sign of increased effort due to exhaustion. This is a preterminal sign and requires prompt intervention.*)
- C (Circulation):
  - Heart rate
  - Pulse volume
  - Capillary refill time (CRT)
  - Blood pressure (*N.B. Hypotension is a preterminal sign.*)
- D (Disability):
  - Level of consciousness (AVPU/Glasgow Coma Score, p. 308)
  - Posture
  - Pupils
  - Blood glucose.

It is essential that appropriate resuscitation is carried out during the primary survey before proceeding to a secondary assessment.

Secondary assessment

This aims to take a focused history and institute further emergency treatment whilst developing a differential diagnosis. It requires a full physical examination from head to toe. If there is any clinical deterioration during this procedure, then the primary assessment must be repeated.

Monitoring and post-resuscitation management

As part of your recognition and management of critically ill children, whatever the underlying diagnosis, you need to make optimal use of the monitoring equipment available to you in the hospital environment. It is important to keep the principles in Box 45.1 in mind at all times.

Outside of the intensive care unit, the high-dependency unit or the emergency department, the following physiological variables should be assessed regularly:

- Respiratory rate
- Heart rate
- Non-invasive blood pressure (NIBP)
- Oxygen saturations
- Electrocardiogram (ECG)
- Temperature.

At the time of initial assessment of a critically ill child it is important to take note of each of these variables and relate them to the standardized airway, breathing, circulation (ABC) approach of resuscitation guidelines.

Clinical observations form an integral part of the assessment (Box 45.2), along with the information yielded from the monitoring equipment. Therefore, whilst assessing 'airway' and 'breathing' using the respiratory rate, you should look at the respiratory

---

BOX 45.1 Principles when using equipment

- Be familiar with the equipment available where you work
- Have basic troubleshooting skills for common equipment
- Always remember that a machine/monitor can give incorrect information
- Be aware that you are more likely to question abnormal results, e.g. accept 'normal BP' on non-invasive blood pressure monitoring, when it is reading falsely high
- Equipment should be fit for its purpose
- Trends are generally more important/useful than spot measurement
- Equipment will not work if it is not plugged in, switched on and connected to the patient
- The most common mistake made is to use the incorrect cuff when measuring non-invasive blood pressure (NIBP)

BOX 45.2 Principle of management

Do not stop looking at the patient when using monitors.

effort, effectiveness of breathing, signs of increased work of breathing and respiratory distress, as well as effect of respiration (resulting oxygen saturation).

The key skill is to relate the initial observations and subsequent trends to normal age-appropriate values (Table 45.1) and to know where to access a reference chart rapidly.

After initial assessment, resuscitation and emergency treatment it is important to keep noting the observations and thinking in terms of the underlying trends, e.g. a respiratory rate that settles or steadily rises. The fail-safe measure is to make sure that there is a way to have the regularly documented observations available for review. If they are displayed electronically, keep checking; if they are charted, keep reviewing. You must constantly ask the question:

- Are things getting better/responding to treatments?
  or
- Are things deteriorating and do I need to escalate treatment and ensure senior involvement?

These principles, together with experience and knowledge, can be combined with the systematic resuscitation training courses (APLS/EPLS/neonatal life support (NLS)) to help clinicians improve their clinical skills and enable them not only to recognize but also to treat the critically ill child safely and effectively (Boxes 45.3 and 45.4).

Acute respiratory distress syndrome

In 1967 Ashbaugh described the clinical syndrome of acute respiratory distress syndrome (ARDS). This is an acute clinical condition of hypoxic respiratory failure rather than a collection of discrete diseases characterized by severe hypoxaemia, tachypnoea and diffuse bilateral pulmonary infiltrates seen on chest X-ray. Though with the advent of modern intensive care it became recognized as a serious problem

BOX 45.3 Specific comments on monitoring the ill child

Saturations

- The technology keeps on advancing; there is less and less artefact or failure to pick up a signal. If you are not able to obtain a signal, be concerned

Respiratory rate

- Abnormal extremes are commonly ignored to everyone's peril

ECG

- Besides noting the rate, consider the rhythm and seek expert advice if uncertain

Capillary refill

- Technique is important. It is best to use the central body (over the sternum). If you use an arm/leg, you must elevate the limb, press firmly for 5 seconds before release and count consistently (use a watch). If you use this technique, a capillary refill time (CRT) > 5 seconds indicates an inadequate cardiac output

Temperature

- Using the axillary temperature as an indicator of central temperature has its pitfalls; true central (oesophageal or rectal) temperature is frequently higher. Tempa Dots miss hypothermia

BOX 45.4 Warning

- Resuscitation training is not a substitute for knowledge and experience
- Clinicians must constantly reflect on their clinical skills, including post-resuscitation management and stabilization

with a high mortality, morbidity and considerable healthcare costs, there was a lack of information as to definition and incidence. In 1992 the American–European consensus conference produced a clearer definition and devised the term 'acute lung injury' (ALI) (Table 45.2). Hypoxaemia is defined using Pa/FiO_2 ratio, the illness must be acute and there must be no left atrial hypertension (low pulmonary capillary

Table 45.1 **Age-appropriate normal values for common physiological variables**

	Newborn	1 month–1 year	2–5 years	5–12 years	> 12 years
Respiratory rate	40–60	30–40	24–30	20–24	12–20
Heart rate	100–180	80–160	60–100	60–90	50–90
Systolic BP	60–90	80–105	95–110	10–110	110–130
Diastolic BP	20–60	50–65	55–65	55–70	65–80
Mean BP	35–50	65–80	65–80	70–85	80–95

Table 45.2 **American–European Consensus Definitions**

	ALI	ARDS
Pa/FiO$_2$ ratio	39.5 kPa (300 mmHg)	< 26.7 kPa (200 mmHg)
Chest X-ray	Bilateral infiltrates	Bilateral infiltrates
Pulmonary capillary wedge pressure	< 18 mmHg	< 18 mmHg

wedge pressure, PCWP) to exclude hypoxaemia due to pulmonary oedema from heart failure. ARDS and ALI account for about 5% of admissions to paediatric intensive care in the UK. ALI covers the milder end of the spectrum of hypoxic respiratory failure.

Pathophysiology

ALI and ARDS are caused by an acute inflammatory reaction in the lungs that is complex and follows either a direct injury to the lungs or an indirect 'non-pulmonary' injury (Box 45.5). The exact process varies depending on the underlying cause; in common there is damage and injury to the alveolar unit at the endothelium, interstitium and epithelium. For the sake of simplicity it is useful to summarize the current knowledge of both conditions as one clinical entity.

BOX 45.5 Conditions associated with or leading to ALI and ARDS

Direct: pulmonary
- Pneumonia
- Aspiration
- Lung contusion
- Inhalation injury
- Near-drowning
- Emboli

Indirect: non-pulmonary
- Sepsis
- Massive transfusion
- Pancreatitis
- Trauma
- Traumatic brain injury
- Post-cardiopulmonary bypass

Endothelium

The endothelium is undoubtedly pivotal to the process and may be damaged and generally activated in a variety of ways. Swollen injured endothelial cells release proinflammatory cytokines, including interleukin (IL)-8. Neutrophils become activated and attracted to the endothelium, passing through the endothelial cell junctions, where gaps have developed into the inter-stitium. The activated endothelium has important functions, including the control of inflammation and coagulation, regulation of local blood flow and control of cell and fluid migration.

Interstitium

The interstitium becomes swollen with a combination of oedematous fluid leaking from the vascular space and increased activated inflammatory cells, particularly migrating neutrophils. These neutrophils are active and produce a range of highly active substances, including proteases such as neutrophil elastase. Fibroblasts also become activated and secrete IL-8 and procollagen into the interstitial space. All of these disrupt the integrity and disturb the normal close relationship of the endothelium to the alveolar space, thus impairing gas exchange.

Epithelium

Type I pneumocytes form the majority of the alveolar surface as a layer of thin cells in close proximity to the basement membrane. In health type II pneumocytes produce and release surfactant that forms a monolayer, facilitating gas exchange. In ARDS and ALI there is accumulation of protein-rich oedema fluid in the alveolar space (pulmonary oedema), and there is necrosis and apoptosis of type I cells and proliferation of type II cells. There is an increase in alveolar macrophages that are activated by migration inhibition factor (MIF). Macrophages release both pro- and anti-inflammatory cytokines, including IL-8, IL-6, IL-10 and IL-1 and growth factors TGF-α. It is thought that macrophages amplify inflammation as well as playing a role in resolution of lung injury via a variety of processes, including binding and internalizing proteases, modulating repair process via transforming growth factor (TGF-α), which stimulates endothelial growth and fibrosis. Neutrophil numbers are massively increased in the alveolar space and, once activated, release leucotrienes, reactive oxidants, proteases and platelet activating factor (PAF). As a result of the inflammation and protein-rich oedema fluid there is inactivation of surfactant and severe impairment of gas exchange.

Prognosis

In adults the mortality has steadily fallen over the last 20 years but is still in the region of 30–40%. In the childhood population mortality is also relatively high and in British paediatric intensive care units (PICUs) it is in the region of 6%.

Management

This is still essentially supportive, despite all the advances in knowledge of the pathophysiology (Boxes 45.6, 45.7

and 45.8). There are no specific treatments as yet available, though identification of the underlying condition is important, especially if it is infective or ongoing, as might occur in aspiration of gastrointestinal contents due to severe reflux.

Coma

Problem-orientated topic:

coma

Cameron, a 9-year-old boy, is brought to the accident and emergency department by ambulance. Earlier that day he saw his GP, complaining of general malaise. A viral illness was diagnosed and symptomatic treatment recommended. Over the afternoon he gradually became less responsive, only partially rousing when spoken to by his mother. She called a 999 ambulance when he became unresponsive.

Q1. What immediate actions should be taken?
Q2. How can you assess conscious level in a child?
Q3. What is the differential diagnosis and what key questions in the history will help you make the diagnosis?
Q4. What key investigations will make the diagnosis?

Q1. What immediate actions should be taken?

Cameron has presented with a decreased level of consciousness and represents a life-threatening emergency. As such the child should be approached with the standard resuscitation techniques, along with some special additional points (Box 45.9).

Q2. How can you assess conscious level in a child?

Unless you assess conscious level on an everyday basis using the Glasgow Coma Score (GCS, Table 45.3), this can be difficult to apply accurately even in adults. It is complicated further in children and various adaptations of the GCS are in use (Adelaide adaptation, Box 45.10). This has lead to the widespread use of the AVPU scale, which offers simplicity and accuracy. In assessing conscious level using either GCS or AVPU, you should also note pupil size and reaction.

In essence, when assessing patients who are in coma, you need to perform a 'rapid neurological assessment' (Box 45.11); this will enable you to make the correct decision regarding intubation (Box 45.12) and to communicate effectively with other relevant specialists.

Table 45.3 **The adapted Glasgow Coma Score**

Activity	Best response	Score
Eye opening	Spontaneous	4
	To verbal stimuli	3
	To pain	2
	None	1
Verbal	Orientated	5
	Confused	4
	Inappropriate words	3
	Non-specific sounds	2
	None	1
Motor	Follows commands	6
	Localizes pain	5
	Withdraws in response to pain	4
	Flexion in response to pain	3
	Extension in response to pain	2
	None	1

Maximum score 15
Minimum score 3
Score ≤ 8 indicates coma needing intubation

BOX 45.10 AVPU Scale

- *A*wake
- Responds to *v*oice
- Responds to *p*ain
- *U*nresponsive
- Pupil size and reaction

BOX 45.11 Rapid neurological assessment

- Assess conscious level: AVPU or GCS
- Posture
- Pupil size + pupil reaction

BOX 45.12 Key levels indicating need for intubation

- P or lower on AVPU scale
- ≤ 8 on GCS

Q3. What is the differential diagnosis and what key questions in the history will help you make the diagnosis?

See Box 45.13.

Q4. What key investigations will make the diagnosis?

The key investigations are those that will help you identify the treatable causes rapidly whilst also looking

---

BOX 45.13 Differential diagnosis of coma

Hypoxic and ischaemic
- Out-of-hospital arrest
- Other event

Vascular
- Sudden-onset headache
- Abrupt loss of consciousness

Traumatic
- Episode of trauma
- Non-accidental injury — suspect

Toxic or poisoning
- Assess drug history, bizarre behaviour

Metabolic
- Polyuria and polydipsia
- Odour in diabetic ketoacidosis

Infective
- Signs and symptoms of infection

Post-ictal
- Seizures

Space-occupying lesion
- Symptoms of early morning headache

BOX 45.14 Key investigations

- Blood glucose: hypo- or hyperglycaemia
- Toxicology
- Blood cultures ± lumbar puncture (*Caution: do not perform if ↑ intracranial pressure*)
- Neuroimaging
- CT scan
- MR scan (MR angiography (MRA) or MR venography (MRV) if evidence of intracranial blood and suspicion of arteriovenous malformation)
- Cerebral angiogram in selected cases

---

for signs of raised intracranial pressure (ICP) that should be managed (Box 45.14).

Head injury

Severe traumatic brain injury (STBI) represents a major cause of childhood deaths. The majority of cases are accidental and therefore by definition are preventable. All paediatricians have a duty to encourage road safety and public education to try to decrease incidence and hence morbidity and mortality (Ch. 17). STBI accounts for 15% of deaths of 1–15-year-olds and 25% in 5–15-year-olds;

along with malignancies, represents the major cause of deaths in teenagers.

The mode of injury (Box 45.15) has a significant influence on the morbidity and mortality, reflecting the force involved in the head injury. For example, the mortality is higher in pedestrian road traffic accidents (RTAs) compared to passenger RTAs. Penetrating injuries are relatively rare in the UK compared to some American cities.

Primary brain injury

During the episode of trauma a large amount of energy is transmitted through the head, including the brain and all its supporting and connective tissues. This produces four main types of injury:
- Cerebral laceration
- Cerebral contusion
- Dural tear
- Diffuse axonal injury.

The pattern and severity (Box 45.16) depend on the forces and the part of the head involved.

Management is outlined in Boxes 45.17, 45.18 and 45.19.

Physiological basis for intracranial pressure (ICP) and cerebral perfusion pressure (CPP): Monro–Kellie Principle (Box 45.20)

The head can be thought of as a 'rigid box' with a fixed potential volume that is made up of the brain, cerebrospinal fluid (CSF), arterial and venous blood and the respective vessels (Fig. 45.1A). Following trauma to the head there can be expansion of the brain volume due to cerebral oedema or there can be 'new

BOX 45.19 Neuroprotection

Standard

- Maintain $PaO_2 > 10$ kPa
- Control $PaCO_2$ 4.5–5.0 kPa
- Paralyse and sedate as necessary
- Maintain CPP
- Control ICP
- Head up 30° in midline
- Maintain normothermia

Unproven

- Moderate hypothermia
- Decompressive craniectomy

BOX 45.20

CPP = MAP – ICP

(CPP = cerebral perfusion pressure; MAP = mean arterial pressure; ICP = intracranial pressure)

matter' that occupies space, e.g. expanding haematoma. There is a limited capacity for compensation for the cerebral oedema or expanding clot by decreasing the amount of CSF or venous blood (Fig. 45.1B). Even whilst this compensation occurs there will be some increase in the ICP towards 20 mmHg. When the capacity to compensate fails, the system becomes non-compliant and further small increases in volume will produce large rapid rises in pressure (Fig. 45.1C). Understanding this helps you appreciate the need for rapid appropriate action, including the rationale for osmotic diuretics and the need to perform definitive surgery within 4–6 hours of injury to remove expanding haematomas. Untreated, either uncal herniation or herniation through the foramen magnum will occur, resulting in brainstem compression and ultimately brain death.

Indications for a CT scan

- ↓ Ventricular size
- Effacement of sulci
- Effacement of basal cistern
- Mass.

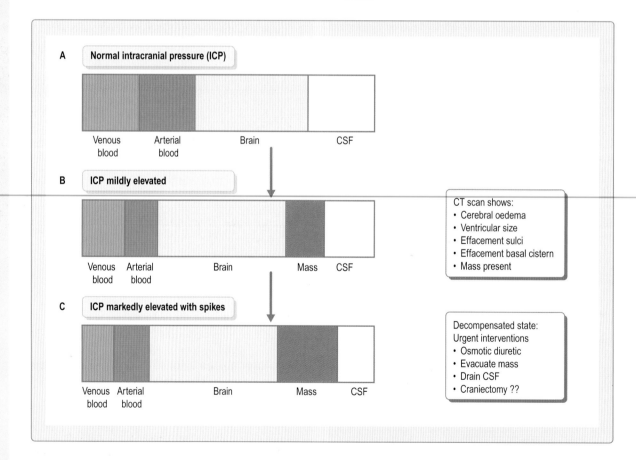

Fig. 45.1 Diagrammatic representation of intracranial volume: relative contribution of each component shown for three situations (Monro–Kellie Principle).
(A) Normal intracranial pressure (ICP); (B) ICP mildly elevated; (C) ICP markedly elevated with spikes. (CSF = cerebrospinal fluid)

Intracranial haemorrhage: non-neonatal

The presentation of intracranial haemorrhage outside the neonatal period depends on the underlying diagnosis. The prognosis is also influenced by this diagnosis, though intracranial haemorrhage, whatever the cause, carries a significant risk of mortality, especially if the child requires intensive care at the time of initial bleed.

The clinical history will in the majority of cases enable you to make a diagnosis rapidly (Box 45.21). In accidental trauma there is rarely any doubt about the diagnosis, but in the case of non-accidental injury (NAI, p. 143) there may be all the classical pointers to the diagnosis, including clear evidence of trauma, absent or inconsistent history, evidence of previous traumatic injuries and even retinal haemorrhages.

The presentation can vary from acute catastrophic loss of consciousness through to a much less acute gradual non-specific neurodegeneration (Box 45.22).

With a simple combination of clinical history and examination, along with initial radiological investigation (CT scan in the majority and MRI in a minority), a diagnosis of intracranial haemorrhage can be reached and the likely cause established. Subsequent investigation as listed in Box 45.23 will usually confirm the cause confidently.

BOX 45.21 Differential diagnosis of intracranial haemorrhage (non-neonatal)

- Trauma:
  - Accidental
  - NAI
- Arteriovenous malformation
- Bleeding disorder:
  - Inherited
  - Anticoagulant treatment
- Acute leukaemia
- Tumour
- Thrombosis
- Infection

BOX 45.22 Modes of presentation

- Acute loss of consciousness
- Gradual-onset coma
- Status epilepticus
- Acute focal neurology
- Acute severe headaches
- Progressive neurological deterioration

BOX 45.23 Investigations of suspected or proven intracranial haemorrhage

Trauma
- CT scan
- Additional appropriate X-rays

NAI
- CT scan
- Skeletal survey
- Expert fundoscopy
- Clotting screen
- Serum copper

AVM
- If suspected on CT scan proceed to cerebral angiography ± MRA or MRV

Inherited bleeding disorder
- Clotting screen
- Platelets
- Specific factor assays as directed by paediatric haematologist

Anticoagulant therapy
- International normalized ratio (INR)
- Seek expert advice rapidly

Acute leukaemia
- White cell count
- Blood film
- Bone marrow aspirate and trephine

Tumour
- Enhanced CT scan

Thrombosis
- MRA, MRV

Infection
- *Do not* carry out lumbar puncture in a hurry

Purpura

Problem-orientated topic:

purpura

Callum, an 8-year-old boy, is referred urgently to the accident and emergency department. He has been unwell for 12 hours with a fever, vomiting, malaise and muscle aches. Examination reveals a widespread petechial rash with a few purpuric areas. He is alert and cooperative but has a tachycardia of 150 beats per minute and a respiratory rate

Continued overleaf

of 20 breaths per minute. Initial assessment of ABC is undertaken.

Q1. What is the most likely diagnosis and what immediate treatments should be given?

Q2. What is the differential diagnosis?

Q3. What clinical signs and laboratory investigations inform the prognosis?

Q4. What is the prognosis?

Q1. What is the most likely diagnosis and what immediate treatments should be given?

The clinical history is highly suggestive of meningococcal septicaemia and therefore the priority is to start appropriate high-dose antibiotics immediately; do not delay whilst trying to confirm diagnosis. The antibiotic can be either intravenous cefotaxime 50 mg/kg or ceftriaxone 80 mg/kg; blood should be taken first for culture and a meningococcal polymerase chain reaction (PCR). Once vascular access is secured and the antibiotics have been given, Callum should be reassessed so his early treatment can be planned.

 http://www.meningitis.org

Meningitis Trust

Q2. What is the differential diagnosis?

See Box 45.24.

Q3. What clinical signs and laboratory investigations inform the prognosis?

See Box 45.25.

Q4. What is the prognosis?

The prognosis of meningococcal septicaemia has steadily improved over the last 15 years. Now the reported mortality from most UK PICUs is less than 10% and is usually in the region of 5%. The reasons for this are undoubtedly multiple and reflect increased public awareness, early and prompt management by GPs, including prehospital antibiotics, improved recognition and resuscitation in hospitals and, to some extent, introduction of early and aggressive intensive care management.

Meningococcaemia

Pathogenesis

Neisseria meningitidis is a Gram-negative diplococcus that is carried in the nasopharynx of 2–5% of the

---

BOX 45.24 Differential diagnosis of purpura

Acute onset with fever and systemic symptoms
- Meningococcal septicaemia
- Viral illness
- Disseminated intravascular coagulation or septic origin
- Acute leukaemia

Less acute onset/absent fever
- Immune thrombocytopenia
- Idiopathic thrombocytopenia
- Thrombotic thrombocytopenia
- Protein C deficiency
- Drugs:
  - Under-production
  - Decreased survival

BOX 45.25 Signs of severe disease suggesting poor prognosis at presentation

- Short history
- Absence of meningism
- Widespread rash at presentation
- Rash that continues to spread despite treatment
- Shock (decompensated > compensated)
- Hyperpyrexial > 40°C
- Low white cell count < 10×10^9
- Low platelet count < 150×10^9

---

population. Group B is the most common serotype. Groups A, C, Y and W now have vaccines, although group C is the only one routinely given. Group A is less common but has caused significant outbreaks in the past. Children usually acquire the organism from colonized adults and the majority develop a bactericidal response. A concurrent viral infection may predispose to mucosal penetration and subsequent bacteraemia.

Septicaemia

Systemic inflammatory response syndrome (SIRS) describes the sequence of events that occurs following infection with meningococcus. It may be defined as:
- Temperature > 38°C
- White cell count > 20 000
- Tachycardia
- Tachypnoea (reduced $PaCO_2$)
  in association with an infective cause.

Clinical features

With the increased awareness of the general public and other health professionals meningococcaemia is being recognized and treatment instituted earlier in its course. It only takes a brief period of working in any PICU, however, to realize how devastating the disease can be. Clinical presentation has classically been divided into acute, subacute and chronic. The acute form is the most dramatic; a child may be sitting up talking to his or her parents one minute and be ventilated on intensive cardiovascular support the next!

Initial symptoms may well be of non-specific fever and malaise, but the presence of a purpuric or morbilliform rash should alert the clinician to the potential diagnosis. Trying to predict which child is going to need full intensive care and which will just require a course of antibiotics has been the subject of much research, and the effect of the infection on the child is most likely to be partly a genetic-mediated response. Continual clinical reassessment of the child is vital, paying particular attention to the cardiovascular system. Features that should alert the clinician include:

- Spreading purpuric rash
- Poor perfusion
- Low blood pressure
- Reduced pulse volume
- Respiratory distress
- Low platelet and neutrophil count
- Abnormal clotting.

The subacute form takes the form of a classical rash that is then accompanied by a localized infection, e.g. meningitis. The chronic form may present with non-specific symptoms and may well be picked up incidentally on cultures.

Investigations

Culture of blood, purpuric lesions and CSF may well identify the organism; however, the early use of antibiotics out of hospital has reduced the success rate. PCR of the blood and CSF has provided an accurate way of identifying meningococcal DNA and the type responsible. It should therefore be performed in all suspected cases.

Management

Early use of antibiotics is essential in eradicating the organism and currently high-dose cefotaxime is often the drug of choice in suspected septicaemia.

Aggressive resuscitation is important if there is haemodynamic compromise. Often large volumes of fluid are required (up to 200 ml/kg!) and therefore early intubation is recommended for its inotropic effect and also to support the almost inevitable pulmonary oedema that follows. Inotropes are often required, with dopamine and dobutamine being used initially, the advantage being they can be given peripherally. Once central access has been obtained these drugs may be changed for noradrenaline (norepinephrine) and

adrenaline (epinephrine) if further support is required. Attention should also be paid to the correction of coagulopathy and electrolyte disturbances, particularly calcium and magnesium. Once initial stabilization has occurred, rapid referral to paediatric intensive care should be arranged for further management.

Public health must be informed of all suspected cases and the patient and close family contacts should be treated with prophylactic antibiotics for invasive disease and nasal carriage.

Prognosis

The mortality of septic shock secondary to meningococcaemia is 20–40%, often within the first 12 hours. If there is coexistent meningitis present the outcome is better, and if there is just meningitis alone mortality is less than 10%. Unfortunately, due to the severe nature of the acute form of presentation, children are still losing limb extremities from vascular occlusion.

Raised intracranial pressure

Problem-orientated topic:

headaches and loss of consciousness

Laura, a 15-year-old girl, is referred to outpatients with a history of headaches worsening over a 3-month period whilst she has been studying for GCSE. Her father, who found her unconscious in her bedroom where she was doing her homework, brings her into the accident and emergency department. Initial assessment reveals a GCS of 8.

Q1. What immediate care should be given?

Q2. What is the differential diagnosis?

Q3. What signs suggest the presence of raised ICP?

Q4. What specific emergency medical treatments can be instituted if raised ICP is suspected?

Q1. What immediate care should be given?

The fact that the GCS is 8 means that the child needs to be urgently intubated. Whilst preparations for this are being made, the ABC should be formally assessed and a rapid neurological assessment should be carried out (p. 308).

Q2. What is the differential diagnosis?

The differential diagnosis is the same as in the coma vignette (p. 307) but in this case the clinical history strongly suggests the possibility of a space-occupying lesion. Once Laura has been intubated and sedated, an urgent CT scan should be organized to confirm or refute this diagnosis. If there is a tumour or other space-occupying lesion the acute loss of consciousness suggests raised ICP, either as a direct mass effect from the lesion or from acute hydrocephalus. These need to be identified to facilitate timely surgical intervention and prevent coning.

Q3. What signs suggest the presence of raised ICP?

Signs of raised ICP (Box 45.26) include:
- Pupils unequal or unreactive
- Hypertension
- Bradycardia (relative)
- Abnormal posture
- Focal neurology
- Abnormal respiratory pattern.

In any patient with a decreased level of consciousness the possibility of raised ICP should be raised; however, most children with decreased level of consciousness do not have raised ICP. The combination of signs and symptoms listed is enough to initiate full management as described.

> **BOX 45.26 Warning: papilloedema in raised intracranial pressure**
>
> Papilloedema is a late sign of raised ICP. Do not be reassured by its absence.

Q4. What specific emergency medical treatments can be instituted if raised ICP is suspected?

See Box 45.27.

Caution. Once the patient is intubated, a formal blood gas should be measured to determine the $PaCO_2$. This should be correlated to an end-tidal CO_2 measurement, allowing you to adjust the ventilation constantly to avoid hyperventilation, which can induce ischaemia, and hypoventilation, which may lead to increased cerebral blood flow and exacerbation of raised ICP.

Steroids are not included in the treatment of raised ICP as there is limited evidence of beneficial effects in most causes. They may have a role if the primary diagnosis is meningitis or tumour. If steroids are given, high-dose types should initially be administered intravenously at 1.5 mg/kg, to a maximum dose of 10 mg.

> **BOX 45.27 Management of raised ICP**
>
> - ABC + oxygen
> - Sedated: analgesia + hypnotic
> - Ventilate
> - Normocapnia ($PaCO_2$ 4.5 kPa)
> - 30° head up in midline
> - Osmotic diuretic:
>   - 0.25–0.5 g/kg mannitol
>   - 2–5 ml/kg 3% saline

All the treatments of a raised ICP are aimed at trying to decrease or limit cerebral oedema and acutely dropping the ICP by creating more space (Monro–Kellie Principle, p. 310).

Encephalopathy

Acute encephalopathy may be described as a sudden onset of diffuse brain dysfunction with or without an associated change in level of consciousness. Whilst it is not a diagnosis in itself it is the manifestation of a significant abnormality and must be recognized and managed in a systematic way to improve outcome.

Causes

The causes of acute encephalopathy can seem endless but may be simply classified:
- Hypoxic–ischaemic
- Infectious
- Haemorrhagic
- Metabolic
- Toxic
- Epileptic.

The hypoxic–ischaemic injury to the brain can result from many clinical situations. The combination of hypoxia leading to anaerobic metabolism and ischaemia leading to accumulation of toxic metabolites results in neuronal cell death and raised ICP. If unchecked, this leads to further ischaemia because of poor cerebral perfusion, then worsening coma and death.

Infectious encephalopathy is caused by organisms able to invade the central nervous system and may result in encephalitis, cerebral oedema, ventriculitis and abscess formation.

Haemorrhagic causes may be accidental or non-accidental and will be discussed elsewhere.

Any buildup of toxic metabolites will cause an impairment of neurological function, be it from a significant electrolyte disturbance, endocrine dysfunction, organ failure or the more uncommon inborn errors of metabolism. One must also remember those toxins that have been ingested deliberately or accidentally.

Seizures may be the manifestation of an encephalopathy as well as the cause. It is therefore important to recognize whether they are new in onset or longstanding.

Management

The initial resuscitation should involve stabilizing the airway, breathing and circulation whilst making an assessment of conscious level (GCS/AVPU). One of the major decisions that needs to be made early is the need for artificial ventilation. The advantages of airway protection and controlling gas exchange are obvious but artificial ventilation also reduces the ability to monitor conscious level and results in other parameters being monitored, e.g. pupils, heart rate, blood pressure etc.

Once the patient has been stabilized, the management can be further divided as follows.

Neuroprotection

To prevent further damage being done to the brain and allow any recovery, it is important that certain factors are addressed:

- *Treatment of infection.* Until a confirmed microbiological diagnosis has been made patients should be started on high-dose antibiotic and antiviral treatment. Specimens must be taken to identify the cause and ideally should include CSF, but raised ICP must first be excluded because of the risk of coning. PCR is now routinely done for both bacterial and viral (herpes simplex) causes.
- *Seizure control.* Unless effectively controlled, seizures result in further hypoxia and ischaemia. Seizure control should be part of the initial resuscitation but looking for further seizure activity is also vital. This can be done clinically but it is not always obvious when the patient is paralysed and sedated. One therefore relies on electroencephalography (EEG) and the cerebral function activity monitor (CFAM) to identify seizure activity. Whilst brief seizures may be managed with benzodiazepines (e.g. lorazepam), prolonged seizure activity often requires intravenous anticonvulsants (e.g. phenytoin) or barbiturate infusions (e.g. phenobarbital, thiopental). APLS has produced recognized protocols for the management of status epilepticus.

 http://www.aplsonline.com

American Academy of Paediatrics APLS learning resources

- *Intracranial pressure.* As the head is a closed box, the blood supply to the brain can be compromised if the brain swells. Unless this is looked for and monitored, the patient with increasing ICP will subsequently present with brainstem herniation, by which time it is often too late. All patients with encephalopathy must therefore have some neuroimaging to make an assessment of ICP. Consideration must also be given as to whether a monitoring device is necessary. The advantage of this device is that an accurate assessment of cerebral perfusion pressure (CPP) can be obtained:

$$CPP = MAP - ICP$$

The control of CPP is paramount in order to prevent cerebral ischaemia and normal values change with age (infant > 50, child > 60, adolescent > 70). Whilst many factors influence CPP, changes in cerebral blood flow will be paramount. As can be remembered the basic science principle is that the flow through a vessel is dependent on the pressure difference and diameter. The diameter of cerebral blood vessels is affected by the $PaCO_2$, low levels causing vasoconstriction and high levels vasodilatation. The pressure difference is dependent on arterial pressure and therefore it is important to maintain blood pressure often to supranormal levels, with inotropes if necessary.

Diagnostic investigations

The sequence of investigation will obviously be dictated by the clinical history and examination but some of the baseline tests that should be considered in all cases are listed in Box 45.28.

Further investigation must be guided by specialist input from a multidisciplinary team. Treatment is then aimed at trying to correct the underlying cause if possible or prevent further damage from being caused.

BOX 45.28 Urine and blood (± gastric aspirate) toxicology

- Full blood count, liver and renal function, laboratory glucose
- Blood, urine and CSF culture, viral serology
- Urine amino and organic acids, plasma amino acids, ammonia, lactate
- Neuroimaging and EEG

Shock

Problem-orientated topic:

septic shock

Verity, a 3-year-old girl, is referred to hospital by her GP with a 12-hour history of fever,

Continued overleaf

vomiting and muscle aches. She is seen on the paediatric admission unit, where examination reveals that she is pale, awake and responsive, but pyrexial at 39.5°C, with a respiratory rate of 40, heart rate of 170 and a CRT of 7 seconds.

Q1. What is Verity's physiological state?

Q2. What important clinical measurement should be taken?

Q3. What immediate treatment should be given and what tests should be performed?

Q1. What is Verity's physiological state?

All resuscitation courses teach you how to recognize and treat failure of the respiratory system, cardiovascular system, a combination of these two and neurological failure. The logic of this is to ensure that you rapidly recognize the life-threatening problem and immediately institute the most appropriate treatment without being distracted by concerns as to the primary underlying diagnosis.

Respiratory failure continues to be the most common reason for children to present with a life-threatening illness, and the outcome following a cardiac arrest remains poor, with less than 10% survival for out-of-hospital arrest and 20–30% for in-hospital arrest.

Using an ABC approach, this child can be classified as being shocked; with the fever this will be due to sepsis. The cardiac output (Box 45.29) is inadequate and compensatory mechanisms to increase it have occurred; the heart rate has increased to maintain cardiac output and systemic vascular resistance has increased in order to maintain blood pressure.

Q2. What important clinical measurement should be taken?

The key clinical measurement that must be recorded is the blood pressure. Without this information you are unable to classify the shock as compensated or decompensated. This is vitally important as, once compensatory mechanisms have failed and the blood pressure is falling, the condition can progress rapidly to irreversible shock and cardiorespiratory arrest with a high probability of death.

BOX 45.29 Cardiac output = heart rate × stroke volume

Compensates when inadequate:
- Increased heart rate
- Increased systemic vascular resistance
- Increased stroke volume (not in younger children)

Q3. What immediate treatment should be given and what tests should be performed?

The principles of management of shock include:
- Administering 100% oxygen; ensuring adequate airway and ventilation
- Securing vascular access × 2 — intra-osseous if necessary
- Blood for culture, blood count and glucose
- Intravenous cefotaxime or ceftriaxone if there is sepsis
- Volume resuscitation as bolus:
  - 10–20 ml/kg colloid or 0.9% saline
  - Reassess and repeat depending on response
- Monitor heart rate, oxygen saturations and urine output (insert catheter).

Observe closely for response and deterioration. Once 40–60 ml/kg fluid resuscitation has been administered and if still signs of shock, then:
- Elective intubation and ventilation:
  - Use most appropriate team
  - Seek expert advice
- Continue fluid resuscitation
- Consider vasoactive infusions:
  - Start dopamine or dobutamine (can be peripheral initially)
  - Adrenaline (epinephrine) if poor response
- Central line access and arterial line
- Look for and treat hypoglycaemia, hypocalcaemia ± acidosis (if poor response)
- Pass nasogastric tube and urinary catheter, if not already done
- Transfer to intensive care unit.

Problem-orientated topic:

non-septic shock

Sophie, a 4-month-old girl, presents to the local paediatric department. She has had poor weight gain for 6 weeks and has been off her feeds for 3 days; she is pale and tachypnoeic at 60 breaths per minute. She is apyrexial, examination of her chest reveals widespread crackles, her heart rate is 190 per minute with a CRT of > 5 seconds and her systolic blood pressure is 50 mmHg.

Q1. What clinical investigation will help make a diagnosis?

Q2. What are the common causes of cardiogenic shock in infancy?

Q3. How should Sophie be managed?

Apparent life-threatening events (ALTEs)

See also page 399.

Problem-orientated topic:

a collapsed and pale infant

James, a 4-month-old boy, is rushed into the emergency department after mum found him pale and unresponsive in his cot. The ambulance crew report that he responded to rescue breaths and has a heart rate of 170/min.

Q1. What is an apparent life-threatening event?

Q2. What is the initial assessment of James?

Q3. What are the possible causes?

Q4. What is the prognosis?

Q1. What clinical investigation will help make a diagnosis?

This child has decompensated shock and, though sepsis is always a concern in young children, the history is more chronic and there is nothing to suggest sepsis strongly. In this situation the picture is highly suggestive of cardiogenic shock; therefore, at the same time as instituting appropriate general management for a shocked child, you should also arrange an urgent chest X-ray and ECG (echocardiogram if available), as these help confirm the diagnosis.

An enlarged heart supports cardiogenic shock and if this is present you are likely to need to give vasoactive agents earlier and to be cautious with fluid resuscitation. The ECG should identify arrhythmias such as supraventricular tachyarrhythmias (p. 226) or a predisposing conduction pathway such as Wolff–Parkinson–White syndrome.

Q2. What are the common causes of cardiogenic shock in infancy?

The more common causes of cardiogenic shock in infancy include:
- Cardiomyopathy:
  - Dilated
  - Hypertrophic
  - Restrictive
- Myocarditis:
  - Infective
  - Autoimmune, e.g. Kawasaki disease
- Arrhythmia
- Congenital heart disease:
  - Obstructive left heart lesion, e.g. aortic stenosis, hypoplastic left heart syndrome, coarctation
  - Other complex heart disease.

Q3. How should Sophie be managed?

Cardiogenic shock in an infant should be referred to the local PICU and the paediatric cardiologist will play a central role in the acute and long-term management. Echocardiography will enable you to place the child in one of the diagnostic groups and direct further investigation and treatment.

Q1. What is an apparent life-threatening event?

An apparent life-threatening event is said to have occurred when an infant has one or more episodes in which there is a combination of cyanosis, marked pallor, apnoea, bradycardia and hyper- or hypotonia. The frequency of presentation to hospital is approximately 1–2/1000 births.

The control of respiration changes during different aspects of sleep. In rapid eye movement (REM) sleep there is loss of postural tone and subsequently increased upper airway resistance. The thermoregulatory system has a marked impact on respiratory drive; decreasing temperature increases minute ventilation. In quiet sleep (QS), however, respiratory effort is controlled by chemoreceptor input and the autonomic nervous system. During the first 6 months of life up to 60% of sleep is REM, falling to 30% by 1 year. Hence temperature control is essential during the first year of life.

Q2. What is the initial assessment of James?

Initial management should be geared to making a primary assessment of the child and, if the patient is presenting acutely, checking a blood glucose and blood gas. A thorough history is essential in order to identify any particular aetiology. Carers must be allowed the chance to describe fully the sequence of events leading up to, during and after the episode. Particular attention should be paid to the relationship to feeds, position in the cot, temperature, family history and associated disorders.

Q3. What are the possible causes?

Recognized causes include:
- Gastro-oesophageal reflux (p. 177)
- Infection (e.g. bronchiolitis, p. 247; meningitis, p. 287)
- Seizures (p. 6)
- Cardiac disorders (e.g. arrhythmias, p. 226)
- Metabolic (e.g. medium-chain acyl CoA dehydrogenase deficiency, MCAD, p. 194)
- Overheating
- Idiopathic (apnoea of infancy).

Up to half of infants with ALTE have no identified cause and it is therefore important that advice is given to carers on trying to avoid further episodes and on how to respond if faced with a similar circumstance.

Q4. What is the prognosis?

The neurodevelopmental outcome obviously depends on the initial severity of presentation, and the risk of recurrence depends on the cause. If there is any associated seizure activity post presentation, this is a bad prognostic factor. Of the 'idiopathic' group with less severe presentation, the majority have no neurological sequelae.

Cardiopulmonary arrest

Problem-orientated topic:

near-drowning

Jane, a 6-year-old girl, is on the way to the accident and emergency department after being found face down in the swimming pool. The paramedics phone ahead to say that she is making no respiratory effort and they cannot feel a pulse.

Q1. What is the initial management of this child?
Q2. What further information do you require?
Q3. What is the likely outcome?

Q1. What is the initial management of this child?

When managing cardiopulmonary arrest it is vital that help is called for straight away. As has been described,

a primary survey of airway, breathing and circulation is essential, as is the continuation of basic life support once cardiopulmonary arrest is confirmed. With all potential trauma, particular attention must be paid to ensuring cervical spine immobilization. The subsequent management depends upon the arrest rhythm identified and following the protocols as detailed in APLS.

Q2. What further information do you require?

In the management of cardiopulmonary arrest, especially out of hospital, it is important to try to ascertain how long it was before basic life support was commenced and for how long resuscitation has continued. This will guide the duration of further resuscitation efforts and give some idea of outcome. As in this case, the patient may well be cold and it is important to measure the core temperature and actively rewarm if this is < 30°C. It is also important to measure the blood glucose and obtain a blood gas so that any metabolic or electrolyte derangements can be corrected.

Q3. What is the likely outcome?

Despite all the improvements in basic and advanced paediatric life support, the outcome of paediatric cardiac arrest is very poor and particularly so when this occurs out of hospital. Survival of out-of-hospital arrests is almost non-existent.

The floppy infant

See also page 16.

Problem-orientated topic:

a pale floppy infant

A 2-month-old boy, Matthew, is referred to the paediatric assessment unit by his GP, who is concerned that all is not quite right. On the child's arrival, the nurse calls you straight away as he is pale and floppy.

Q1. What is the first diagnosis to consider?
Q2. What further information will help make this diagnosis?
Q3. What alternative diagnoses should be considered?

Q1. What is the first diagnosis to consider?

When faced with an ill-looking infant, the reflex response tends to be to manage as sepsis. In the majority of cases this will be correct but it must be remembered that other treatable causes do exist.

Q2. What further information will help make this diagnosis?

In order to make the diagnosis of sepsis supportive information should be obtained from the history, such as symptoms of tiredness, irritability, vomiting and fever over a few days. Examination may well reveal a tachycardia, tachypnoea and poor peripheral perfusion. Whilst investigations such as cultures can be very useful in confirming the diagnosis they can take 1–2 days and the full blood count and C-reactive protein are not always helpful. A pragmatic approach tends to be to treat for possible sepsis whilst awaiting cultures and considering other diagnoses.

Q3. What alternative diagnoses should be considered?

Other possible causes of apparent sepsis in an infant can be approached in a systematic way:
- Cardiovascular:
  - Congenital heart disease
  - Arrhythmias
  - Myocarditis and pericarditis
- Gastrointestinal:
  - Severe dehydration
  - Pyloric stenosis
  - Intussusception
- Metabolic:
  - Electrolyte abnormalities
  - Inborn errors
  - Hypoglycaemia
- Endocrine:
  - Congenital adrenal hyperplasia
- Neurological:
  - Intracranial haemorrhage (consider NAI).

Spinal muscular atrophy

Spinal muscular atrophy (SMA) covers a spectrum of inherited neuromuscular diseases caused by degeneration of the anterior horn cells. Separation according to diagnostic groups is in part based on the age of presentation/onset of symptoms (Box 45.30). Diagnostic groups are still clinical and the disease is not classified on a genetic basis.

> **BOX 45.30 Diagnostic groups in spinal muscular atrophy**
>
> **SMA type I**
> - Weakness before 6 months
>
> **SMA other**
> - Later onset
> - Slower progression
> - Respiratory symptoms may not arise until teenager or adult
>
> **Clinical features**
> - Unexplained 'flatness' at birth
> - Poor respiratory effort
> - Recurrent apnoeas
> - ALTE: hypoxic–ischaemic brain injury
> - Chest infection
> - Floppy/generalized muscle weakness
> - Feeding difficulties.
>
> **Management**
> - Non-invasive ventilation
> - Intubation and ventilation
> - Tracheotomy and long-term support
> - Palliative care.
>
> There are marked differences in treatments offered at different centres. Until recently in the UK only palliative care was offered; ventilatory support was not offered with a prediction of death within 2 years. In Japan children with SMA type I have routinely been treated with ventilatory support and the morality of the Western European practice is questioned.
>
> **Ethical and legal considerations**
> Principles based on 'best interests' should be used:
> - Disparity of offered treatments; contrast:
>   - Duchenne muscular dystrophy
>   - Spinal cord injury
>   - Hypoplastic left heart syndrome
> - Imbalance of opinions:
>   - Medical
>   - Family
> - Non-invasive ventilation:
>   - Increases survival
>   - Significant cost of home ventilation
>   - Internet's powerful effect on family expectations.
>
> http://www.mda.org/disease/sma1.aspx
>
> Further information about spinal muscular atrophy type 1

Sabita Uthaya   Neena Modi

Neonatology I: Problems of the prenatal and perinatal period

LEARNING OUTCOMES

By the end of this chapter you should:

- Be able to recognize high-risk obstetric situations and anticipate likely problems in the newborn
- Be able to obtain and understand the importance of a comprehensive clinical history
- Understand the fundamentals of physiological support in the newborn
- Understand the relevance of informing and involving parents
- Be familiar with standard definitions in neonatal medicine
- Ensure that you are trained in newborn resuscitation
- Ensure that you are able to examine a newborn infant objectively.

Fetal physiology, growth and development

(See also Chs 22 and 48.)

Growth and development of the placenta

The placenta is a metabolically active organ and is an important determinant of the growth and wellbeing of the fetus. It regulates two-way transport between mother and fetus. Disruption of placental development results in a range of problems, including intrauterine growth restriction (IUGR) and death, and may lead to preterm birth.

Placentation begins with the implantation of the blastocyst in the decidua, the uterine mucosal lining. Following contact with the endometrium, the blastocyst becomes surrounded by an outer layer known as the syncytiotrophoblast and an inner layer of cytotrophoblast.

The trophoblast differentiates into villous or extravillous trophoblast. Extravillous trophoblast invades the maternal tissues and modifies the maternal spiral arteries to accommodate the increase in blood flow to the implantation site. The villous trophoblast comes into contact with maternal blood in the intervillous space and is involved in transport across the placenta. Beginning at around day 18 post conception and carrying on to term, placental blood vessels form by vasculogenesis inside the placental villi, leading to the tertiary villi that make up the villous trees of the placenta until the end of pregnancy. Terminal villi are responsible for gas and nutrient exchange.

Uteroplacental insufficiency results from defective extravillous invasion and failure to modify the maternal spiral arteries.

Fetal growth and development

The most rapid growth rate occurs during fetal life, followed closely by that in the postnatal period.

Assessment of fetal growth

The clinical assessment of uterine size correlates poorly with fetal growth. Fetal size is best measured using ultrasound. Standard measurements are fetal biparietal diameter, abdominal circumference and head to abdominal circumference ratios. Fetal weight may also be estimated with good accuracy. Measurements are plotted on population-based centile charts that may be used for monitoring fetal growth over time.

The term small for gestational age (SGA) is used to describe a baby whose birth weight lies below the 10th centile for gestational age. The term intrauterine growth restriction (IUGR) is applied to an infant in whom there has been a decline in growth velocity in utero.

Fetal growth restriction is considered 'symmetrical' when head size and weight are proportionately reduced or 'asymmetrical' when weight is affected to a greater extent than head size. Symmetrical growth restriction arises when growth declines early in pregnancy, while third-trimester restriction leads to 'head sparing' and disproportionate growth.

Aberrant fetal growth

IUGR results from limitation of fetal growth by one or more pathological processes. These include congenital infections, chromosomal abnormalities and 'uteroplacental insufficiency', in which failure of the extravillous trophoblast invasion results in high uteroplacental resistance and reduced uterine artery blood flow. High uteroplacental resistance is indicated by abnormal Doppler waveforms in the fetal umbilical arteries with absent or reversed end-diastolic flow. Intrauterine growth may also be constrained by poor maternal health or small maternal size.

Fetal macrosomia is a term used to describe a fetus growing above the 90th centile. The most common cause is poorly controlled maternal diabetes and the finding of macrosomia may be an indication to investigate the mother. Alternatively, a constitutionally large fetus is a possibility. Shoulder dystocia is a potential problem and must be anticipated to avoid complications during delivery.

The perinatal outcome of infants with growth restriction secondary to problems of placentation tends to be poorer than in infants where placental function has been normal. The management of pregnancies where there is abnormal placental function is based on close surveillance with longitudinal assessment of fetal growth and Doppler waveforms. The aim is to plan the optimal time for delivery by balancing the risks of prematurity with those of fetal demise and compromise in an unfavourable uterine environment. If there is evidence of decompensation, delivery by caesarean section after administration of antenatal steroids is indicated if the infant is at a gestational age less than 32 weeks. Where uncertainty exists over management, early delivery has been shown in a randomized controlled trial to make no difference to overall perinatal mortality when compared with delayed delivery. However, neurodevelopmental morbidity was greater in the more premature infants who were delivered early. Where the infant is above 34 weeks' gestation, the risks of prematurity are outweighed by those of delayed delivery. Assessment of fetal wellbeing is summarized in Table 46.1.

The effect of labour and delivery on the neonate

There are around 650 000 births each year in the UK. Of these babies, the overwhelming majority are born healthy and at term. The outcomes of pregnancy can be summarized in the rates of stillbirth and perinatal, neonatal and infant mortality (Table 46.2). It is important to recognize the factors that contribute to variations in these rates over time, between countries and between different areas and populations within countries. In 1992 the legal definition of viability was reduced from 28 to 24 weeks' gestational age.

Care during labour and delivery can have profound effects on infant wellbeing. Labour that is delayed or complicated and births that are unsupervised or supervised by unskilled attendants characterize maternal care in many parts of the world and lead to high rates of mortality and morbidity. With improvements in obstetric care, rates of birth trauma, asphyxia, infection and congenital malformations decline and the proportion of mortality and morbidity attributable to preterm birth increases.

Table 46.1 Assessment of fetal wellbeing

Method	What it involves	Comments
Fetal movements	Maternal counting of movements over a given time	Decrease in fetal movements is associated with increased mortality and fetal compromise
Liquor volume assessment	Clinical assessment by palpation verified by ultrasound assessment of deepest liquor pool or amniotic fluid index	Oligohydramnios is a sign of placental insufficiency and polyhydramnios is associated with high perinatal loss rate
Doppler studies	Umbilical artery Doppler measurement of resistance to blood flow	Reversed and absent end-diastolic flow indicate impaired placental function
Antenatal cardiotocography	Fetal heart rate record	Of value when combined with other measures
Biophysical profiles	Ultrasound scanning for fetal movements, fetal muscular tone, fetal breathing movements, amniotic fluid volume, fetal heart rate record. Combination of all to produce single score	Time-consuming and superseded by Doppler studies

Table 46.2 Stillbirth and perinatal, neonatal and infant mortality rates

Rate	Definition
Stillbirth	The number of babies born without signs of life after 24 weeks' gestation per 1000 total (live and still) births
Perinatal mortality	The number of stillbirths and deaths within the first 7 days of postnatal life per 1000 total (live and still) births
Early neonatal mortality	The number of deaths within the first 7 days of postnatal life per 1000 live births
Late neonatal mortality	The number of deaths between 8 and 28 days of postnatal life per 1000 live births
Neonatal mortality	The number of deaths up to 28 days of postnatal life per 1000 live births
Post-neonatal mortality	The number of deaths from 28 days to 1 year per 1000 live births
Infant mortality	The number of deaths in the first year per 1000 live births

Infants with IUGR tolerate labour and delivery less well than appropriately grown infants. However, the evidence to support the routine delivery of IUGR infants by caesarean section is not conclusive.

Birth trauma

Fractures may occur at the time of birth. They are seen more often with large babies. They may involve any long bones but are most commonly seen involving the clavicle. Clavicular fractures do not require treatment, unlike those involving the femur and humerus. The infant may present with a swollen and tender limb and avoid voluntary movement of the particular limb.

Brachial plexus injuries

These are described in association with shoulder dystocia when the head is delivered and traction is applied in order to deliver the rest of the body, in cases of breech delivery when attempting to deliver the head following delivery of the trunk, and also in the absence of a history of difficult delivery. The resulting paralysis is dependent on which nerve roots are involved. Erb's palsy involves a lesion of C5–6 with denervation of the deltoid, supraspinatus, biceps and brachioradialis. The infant holds the arm with the shoulder internally

BOX 46.1 Causes of hypovolaemic shock in the perinatal period

- Maternal antepartum haemorrhage (placenta praevia, abruption placenta, uterine rupture)
- Feto–maternal or feto–fetal haemorrhage
- Ruptured vasa praevia
- Traumatic delivery resulting in haemorrhage (subcapsular haematoma of the liver, intraventricular haemorrhage, subdural haemorrhage, subaponeurotic haemorrhage, extensive bruising)
- Early cord clamping
- Cord accidents

rotated, and the forearm pronated with extension of the elbow and flexion of the wrist (the 'waiter's tip position'). In this condition the Moro reflex is asymmetrical. In the majority of cases there is recovery of function but this may take several months.

Shock

Hypovolaemic shock now rarely results from traumatic delivery (Box 46.1). The hallmark of neonatal shock is profound pallor. The peripheral pulses are weak and thready but the baby, especially if mature, may have a weak cry and show respiratory movements.

The immediate management of hypovolaemic shock is shown in Box 46.2.

Asphyxia

See page 365.

Infection

See page 376.

High-risk pregnancy and its outcome

A pregnancy is described as high-risk if there are maternal or fetal conditions that pose a threat to the health of the fetus and/or the mother (Box 46.3).

Once a pregnancy is identified as high-risk, close monitoring of the fetus and the mother is required. The parents need to be counselled on the plan of management and possible outcomes. If appropriate, termination of pregnancy may be offered. Management plans should be made jointly by obstetricians, neonatologists and other appropriate specialists such as surgeons and geneticists. The plan of management will include treatment of the mother, the timing of delivery, the mode and place of delivery and the subsequent management of the infant. If indicated, the need for a paediatrician to be present at the time of delivery or to be informed of the birth once it has occurred should be clearly documented. Good communication between the various professionals involved is vital.

Following delivery further management must be discussed with a senior colleague, even if a plan has

been made antenatally. The baby must be examined carefully to confirm antenatal assessments (Table 46.3).

Management of threatened preterm delivery (Box 46.4)

The aim of managing threatened preterm delivery is to allow adequate time for the administration of antenatal steroids to the mother while balancing the risks of delayed delivery with those of prematurity. Tocolytics are only indicated in preterm labour between 25 and 34 weeks of gestation. The reason for using tocolytics is to allow sufficient time for the administration of antenatal steroids and not to delay delivery indefinitely.

Immediate or early delivery may be indicated if the risks of continuing pregnancy outweigh the risks of prematurity, as may be the case, for example, with frank chorioamnionitis. Alternatively, allowing the pregnancy to continue may place the health of the mother at risk, as in severe pre-eclampsia.

Twin pregnancy

The twinning rate in the last two decades has risen largely as a result of the new reproductive technologies. Twins have a higher perinatal mortality rate than singletons. This is due to the higher rate of prematurity and growth restriction. Growth restriction in twins occurs after the second trimester.

Table 46.3 Characterizing the newborn baby

Description	Definition	Comments
Low birth weight baby Very low birth weight baby Extremely low birth weight baby	A baby weighing less than 2.5 kg at birth A baby weighing less than 1.5 kg at birth A baby weighing less than 1.0 kg at birth	Low birth weight may be attributable to preterm delivery or IUGR Low birth weight rates vary around the world About 7% of births in the UK are of low birth weight Less than 1% of births in the UK are of very low birth weight
Preterm baby	A baby born before 37 completed weeks after the first day of the last menstrual period	In the UK approximately 1 in 6 preterm babies is born below 32 weeks' gestation
Small for gestational age (SGA) baby Large for gestational age (LGA) baby Intrauterine growth restriction (IUGR)	A baby whose birth weight is less than the 10th centile for gestational age A baby whose birth weight is greater than the 90th centile for gestational age The slowing of fetal growth velocity	The 10th and 90th centiles for gestational age differ between boys and girls and between different ethnic groups SGA and LGA are statistical terms; a baby may have suffered IUGR and still have a birth weight above the 10th centile Third-trimester IUGR results in a characteristic clinical phenotype: asymmetric growth, scaphoid abdomen, reduced subcutaneous adipose tissue

---

BOX 46.4 Paediatrician checklist in the event of threatened preterm delivery

- Get a good history and establish the gestation accurately
- Alert colleagues
- If delivery is extremely preterm, a senior doctor must speak with the parents. They must be counselled on what to expect in terms of outcome, as well as on what will happen at delivery. In cases of borderline viability their views on resuscitation must be sought
- Invite parents to visit the neonatal unit, if time permits
- Check the resuscitaire and equipment
- Ensure the delivery room is warm
- Ensure that the various members of the team know their role

Types of twinning

Two sperm fertilizing two ova produce dizygotic twins. Separate amnions, chorions and placentas are formed in dizygotic twins. The placentas in dizygotic twins may fuse if the implantation sites are close to each other.

Monozygotic twins develop when a single fertilized ovum splits during the first 2 weeks after conception. Monozygotic twins also are called identical twins. An early splitting (i.e. within the first 2 days after fertilization) of monozygotic twins produces separate chorions and amnions (dichorionic/diamniotic). Dichorionic twins have different placentas but these may be separate or fused. Approximately 30% of monozygotic twins have dichorionic/diamniotic placentas.

Later splitting (i.e. during days 3–8 after fertilization) results in monochorionic/diamniotic placentation. Approximately 70% of monozygotic twins are monochorionic/diamniotic. If splitting occurs even later (i.e. during days 9–12 after fertilization), then monochorionic/monoamniotic placentation occurs. If twinning occurs beyond 12 days after fertilization, then the monozygotic pair only partially split, resulting in conjoined twins.

Twin-to-twin transfusion syndrome (TTTS)

This occurs in 15% of monochorionic twin pregnancies. If untreated, the mortality is high and results in significant neurodevelopmental impairment. TTTS results when there is unbalanced transfusion from a net donor twin to a net recipient twin via placental arteriovenous anastomoses in the absence of bidirectional superficial anastomoses. The diagnosis is made on serial ultrasounds. The characteristic picture is that of a recipient twin with hypervolaemia, polyhydramnios, cardiac enlargement and/or failure, abnormal umbilical venous Doppler waveforms and, in terminal cases, fetal hydrops. The donor twin tends to be 'stuck' with oligohydramnios, oliguria, growth restriction and abnormal umbilical arterial Doppler waveforms.

Although traditionally weight and haemoglobin discordance were used to diagnose TTTS, this is unreliable and should no longer be used. The diagnosis rests on the finding of arteriovenous anastomoses, the fetal observations described above and the presence or absence of compensatory arterio-arterial anastomoses.

There is a high incidence of prematurity in TTTS. Premature TTTS twins tend to do worse than those without TTTS. The donor twin is more likely to die in utero. When one twin dies, although there is improvement in TTTS, the surviving twin has a high risk of death and long-term neurological morbidity. This is irrespective of which twin has died.

Postnatally, the main problems following TTTS are growth restriction and renal impairment in the donor and cardiac dysfunction in the recipient. Management of the condition during pregnancy depends on the severity. Various methods that exist include serial amnioreduction, selective laser ablation, selective feticide and septostomy.

Management of antenatally detected congenital malformations

With advances in ultrasound technology, the diagnosis of structural abnormalities in the fetus has improved. Additionally, the availability of invasive procedures such as chorionic villus sampling, and biochemical and DNA analysis has made antenatal diagnosis more accurate, allowing for better counselling of parents (Box 46.5).

BOX 46.5 Antenatal detection of congenital malformation

Use of ultrasound for antenatal diagnosis
- Neurological conditions (neural tube defects, hydrocephalus)
- Cardiac defects (congenital heart disease)
- Gastrointestinal malformations (congenital diaphragmatic hernia, anterior abdominal wall defects)
- Renal tract anomalies (hydronephrosis, multicystic kidneys)
- 'Soft' markers of aneuploidy (choroid plexus cysts, increased nuchal translucency)
- Skeletal dysplasias

Use of invasive procedures
- Chorionic villus sampling, after 10 weeks of gestation (genetic diagnosis)
- Amniocentesis, 14–16 weeks (karyotyping)
- Fetal blood sampling

Physiological adaptations at birth

During fetal life there is high pulmonary vascular resistance and a low-resistance placental component of the systemic communication. Owing to this and the presence of a patent ductus arteriosus, only a small amount of blood flows into the pulmonary circulation.

At birth two events occur that alter this pattern. Firstly, the umbilical cord is clamped and secondly the lungs fill with air. When the umbilical cord is clamped, venous return to the right atrium from the placenta is reduced. This has the effect of closing the foramen ovale due to the resultant low right atrial pressure, coupled with the rise in left atrial pressure secondary to increased pulmonary venous return. Additionally, the ductus venosus closes due to the reduced umbilical venous return.

The second event, lung aeration, results in decreased pulmonary vascular resistance. This is mediated by the mechanical effects of ventilation, raised arterial oxygen tension and lowered arterial carbon dioxide tension.

Other endogenous factors also contribute towards regulating pulmonary vascular resistance. Nitric oxide and prostaglandin I_2 (PGI_2) both reduce pulmonary vascular resistance. PGI_2 production increases after birth as a result of pulmonary tissue stretch. Bradykinin increases PGI_2 as well as nitric oxide production. Nitric oxide acts by causing smooth muscle cell relaxation.

Factors that increase pulmonary vascular resistance and interfere with the adaptation process after birth include acidosis, hypoxia, under-inflation of the lung, pulmonary hypoplasia and ventricular dysfunction.

Problem-orientated topic:

assessment at birth

Janine, a 25-year-old healthy primigravida, delivers a newborn boy weighing 1.8 kg. The baby cries at birth and appears lusty and vigorous. The midwife dries and wraps him, gives him to his mother and calls you to see him.

Q1.   What immediate assessment should be made?
Q2.   What are the causes of low birth weight?
Q3.   To what problems are low-birth weight babies vulnerable?
Q4.   What investigations do you carry out and what management do you initiate?

Q1. What immediate assessment should be made?

The principles of newborn care at delivery are the same in every setting and for every baby. The World Health Organization publication, 'Pregnancy, Childbirth, Postpartum and Newborn Care', contains clear guidance.

http://www.who.int/reproductive-health/
publications/popnc/pcpnc.pdf

Large PDF WHO publication on pregnancy, perinatal
and post-partum care

Immediate assessment should indicate whether a newborn baby is in need of assistance. If the baby is pink, lusty, vigorous and breathing regularly, no respiratory intervention is necessary. The baby should be kept warm and allowed to stay in skin-to-skin contact with his or her mother.

Oxygen should not be given as a matter of routine but only if indicated by cyanosis. Accumulating evidence suggests that air resuscitation is safe and effective.

Immediate assessment will also indicate whether the baby is preterm. A full examination should be performed. Where there is uncertainty a formal estimate of gestational age can be made using a structured system such as the Dubowitz or Parkin assessments.

Clinical history

It is vital that a thorough and complete history is obtained on any baby either on the postnatal ward prior to carrying out a newborn examination, or on the neonatal unit if he or she has required admission (Box 46.6). This is best obtained by speaking to the parents rather than looking at someone else's notes!

BOX 46.6 Clinical history

- Maternal history: medical, social
- Family history: including history of consanguinity
- Previous obstetric history
- Antenatal history: including results of screening, ultrasounds, medications, admissions and illnesses, antenatal steroids
- Labour: onset, duration of each stage, analgesia, meconium-stained liquor, complications
- Delivery: mode, anaesthetic, resuscitation

Q2. What are the causes of low birth weight?

Maternal associates

- Younger and older age
- Poor socioeconomic status
- Certain ethnic groups
- Small mother
- Maternal illnesses (essential hypertension, pre-eclampsia, renal disease)
- Alcohol/drug abuse/smoking
- Multiple pregnancy.

Fetal associates

- Constitutionally small
- Chromosomal anomaly

- Metabolic disorders
- Congenital infection
- Exposure to toxins early in pregnancy (drugs, alcohol).

Q3. To what problems are low-birth weight babies vulnerable?

IUGR babies are at risk of:
- Hypothermia
- Hypoglycaemia
- Polycythaemia
- Neutropenia
- Thrombocytopenia
- Infection
- Enteral intolerance
- Necrotizing enterocolitis.

Q4. What investigations do you carry out and what management do you initiate?

- Confirm gestational age and carry out a clinical assessment of gestational age if dates are uncertain.
- Obtain a karyotype if the baby has dysmorphic features or congenital abnormalities.
- Consider screening for congenital infection.
- Initiate early, regular and frequent feeds.
- Monitor temperature and blood glucose levels.
- Check a free-flowing venous haematocrit.

Principles of homeostatic support in very immature sick newborns

---

Problem-orientated topic:

preterm delivery

You are called to the delivery suite where Lucy, a 17-year-old primigravida, is in advanced preterm labour. A baby believed to be 24 weeks' gestational age is delivered as you arrive. You successfully resuscitate the baby and arrange transfer to the neonatal unit.

Q1. What are the problems the infant is likely to face in the subsequent 48 hours?

Q2. How would you attempt to prevent or ameliorate these?

Q1. What are the problems the infant is likely to face in the subsequent 48 hours?

- Thermoregulation
- Fluid and electrolyte balance
- Avoidance of hypo- and hyperglycaemia
- Establishment of feeds (Ch. 4)
- Lung diseases (Ch. 47)
- Intracranial lesions (Ch. 48)
- Infection (Ch. 48).

Q2. How would you attempt to prevent or ameliorate these?

The following are described below:
- Thermoregulation
- Fluid and electrolyte balance
- Glucose homeostasis
- Acid–base balance.

Thermoregulation (Box 46.7)

Newborn infants, particularly if born preterm, differ from adults and older children in their ability to maintain body temperature. Their large surface area to body weight ratio results in heat loss that is greater relative to heat production. Infants also lack the behavioural and physiological responses to warm and cold environments that older age groups possess. Heat production is dependent on basal metabolic rate. Babies are incapable of shivering in response to cold. Catecholamine release during cooling leads to heat production, through the activation of 'brown adipose tissue'. This is metabolically distinct from white adipose tissue. Brown adipose tissue is found in many depots within the body. The main areas are the perirenal, interscapular, cervical and peri-aortic depots. These sites account for 90% of the total stores. Premature infants lack the ability to recruit brown adipose tissue for heat generation. This, coupled with their large surface area to volume ratio and propensity for heat loss, places them at higher risk of hypothermia.

Infants who become cold are more likely to die and suffer morbidities. Hypothermia can exacerbate surfactant depletion, oxygen uptake and hypoglycaemia

BOX 46.7 Definition of mild, moderate and severe hypothermia	
Normal	36.5–37.5°C
Mild	36.0–36.4°C
Moderate	32.0–35.9°C
Severe	< 32.0°C

BOX 46.8 Heat loss

Convection
- Loss of heat to the surrounding air, determined by the difference in temperature between the baby and the surrounding air
- Avoiding draughty rooms helps prevent loss of heat by this means

Conduction
- Loss of heat to surfaces that the infant is in contact with
- Ensuring the baby is wrapped in warm towels avoids heat loss in this way

Radiation
- Loss of heat to the surrounding surfaces
- Using double-walled incubators protects against radiation heat loss; radiant warmers may be used to keep babies warm

Evaporation
- Evaporation of water through the skin and respiratory tract
- This is especially a problem with extremely premature infants whose skin is thin and whose stratum corneum is not keratinized; this results in large transepidermal water loss
- Each ml of water that evaporates from the skin is accompanied by the loss of 560 calories of heat, and so it is also difficult to keep a baby with a high transepidermal water loss warm

and lead to the increased utilization of calorific reserves and tissue acidosis. Temperature control is therefore extremely important in newborn babies (Boxes 46.8 and 46.9).

Measurement of temperature

Temperature measured in the rectum, axilla and skin over the abdomen reflects the core temperature. Rectal temperature may be measured using either a mercury thermometer or a flexible thermocouple. If the former is used, it is inserted to 3 cm in a term infant and 2 cm in a preterm infant. If the latter is used, the probe is inserted to 5 cm. The normal rectal temperature varies between 36.5 and 37.5°C.

Fluid and electrolyte balance

Postnatal alterations in body water compartments

Disturbances in electrolyte and water balance are not uncommon in newborn infants. Loss of body

- A warm, draught-free delivery room (at least 25°C)
- A warm surface to receive, dry and wrap baby
- Immediate drying
- Mother–infant skin-to-skin contact
- Putting a warm cap on baby's head
- Covering baby and mother together
- Delayed washing and bathing
- Do not remove vernix
- Warm transport incubator if transfer to the neonatal unit is anticipated
- Babies < 29 weeks or with estimated birth weight of < 1000 g may be placed in a plastic bag up to the neck without prior drying, and covering the head but not the face. This prevents heat loss through evaporation, a major contribution to hypothermia

water is an integral part of the physiology of postnatal adaptation and the transition from an aqueous intra-uterine environment to a gaseous environment. The postnatal loss of body water derives principally from the extracellular compartment and this accounts for the major part of postnatal weight loss. As sodium is the principal electrolyte in extracellular fluid, negative sodium balance is the physiological norm during the period of postnatal adaptation. The timing of the loss of extracellular fluid is closely linked to cardiopulmonary adaptation and is delayed in infants with respiratory distress syndrome.

Water balance

In very immature babies the principal determinant of water balance in the first days after birth is the magnitude of insensible water loss. Every effort should be made to reduce this to a minimum. Water should be provided in an intake sufficient to allow the excretion of a relatively small initial renal solute load and to maintain tonicity in the face of initially high, but rapidly falling, transepidermal losses. Skin maturation, unlike the maturation of renal function, is accelerated by birth. After 32 weeks' gestation water loss through the skin has fallen to around 12 ml/kg/day. Extremely immature preterm babies, in whom minimum urine osmolality is of the order of 90 mosm/kg, will be able to achieve a maximum urine flow rate of around 7 ml/kg/hr.

Sodium balance

Preterm neonates have a limited ability to excrete and retain a sodium load. In neonates, a smaller proportion of filtered sodium is absorbed in the proximal tubule and a correspondingly larger proportion delivered distally. Distal tubular sodium reabsorption is regulated via the renin–angiotensin–aldosterone system (RAAS). Poor sodium retention is due to impaired reabsorption at the proximal tubule, resulting in a higher distal sodium delivery, and to limited aldosterone responsiveness at the distal tubule. Intestinal absorption is also limited. Sodium is not lost through the skin because babies born below 36 weeks' gestation do not sweat, though this develops within the first 2 weeks after birth. Both preterm and full-term neonates have a limited capacity to excrete a sodium load. This is because acute sodium loading results in only a blunted fall in RAAS activity and a limited natriuretic response. Excessive sodium administration in the immediate postnatal period will delay the postnatal loss of extracellular fluid, including loss of pulmonary interstitial fluid, and exacerbate respiratory distress.

Management of neonatal fluid balance is outlined in Box 46.10.

Glucose homeostasis

Neonatal glucose metabolism

During fetal life glucose is transported across the placenta by a process of facilitated diffusion. The fetal brain is able to utilize ketones in addition to glucose. Glucose is the predominant energy source for the fetus and only negligible amounts of fetal glucose are produced, if any. At birth, the constant supply of glucose is interrupted and the newborn has to make adaptations to mobilize glucose and other substrates in order to meet its energy requirements.

At birth there is an increase in adrenaline (epinephrine), noradrenaline (norepinephrine) and glucagon, whereas the concentration of insulin decreases. The level of glucose falls and reaches its nadir at 1 hour of postnatal age, followed by a gradual rise at 2–4 hours of age. The result of the hormonal surges is that glycogen and fatty acid levels rise. Adipose tissue stored in the third trimester is a protective mechanism against postnatal decline in glucose concentration. The insulin/glucagon molar ratio is high in the fetus at term and then declines rapidly after birth, promoting glycogenolysis and gluconeogenesis.

Prevention and anticipation of hypoglycaemia (Box 46.11)

Hypoglycaemia is defined as a blood glucose < 2.6 mmol/l. Severe hypoglycaemia (blood glucose < 1.5 mmol/l) is a potentially serious condition and should be treated immediately. Good practice centres

1. Minimize insensible water loss through adequate humidification of inspired gases, maintenance of high ambient humidity and meticulous skin care

2. What is the infant's estimated transepidermal water loss? Base your estimate on gestational age, postnatal age and ambient humidity

3. Calculate initial fluid requirement as 'estimated insensible water loss PLUS allowance for urine output'

4. Avoid or minimize parenteral sodium intake until the period of postnatal contraction of the extracellular fluid compartment is over; this is marked by stabilization of postnatal weight loss

5. Optimize renal perfusion; monitor core–peripheral temperature gap, capillary refill time and blood pressure; provide volume and/or inotrope support as necessary

6. Review regularly; monitor urine output and serum sodium, potassium and creatinine

7. Urine output should be > 1 ml/kg/hr; if not, administer a fluid challenge followed by a single dose of furosemide 2 mg/kg

8. If the serum sodium falls below 134 mmol/l, decrease the intravenous volume administered; if the serum sodium rises above 142 mmol/l, increase intravenous intake

9. The blood urea is of little value in the assessment of renal function in the newborn as it is influenced by numerous non-renal factors

10. Successful management is marked by steady fall in serum creatinine, stable electrolytes and weight gain of around 12–16 g/kg/day after the period of initial weight loss

---

Box 46.11 Risk factors for hypoglycaemia

- Small for gestational age
- Postmaturity
- Infant of diabetic mother
- Prematurity
- Severe rhesus alloimmunization
- Polycythaemia
- Seizures
- Septicaemia
- Hypothermia
- Hypoxic–ischaemic encephalopathy
- Maternal therapy with tolbutamide or β-blockers
- Inborn errors of metabolism:
  - Glycogen storage disease (type 1)
  - Galactosaemia
  - Fructose 1–6 diphosphatase deficiency
  - Hereditary fructose intolerance
  - Adrenocortical deficiency
  - Proprionic acidaemia
  - Fatty acid oxidation defects, e.g. medium-chain acyl CoA dehydrogenase deficiency (MCAD)
- Beckwith–Wiedemann syndrome
- Primary islet cell disorders (hyperinsulinism)
  - Hyperplasia
  - Adenoma
  - Persistent hyperinsulinaemic hypoglycaemia of infancy
- Pituitary insufficiency

---

on the anticipation and prevention of hypoglycaemia and the early establishment of enteral feeds. Healthy well-grown term infants do not require screening for hypoglycaemia. Persistent hypoglycaemia, especially in the presence of symptoms (floppiness, jitteriness, poor feeding and lethargy, rarely seizures and coma), must be treated as an emergency, as it is associated with adverse neurological outcome. Infants who are symptomatic need admission to the neonatal unit and further investigation. Always remember that a baby who is sleepy and feeding poorly may have an infection or be hypothermic or hypoglycaemic and that these conditions may coexist.

Prevention of hypoglycaemia

Infants at risk of hypoglycaemia should be identified and a plan of management drawn up. At-risk infants should be fed within 1 hour of birth and the blood glucose checked at 3–4 hours of age before the second feed. There is no need for a blood glucose measurement before this time. The baby with a blood glucose measurement < 3 mmol/l at 3–4 hours of age should be fed every 3 hours until the prefeed blood glucose is at least 3 mmol/l on two consecutive occasions.

If the blood glucose remains low and the baby remains asymptomatic, increase the feed frequency and volume. Breastfed babies can have formula top-ups either by cup or by nasogastric tube. If the glucose measurement is < 2.6 mmol/l, check a true blood glucose using a blood gas machine or send a sample to the laboratory in a fluoride oxalate tube.

If the true whole blood glucose concentration is < 2.6 mmol/l, close surveillance should be maintained and intervention is recommended if whole blood glucose remains below this level despite frequent appropriate volume feeds or if abnormal clinical signs develop.

Admit the baby if frequency of feeds needs to be increased to 2-hourly. Continue feeding with breast milk whenever it is available, as there is evidence that breast milk helps in the earlier achievement of a normal blood glucose level. If additional milk is required, use a preterm formula. Early referral to a specialist centre is indicated in cases of hyperinsulinaemic hypoglycaemia.

Management of infants with intravenous glucose

- Any baby who has persistent symptoms, is not tolerating enteral feeds, or is unable to maintain normoglycaemia with appropriate enteral feeds alone should be commenced on an intravenous infusion of 10% glucose.
- Babies on i.v. glucose should still receive breast or enteral feeds, if appropriate.
- Normal neonatal hepatic production rate of glucose is between 4 and 6 mg/kg/min.
- Large volumes of enteral feed may not be tolerated.
- I.v. bolus 3 ml/kg 10% glucose should only be given if whole blood glucose measured on blood gas machine is < 1.5 mmol/l and the baby has not responded to previous treatment or there are severe symptoms. Always increase the concentration of glucose infusion as well.
- If the blood glucose is not maintained, increase the concentration of glucose rather than the volume. A central line will be necessary if glucose concentrations exceeding 15% are required.
- Consider glucagon early (see below).
- Discuss all babies with persistent hypoglycaemia with a senior colleague.

Management of persistent hypoglycaemia
(Boxes 46.12 and 46.13)

- If a baby requires glucose infusion rates of greater than 8 mg/kg/min, insert a central line (long line/umbilical venous catheter).
- If the baby remains hypoglycaemic despite increasing glucose infusion rate to 12 mg/kg/min, draw blood at the time baby is hypoglycaemic for:
  – Blood glucose
  – Insulin
  – Cortisol
  – Growth hormone.
- The presence of insulin in the face of hypoglycaemia is indicative of hyperinsulinism. Urine will be found to be negative for ketones. Consider the diagnosis of hyperinsulinism if a history of maternal diabetes is not forthcoming. This will require early referral to a specialist centre for further management.

BOX 46.12 Emergency treatment of hypoglycaemia

If the baby has major clinical signs (convulsions, coma) or the blood glucose (BG) is < 1.0 mmol/l:

- Take a sample for confirmatory BG but do not wait for result
- Give an intravenous bolus of 3 ml/kg 10% glucose followed by an infusion of at least 3 ml/kg/hr
- Hypoglycaemia may need to be treated with glucagon (100 μg/kg given intramuscularly or intravenously) if there is difficulty in securing intravenous access in the presence of clinical signs or there is persistent hypoglycaemia despite increasing the glucose infusion rate
- Check BG hourly until > 2.0 mmol/l

BOX 46.13 Investigation of severe or persistent hypoglycaemia

Conditions
- See Box 46.12

Blood
- pH, lactate, ketone bodies, fatty acids, insulin, glucagon, catecholamines, cortisol, growth hormone, amino acid profile

Urine
- Organic acid profile

Acid–base balance

Blood gas measurements are frequently made in neonatal medicine. During aerobic metabolism carbon dioxide is produced. In the presence of carbonic anhydrase CO_2 combines with H_2O to form carbonic acid, which in turn dissociates to form HCO_3^- and H^+. CO_2 is excreted through the lungs and H^+ through the kidneys.

$$CO_2 + H_2O \longleftrightarrow H_2CO_3 \longleftrightarrow H^+ + HCO_3^-$$

The regulation of acid–base balance involves buffers, respiratory function and renal function. In the proximal renal tubular cells H^+ ions are actively pumped into the tubular lumen and combine with filtered bicarbonate to form carbonic acid, which dissociates to water and CO_2. The CO_2 then diffuses back into the tubular cell to repeat the cycle. The net effect is that for each hydrogen ion excreted, one bicarbonate ion is retained, so that bicarbonate reserves are continuously regenerated.

A metabolic acidosis is due to an increase in acid or a decrease in base. The most common cause of metabolic acidosis in neonatal intensive care is tissue hypoxia leading to lactic acidosis. Metabolic acidosis occurs with sepsis, renal failure, amino acid intolerance during parenteral nutrition and in inborn errors of metabolism. A metabolic acidosis is marked by a low pH, PCO_2 and bicarbonate and a high negative base excess. If respiratory compensation occurs, the pH normalizes as the PCO_2 falls.

A respiratory acidosis is characterized by a high PCO_2. Sodium bicarbonate will exacerbate the condition and further raise the PCO_2. As renal compensation occurs, the plasma bicarbonate will rise.

The most common cause of a metabolic alkalosis is excessive administration of bicarbonate or loss of gastric acid with vomiting or in nasogastric aspirates. A respiratory alkalosis results from over-ventilation, whether iatrogenically during mechanical ventilation or spontaneously in neurologically damaged infants.

The correct management of disordered acid–base balance should always begin with consideration of the cause.

Congenital malformations

Examination of the newborn

(This is described in more detail in Chapter 8.)

Aims

The purpose of the first-day routine postnatal check is to:
- Identify any antenatal issues that may be relevant for the infant's health
- Identify any abnormalities in the baby
- Identify abnormalities where early referral impacts on outcome (cataracts, hips, cleft palate)
- Deal with parental concerns/questions
- Investigate/refer any abnormalities found.

How to examine a newborn

- Adopt a top-to-toe approach.
- Follow the sequence: look, feel, listen, measure.
- Check general appearance (dysmorphic features, skin).
- Plot anthropometric indices (weight, head circumference, length).
- Neurological:
  - Check movements, tone, reflexes, posture, alertness, visual orientation.
- Cardiovascular:
  - Look at the precordium, look for cyanosis; feel apex beat and femoral pulses; listen for murmurs.
- Abdominal:
  - Examine liver, spleen, kidneys, testes, genitalia.

- Inspect anus and establish patency.
- Respiratory:
  - Look for recession, indrawing, nasal flaring, cyanosis; listen for air entry, stridor, wheeze; measure respiratory rate.
- Eyes:
  - Seek red reflexes, colobomas, squint; check the orbit.
- Examine the palate (soft and hard).
- Hip examination:
  - Are hips stable, subluxable or dislocated? Are hips relocatable if dislocated?
- Musculoskeletal:
  - Look for talipes, brachial plexus injury, fractures, spine.

Problem-orientated topic:

abdominal masses

Whilst carrying out first-day checks on the postnatal ward you discover a baby has bilateral masses on abdominal examination. The baby appears well and the parents are anxious to go home.

Q1. What is your differential diagnosis?
Q2. What do you do?

Q1. What is your differential diagnosis?

- Renal dysplasia (multicystic kidney diseases)
- Polycystic kidney disease
- Hydronephrosis (dilatation of the renal pelvis due to functional or anatomical obstruction along the urinary tract); if bilateral, may be indicative of posterior urethral valves in a male
- Tumours.

Q2. What do you do?

Bilateral abdominal masses are suggestive of a renal abnormality. Examine the baby carefully for any other abnormalities. Explain to the parents what you have found and the need for further tests. Discuss with a senior colleague. Request an urgent renal ultrasound. Monitor urine output and check baseline serum creatinine and electrolytes.

Care of the parents (Box 46.14)

The arrival of a new baby is an emotional time for parents and can be extremely stressful if the baby is

- Courtesy is important: take the trouble to establish the names of the parents at the first meeting
- Take a clinical history from the parents, not from someone else's notes!
- Social factors are relevant to newborn health and wellbeing: take a social history, politely but meticulously
- Avoid jargon
- Listen to parents' concerns but do not be tempted to make promises you cannot keep ('I'm sure he'll be fine')
- If you cannot answer a question, say so and explain that you will find out or ask someone more senior to speak to them
- Document a summary of your discussion

unwell. A neonatal unit can be a bewildering place. Information must be obtained from parents and imparted to them. Introduce yourself and explain that you are one of a large team of staff who may be involved in the care of their baby. Take a careful clinical history as soon as possible. Social factors are relevant to newborn health and wellbeing. It is wise to take an objective social history as a matter of admission routine. Explain what their baby's problem is in simple terms and describe what is being done. Make it clear that this is the first of many discussions. No matter how busy, staff must keep parents informed.

Supporting parents of a sick newborn baby

Parents have greatly differing needs. They may require practical, emotional and financial support. A parent may be an unsupported teenager or a senior healthcare professional. A parent may attempt to cope by staying away from the hospital or by attempting to control every detail of his or her baby's care.

Explain the working practices of the unit and provide written information. A careful social history obtained at the outset will help direct support as appropriate. Nursing and medical staff are inevitably most closely involved but additional support may be drawn from social workers, psychologists, counsellors, religious advisors, support and self-help groups, GPs, relatives and friends.

It can be difficult to retain information, especially in a stressful situation, and information may have to be given to parents repeatedly. It can be helpful to begin each update by asking parents to tell you what they were last told. Documentation and team debriefings are important to ensure that information is shared.

Many sick newborn babies require prolonged hospitalization. Parents have to live through lengthy uncertainty while continuing to deal with the ongoing requirements of daily life. This can take its toll and staff may find themselves used as 'punch bags'. Staff, particularly if junior or inexperienced, may have to be supported themselves. They should be made aware of normal human responses when confronted with bad news and the progression from denial to anger and ultimately to acceptance.

Every parent wants to know what the future holds for his or her baby. A prognosis may be clear-cut or uncertain, very good or very poor. It can be easy for staff to forget that what may seem obvious to them — for example, that the prognosis for physiological jaundice is excellent — may not be obvious to a parent. A guarded prognosis can be difficult to impart and should be undertaken by a consultant.

Assessment of home care

An introduction to parenting skills is usually included in antenatal and postnatal classes. For the majority of parents with healthy mature babies, this, along with the support they receive from family and friends, is sufficient. Maternity units try to provide access to breastfeeding counsellors, who are skilled at supporting new mothers and offering practical advice. Every mother–baby dyad is different and helping a new mother gain confidence in caring for her baby is an important part of the professional role. All parents need information on how to minimize the risks of sudden infant death and on immunization schedules.

If a baby has special requirements or is going home after a long period of hospitalization, or if parents have difficulties of their own to contend with, extra assessment and support are likely to be necessary. Parents will need training if their baby has specific requirements. This may be in nasogastric tube or gastrostomy feeding, in physiotherapy exercises, in the management of convulsions, or in feeding technique and positioning for gastro-oesophageal reflux. If a baby requires continuing oxygen therapy, a home visit by the community support team is necessary to assess pushchair access with heavy cylinders, installation of suction equipment and general suitability. Single parents or very young parents may need early support from their health visitor. Terminal care at home will require multidisciplinary input. Families with social difficulties will require the assistance of a social worker.

A good family and social history on admission will indicate areas where extra help may prove necessary.

Regular ongoing discussions with parents and a team approach with good communication will identify needs as they arise. As discharge approaches, a checklist of requirements should be drawn up.

Bereavement

Death may occur suddenly and unexpectedly or after a prolonged and difficult period of intensive care. The care of parents does not stop with the death of a baby. A senior member of the medical staff, usually a consultant, should explain the process of the post-mortem examination and ask for parental permission to perform this. Most hospitals or neonatal units are able to call upon the services of a bereavement support coordinator, who is able to explain the death registration procedure to parents and help them make arrangements for the funeral or cremation. Parents often form close bonds with staff, particularly if their baby has spent many weeks in hospital. Many parents appreciate staff attending the funeral. They may be comforted by being able to talk to staff about their baby, particularly as friends and relatives may find this difficult to do. After a period of about 4–6 weeks, an appointment is usually made with a consultant and nurse. This provides an opportunity to discuss unresolved questions, explain autopsy findings and come to terms with what has happened.

Further reading

Dubowitz LMS, Dubowitz V, Mercuri E 2000 The neurological assessment of the preterm and full-term newborn infant, 2nd edn. MacKeith, Cambridge

Neonatology II: Respiratory and cardiac disorders

LEARNING OUTCOMES

By the end of this chapter you should:

- Know how to diagnose the common and important causes of respiratory distress in term and prematurely born babies
- Understand the basic science of respiratory disorders in the neonate and how this relates to their presentation and management
- Know how to diagnose common cardiac disorders presenting in the neonatal period
- Know how to manage common neonatal respiratory and cardiac disorders
- Be able to interpret arterial blood gas measurements appropriately
- Be able to recognize the chest radiograph abnormalities of common neonatal respiratory disorders.

Neonatal respiratory disorders

Basic science

Fetal lung fluid

- In fetal life, the lung is filled with liquid, increasing from 4 to 6 ml/kg body weight at mid-gestation to about 20 ml/kg near term.
- Compared to either amniotic fluid or plasma, lung liquid has a high chloride but a low bicarbonate and protein concentration.
- The secondary active transport of chloride ions from the interstitial space into the lung is the main force for lung liquid secretion, sodium ions and water following passively down electrical and osmotic gradients.
- The presence of lung liquid is essential for normal lung development; chronic drainage results in pulmonary hypoplasia.

- During labour and delivery, the concentration of adrenaline (epinephrine) increases, the chloride pump responsible for lung liquid secretion is inhibited and lung liquid secretion ceases.
- Lung liquid resorption commences as the raised adrenaline levels stimulate sodium channels on the apical surface of the pulmonary epithelium, via which fetal lung liquid absorption occurs.
- Thyroid hormone and cortisol are necessary for maturation of the normal response of the fetal lung to adrenaline. Exposure to postnatal oxygen tensions increases sodium transport across the pulmonary epithelium.
- Although some liquid is squeezed out under the high vaginal pressure during the second stage of labour, the majority is absorbed into the pulmonary lymphatics and capillaries.
- Delayed lung liquid clearance, as occurs following delivery without labour, results in transient tachypnoea of the newborn (TTN) or 'wet lungs'.

Surfactant

Surfactant synthesis increases with increasing gestational age and, as respiratory distress syndrome (RDS) is due to surfactant deficiency, the incidence is inversely related to maturity at birth.

Surfactant composition
- Surfactant is a complex mixture of phospholipids; 70–80% is phosphatidylcholine (PC) and 5–10% is phosphatidylglycerol (PG).
- Approximately 60% of the PC is formed from saturated fatty acids; the primary saturated fatty acid is palmitic acid and the largest component of the phospholipids is dipalmitoyl phosphatidylcholine (DPPC).
- Surfactant proteins (SP-A, B, C and D) constitute 5–10% of surfactant by weight.

Surfactant function
- Surface tension reduction
- Stability of the alveoli and prevention of atelectasis
- Prevention of transudation of fluid.

Surfactant proteins
- SP-B is essential for surfactant surface activity and can also protect the pulmonary surfactant film from inactivation by serum proteins.
- SP-C enhances surface absorption and spreading of phospholipids.
- SP-A and SP-D are collectins and, as such, have important roles in the host defence against infection. They target the carbohydrate structures of invading microorganisms.

Lung hypoplasia

Primary pulmonary hypoplasia usually occurs with other associated anomalies, particularly of the renal and urological tract and the diaphragm. Some apparently idiopathic cases may have a genetic basis. Secondary pulmonary hypoplasia is more common and occurs if there has been reduced amniotic fluid or intrathoracic space or inadequate fetal breathing movements:
- The timing of onset of the oligohydramnios in pregnancies complicated by ruptured membranes is critical; pulmonary hypoplasia occurs only if the onset is prior to 26 weeks of gestation but is not an invariable consequence.
- Reduction in amniotic fluid production occurs in fetal renal anomalies — for example, Potter's syndrome and uteroplacental insufficiency.
- Reduction in intrathoracic space — for example, in small chest syndromes (e.g. asphyxiating thoracic dystrophy or Jeune's syndrome), cystic

adenomatoid malformation/sequestration of the lung, congenital diaphragmatic hernia (CDH) and pleural effusions — can result in pulmonary hypoplasia due to compression. In fetuses that are hydropic due to rhesus isoimmunization, pulmonary hypoplasia is a consequence of the pleural effusions but there is also an immune mechanism.
- In neurological or neuromuscular diseases that present in utero — for example, Werdnig–Hoffmann disease and myotonic dystrophy inherited from the mother — impaired fetal breathing movements result in abnormal lung growth.
- Infants with trisomy 18 or 21 are at increased risk of pulmonary hypoplasia.

Problem-orientated topic:

a premature infant with respiratory distress from birth

A male infant, Paul, is born by spontaneous vaginal delivery at 28 weeks of gestation weighing 0.946 kg; antenatal steroids were not given. The membranes ruptured at 22 weeks of gestation. Paul has poor respiratory effort at birth and is therefore intubated and transported to the neonatal unit, supported by mechanical ventilation. An umbilical arterial catheter is inserted and the first blood gas demonstrates pH 7.15, $PaCO_2$ 8 kPa and PaO_2 6 kPa; at this time the baby is receiving 80% oxygen and peak inspiratory pressure (PIP) and positive end-expiratory pressure (PEEP) of 20/4 and a rate of 60/min.

Q1. Does the baby have RDS?

Q2. What further information would help you to be sure?

Q3. What differentials should be considered when a prematurely born infant develops respiratory difficulties at birth and has an ongoing respiratory support requirement?

Q4. Are any of the differentials likely here?

Q5. How would this influence your management?

Q1. Does the baby have RDS?

Paul has been born very prematurely and antenatal steroids were not given. The arterial blood gases are compatible with severe RDS.

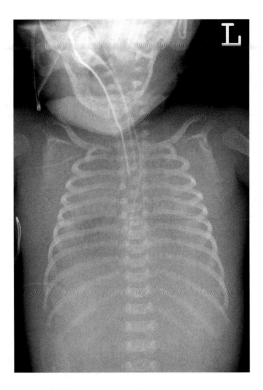

Fig. 47.1 Severe respiratory distress syndrome: 'a white-out'.
Note the infant is ventilated and the nasogastric tube is misplaced, the tip being in the oesophagus.

Table 47.1 **Lung function abnormalities in neonatal respiratory disorders**

	Compliance	Resistance	Lung volume
Respiratory distress syndrome (RDS) (severe)	↓↓	Normal	↓↓
Transient tachypnoea of the newborn (TTN)	↓	Normal	↓
Pulmonary hypoplasia	↓↓	Normal	↓↓
Meconium aspiration syndrome (MAS)	↓	↑	↑↓
Bronchopulmonary dysplasia (BPD)	↓	↑	↑↓

> **BOX 47.1 Differential diagnosis of a baby born prematurely with respiratory difficulties from birth**
>
> - Respiratory distress syndrome
> - Infection: congenital pneumonia/group B streptococci
> - Transient tachypnoea of the newborn
> - Air leak
> - Coexistent pulmonary hypertension
> - Pulmonary hypoplasia

Q2. What further information would help you to be sure?

A chest radiograph in an infant with RDS shows a symmetrical picture of reticulogranular shadowing and air bronchograms to the outer thirds of the lung fields (Fig. 47.1), but importantly does not exclude infection due to group B streptococcus (GBS). A radiograph is essential to exclude other causes of respiratory distress, in this case pulmonary hypoplasia in particular, given that the infant was born following prolonged and premature rupture of the membranes.

Lung function measurements would demonstrate an infant with RDS as having non-compliant lungs and a low functional residual capacity (lung volume); similar results, however, would also be found in an infant with pulmonary hypoplasia (Table 47.1).

Pulmonary maturity can be assessed by measurement of lecithin to sphingomyelin (L:S) ratio in amniotic fluid or in fluid from the baby's pharynx or stomach, but such tests are not part of routine clinical practice.

An echocardiograph examination would be necessary to determine whether the infant has pulmonary hypertension as a cause of the high supplementary oxygen requirements.

Q3. What differentials should be considered when a prematurely born infant develops respiratory difficulties at birth and has an ongoing respiratory support requirement?

In any prematurely born baby who develops respiratory difficulties, infection must be considered (Box 47.1).

Q4. Are any of the differentials likely here?

- The mother has gone into preterm labour at 28 weeks of gestation and infection is a cause of preterm labour; hence infection must be considered as a possible or contributory cause to this infant's respiratory distress.
- The infant has a raised carbon dioxide level and thus has lung disease, but it is possible that the infant has coexisting pulmonary hypertension. Pulmonary hypertension is common in infants with RDS, affected infants often having a poor response to exogenous surfactant therapy. Pulmonary hypertension is more common in infants who have had birth depression.
- The infant was born following preterm and prolonged rupture of the membranes and

pulmonary hypoplasia is more likely in such infants.

- Air leak and other congenital abnormalities would be excluded by the chest radiograph appearance.
- The infant was born following labour and had a vaginal delivery, making transient tachypnoea of the newborn unlikely.

Q5. How would this influence your management?

- In addition to his respiratory support being optimized, Paul should receive treatment with a natural surfactant.
- Antibiotics should be given.
- If the infant's oxygen requirement was out of proportion to the severity of lung disease, after optimizing lung recruitment by either increasing the PEEP level or transferring him to high-frequency oscillation and increasing the mean airway pressure, pulmonary hypertension should be considered and an echocardiograph examination undertaken.

Respiratory distress syndrome (RDS)

Approximately 1% of infants develop RDS. Many factors influence the development of RDS (Box 47.2).

Clinical features
- Infants with RDS present within 4 hours of birth; they are tachypnoeic (respiratory rate > 60 breaths/

BOX 47.2 Factors influencing the development of respiratory distress syndrome

Positive
- Cortisol
- Thyroxine
- Beta-adrenergic drugs
- Epidermal growth factor
- Prolactin?

Negative
- Prematurity
- Male gender
- Ethnicity (Caucasian)
- Genetic predisposition
- Insulin
- Hypoxia
- Hypothermia
- Acidosis
- Hypotension

---

min) and have intercostal and subcostal indrawing, sternal retraction, nasal flaring and an expiratory grunt.
- In the absence of surfactant therapy, the dyspnoea worsens over the first 24–36 hours after birth, due to the disappearance of the small quantities of surfactant present in an infant with RDS and the inhibitory effect of plasma proteins on surfactant, which leak on to the alveolar surface in the early oedematous stage of lung damage.
- At approximately 36–48 hours of age, endogenous surfactant synthesis commences and the infant's respiratory status improves; this is associated with a spontaneous diuresis.
- Nowadays, the classical presentation is unusual, as exogenous surfactant is given and relatively mature infants so treated are frequently in room air by 48 hours of age.

Chest radiograph appearance
- There is symmetrical diffuse atelactasis resulting in fine granular opacification in both lung fields and on air bronchogram the air-filled bronchi stand out against the atelectatic lungs.
- If the disease is severe, there may be 'white-out', the lungs appearing so opaque that it is not possible to distinguish between the lung field and the cardiothymic silhouette (Fig. 47.1).
- If the radiograph is taken in the first 4 hours, interpretation may be difficult because of retention of fetal lung fluid.

Assessment of lung maturity
- Antenatally, fetal lung maturity can be assessed by sampling amniotic fluid because, as the fluid secreted by the fetal lung moves out into the amniotic fluid, it carries with it surfactant.
- As the lung matures, the amount of DPPC (lecithin, L) in the amniotic fluid increases, but the amount of sphingomyelin (S) remains unchanged throughout gestation; thus lung maturity can be assessed from the ratio of lecithin to sphingomyelin (L:S ratio).
- An L:S ratio greater than 2.0 is usually associated with lung maturity and in 95% of cases will predict the absence of RDS. However, a mature L:S ratio can be associated with RDS in the infants of diabetic mothers or those with rhesus disease, as in such cases the abnormality is deficiency of phosphatidyglycerol.
- The lower the L:S ratio, the more likely the infant is to develop RDS, but an L:S ratio less than 2.0 predicts RDS with an accuracy of only 54%.

Differential diagnosis

- It is impossible to differentiate severe early-onset septicaemia from RDS.
- Infants with RDS may have coexistent pulmonary hypertension, their oxygen requirement will be out of proportion to their chest radiograph appearance and they frequently have a poor response to surfactant therapy.
- Respiratory distress presenting after 4–6 hours of age is usually due to pneumonia.
- Consider air leak (tension pneumothorax etc.).

Preventative strategies

Antenatal corticosteroids (Box 47.3) may be used:

- Antenatal steroids mature the fetal lung, inducing the enzymes for surfactant phospholipid synthesis and the genes for the surfactant proteins.
- Randomized trials have demonstrated that antenatal administration of dexamethasone or betamethasone to pregnant women reduces the incidences of RDS (OR 0.63, CI 0.44–0.82), neonatal death (OR 0.60, CI 0.48–0.75), cerebral haemorrhage (OR 0.48, CI 0.32–0.72) and necrotizing enterocolitis (OR 0.58, CI 0.32–1.09).
- Benefit is maximal in infants delivered between 24 and 168 hours of maternal therapy being started; a smaller benefit is seen in infants whose mothers have received less than 24 hours of treatment.
- The safety and efficacy of multiple versus single courses are currently being investigated in randomized trials.

Other antenatal strategies include the following:

- Thyrotrophin-releasing hormone (TRH), unlike T_4 (thyroxine), T_3 (tri-iodothyronine) or thyroid-stimulating hormone (TSH), crosses the placenta.

Meta-analysis of the results of randomized trials examining the efficacy of antenatal administration of TRH, however, have demonstrated that it does not reduce the risk of neonatal respiratory distress or bronchopulmonary dysplasia (BPD), but may have adverse effects.

- The effect of antenatal β-mimetics appears to be small.
- Benefit from ambroxol has been reported but this is not a consistent finding.

Management

Practice differs in the labour suite as to whether preterm babies at risk of RDS are placed immediately on nasal continuous positive airway pressure (CPAP) or intubated and given surfactant. Once surfactant is given, again practice varies, some clinicians immediately extubating the infant on to nasal CPAP while others keep the infant intubated until further assessment takes place on the neonatal intensive care unit (NICU). Others will delay giving surfactant until the infant is on the NICU.

Surfactant therapy is as follows:

- Commercially available surfactant preparations are described as 'natural' (derived from animals' lungs) or synthetic surfactants.
- Meta-analysis of data from randomized trials demonstrated that administration of natural rather than synthetic surfactant was associated with reductions in mortality and pneumothorax.
- Surfactant is usually given prophylactically, within the first hour of birth, as such a policy is associated with significant reductions in neonatal mortality, BPD and death, and in pneumothorax.
- Surfactant given as 'rescue' therapy — that is, to infants with established RDS — results in reductions in pneumothorax, mortality and the combined outcome of mortality and BPD.
- Although beneficial effects are seen after a single dose of surfactant, better results are obtained with more than one dose. Many clinicians usually now give two doses of a natural surfactant.
- Not all babies respond to surfactant, including those with a patent ductus arteriosus (PDA), cardiogenic shock, pulmonary hypertension or an air leak; failure to respond marks out a group of babies with a poorer prognosis.

Mortality and morbidity

- Overall the mortality from RDS is between 10 and 15%; the mortality rate is inversely proportional to gestational age.
- Acute complications of RDS include air leaks, PDA and pulmonary haemorrhage. Infants with RDS may suffer an intracerebral haemorrhage or periventricular leucomalacia, both conditions

---

BOX 47.3 Guidelines for antenatal steroid usage

- Should be considered for all women at risk of preterm labour between 24 and 36 weeks
- Betamethasone (two doses 24 hours apart) is preferred to dexamethasone (four doses 12 hours apart). In an observational study, betamethasone was associated with a lower occurrence of cystic periventricular leucomalacia
- Corticosteroids should be given unless immediate delivery is anticipated
- In the absence of chorioamnionitis, antenatal corticosteroids are recommended in pregnancies complicated by preterm and prolonged rupture of the membranes and in other complicated pregnancies, unless there is evidence that corticosteroids will have an adverse effect on the mother

increasing the risk of adverse neurodevelopmental outcome.

- BPD, defined as oxygen dependency beyond 36 weeks' postmenstrual age, develops in more than 50% of infants born prior to 29 weeks of gestation.

Types of respiratory support

- *Warm humidified supplementary oxygen.* This may be all that infants with mild RDS require.
- *Continuous positive airway pressure (CPAP).* This prevents atelectasis and can improve oxygenation.
- *Conventional mechanical ventilators.* These deliver intermittent positive pressure inflations and positive end-expiratory pressure (PEEP). The ventilator inflations are delivered at a preset rate.
- *Patient-triggered ventilation (PTV).* This can be delivered as assist/control (A/C); that is, every spontaneous breath can trigger a positive pressure inflation at preset peak and PEEP levels and as synchronous intermittent mandatory ventilation (SIMV) in which only a predetermined number of positive pressure inflations can be triggered regardless of the number of spontaneous breaths that exceed the critical trigger level.
- *High-frequency jet ventilation (HFJV).* High-velocity 'bullets' of gas are fired at rates of 200–600 per minute and this entrains gas down the endotracheal tube.
- *High-frequency oscillatory ventilation (HFOV).* Small tidal volumes are usually delivered at frequencies between 10 and 15 Hz.

During conventional mechanical ventilation:

- Oxygenation is controlled by the inspired oxygen concentration and the mean airway pressure (MAP).
- The MAP is controlled by the PIP, inspiratory time (Ti) and PEEP. Increased PEEP is the most effective method of increasing oxygenation.
- Carbon dioxide elimination is controlled by the minute ventilation (= tidal volume × rate); tidal volume is determined by the difference between PIP and PEEP.
- Ventilator settings should be altered according to the blood gas abnormality (Table 47.2).

Transient tachypnoea of the newborn (TTN)

TTN occurs in between 4 and 6 per 1000 term-born infants. TTN may be more common in prematurely born infants but coexisting RDS may mask the presentation.

Table 47.2 Adjustments to ventilator settings according to blood gas values

PaO_2 result	$PaCO_2$ result	Suggested changes in ventilation
Low PaO_2	Normal $PaCO_2$	↑ FiO_2 ↑ MAP by ↑ PEEP (not ↑ PIP, which will ↓ $PaCO_2$)
Low PaO_2	High $PaCO_2$	↑ PIP (which will increase MAP and increase delivered volume)
Normal PaO_2	High $PaCO_2$	Keep MAP constant ↓ PEEP or ↑ rate

(MAP = mean arterial pressure; PEEP = positive end-expiratory pressure; PIP = peak inspiratory pressure)

Pathogenesis

TTN is more common in infants who are born by caesarean section without labour, in male infants and in those with a family history of asthma.

Clinical features

Infants with TTN are tachypnoeic with respiratory rates of up to 100–120 breaths/min, but rarely grunt. Peripheral oedema is often present and affected babies lose weight more slowly than controls. There is usually only a mild hypoxia and rarely a marked respiratory or metabolic acidosis.

Chest radiograph appearance

There is hyperinflation and prominent perihilar vascular markings due to engorgement of the periarterial lymphatics, oedema of the interlobar septae and fluid in the fissures.

Management

- Supplementary oxygen may be required, but rarely high concentrations of oxygen or even mechanical ventilation are needed.
- Intravenous antibiotics should be administered until infection has been excluded.
- Nasogastric tube feeds should be withheld until the respiratory rate settles.
- Diuretics are not of benefit.

Mortality and morbidity

- TTN is self-limiting and affected infants have usually made a complete recovery within a few days of birth.
- Complications are rare, but air leaks may occur if the infant has required CPAP or mechanical ventilation.
- Infants who have had TTN are more likely to wheeze at follow-up.

- Prolonged rupture of the membranes
- Premature labour
- Organisms present in the vagina
- Chorioamnionitis
- Prolonged labour
- Frequent pelvic examinations in labour
- Mothers who, despite having GBS in their
  vagina, have little or no circulating anti-GBS
  immunoglobulin
- Food, especially dairy products, contaminated
  with *Listeria monocytogenes* by infected farm
  animals

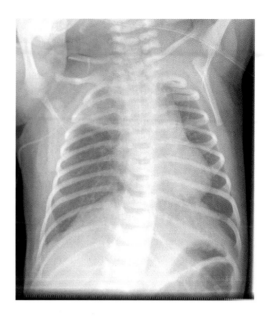

Fig. 47.2 **Lobar pneumonia with right upper lobe changes**

Pneumonia

Early-onset pneumonia

Early-onset pneumonia (Box 47.4) is acquired trans-placentally or during labour or delivery:

- Transplacentally acquired organisms include *Listeria monocytogenes, Mycobacterium tuberculosis, Treponema pallidum,* rubella virus, cytomegalovirus (CMV), herpes simplex virus (HSV), adenovirus and influenza A virus.
- In ascending infection causing pneumonia, 60–70% of cases are due to *Streptococcus agalactiae* (group B streptococcus, GBS). *Escherichia coli* (*E. coli*) is the second most common cause of early neonatal sepsis.
- Other organisms that cause ascending infection include *Haemophilus influenzae, Strep. pneumoniae, Listeria monocytogenes, Klebsiella pneumoniae, Candida albicans,* adenovirus, CMV, HSV and echovirus.

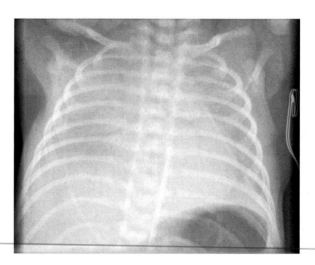

Fig. 47.3 **Diffuse group B streptococcal pneumonia with changes mimicking respiratory distress syndrome**

Clinical features

- Infants with transplacentally acquired infection present at birth and those infected with organisms acquired from the birth canal present within the first 48 hours after birth.
- The infant typically suffers progressive respiratory distress and has signs of systemic sepsis, which develop within a few hours of birth. There may be fever or hypothermia, or non-specific signs such as poor feeding and irritability.
- Infants with congenitally acquired listerial infection are often extremely ill at birth with severe pneumonia and hepatomegaly. Diarrhoea and an erythematous skin rash may occur. Characteristically, affected infants have small pinkish-grey cutaneous granulomas; these

granulomas are widespread in lung, liver and nervous system.

Chest radiograph appearance

The appearance is varied; there can be lobar (Fig. 47.2) or segmental consolidation, atelectasis or diffuse haziness or opacification (Fig. 47.3). Pleural effusions may occur, particularly if the pneumonia is the result of bacterial or fungal infection. Abscess or pneumatoceles occur with staphylococcal or coliform pneumonia.

Management

- Initial treatment for early-onset pneumonia should be a combination of ampicillin or benzylpenicillin and an aminoglycoside. Modification to that regimen may be necessary once the culture results are known:

- *H. influenzae* with ampicillin resistance is emerging and cefotaxime should be added.
- Cefotaxime and ceftriaxone are used for *E. coli* sepsis.
- For *Listeria*, the most effective antibiotic therapy is ampicillin plus gentamicin; *Listeria* is resistant to all third-generation cephalosporins.

- Antibiotic therapy should continue for at least 10 days, and for 3 weeks if the pneumonia is due to *Staphylococcus aureus*.
- Long-term intravenous therapy should be given if there is abscess formation.
- Empyemas should be drained and intravenous antibiotics administered for at least 2 weeks.
- It is important to prevent vertical transmission of GBS by giving intrapartum antibiotic prophylaxis (penicillin or ampicillin) to women identified by screening in pregnancy as carrying GBS and/or having risk factors:
  - A previous infant with GBS disease
  - GBS in the maternal urine during pregnancy
  - Preterm labour
  - Ruptured membranes for more than 18 hours prior to delivery
  - Intrapartum fever.

Late-onset pneumonia

- The most commonly responsible bacteria are coagulase-negative staphylococci, *Staph. aureus* and Gram-negative bacilli, including *Klebsiella*, *E. coli* and *Pseudomonas*.
- Viruses can also cause late-onset pneumonia, including respiratory syncytial virus (RSV), influenza virus, parainfluenza virus, adenovirus and rhinovirus.
- Fungal infections can occur in infants who have had prolonged exposure to antibiotics, particularly third-generation cephalosporins.

Clinical features
There is an increasing requirement for ventilatory support and/or supplementary oxygen.

Management
- Initial antibiotic treatment should be guided by local microbiological data.
- If the infant is already on antibiotics, the regimen should usually be changed and the spectrum of cover broadened.

Pulmonary hypoplasia

Clinical features
- Infants with mild pulmonary hypoplasia may be apparently asymptomatic but on inspection are tachypnoeic.
- Those more severely affected require ventilatory support from birth.
- Infants with pulmonary hypoplasia have small-volume, non-compliant lungs and their chest wall is disproportionately small with respect to the abdomen.
- Infants with secondary pulmonary hypoplasia may have associated congenital anomalies: for example, diaphragmatic hernia/eventration, an anterior abdominal wall defect, a dislocated hip and/or talipes. They may also have the features of neuromuscular diseases such as Werdnig–Hoffmann disease or congenital dystrophia myotonica.

Diagnosis
- On the chest radiograph, the ribs may appear crowded with a low thoracic to abdominal ratio and a classically bell-shaped chest, but the lung fields are clear unless there is coexisting RDS.
- Pneumothorax or other forms of air leak are frequently present.

Differential diagnosis
The 'dry lung syndrome' has been described following oligohydramnios due to premature rupture of the membranes and is likely to be due to functional compression. Affected infants are difficult to resuscitate, requiring high peak inflating pressures; the requirement for high pressures may continue for 48 hours but then the infants make a spontaneous recovery, indicating that they have no structural abnormality.

Pathology
Pulmonary hypoplasia is diagnosed if the lung weight to body weight ratio is less than 0.015 in infants born before 28 weeks of gestation and less than 0.012 in infants born after 28 weeks of gestation; in addition there is a radial alveolar count of less than 4%.

Management
Antenatal measures are as follows:
- Pleural effusions can be chronically drained by thoraco-amniotic shunts, which will facilitate ease of resuscitation.
- In utero surgery has been undertaken for infants with CDH but this has been problematic. The efficacy of reversible tracheal 'obstruction' is being investigated in cases predicted to be at high risk of fatal pulmonary hypoplasia.

Postnatal measures are as follows:

- The minimum ventilator pressures compatible with acceptable gases should be used, as these infants are at high risk of air leaks.
- Low-pressure, fast-rate ventilation or high-frequency oscillatory ventilation (HFOV) can be helpful in some infants, but extra-corporeal membranous oxygenation (ECMO) would usually be contraindicated as the infants do not have a reversible condition.
- Pulmonary vasodilators can be useful if there is coexisting pulmonary hypertension.
- Home oxygen therapy allows early discharge, but parents need to be counselled that supplementary oxygen may be required for many months.
- Every attempt should be made to reduce further compromise to the lungs; full immunization is essential and RSV prophylaxis should be considered.

Mortality and morbidity

- Infants with Potter's syndrome (renal agenesis, large low-set ears, prominent epicanthic folds and a flattened nose) and postural limb defects die in the neonatal period.
- There is also 100% mortality rate in infants with the oligohydramnios syndrome (pulmonary hypoplasia, abnormal facies and limb abnormalities) due to prolonged rupture of the membranes. In less severely affected infants, the perinatal mortality rate is approximately 50% if membrane rupture occurs between 15 and 28 weeks.
- Infants with pulmonary hypoplasia who remain on high-pressure ventilation and high inspired oxygen concentrations at the end of the first week are in an extremely bad prognostic group, rarely surviving to discharge; those that do survive require home oxygen therapy and many die in the first 2 years following infection.
- Infants born following oligohydramnios can suffer limb abnormalities due to the compression, the reported incidence varying from 27 to 80%.
- Neurological or developmental deficits are common, being reported in 28% of infants born after preterm rupture of the membranes prior to 26 weeks of gestation.

Problem-orientated topic:

a term baby with respiratory distress from birth

A female infant (birth weight 4.1 kg) is delivered at 42 weeks of gestation by emergency caesarean section for fetal distress. The infant is covered with meconium, makes no respiratory effort at birth and has a heart rate of 40 beats/min. The infant is intubated and no meconium is seen below the cords. The infant responds rapidly to positive pressure inflations and is extubated at 5 minutes. At 1 hour, however, the infant is still tachypnoeic and is then noted to have an oxygen saturation of 80% in air.

Q1. Does the baby have meconium aspiration syndrome (MAS)?

Q2. What further information would help you to be sure?

Q3. What differentials should be considered?

Q4. Are any of the differentials likely and, if so, how would this influence your management?

Q1. Does the baby have meconium aspiration syndrome (MAS)?

The baby was born post-term and MAS is more common in post-mature babies. In addition, she has fetal distress and is covered in meconium at delivery. There is, however, no meconium below the vocal cords when the infant is intubated.

Q2. What further information would help you to be sure?

The chest radiograph in MAS demonstrates widespread patchy infiltration and over-expansion (Fig. 47.4); small pleural effusions occur in approximately 20% of patients. A radiograph facilitates exclusion or diagnosis of other causes of respiratory distress such as air leak, infection or a congenital abnormality (e.g. a diaphragmatic hernia or cystic adenomatoid malformation). It also demonstrates whether an infant has RDS, which would be very uncommon in a mature infant; when it does occur, there is often a family history. Acute respiratory distress syndrome (ARDS) is more likely than RDS and occurs in infants who have suffered birth depression.

In this case, there is no patchy infiltrate but bilateral pneumothoraces.

Q3. What differentials should be considered?

In any baby with respiratory problems, infection must be considered (Box 47.5).

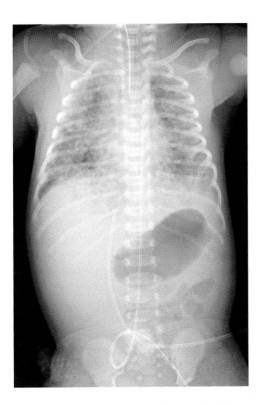

Fig. 47.4 Meconium aspiration syndrome with diffuse bilateral patchy infiltrates

---

BOX 47.5 Causes of respiratory distress from birth in a term infant

- Meconium aspiration syndrome
- Congenital pneumonia/sepsis
- Transient tachypnoea of the newborn
- Air leak
- Respiratory distress syndrome
- Acute respiratory distress syndrome
- Congenital abnormalities

Q4. **Are any of the differentials likely and, if so, how would this influence your management?**

- In the absence of any rapid reliable diagnostic test for infection, any infant with respiratory distress should receive intravenous antibiotics until blood culture results are available at 48 hours.
- This infant required positive pressure resuscitation and this increases the risk of air leak; whether an air leak requires intervention, such as a drainage procedure, is determined by the size of the air leak and the magnitude of the infant's respiratory distress.
- This infant's respiratory status deteriorated and she required 60% supplementary oxygen to maintain

appropriate oxygen saturation levels. The bilateral pneumothoraces were drained by placement of chest tubes and underwater-sealed drains.

Meconium aspiration syndrome (MAS)

- Meconium staining of the amniotic fluid occurs in 8–20% of pregnancies.
- Five percent of babies born through meconium-stained amniotic fluid develop MAS.
- Meconium aspiration is a disease of term or post-term babies; if meconium staining of the liquor occurs in a preterm pregnancy, it suggests infection.

Pathophysiology

Prolonged severe fetal hypoxia can stimulate fetal breathing with inhalation of amniotic fluid containing meconium or the inhalation occurs perinatally if the airway contains meconium-stained amniotic fluid. Meconium inhalation causes a number of problems:

- Meconium is irritant and inflammatory cells and mediators are released in response to the presence of the meconium in the airways. An inflammatory pneumonitis with alveolar collapse develops.
- The pulmonary artery pressure is increased, as the inflammatory response results in release of substances that cause vasoconstriction.
- Although meconium is initially sterile, because of its organic nature, its presence in the airway predisposes to pulmonary infection, particularly with *E. coli*. In addition, as meconium may inhibit phagocytosis and the neutrophil oxidative burst, bacteria can grow in meconium-stained amniotic fluid.
- Meconium (particularly the chloroform-soluble phase: free fatty acids, triglycerides and cholesterol) inhibits surfactant function and production in a concentration-dependent manner.
- Meconium is sticky and composed of inspissated fetal intestinal secretions. When it is inhaled it creates a ball valve mechanism in the airways; air can be sucked in but cannot be exhaled. The result is gas trapping and lung over-distension, predisposing to air leaks.

Clinical features

- Infants with MAS are tachypnoeic and have intercostal and subcostal recession.
- They are frequently hypoxic due to ventilation–perfusion mismatch and pulmonary hypertension.
- The meconium in the airways causes widespread crackles and, due to air trapping, affected infants have an over-distended chest.

- In mild cases recovery may occur within 24 hours.
- Infants who require ventilation are frequently still symptomatic at 2 weeks of age and may remain oxygen-dependent beyond the neonatal period.

Chest radiograph appearance

- Early radiographs demonstrate widespread patchy infiltration and over-expansion (Fig. 47.4); small pleural effusions occur in approximately 20% of patients.
- In severe cases, by 72 hours of age the appearance is of diffuse and homogeneous opacification of both lung fields because of pneumonitis and interstitial oedema.
- In severe cases the chest radiograph appearance may merge into the pattern seen in BPD.

Management

- Broad-spectrum antibiotics, such as penicillin and gentamicin, should be given.
- Sufficient supplementary oxygen should be given to maintain the arterial oxygen saturation levels at 95% or arterial oxygen level greater than 10 kPa. Warmed humidified oxygen should be delivered into a head box, even if the infant requires an oxygen concentration of up to 80%, providing there is no respiratory acidosis.
- CPAP may improve oxygenation but will increase the risk of pneumothorax and thus is not recommended in MAS.
- Intubation and ventilation are indicated if the $PaCO_2$ rises above 8 kPa (60 mmHg), particularly if the infant is hypoxic. If, however, the infant has hypoxic–ischaemic encephalopathy more rigid control of the blood gases is required.
- Babies with MAS can be very difficult to ventilate; theoretically, a long expiratory time and a low level of PEEP should be used, but elevation of PEEP may be necessary to improve oxygenation.
- A neuromuscular blocking agent should be administered, as infants with MAS often 'fight' the ventilator, thus increasing their risk of an air leak.
- In infants with severe disease and pulmonary hypertension, HFOV, particularly if used with nitric oxide, can improve oxygenation and reduce the need for ECMO.
- Meta-analysis of the results of two randomized trials demonstrated that surfactant administration also reduces the risk of requiring ECMO. Administering the surfactant by dilute surfactant lavage may be particularly effective in improving gas exchange.

Preventative strategies

- A meta-analysis of the results of four randomized trials showed no significant benefit of routine endotracheal intubation and suctioning at birth over routine resuscitation, including oropharyngeal suctioning of vigorous term meconium-stained babies.
- On the evidence to date, intubation and suctioning should be restricted to newborns who are depressed: that is, they have a heart rate less than 100 beats/min, poor respiratory effort and poor tone.
- Compression of the neonatal thorax is not recommended, as it is unlikely to prevent gasping and can stimulate respiratory efforts.
- Aspiration of the stomach is frequently undertaken to prevent subsequent inhalation following vomiting or reflux of previously swallowed meconium.

Mortality and morbidity

- Mortality rates are between 4 and 12%; the majority of deaths are from respiratory failure, pulmonary hypertension or air leaks.
- Fifty percent of babies who require mechanical ventilation because of MAS suffer an air leak.
- Bronchopulmonary dysplasia is a rare complication of MAS.
- Neurological sequelae occur in infants with coexisting HIE.
- Lung function abnormalities, including increased bronchial hyper-reactivity, have been reported and up to 40% of those who have had severe MAS go on to develop asthma at school age.

Pulmonary hypertension of the newborn

Clinical features

- Infants with persistent pulmonary hypertension of the newborn (PPHN) usually present within 12 hours of birth.
- Affected infants are cyanosed but have only mild respiratory distress, unless they have an underlying disorder such as GBS infection or CDH.

Diagnosis

- Hypoxaemia is disproportionately severe for the radiological abnormalities.
- There is a right-to-left ductal shunt with a lower level of oxygenation in the distal aortic blood (obtained from an umbilical artery catheter) compared to the preductal blood (obtained from the right radial artery).
- The echocardiograph demonstrates a structurally normal heart.

Chest radiograph appearance

The chest radiograph changes may be minimal in primary pulmonary hypertension and in secondary pulmonary hypertension the appearance is that of the underlying lung disease.

Investigations

- The response to ventilation with 100% oxygen can help to distinguish between PPHN and cyanotic heart disease; in some infants with pulmonary hypertension, the arterial oxygen level will increase to above 13 kPa (100 mmHg), whereas in cyanotic congenital heart disease it will not rise above 5–6 kPa (37.5–45 mmHg).
- Not all neonates with pulmonary hypertension, however, especially those with sepsis or a CDH, have a large improvement in oxygenation in response to 100% oxygen.
- Echocardiography is important, not only to establish the diagnosis but also to exclude cyanotic congenital heart disease.

Management

- It is easy to precipitate severe hypoxaemia in infants with pulmonary hypertension; thus minimal handling is important.
- Aggressive therapy should be used to achieve an appropriate systemic blood pressure, as the size of the right–left shunt is in part dependent on the systemic blood pressure.
- To maximize oxygen transport to the tissues, the haemoglobin level should be kept greater than 13 g/dl (packed cell volume (PCV) 40%). If the infant is polycythaemic (central PCV greater than 70%), a dilutional exchange transfusion should be undertaken.
- Broad-spectrum antibiotic cover should be given. Infants should be ventilated if their PaO_2 is less than 5–6 kPa (37–45 mmHg) in 70% oxygen. Hyperventilation to reduce the $PaCO_2$ to 2.5–3.5 kPa is no longer recommended, as this has adverse effects.
- Alkalosis can promote pulmonary vasodilatation, but prolonged alkalosis should be avoided as this increases the hypoxic reactivity of the pulmonary vasculature.
- ECMO is an effective rescue therapy for infants with pulmonary hypertension.
- A number of vasodilator drugs have been used to treat pulmonary hypertension in the neonate.
- Unfortunately, neither tolazoline nor epoprostenol (prostacyclin) is a specific vasodilator and their administration can result in systemic hypotension; in addition they are not always effective, only between 25 and 50% of affected babies responding to tolazoline.

- Magnesium sulphate administration also can improve oxygenation, but levels must be carefully monitored, as hypermagnesaemia can cause hyporeflexia, hypotension and calcium and potassium disturbances.
- Inhaled nitric oxide (NO) is a specific pulmonary vasodilator. When NO is inhaled, it diffuses across the capillary membrane and activates guanylate cyclase in the pulmonary arteriolar smooth muscle; the resulting increase in cyclic guanosine monophosphate (cGMP) causes smooth muscle relaxation. NO then binds rapidly to haemoglobin; once bound, it is inactivated and therefore produces no systemic effects.
- In term infants 5 ppm of iNO appears as effective as higher doses.
- In term-born babies, meta-analysis of the results of randomized trials demonstrated that inhaled NO results in an improvement in oxygenation and a reduction in the combined outcome of death or need for ECMO; the effect is due to a reduction in the need for ECMO.
- Inhaled NO works best if given in association with a volume recruitment ventilation strategy.
- No significant long-term benefits of inhaled NO have been demonstrated in babies with CDH and its use in preterm infants remains experimental.
- NO does have side-effects related to nitrogen dioxide and methaemoglobin formation and its administration has been associated with an increased bleeding time.

Mortality

The mortality rates are between 10 and 20% in infants who require ECMO because of primary pulmonary hypertension or pulmonary hypertension complicating RDS or MAS. In babies with GBS sepsis, the mortality rate ranges from 10 to 50%.

Problem-orientated topic:

respiratory deterioration in an older premature infant

A 26-week gestation infant, Jenny, has been ventilator- and oxygen-dependent since birth. At 3 weeks of age she develops gradually increasing respiratory support requirements.

Q1. Does the infant have bronchopulmonary dysplasia?

Q2. What is the most likely cause of the infant's condition?

Continued overleaf

Q3. What is the differential diagnosis of the deterioration?

Q4. What further information would help you to be sure?

Q1. Does the infant have bronchopulmonary dysplasia?

Bronchopulmonary dysplasia (BPD) is diagnosed in an infant with or without ventilator dependence who is chronically oxygen-dependent beyond at least 28 days after birth. As Jenny is only 3 weeks old, she does not yet fit the definition of BPD but is at high risk of developing the condition.

Q2. What is the most likely cause of the infant's condition?

Ventilator-dependent prematurely born infants are at increased risk of nosocomial infection and this is a frequent cause of deterioration in such babies. Organisms isolated from the endotracheal tube may not be responsible for the infection and could reflect colonization only. Viral infections should also be considered as a cause of the deterioration and the appropriate samples sent to the laboratory, including a nasopharyngeal aspirate to exclude RSV and other respiratory viruses.

Q3. What is the differential diagnosis of the deterioration?

- Infection
- PDA
- Gastro-oesophageal reflux with aspiration.

Q4. What further information would help you to be sure?

- A new or worsening PDA murmur would suggest this to be the cause of the deterioration; this should then be investigated by an echo examination.
- A chest radiograph demonstrating new abnormalities would be suggestive of infection.
- If there were abnormalities in the right upper lobe on the chest radiograph, this would be suggestive of aspiration, particularly if there was a history of obtaining milk on suctioning. A pH study would determine if there was acid reflux.

Bronchopulmonary dysplasia (BPD)

Northway et al (1967) originally described four stages of BPD, based on a sequence of chest radiograph changes. A more functional definition has been recommended at a workshop sponsored by the National Institutes of Health (NIH):

- Infants are considered to have BPD if oxygen-dependent for at least 28 days.
- They are then classified as suffering from mild, moderate or severe BPD according to their respiratory support requirement at a later date:
  - Mild BPD if they were breathing air
  - Moderate BPD if they required less than 30% supplementary oxygen
  - Severe BPD if they needed more than 30% oxygen and/or intermittent positive pressure ventilation (IPPV) or CPAP.
- Immature infants (less than 32 weeks of gestational age) are assessed at 36 weeks post-menstrual age (PMA) or at discharge home, whichever comes first.
- Infants born at 32 weeks of gestation or more are assessed at 56 days' postnatal age or discharge home, whichever comes first.

Pathogenesis

- There is an inverse relationship between the incidence of BPD and gestational age.
- BPD most commonly occurs in prematurely born infants who have had RDS, but can occur in immature infants who had no initial lung disease.
- Infants born at term may also develop BPD, particularly if they suffered severe initial lung disease, as evidenced by a requirement for ECMO.
- BPD was originally ascribed to oxygen toxicity. Oxygen toxicity is caused by the increased production of cytotoxic oxygen free radicals, which overwhelm the antioxidant defences. Prematurely born infants are particularly vulnerable, as they have incomplete development of their pulmonary antioxidant enzyme systems and low levels of antioxidants, such as vitamins C and E.
- Baro- or volutrauma is incriminated and there is an inverse relationship between hypocarbia during mechanical ventilation and BPD development. Volutrauma may occur at resuscitation if rapid lung expansion is attempted.
- Pulmonary interstitial emphysema (PIE) has been associated with a high incidence of BPD; respiratory function is compromised by air dissection into false air spaces.
- Fluid overload may explain the association of PDA and BPD, as it causes congestive heart failure and hence deterioration in lung function. The

association of PDA and an increased risk of BPD is potentiated by infection, particularly if temporally related.

- Antenatal infection, chorioamnionitis and postnatal infection may predispose to BPD development.
- BPD has been associated with persisting surfactant abnormalities; the L:S ratio increases slowly in BPD infants and there is late appearance of PG. Abnormalities related to surfactant proteins, particularly SP-A, have also been associated with BPD.

Pathophysiology
During the acute phase of lung injury, a host response is initiated that persists in infants who develop BPD:

- Proinflammatory cytokines (interleukins (IL) IL-1, IL-6 and soluble intercellular adhesion molecule (ICAM)-1) are demonstrated in the lung lavage from day 1, reaching a peak in the second week. ICAM-1 is a glycoprotein that allows cell-to-cell contact.
- Direct contact between activated cells leads to further production of proinflammatory cytokines and other mediators.
- IL-1β activity also increases during the first week, inducing the release of inflammatory mediators, activating inflammatory cells and upregulating adhesion molecules on endothelial cells.
- There is release of the α-chemokine, IL-8, which induces neutrophil chemotaxis, and the β-chemokine macrophage inflammatory protein (MIP)-1-α, which is chemotactic for monocytes and macrophages.
- The activated neutrophils mediate endothelial cytotoxicity, inhibit phosphatidylcholine synthesis and release elastase. There are also raised levels of collagenase and phospholipase A2.
- Inactivation of α-1-antiprotease by oxidative modification further compromises the protease–antiprotease imbalance.
- Leucotrienes, present in high levels in the lungs of infants developing BPD, cause bronchoconstriction, vasoconstriction, oedema, neutrophil chemotaxis and mucus production in the lung.
- The inflammatory infiltration is associated with loss of endothelial, basement membrane and interstitial sulphated glycoaminoglycans, which are important in restricting albumin flux and inhibiting fibrosis.
- Tumour necrosis factor-alpha (TNF-α) activity increases late; TNF-α and IL-6 induce fibroblast and collagen production and cause pulmonary fibrosis in animal models.

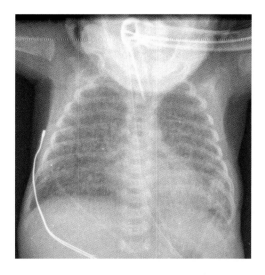

Fig. 47.5 Bronchopulmonary dysplasia with diffuse fibrotic shadows

Clinical features
- The majority of cases have been dependent on oxygen supplementation and often mechanical ventilation since birth. Some, however, may have had minimal or no initial respiratory distress, but then deteriorate and become chronically oxygen-dependent.
- Infants with BPD frequently fail to thrive. Feeding difficulties and aspiration are common, due to bulbar dysfunction or gastro-oesophageal reflux.
- They are at high risk of deterioration related to recurrent respiratory infections. Copious endotracheal secretions, persistent atelectasis, lobar hyperinflation and tracheomalacia and/or bronchomalacia are common.
- The most severely affected infants develop right heart failure, and cor pulmonale develops in those who are chronically hypoxaemic.
- Osteopenia is common and fractures may occur.

Chest radiograph appearance
- Infants with the most severe BPD have hyper-expansion, streaks of abnormal density (Fig. 47.5), areas of emphysema and cystic abnormalities more marked at the lung bases; this picture is consistent with 'Northway BPD type IV'.
- The majority of prematurely born infants have non-specific abnormalities, which include small-volume hazy lung fields.

Computed tomography (CT)
CT scans, rather than chest radiographs, give more detailed information. Common findings on CT are multi-focal areas of hyperaeration, and linear and triangular subpleural opacities.

Pathology

- Histological examination of the lungs demonstrates areas of emphysema, which may coalesce into larger cystic areas surrounded by areas of atelectasis.
- Florid obliterative bronchiolitis occurs, particularly if high peak inflating pressures have been used. This results in occlusion of the airway lumen and distal pulmonary collapse.
- In older infants, there is airway injury, smooth muscle hypertrophy, squamous metaplasia of the respiratory epithelium, glandular hyperplasia, fibrosis alternating with areas of emphysema and hypertrophy of the pulmonary arterial smooth muscle.
- In 'new' BPD there is dilated distal gas exchange structures, decreased alveolarization, minimal small airway injury and less prominent inflammation and fibrosis. As a consequence, it has been proposed that the 'new' BPD is not primarily the injury/repair paradigm of traditional BPD, but rather a maldevelopment sequence resulting from interference/interruption of normal developmental signalling for terminal maturation and alveolarization of the lungs of very preterm infants.

Management

- The peak inspiratory pressures and inspired oxygen concentrations should be kept to the minimum compatible with appropriate blood gases (a PaO_2 of 6.7–9.3 kPa and no evidence of a respiratory acidosis (pH < 7.20)).
- Results of recent randomized trials have demonstrated that there is no overall advantage in keeping oxygen saturation levels above 92%, but in infants with evidence of pulmonary hypertension the oxygen saturation level should be maintained at 95% at least.
- After the first week, increasing the PEEP level to 6 cmH$_2$O can improve oxygenation without adversely affecting CO_2 elimination, but this strategy may not be successful in infants with severe 'cystic' BPD.
- Inhaled NO can improve oxygenation in infants with developing or established BPD; randomized trials are required to determine whether inhaled NO will improve long-term outcome.
- Certain infants, despite appropriate respiratory support, suddenly become grey, pale, sweaty and cyanosed, frequently associated with poor chest wall expansion. These episodes seem to occur in agitated infants and sedation can help to reduce the number of episodes, but if they are very frequent and troublesome it may be necessary to paralyse affected infants.
- Infants with BPD may require prolonged ventilation, and tracheostomy should be considered for infants who remain fully ventilated after 3 months of age.
- Frequent attempts should be made to wean the infant from the ventilator.
- Methylxanthines may be useful to hasten weaning but have only been of proven value in infants less than 1 month old.
- No long-term positive effects of bronchodilator administration to infants on the neonatal unit have been demonstrated and their use should be restricted to infants whose respiratory status is compromised by reversible airways obstruction.
- The timing of administration of systemic corticosteroids influences the impact of their efficacy and they have numerous side-effects:
  - Commenced in the first 96 hours after birth, corticosteroids reduce the risk of BPD at both 28 days and 36 weeks PMA, lower the risk of PDA and pulmonary air leak and promote earlier extubation, but adverse neurodevelopmental outcome is increased.
  - Given in the second week after birth, corticosteroids significantly reduce BPD at 28 days and 36 weeks post-conceptual age (PCA), but also lower mortality at 28 days.
  - If started after 3 weeks of age, there is a significant reduction in BPD at 36 weeks PCA and a reduction in failure to extubate by 28 days and in need for late-rescue dexamethasone and home oxygen therapy.
  - Inhaled compared to systemic administration of corticosteroids has a slower onset of action and a smaller magnitude of effect; inhaled steroid therapy initiated in the first 2 weeks after birth results in a reduction in requirement for rescue systemic steroids and facilitates extubation.
- Chest infections occur frequently in infants with BPD and should be treated with antibiotics or antiviral therapy as appropriate.
- Infants with severe BPD will not usually tolerate more than 150 ml/kg/24 hr. If their weight gain is greater than 20 g/kg/24 hr on such a regimen, this may indicate heart failure and regular diuretics should be considered. If chronic diuretic therapy is given, acid–base balance, chloride and calcium levels must be carefully monitored and regular renal ultrasounds performed to check for the development of nephrocalcinosis.
- Meta-analysis of randomized trials has demonstrated that chronic administration of

diuretics results in no long-term benefits and can result in side-effects; thus diuretics should be reserved for infants with acute fluid overload or who are in incipient heart failure.

- Infants with BPD require a calorie intake approximately 20–40% greater than age-matched infants without respiratory embarrassment. Energy requirements above 150 kcal/kg are rare and usually associated with malabsorption. Large-volume, enterally administered feeds are poorly tolerated and restriction to 120 ml/kg/day, using either a concentrated preterm feed or calorie supplementation, is preferable. A milk fortifier may be needed if the infant is receiving human milk.
- Parental support is essential as affected infants have prolonged admissions.
- Routine immunizations should be given once BPD infants reach 2 months of age, but a killed polio vaccine should be used if they are still on the NICU. Immunization against influenza should also be considered, especially for infants receiving home oxygen therapy. Immunoprophylaxis against RSV should be given for infants discharged home on supplementary oxygen and considered for other BPD infants.
- Home oxygen therapy should be considered for infants who have no medical problem other than their increased inspired oxygen requirement or, if there is appropriate community support, tube feeding.

Mortality and morbidity
- Mortality is usually caused by intercurrent infection, cor pulmonale or respiratory failure.
- BPD infants may require many months, if not years, of supplementary oxygen at home.
- BPD infants suffer frequent respiratory deteriorations and require on average two rehospitalizations in the first 2 years. Rehospitalization is more likely in those who require supplementary oxygen at home and/or have an RSV infection.
- Pulmonary function abnormalities in the first year are common and include a high airways resistance, low dynamic pulmonary compliance, reduced functional residual capacity and abnormal gas exchange. Lung function usually improves with age but may still be abnormal, with reduced exercise tolerance and increased airway hyper-reactivity, in school-age children.
- Infants with severe BPD suffer growth failure and, although growth accelerates as respiratory symptoms improve, those with severe BPD may still be of small stature as adults.

- Poor developmental outcome is more common in those requiring a prolonged hospitalization.

Apnoea

Apnoea is a common problem in prematurely born infants and the incidence is inversely related to gestational age. There are three types of apnoea:
- *Central.* There is total cessation of inspiratory efforts with no evidence of obstruction.
- *Obstructed.* Infants have chest wall movement but no nasal airflow, as they try to breathe against an obstructed airway.
- *Mixed.* Obstructed respiratory efforts are usually followed by central apnoeas.

Infants may also have periodic breathing: regular cycles of breathing of 10–18 seconds' duration interrupted by pauses in respiratory activity of at least 3 seconds in duration, that pattern occurring for at least 2 minutes.

Causes
- Immaturity of the respiratory centre
- Intracranial bleed
- Hydrocephalus
- Infection
- Anaemia
- Metabolic disturbances
- Temperature instability
- Medications, e.g. opiates.

Management
- Stimulation
- CPAP, which may be of benefit in infants who have frequent troublesome apnoeas
- Severe refractory apnoea: intubation and ventilation
- Pharmacological treatment:
  - Caffeine, preferred to theophylline as it has a higher therapeutic index and is 'once a day'
  - Doxapram for refractory cases.

Air leaks

Pneumothorax

Pathogenesis
- Spontaneous pneumothoraces occur immediately after birth due to the high transpulmonary pressure swings generated by the first spontaneous breaths.
- Pneumothoraces more usually occur as a complication of respiratory disease or a congenital malformation, particularly if there is uneven ventilation, alveolar over-distension and air trapping and the infant is receiving ventilatory support.

349

- Approximately 5–10% of ventilated babies develop air leaks; they are particularly likely to occur in babies who 'fight' the ventilator and actively exhale during ventilator inflation (active expiration).
- Rarely, pneumothoraces occur as a result of a direct injury to the lung: for example, by perforation by suction catheters or introducers passed through the endotracheal tube or by central venous catheter placement.

Clinical features

- Small pneumothoraces may be asymptomatic.
- Large pneumothoraces are associated with dramatic deterioration and marked respiratory distress, desaturation, pallor and shock.
- A tension pneumothorax results in a shift of the mediastinum and abdominal distension due to displacement of the diaphragm.
- Pneumothorax can aggravate intracerebral haemorrhage in preterm infants.

Chest radiograph appearance

- A large pneumothorax is associated with absent lung markings and a collapsed lung on the ipsilateral side.
- If the pneumothorax is under tension, there will also be eversion of the diaphragm, bulging intercostal spaces and mediastinal shift (Fig. 47.6).
- A small pneumothorax, however, may only be recognized by a difference in radiolucency between the two lung fields (Fig. 47.7).
- A lateral chest radiograph (Fig. 47.8) can be useful to demonstrate the free air and to identify whether the tip of the chest drain is optimally placed.

Differential diagnosis

Unusually the appearance of either lobar emphysema or cystic adenomatoid malformation of the lung may resemble a pneumothorax. In a preterm infant with a thin chest wall, transillumination with an intense beam from a fibreoptic light will demonstrate an abnormal air collection by an increased transmission of light, but pulmonary interstitial emphysema can give a similar appearance.

Management

- Asymptomatic pneumothoraces do not require treatment, but the infant should be monitored until the pneumothorax has resolved.
- Nursing an infant with a pneumothorax in an inspired oxygen concentration of 100% favours resorption of the extra-alveolar gas, but this strategy should not be used in infants at risk of retinopathy of prematurity.
- If the infant is symptomatic or has a tension

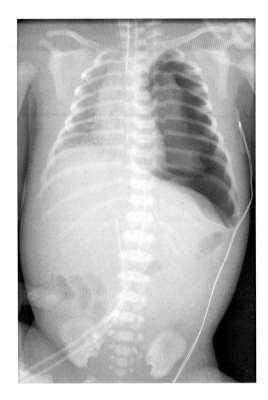

Fig. 47.6 Tension left-sided pneumothorax with mediastinal displacement and eversion of the ipsilateral diaphragm

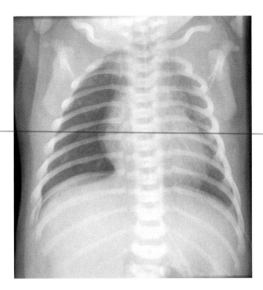

Fig. 47.7 Small right-sided pneumothorax demonstrated by the discrepancy in the translucency of the lung fields and a small rim of basal free air

pneumothorax, the pneumothorax must be drained. If the infant is in extremis and there is no time for insertion of a chest drain, emergency aspiration should be undertaken with a butterfly needle (18-gauge).

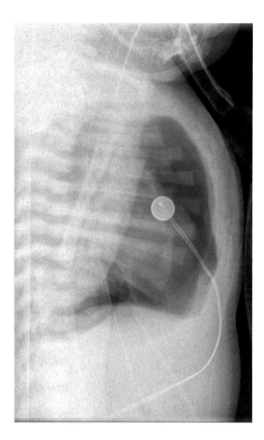

Fig. 47.8 Lateral chest radiograph demonstrating a large pneumothorax

- A chest tube (French gauge 10–14) should be inserted under local anaesthesia through either the second intercostal space just lateral to the mid-clavicular line or the sixth space in the mid-axillary line. The tip of the chest tube should be retrosternal to achieve the most effective drainage. A lateral chest radiograph should be obtained to determine whether the drain has been positioned correctly.
- Once inserted, the tube should be connected to an underwater seal drain with suction of 5–10 cmH$_2$O. Heimlich valves are useful during transport but, as they can become blocked, they should not be used for long-term drainage. The chest drain can be removed 24 hours after there is no further bubbling of air into the water seal.
- Complications of chest drains include traumatization of the lung, the thoracic duct resulting in a chylothorax, cardiac tamponade due to a haemorrhagic pericardial effusion and phrenic nerve injury.

Preventative strategies
- Neuromuscular blocking agents can be given to stop infants breathing out of phase with the ventilator (active expiration or asynchrony).

- Analgesics and/or sedatives are also given to try to suppress respiratory activity but have not been demonstrated in randomized trials to reduce the pneumothorax rate.
- An alternative approach is to use a form of ventilatory support that encourages the infant to breathe synchronously with the ventilator: that is, inspiration and inflation coinciding. Use of a faster (60/min) rather than a slower (30–40/min) ventilator rate and rescue high-frequency oscillation, but not patient-triggered ventilation, has been associated with a lower pneumothorax rate.
- Surfactant administration is associated with a lower risk of pneumothorax development.

Pulmonary interstitial emphysema (PIE)

The incidence of PIE is inversely related to birth weight. It occurs in neonates with respiratory distress supported by positive-pressure ventilation and exposed to high-peak inspiratory pressures and/or malpositioned endotracheal tubes. PIE commonly involves both lungs but may be lobar in distribution. It frequently occurs with either a pneumothorax or a pneumomediastinum.

Pathogenesis
In surfactant-deficient infants, rupture of the small airways can occur distal to the termination of the fascial sheath; gas then dissects into the interstitium and becomes trapped within the perivascular sheaths of the lung, resulting in PIE. The trapped gas reduces pulmonary perfusion by compressing the vessels and interfering with ventilation; as a result, affected infants are profoundly hypoxaemic and hypercarbic.

Chest radiograph appearance
The chest radiograph demonstrates hyperinflation and a characteristic cystic appearance (Fig. 47.9).

Management
If the PIE is localized:
- The infant should be nursed in the lateral decubitus position with the affected lung dependent and hence under-ventilated; this promotes partial or complete atelectasis.
- Selective bronchial intubation to bypass the affected lung for 24–48 hours may also be associated with resolution of the PIE.
- If the PIE persists and compresses adjacent normal lung parenchyma despite such manoeuvres, resection of the affected area may be necessary to alleviate respiratory distress.

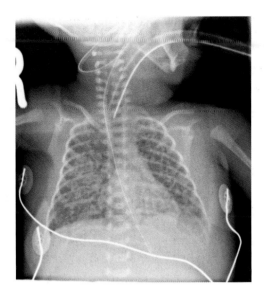

Fig. 47.9 Diffuse pulmonary interstitial emphysema

If the infant has widespread PIE:

- The ventilator pressures should be reduced to the minimum compatible with acceptable gases.
- Transfer to high-frequency jet, flow interruption or oscillatory ventilation may improve gas exchange.
- If the infant is in extremis, linear pleurotomies, scarifing the lung through the chest wall to create an artificial pneumothorax, may help to decompress the PIE.

Mortality and morbidity

The mortality from diffuse PIE is high and survivors frequently develop BPD.

Pneumomediastinum

Pneumomediastinum occurs in approximately 2.5 per 1000 live births. An isolated pneumomediastinum rarely causes severe symptoms, but pneumomediastinum usually occurs with multiple air leaks in severely ill ventilated babies.

Chest radiograph appearance

On the chest radiograph, a pneumomediastinum appears as a halo of air adjacent to the borders of the heart, and on lateral view there is marked retrosternal hyperlucency. The mediastinal gas may elevate the thymus away from the pericardium, resulting in a crescentic configuration resembling a spinnaker sail.

Management

An isolated pneumomediastinum usually requires no treatment. Drainage of a pneumomediastinum is difficult; multiple needling and tube drainage may be required, as the gas is in multiple independent lobules.

Acute respiratory distress syndrome (ARDS) (see also p. 305)

Pathogenesis

ARDS can occur following asphyxia, shock, sepsis or MAS. Asphyxia results in damage to the myocardium and the associated severe metabolic acidaemia in depressed myocardial contractility; this leads to heart failure and pulmonary oedema. Asphyxia also damages the pulmonary blood vessels and ARDS develops if there is a large leak of protein-rich fluid on to the alveoli.

Clinical features

ARDS is a disease of term babies. In the first hours after birth affected infants usually present with tachypnoea (respiratory rate of at least 100/min) rather than with retraction or grunting. Respiration is stimulated by the metabolic acidaemia, by damage to the central nervous system and/or by pulmonary oedema. Infants with ARDS are severely hypoxaemic.

Chest radiograph appearance

This demonstrates diffuse pulmonary infiltrates and in severe cases there will be a 'white-out'.

Management

- Surfactant administration can improve oxygenation in ARDS and is most effective if administered early and in larger doses than used in RDS.
- In adults and children with ARDS, prone positioning has been shown to improve oxygenation.
- A high level of PEEP should be used in an attempt to restore the functional residual capacity to normal values; this will also increase the MAP level and hence oxygenation.
- High-volume strategy HFOV can also improve oxygenation, particularly in those patients who had a positive response to PEEP elevation.
- Fluid intake should initially be restricted to 40 ml/kg/24 hrs, and if heart failure is present, furosemide should be administered.
- Broad-spectrum antibiotics should be administered, but aminoglycoside levels should be monitored for toxicity.

Mortality and morbidity

The mortality of ARDS is high, particularly in infants who develop secondary infection or do not respond to elevation of their PEEP level. Air leaks and infection are commonly seen in infants with ARDS.

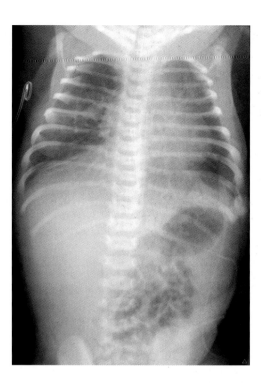

Fig. 47.10 **Congenital cystic adenomatoid malformation.** Note the delayed lung fluid clearance on the right and displacement of the mediastinum to the left.

Other congenital anomalies of the lung

- Pulmonary agenesis
- Sequestration
- Congenital cystic adenomatoid malformation of the lung (CCAM, Fig. 47.10)
- Congenital lung cysts
- Congenital lobar emphysema
- Immotile cilia syndrome
- Congenital pulmonary lymphangiectasia
- Alveolar capillary dysplasia.

Diaphragmatic abnormalities

Congenital diaphragmatic hernia (CDH) is described on page 386; other anomalies include eventration and paralysis.

Upper airway obstruction

There can be nasal, pharyngeal or laryngeal obstruction (Box 47.6).

Clinical features

- If the obstruction is partial, the only sign may be tachypnoea.

- Infants more severely affected will be obviously working hard to breathe against the obstruction and have a respiratory acidosis.
- Stridor occurring immediately after birth should raise the suspicion of a laryngeal lesion.
- Infants with complete upper airway obstruction will have severe respiratory failure, which will be fatal if unrelieved.

Investigations

- ENT opinion
- CT scan: choanal atresia
- Chest radiograph or a penetrated filtered (Cincinnati) view: laryngotracheobronchial lesions
- MRI: extrinsic laryngeal lesions
- Laryngoscopy
- Rigid laryngotracheobronchoscopy.

Management

- Nasal causes of obstruction are relieved by an oral airway.
- Surgical intervention is required for choanal atresia.
- If the tongue is causing the obstruction because it is too large or displaced posteriorly, the infant should be nursed prone.
- Laryngeal obstruction is relieved by intubation but not by an oral airway.
- Vocal cord palsy resulting from a birth injury usually resolves spontaneously.

- Bilateral cord lesions associated with a neurological lesion do not respond spontaneously and a tracheostomy and feeding gastrostomy will be required.
- Subglottic oedema requires pre-extubation corticosteroids and adrenaline (epinephrine) nebulizers.
- Subglottic stenosis may require a cricoid split or laryngeal reconstruction using rib cartilage.
- Laryngomalacia usually resolves over 12–24 months.

Pulmonary haemorrhage

Pulmonary haemorrhage is a severe form of pulmonary oedema, where there has also been leakage of red cells giving haemorrhagic pulmonary oedema. Pulmonary haemorrhage can occur:

- At birth, following severe birth depression
- Most commonly in very low birth weight infants who have heart failure secondary to elevated pulmonary blood flow because of a PDA
- If a synthetic surfactant is given, particularly if used prophylactically
- In infants with:
  - Heart failure
  - Sepsis
  - Fluid overload
  - Clotting abnormalities
  - Intrauterine growth retardation.

Clinical features

- If the pulmonary haemorrhage is large, the infant will deteriorate suddenly with copious bloody secretions appearing from the airway.
- Spontaneously breathing infants are dyspnoeic and cyanosed; those who are ventilated will desaturate.
- The infant may be hypotensive due to blood loss and heart failure.
- On examination, the infant may be limp and unresponsive with reduced air entry and widespread crackles in the lungs.

Chest radiograph appearance

- If severe, there will be a 'white-out' with air bronchograms.
- Less commonly there is a lobar pattern of consolidation.

Management

- Infants should be intubated and ventilated; high peak pressures may be required. A high PEEP level should be used to help redistribute fluid back into the interstitial space.

- Broad-spectrum antibiotics should be used.
- Neuromuscular blockade should be given until the haemorrhage has stopped.
- Blood transfusions may be required.
- The infant should be fluid-restricted.
- There is some evidence to suggest a single dose of surfactant may improve oxygenation.

Mortality and morbidity

- The mortality may be as high as 40%.
- High-pressure ventilation puts the infant at increased risk of BPD.
- The incidence of cerebral bleeds is doubled.

Neonatal cardiac disorders

The common disorders are listed in Box 47.7.

Problem-orientated topic:

a prematurely born infant who cannot be weaned from the ventilator

A female infant, Helen, is born at 24 weeks of gestation and with a birth weight of 0.55 kg following spontaneous-onset labour. She has been ventilated since birth. After 2 weeks of mechanical ventilation, attempts to wean the baby from ventilation fail. On examination Helen is hypotensive, with a wide pulse pressure. She has an active precordium and a systolic murmur of grade 3/6, with maximum intensity in the left second intercostal space. Her peripheral pulses are easily palpable.

Q1. Does the baby have a patent ductus arteriosus?

Q2. What are the other possible causes of failure to wean this baby from the ventilator?

Q3. What would you expect the chest radiograph to demonstrate?

Q4. How would you confirm your diagnosis and what would you expect to find?

Q5. What is the appropriate management?

Q1. Does the baby have a patent ductus arteriosus (PDA)?

- Yes, she does. Infants with a haemodynamically significant PDA have tachycardia, bounding pulses, an active precordium and a murmur, although this might be absent.

Acyanotic heart disease

- Lesions with systemic outflow obstruction:
  - Coarctation of aorta
  - Severe aortic stenosis
- Lesions with left-to-right shunt:
  - Ventricular septal defect (VSD)
  - Atrial septal defect (ASD)
  - Atrioventricular septal defect (AVSD)
  - Patent ductus arteriosus (PDA)

Cyanotic heart disease

- With pulmonary oligaemia:
  - Tetralogy of Fallot
  - Pulmonary atresia with or without septal defects
  - Tricuspid atresia with pulmonary stenosis
  - Ebstein's anomaly
  - Double-outlet right ventricle with pulmonary stenosis
  - Persistent pulmonary hypertension of the newborn (PPHN)
- With pulmonary plethora:
  - Double-outlet right ventricle without pulmonary stenosis
  - Transposition of great arteries with large VSD
  - Truncus arteriosus
  - Single ventricle

Lesions presenting with heart failure

- AVSD
- Total anomalous pulmonary venous return
- Duct-dependent left ventricular outflow tract obstruction
- Hypoplastic left heart syndrome

Lesions with systemic outflow obstruction

- Coarctation of aorta
- Aortic arch anomalies

Lesions with left-to-right shunt

- VSD
- ASD
- PDA
- Rhythm disturbances:
  - Supraventricular tachycardias
  - Congenital complete heart block
- Cardiac muscle dysfunction:
  - Cardiomyopathy
  - Pompe's disease
  - Asymmetric septal hypertrophy (infant of diabetic mother)
  - Viral myocarditis
  - Severe perinatal asphyxia

- The typical ductal murmur is systolic in about 75% of cases, but can be continuous and is best heard at the upper left sternal edge, under the clavicle.
- As the pulmonary vascular resistance falls, the left-to-right shunt through the ductus increases and the peripheral pulses become bounding. This reflects the widened pulse pressure due to the 'steal' of blood being shunted from the high-pressure systemic circulation into the lower-pressure pulmonary circulation.

Q2. What are the other possible causes of failure to wean this baby from the ventilator?

- Helen may have an increased work of breathing related to either residual lung disease or pulmonary congestion secondary to another cardiac lesion. The latter is unlikely, as the murmur has appeared only at 2 weeks of age.
- The baby may also have weakness of her respiratory muscles related to extreme prematurity and/or prolonged ventilation.

Q3. What would you expect the chest radiograph to demonstrate?

The radiograph would show cardiomegaly and increased pulmonary vascularity. There may be additional residual lung disease or evidence of evolving BPD.

Q4. How would you confirm your diagnosis and what would you expect to find?

Echocardiography would confirm typical findings of a PDA (see below) and exclude other cardiac lesions.

Q5. What is the appropriate management?

- Initial treatment is fluid restriction.
- Diuretics may be needed if the infant is in heart failure, but theoretically furosemide might promote ductal patency via its effect on renal prostaglandin synthesis.
- Closure of the PDA can be attempted by using prostaglandin inhibitors such as indometacin or ibuprofen.
- Surgical ligation of the duct is indicated if medical management fails and it is not possible to wean the baby from the ventilator.

Patent ductus arteriosus (PDA)

(see also p. 221)

- In fetal life, blood is shunted from the right heart via the pulmonary artery through the ductus arteriosus to the aorta and the lungs are 'bypassed'.
- At birth, the ductus arteriosus begins to constrict with the onset of breathing.
- In the majority of infants, the ductus arteriosus has closed by 24 hours of age and in 90% will have closed by 60 hours of age.
- Ductal closure is delayed in infants with pulmonary hypertension and respiratory failure as a consequence of acidosis or persistence of low oxygen tensions; in such circumstances prostaglandin E_2 levels remain high.
- The incidence of PDA is inversely related to gestational age, reflecting the association between maturity at birth and RDS.

Clinical features

- Infants with a haemodynamically significant PDA have tachycardia, bounding pulses, an active precordium and a murmur, although the latter might be absent.
- The typical ductal murmur is systolic (in about 75% of cases), but can be continuous and is best heard at the upper left sternal edge, under the clavicle.
- As the pulmonary vascular resistance falls, the left-to-right shunt through the ductus increases and the peripheral pulses become bounding, reflecting the widened pulse pressure due to the 'steal' of blood being shunted from the high-pressure systemic circulation into the lower-pressure pulmonary circulation.
- The left-to-right shunt means higher blood flow in the lungs and affected infants are tachypnoeic with crackles at the lung bases.
- The increased pulmonary blood flow results in a decrease in lung compliance, and thus a PDA can present as failure of improvement in an infant with RDS or an acute deterioration necessitating an increase in respiratory support.

Chest radiograph appearance

The chest radiograph demonstrates cardiomegaly, pulmonary plethora and a wide angle between the left and right main bronchi due to left atrial dilation.

Investigations

- Typical echocardiographic findings of a moderate to large left-to-right ductal shunt are bowing of the interatrial septum to the right with enlargement of the left atrium and ventricle, and left atrium enlargement with a left atrial:aortic root (LA:Ao)

ratio greater than 1.4:1 and an increased ductal diameter (usually 2–3 mm).
- Colour Doppler examination reveals a continuous flare in the main pulmonary artery from the arterial duct.
- The size of the shunt can be determined from the ductal size on colour Doppler examination and the LA:Ao ratio; if the shunt is large, diastolic flow in the descending aorta is reversed throughout diastole.

Management

- Initial management of an infant with a PDA usually includes fluid restriction.
- Diuretics may be needed if the infant is in heart failure, but theoretically furosemide might promote ductal patency via its effect on renal prostaglandin synthesis.
- If there is no improvement following fluid restriction for 24 hours and there are no contraindications, such as poor renal function or a low platelet count, a prostaglandin inhibitor (indometacin or ibuprofen) can be given.
- Ductal closure is achieved with indomethacin treatment in 48 hours in approximately 70% of infants.
- Surgical ligation of the duct is indicated if medical management fails and it is not possible to wean the baby from the ventilator.

Morbidity

- BPD is significantly increased in infants who have had a PDA, particularly if they have also suffered nosocomial infection.
- If there is a large PDA, there is a diastolic steal and retrograde diastolic flow in the cerebral circulation, the descending aorta and renal and mesenteric blood vessels. This compromises gastrointestinal blood flow and hence the incidence of necrotizing enterocolitis is increased in infants who have had a PDA.

Problem-orientated topic:

a baby born at term with cyanosis

A male infant, birth weight 3.3 kg and born at term, is noticed to be blue soon after birth. He is the first child of unrelated parents. The mother recently flew into the UK from Africa and has not received any antenatal care. Examination reveals the baby to be centrally cyanosed, but without signs of respiratory distress or dysmorphic features. The apical impulse is in the left fourth intercostal space and there is no increased precordial activity. The first and second heart sounds are normal and there are no murmurs. The femoral pulses are felt and there is no discrepancy in the four limb blood pressures. The baby has oxygen saturation levels of 80% in all four limbs.

Q1. Does this infant have cyanotic congenital heart disease?

Q2. What are the differential diagnoses?

Q3. What investigations would you undertake to make the diagnosis?

Q4. How should this infant be managed?

Table 47.3 **Examples of syndromes with associated cardiac conditions**

Syndrome	Cardiac condition
CHARGE	VSD, AVSD, ASD
CATCH 22	Aortic arch anomalies and tetralogy of Fallot
Down's	AVSD, VSD
Noonan's	Valvular pulmonary stenosis
Turner's	Coarctation of aorta
Williams'	Supravalvular aortic stenosis

(ASD = atrial septal defect; AVSD = atrioventricular septal defect; CATCH 22 = cardiac defects, abnormal facies, thymic hypoplasia, cleft palate, hypocalcaemia, variable deletion on chromosome 22; CHARGE = coloboma, heart defects, atresia of the choanae, retardation of growth and/or development, genital and/or urinary abnormalities, ear abnormalities and deafness; VSD = ventricular septal defect)

Q1. Does this infant have cyanotic congenital heart disease?

Yes, the infant has an atrioventricular septal defect (AVSD). The mother has had no antenatal care, so any major cardiac abnormality will not have been detected during the pregnancy.

Q2. What are the differential diagnoses?

- Persistent pulmonary hypertension of the newborn (PPHN) should be considered, but is unlikely given the similar saturation levels in all four limbs.
- The lack of respiratory distress also makes a primary respiratory disease unlikely.
- Rarely, infants with a myopathy or spinal muscular atrophy can present with cyanosis, but are also usually floppy.
- Babies with methaemoglobinaemia have normal arterial oxygen tensions despite central cyanosis.
- The lack of dysmorphic features makes an underlying syndrome (Table 47.3) unlikely.

Q3. What investigations would you undertake to make the diagnosis?

- An arterial blood gas from pre- and post-ductal arteries should be taken; similarity in the PaO_2 will exclude pulmonary hypertension and a normal CO_2 level significant respiratory disease.
- Chest radiograph (Fig. 47.11) and 12-lead ECG will give further clues to the aetiology of cyanosis in this infant (Box 47.8 and Table 47.4 below).

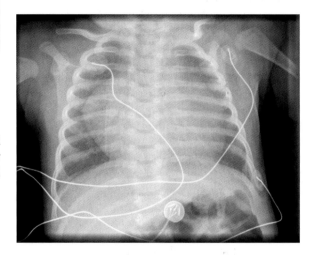

Fig. 47.11 **Atrioventricular septal defect. Note the large heart.**

- Echocardiography will confirm the exact nature of cardiac defect.

Q4. How should this infant be managed?

- A hyperoxia test should be done, with the infant breathing 100% oxygen via a face mask for 15 minutes.
- A further post-ductal arterial blood gas should then be obtained. If the PaO_2 has risen above 33 kPa, congenital heart disease is extremely unlikely and primary pulmonary hypertension is the most likely cause of central cyanosis.
- If the PaO_2 fails to rise above 5 kPa, cyanotic congenital heart disease is more likely. A prostin infusion should be started after consultation with the regional paediatric cardiology unit prior to transfer for possible surgical intervention (Box 47.8).

BOX 47.8 Surgical procedures for congenital heart disease

Balloon atrial septostomy (Rashkind procedure)
- Creates an interatrial opening to allow mixing of blood in the atria
- Used for transposition of the great arteries, tricuspid atresia

Palliative systemic to pulmonary artery shunts
- Use systemic arterial flow to improve pulmonary blood flow in cardiac lesions with impaired pulmonary perfusion
- Used for tetralogy of Fallot, hypoplastic right heart, tricuspid atresia
  - Modified Blalock–Taussig shunt (subclavian and ipsilateral pulmonary artery anastomosis)
  - Waterston–Cooley shunt (ascending aorta and right pulmonary artery)
  - Potts shunt (descending aorta and left pulmonary artery anastomosis)

Palliative cavopulmonary shunt (Glenn shunt)
- Anastomosis of the superior vena cava to the right pulmonary artery
- An intermediate procedure in patients awaiting Fontan procedure, which allows systemic venous flow to go directly into the pulmonary circulation

Fontan procedure
- Redirection of the flow from the inferior vena cava to the right pulmonary artery with functionally univentricular heart
- Used in tricuspid atresia, hypoplastic left heart syndrome

Norwood procedure
- Stage 1: anastomosis of proximal main pulmonary artery to aorta with aortic arch reconstruction and transection and patch closure of distal main pulmonary artery (MPA), modified Blalock–Taussig shunt and creating atrial septal defect (ASD)
- Stage 2: bidirectional redirection of the flow from the inferior vena cava to the right pulmonary artery (Glenn shunt and modified Fontan)
- Stage 3: total cavopulmonary connection (Fontan)

Ross procedure
- Pulmonary root autograft for aortic stenosis

Cyanotic congenital heart disease

- Cyanosis in congenital heart disease (Table 47.4) is caused by either an obstruction to the pulmonary blood flow or mixing of the pulmonary venous and systemic venous returns in the heart or major arterial trunks with a right-to-left shunt or abnormal arterial connections.

- Infants with PPHN have right-to-left shunts at the level of the ductus arteriosus and the foramen ovale.
- PPHN was previously called persistent fetal circulation but that term is inaccurate, as the high-flow, low-resistance circuit through the placenta present in the fetal circulation is missing.
- Pulmonary hypertension in the neonate may also be secondary to a number of conditions, including severe intrapartum asphyxia, infection, pulmonary hypoplasia, drug therapy (for example, the use of prostaglandin synthetase inhibitors before delivery), congenital heart disease or over-ventilation.
- The neonatal pulmonary vasculature is extremely sensitive to changes in pH, PaO_2 and $PaCO_2$. A rise in the haematocrit can also cause pulmonary hypertension.
- When pulmonary hypertension occurs due to failure of the normal decrease in pulmonary vascular resistance after birth, affected infants have a normal arteriolar number and muscularization.
- In other conditions, there are varying degrees of vascular remodelling and a decreased arteriolar number.
- Following chronic hypoxia in utero, excessive muscularization of the pulmonary arterioles is found and muscle extends into the normally muscle-free intra-acinar arteries; such changes are seen in extremely small for dates infants.
- The pulmonary hypertension seen in infants with CDH or in other conditions associated with pulmonary hypoplasia is due to a reduction in the number of intralobar arteries and increased muscularity of the arteries.
- PPHN may also be due to alveolar capillary dysplasia with congenital misalignment of the pulmonary veins.

Clinical features

Cyanotic heart disease presents with cyanosis and in addition with a murmur, heart failure or shock:
- A murmur in the pulmonary area suggests the presence of pulmonary stenosis and makes the diagnosis of Fallot's tetralogy more likely, whereas the absence of a murmur suggests transposition of the great arteries.
- Cyanotic heart diseases with normal or increased pulmonary circulation, transposition of great arteries, single-chamber lesions (univentricular heart) and total anomalous pulmonary venous return and truncus arteriosus present with a combination of heart failure and cyanosis. If there is associated pulmonary stenosis, however, this is protective against heart failure and affected infants present with cyanosis alone.

Table 47.4 Cyanotic congenital heart diseases (CHD)

CHD	Clinical presentation	Age at presentation	Examination	Chest radiograph	ECG	Management
Transposition of great arteries	Cyanosis in the first week Degree of cyanosis is variable: can be very severe, or very mild and may be missed	Around 48–72 hours of age, usually when duct is closing	Single second sound No murmurs	Normal or increased pulmonary blood flow Narrow mediastinum and cardiac silhouette showing 'egg on side' appearance	May be normal Right ventricular hypertrophy	Prostaglandin infusion Balloon atrial septostomy Arterial switch operation
Tetralogy of Fallot	Mild cyanosis in the newborn Degree of cyanosis depends upon degree of right ventricular outflow tract (RVOT) obstruction	Variable depending upon degree of pulmonary stenosis May be symptom-free until 6 months of age	Single second sound Ejection systolic murmur in the second space	Pulmonary oligaemia Upturned apex giving boot-shaped appearance	Right ventricular hypertrophy Right axis deviation	Primary repair of RVOT at 3–4 months of age if anatomy is favourable
Tricuspid atresia	Severe cyanosis since birth Associated tachypnoea	Usually in the first 2 weeks of life	Single second sound Systolic murmur in lower left sternal border	Normal or slightly enlarged Decreased pulmonary blood flow	Left ventricular hypertrophy Left axis deviation	Prostaglandin infusion and balloon atrial septostomy for neonates with severe cyanosis Palliative shunt (Blalock–Taussig) followed by Fontan procedure
Total anomalous venous return with obstruction	Symptoms of heart failure Marked respiratory distress Cyanosis variable	Usually in the first week of life	No murmurs Wide fixed splitting of second heart sound Hepatomegaly	Pulmonary venous congestion/pulmonary oedema with small cardiac size Snowman appearance in supradiaphragmatic obstruction	Right ventricular hypertrophy	Surgical correction of pulmonary venous drainage
Truncus arteriosus	Cyanosis and heart failure in the first few weeks	First 2 weeks of life	Continuous ejection systolic murmur Single second sound	Cardiomegaly Increased pulmonary vascularity	Combined ventricular hypertrophy	Surgical repair
Ebstein's anomaly	Cyanosis and heart failure in the first week of life	First week	Characteristic triple or quadruple rhythm with soft systolic murmur on lower left sternal edge	Extreme cardiomegaly in severe cases Mild cases have normal-sized heart	Right bundle branch block and right atrial enlargement First degree AV block may be present	Surgical repair of tricuspid valve

- Infants with severe pulmonary obstruction present with severe cyanosis and shock when the ductus arteriosus closes; in such infants patency of the ductus arteriosus is vital for blood to reach the pulmonary circulation.

Chest radiograph appearance
The shape of the heart may give a clue to the underlying heart lesion:
- A boot-shaped heart is said to be characteristic of tetralogy of Fallot.
- An egg-shaped heart with a narrow mediastinum is characteristic of transposition of the great arteries.
- A snowman or figure of eight appearance is characteristic of supracardiac total anomalous pulmonary venous return.
- A scimitar appearance over the right lower lung field is sometimes seen in infradiaphragmatic anomalous pulmonary venous return.
- The presence of a small heart and increased pulmonary vascularity can be a feature of obstructed pulmonary venous return.
- Lesions associated with pulmonary oligaemia include tetralogy of Fallot, various forms of single ventricle with pulmonary stenosis and tricuspid atresia.
- Pulmonary plethora can occur in transposition of the great arteries, single-chamber lesions (univentricular heart), total anomalous pulmonary venous return and truncus arteriosus.

Electrocardiogram appearance
A superior axis on the ECG is seen if there is an AVSD or tricuspid atresia. A conduction abnormality is commonly associated with Ebstein's anomaly.

Acyanotic congenital heart disease

Common acyanotic congenital heart diseases are listed in Table 47.5.

Clinical features
The presentation depends on whether the lesion produces predominantly volume overload or pressure overload:

Lesions causing volume overload tend to remain asymptomatic in the neonatal period unless severe:
- Left-to-right shunt lesions such as atrial septal defect (ASD), ventricular septal defect (VSD) and patent ductus arteriosus (PDA)
- Regurgitant lesions like congenital mitral regurgitation and cardiomyopathy.

Lesions causing pressure overload tend to present with symptoms of heart failure (Box 47.9) or shock with decreased peripheral perfusion:

> **BOX 47.9 Causes of heart failure in the newborn according to age at presentation**
>
> **At birth**
> - Severe hypoplastic left heart syndrome
> - Severe tricuspid and pulmonary insufficiency
> - Large systemic arteriovenous fistula
>
> **The first week**
> - Transposition of great arteries
> - Hypoplastic left heart syndrome
> - Total anomalous pulmonary venous return
> - Critical aortic and pulmonary stenosis
>
> **Between 7 and 28 days**
> - Coarctation of aorta
> - Critical aortic stenosis
> - AVSD with large left-to-right shunt and low pulmonary vascular resistance

- Lesions with outflow tract obstruction such as coarctation of aorta, aortic arch anomalies and valvular pulmonary stenosis.

Neonatal arrhythmias

Supraventricular tachycardia (SVT)

Clinical features
This is the most common symptomatic arrhythmia in the neonatal period. Affected infants can present antenatally with hydrops fetalis or postnatally with heart failure. The heart rate is usually faster than 200 beats/min.

Pathogenesis
SVT in neonates is usually due to an accessory atrioventricular pathway. It can be associated with underlying structural heart disease such as Ebstein's anomaly, tricuspid atresia or corrected transposition of great arteries.

Investigations
The ECG shows narrow QRS complexes, with a heart rate in the range of 180–300 beats/min. The P wave is often difficult to see, but when present usually has an abnormal axis or morphology.

Management
SVT usually responds to intravenous adenosine. Infants who are in shock may need DC cardioversion with 1–2 joules/kg. It is important to liaise with the regional cardiology team with regard to choice of maintenance treatment.

Table 47.5 Common acyanotic congenital heart diseases

CHD	Clinical presentation	Age at presentation	Examination	Chest radiograph	ECG	Management
Ventricular septal defect (VSD) (p. 214)	Usually asymptomatic in the neonatal period	Infancy	Pansystolic murmur in the lower left sternal edge	Cardiomegaly and increased pulmonary vascularity if large left-to-right shunt	Normal or left ventricular hypertrophy	Small VSDs close spontaneously Large VSDs need closure
Atrial septal defect (ASD) (p. 220)	Asymptomatic	Childhood	Ejection systolic murmur with wide fixed split second heart sound	Normal or enlarged heart Increased pulmonary vascularity	Right axis deviation and right bundle branch block	Closure surgical or catheter
Atrioventricular septal defect (AVSD) (p. 215)	Symptoms of heart failure usually after 4 weeks of age Cyanosis	Usually after 4 weeks of age	Hyperdynamic precordium Pansystolic murmur	Cardiomegaly with increased pulmonary vascularity	Left axis deviation or superior QRS axis Biventricular hypertrophy	Pulmonary artery banding Surgical closure
Coarctation of the aorta (p. 216)	Symptoms of heart failure Poorly felt femoral pulses on routine examination	Usually symptomatic after 1 week of age	Ejection systolic murmur at upper left sternal border with radiation to interscapular area Discrepancy in upper and lower limb BP	Cardiomegaly and pulmonary venous congestion	Right ventricular hypertrophy with right bundle branch block	Repair of coarctation
Hypoplastic left heart syndrome	Shock and heart failure	Usually within 72 hours of age	Loud and single second heart sound No murmurs	Pulmonary venous congestion Cardiomegaly	Right ventricular hypertrophy	Prostaglandin infusion Balloon atrial septostomy Staged repair using Norwood-type procedure

Congenital complete heart block

Clinical features

Affected fetuses may be detected by the presence of bradycardia at routine ultrasound examination or during labour. Neonates with congenital heart block can be asymptomatic or present with heart failure or Stokes–Adams attacks. Infants may have underlying congenital heart disease such as septal defects. It is important to exclude maternal systemic lupus erythematosus or collagen vascular disease.

Management

In symptomatic infants or in those with heart rates of less than 40 beats/min, artificial pacing may be needed. Isoprenaline infusion is used occasionally in infants to raise the heart rate temporarily in an acute situation.

Approach to a neonate with a suspected cardiac problem

History

- Family history of congenital heart disease
- Exposure to intrauterine infections or teratogens
- Symptoms of heart failure: difficulty to manage sucking while feeding, forehead sweating and tachypnoea, increased precordial activity.

Examination

- General examination to look for any evidence of dysmorphism
- Evidence of cyanosis?
- Peripheral pulses, femoral pulses, brachial femoral delay
- Signs of heart failure: hepatomegaly and intercostal and subcostal recessions
- Precordial activity
- Auscultation of the heart and heart sounds and determining the presence of murmurs
- Blood pressure in all four limbs
- Pre- and post-ductal oximetry.

Investigations

- Chest radiograph:
  - Size and shape of the heart
  - Vascularity of lung fields
  - Exclusion of any primary or coexistent respiratory problem (important)
  - Anomalies of ribs and vertebrae.
- Electrocardiogram:
  - ECG is important, particularly if there are ischaemic and rhythm disturbances of the heart.
- Echocardiography:
  - This is mandatory in a neonate with a suspected congenital cardiac problem.
- Cardiac catheterization:
  - A cardiac centre may be needed in more difficult cases.
- MRI.

Management

- It is important to liaise with a paediatric cardiac centre regarding the management of all infants with suspected serious congenital cardiac problems to facilitate stabilization and transfer of such infants.
- Apply the basic principles of stabilization of the airway, breathing and circulation.
- It is essential to keep the duct patent in conditions suspected of being duct-dependent; this is achieved by a continuous infusion of prostaglandins (5–10 ng/kg/min).
- Management of heart failure depends upon the underlying aetiology and includes strategies to improve preload and afterload and increase cardiac contractility.
- Many cardiac disorders require surgical intervention (Table 47.5).

References and further reading

Aghajafari F, Murphy K, Matthews S et al 2002 Repeated doses of antenatal corticosteroids in animals: a systemic review. American Journal of Obstetrics and Gynaecology 186(4):843–849

Baud O, Foix-L'Helias L, Kaminski M et al 1999 Antenatal glucocorticosteroid treatment and cystic periventricular leukomalacia in very premature infants. New England Journal of Medicine 341:1190–1196

Cooke L, Steer P, Woodgate D 2004 Indomethacin for asymptomatic patent ductus arteriosus in preterm infants (Cochrane Review). In: Cochrane Library, issue 3

Costeloe K, Hennessy E, Gibson AT et al for the Epicure Study Group 2000 The EPICure study: outcomes to discharge from hospital for infants born at the threshold of viability. Pediatrics 106:659–671

Crowley P 2004 Prophylactic corticosteroids for preterm birth (Cochrane Review). In: Cochrane Library, issue 3

Crowther CA, Alfirevic Z, Haslann RR 2004 Thyrotropin-releasing hormone added to corticosteroids for women at risk of preterm birth for preventing neonatal respiratory disease (Cochrane Review) In: Cochrane Library, issue 3

Greenough A 2002 Update on modalities of mechanical ventilators. Archives of Disease in Childhood, Fetal and Neonatal Edition 87:F3–6

Greenough A, Milner AD, Dimitriou G 2004 Synchronised mechanical ventilation for respiratory support in newborn infants (Cochrane Review). In: Cochrane Library, issue 3

Halliday HL 2004 Endotracheal intubation at birth for preventing morbidity and mortality in vigorous, meconium-stained infants born at term (Cochrane Review) In: Cochrane Library, issue 3

Lewis V, Whitelaw A 2004 Furosemide for transient tachypnoea of the newborn (Cochrane Review). In: Cochrane Library, issue 3

Northway WHJ, Rosan RC, Porter DY Pulmonary disease following respiratory therapy of hyaline membrane disease: bronchopulmonary dysplasia. New Eng J Med 1967; 276:357–368

Ohlsson A, Walia R, Shah S 2004 Ibuprofen for the treatment of a patent ductus arteriosus in preterm and/or low birthweight infants (Cochrane Review). In: Cochrane Library, issue 3

Schreiber MD, Gin-Mestan K, Marks JD et al 2003 Inhaled nitric oxide in premature infants with respiratory distress syndrome. New England Journal of Medicine 349:2099–2107

Soll RF, Blanco F 2004 Natural surfactant extract versus synthetic surfactant for neonatal respiratory distress syndrome (Cochrane Review). In: Cochrane Library, issue 3

Soll RF, Dargaville P 2004 Surfactant for meconium aspiration syndrome in full term infants (Cochrane Review). In: Cochrane Library, issue 3

Soll RF, Morley CJ 2004 Prophylactic versus selective use of surfactant for preventing morbidity and mortality in preterm infants (Cochrane Review). In: Cochrane Library, issue 3

UK Collaborative ECMO Trial Group 1996 UK collaborative randomized trial of neonatal extracorporeal membrane oxygenation. Lancet 348:75–82

Wiswell T, Knight GR, Finer NN et al 2002 A multicentre randomized controlled trial comparing Surfaxin (Lucinactant) lavage with standard care for treatment of meconium aspiration syndrome. Pediatrics 109:1081–1087

Janet M. Rennie

Neonatology III: Neurology, haematology, metabolism and sepsis

LEARNING OUTCOMES

By the end of this chapter you should:

- Be able to describe the features of neonatal encephalopathy
- Be able to explain the mechanisms of brain injury in full-term and preterm infants
- Know how to initiate the management of neonatal encephalopathy
- Know the common causes and management of neonatal anaemia and thrombocytopenia
- Be able to discuss the differential diagnosis, investigation and management of haemolysis and jaundice in the newborn
- Have an understanding of glucose and calcium metabolism in the newborn
- Have an understanding of the pathophysiology of sepsis and its presentation in the newborn.

Neurology

Basic science

Brain development

During intrauterine and early neonatal life the baby's brain is developing extremely fast. At 20 weeks the brain is almost completely smooth, and although neuronal formation is complete myelination has not begun, nor has glial cell differentiation (Fig. 48.1). In the second and third trimester the rapid pace of development continues, with the formation of sulci and gyri and continued organization of the central nervous system (CNS). Interference with the normal process of development can occur and modern neuroimaging has made the diagnosis of such disorders much easier

(examples are schizencephaly, polymicrogyria and lissencephaly).

Cerebral blood flow

Cerebral blood flow (CBF) is relatively low in the newborn compared to later in life and the major determinant of CBF is blood pressure. Other factors that affect CBF are carbon dioxide concentration and intracranial pressure (ICP). Babies are not as good as older children at 'autoregulating' CBF; autoregulation means that CBF is kept constant over a range of blood pressure, thus protecting the brain from fluctuations in blood pressure. The concept of loss of autoregulation is important in understanding why brain injury occurs when there is cerebral oedema (ICP) and in preterm brain injury

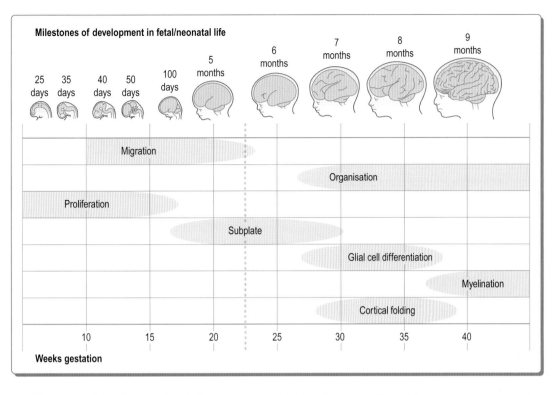

Fig. 48.1 **Milestones of development in relation to the neonatal intensive care unit (NICU)**

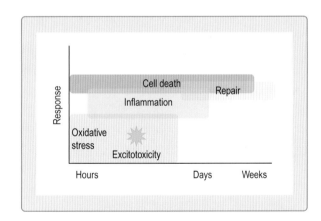

Fig. 48.2 **Mechanisms of brain injury in the term neonate** (From: Ferriero 2004 DM Neonatal brain injury. New England Journal of Medicine 351:1985–1995)

(lost autoregulation, fluctuating blood pressure, and high carbon dioxide levels in respiratory failure).

Mechanisms of neonatal brain injury

A reduction in CBF and brain energy supply sufficient to cause damage initially causes some cell death but the damaging process continues long after CBF is restored (Fig. 48.2). The key processes in ongoing damage are:

- Oxidative stress
- Apoptosis
- Excitotoxicity
- Cytokine damage.

Some cells appear to commit cell suicide ('apoptosis') because of upregulation of genetic triggers; others are damaged by excitotoxicity due to glutamate release, or die from free radical oxidative stress or from cytokine release as a consequence of inflammation. Understanding of the ongoing process of cell death and damage has led to an understanding of a 'therapeutic window' lasting some hours immediately after the injury. There is hope that appropriate intervention during this window can ameliorate some of the ongoing damage, and currently there is much interest in brain cooling as an intervention in full-term infants.

Problem-orientated topic:

abnormal movements

Jack, a 2-day-old baby of an 18-year-old single primiparous woman who works in a nightclub, is noticed to make repetitive jerky movements of his arms and to be slightly blue. The whole episode lasts less than 1 minute. Jack was born by ventouse and had previously been feeding well from the breast.

Continued overleaf

Q1. What other information from the history would be helpful?

Q2. What emergency investigations are indicated?

Q3. What management are you going to arrange?

Q1. What other information from the history would be helpful?

Babies with encephalopathy are characteristically lethargic and floppy, with a reduced level of spontaneous activity at first. They then become irritable, with seizures, which are the hallmark of the disease. Babies who have seizures without encephalopathy are likely to have suffered a stroke. The most common cause of an early neonatal encephalopathy with seizures in a term baby is hypoxic–ischaemic encephalopathy (Box 48.1). Neonatal encephalopathy is a serious condition, occurring in 1–6 per 1000 births at term. The mortality is around 15%, and 25% of survivors will suffer significant neurological disability.

Q2. What emergency investigations are indicated?

See Box 48.2.

Q3. What management are you going to arrange?

- Admit the baby to the intensive care unit; establish monitoring.
- Get urgent glucose and blood gas.
- Establish intravenous and ventilatory support, if required.
- Arrange first-line investigations, including lumbar puncture (LP), promptly.
- Consider initiating treatment with a loading dose of phenobarbital if seizures quickly recur or if a single seizure is very prolonged (rare in the newborn).
- Restrict fluid in babies thought to have HIE but maintain glucose levels.
- Explain seizure to the parents but do not try to prognosticate too early; the prognosis varies considerably according to the cause and accurate prognosis requires information from EEG and MRI.

Preterm brain injury

Germinal matrix-intraventricular haemorrhage

The preterm brain is particularly vulnerable to injury because autoregulation of CBF is often impaired, asso-

BOX 48.1 Differential diagnosis of neonatal seizures

Hypoxic–ischaemic encephalopathy
- Seizures within 24 hours of birth, history of fetal distress and birth depression, often with early metabolic acidosis
- Baby is encephalopathic; altered CNS state

Focal infarction (stroke)
- Seizures often occur on day 2 or 3 and can be focal
- Baby usually still feeding and alert between seizures — not encephalopathic

Meningitis
- There may be a history of prolonged membrane rupture or of maternal pyrexia in labour
- Fontanelle often full; baby systemically ill
- Remember to ask about maternal genital herpes

Neonatal abstinence syndrome
- History of maternal drug use, including methadone programmes
- Babies often sleep poorly, feed avidly and scratch their faces

Withdrawal from maternal medication
- E.g. selective serotonin reuptake inhibitors (SSRIs)
- Take a good history of maternal therapeutic drug use in all cases of neonatal seizure

Hypoglycaemia
- There can be a history of poor feeding or maternal diabetes
- Diagnosis depends on performing urgent glucose estimation on all babies with seizure

Inborn error of metabolism
- Worsening metabolic acidosis and seizures difficult to control
- Diagnosis depends on careful investigation

Intracranial haemorrhage (subdural or intraparenchymal)
- More common after instrumental delivery, particularly if multiple attempts or failed instrumental delivery
- Baby may be pale and may not have received vitamin K prophylaxis
- This is the most common cause of seizure in preterm babies

ciated illness causes changes in CBF and blood pressure, and the developing brain contains the germinal matrix, which is situated over the head of the caudate nucleus in the floor of the lateral ventricle. The germinal matrix has thin-walled vessels and is often the site of bleeding. Blood clot in the germinal matrix can obstruct the draining vein of the adjacent brain parenchyma, leading to further damage from haemorrhagic venous infarction. This pattern of bleeding is called germinal matrix-intraventricular haemorrhage (GMH-IVH). Bleeding into the substance of the brain is often called haemorrhagic periventricular infarction (HPI) or intraparenchymal lesion (IPL). Older books use the Papile classification for IVH (Box 48.3), but more modern thinking is that this implies a hierarchy that does not exist and fails to take into account the fact that some lesions in the parenchyma of the brain can be ischaemic.

Periventricular leucomalacia

In addition to bleeding into the parenchyma of the brain, preterm babies are vulnerable to injury to the area in which white matter will form. This tends to occur in the periventricular area and is termed periventricular leucomalacia (PVL). In preterm babies the predominant cell type in this area of the brain is the oligodendrocyte precursor. These cells eventually mature and make myelin, which begins to form at around term. The oligodendrocyte precursor cell is exquisitely vulnerable to damage from free radicals and cytokines. Areas of damaged cells remain demyelinated in the long term, and babies with extensive white matter injury usually have cerebral palsy as a result. MRI reveals far more white matter damage in groups of preterm babies than was previously suspected with ultrasound diagnosis alone, and the importance of subtle changes in the white matter remains to be determined. There is concern that even subtle white matter injury leads to altered connectivity in the brain, with effects on the cortical and central grey matter. This may be the reason why short attention span and learning difficulties are commonly seen in very preterm survivors.

Key points: preterm brain injury

- Preterm brain injury is usually diagnosed with ultrasound screening in the nursery in a baby with no clinical signs. Occasionally presentation may be with anaemia, seizures and a tense fontanelle.
- GMH-IVH is tightly linked with gestational age (large haemorrhages are more common in very preterm babies, particularly below 28 weeks of gestation).
- Hypercarbia, acidosis and bruising are associated with GMH-IVH.
- PVL is less tightly linked with gestational age than GMH-IVH but is rare after 34 weeks.
- Hypocarbia and maternal chorioamnionitis are associated with PVL.
- Severe PVL that is cystic is associated with the development of cerebral palsy.
- Subtle white matter damage is very common in preterm babies but can only be diagnosed with MRI; early research suggests that this may be linked to the neurocognitive and behavioural problems that are common in preterm survivors who do not have cerebral palsy.

Hydrocephalus

The occipito-frontal head circumference should be measured in all babies at birth, and should be measured again whenever a baby presents with an illness. Measuring the infant's head is also part of child health surveillance undertaken by GPs and health visitors in the UK. The measurements should be plotted on a centile chart; any deviation from the expected trajectory along the centile line established at birth should be taken seriously. A baby with an enlarging head requires investigation, initially with a cranial ultrasound scan, although CT or MRI should be performed if the diagnosis is not quickly apparent.

Not all babies with enlarging heads have raised CSF pressure due to hydrocephalus. Other diagnoses are important, such as subdural haematoma and benign enlargement of the subarachnoid space. Babies tolerate raised ICP better than adults because the skull is not fused, but eventually signs will develop. These include sunsetting of the eyes, bulging fontanelle, prominent scalp veins and vomiting. Neurosurgical help should be sought but in an emergency CSF can be drained via an LP or a ventricular tap.

Neonatal abstinence syndrome

Neonatal abstinence syndrome can present at any time in the first 2 weeks of life, but in general signs are present in the first 2–3 days and include irritability, tremor, vomiting, diarrhoea, sweating and fever. The drugs of abuse most likely to be followed by neonatal abstinence syndrome are opioids, including methadone. Babies are often snuffly and scratch their faces. Seizures can occur but should be avoided by early diagnosis and effective treatment. Assessment of the severity of neonatal abstinence syndrome can be made with a scoring system and there are a number in common use around the UK. These vary in complexity and only one (the Finnegan chart) has been shown to reduce treatment duration when compared to subjective assessment alone. None of the charts has been validated against a population of normal babies. Treatment is usually started with an oral opioid, usually morphine up to a total daily dose of 0.5 mg/kg, and few would now consider treatment with sedative agents alone to be adequate. Treatment is often required for around a month, occasionally longer.

Haematology

Basic science

The production of blood cells and platelets from a stem cell line is referred to as haematopoiesis and the cells produced are known as haematopoietic cells (Fig. 48.3). The 'mother' of all stem cells is, of course, the fertilized oöcyte, but stem cells are defined as cells that can self-renew and can differentiate into one or more of the 200 cell types found in the body. There is currently great interest in harvesting stem cells from umbilical cord blood for use in bone marrow transplantation, which is a rich source of haematopoietic stem cells.

In older children and adults haematopoiesis takes place in the bone marrow, but in the fetus the process begins as early as the sixth week of pregnancy, in the liver. The liver remains an important site of haematopoiesis until term. Haematopoiesis is under the control of cytokines; red blood cell production is stimulated by erythropoietin, white cells by different colony stimulating factors (e.g. granulocyte colony stimulating factor, G-CSF) and platelets by thrombopoietin. The production of red cells and haemoglobin falls dramatically after birth, probably because of the sudden increase in tissue oxygenation. Production gradually increases so that by 3 months a healthy baby can produce around 2 ml of red cells each day. However, the reduced capacity for formation in the early weeks, combined with a shortened red cell survival and a need for frequent blood tests, leads to anaemia in preterm babies. In fetal life the predominant haemoglobin is haemoglobin F, which has a greater affinity for oxygen than haemoglobin A.

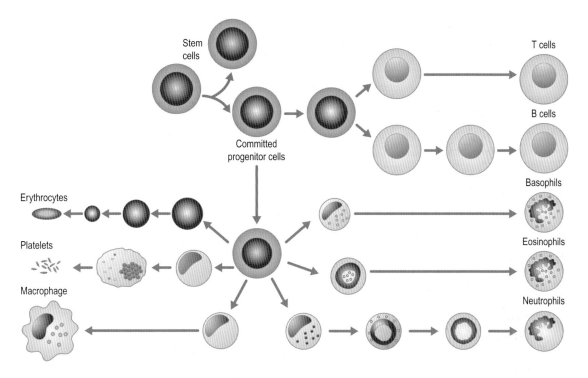

Fig. 48.3 Haematopoiesis

Production of haemoglobin A remains at low levels until after 30–32 weeks of pregnancy, and forms about 20–25% of total haemoglobin at term.

Anaemia

Problem-orientated topic:

pallor

Chloe is born by emergency caesarean section at term. Her mother, a 35-year-old physician, presented to the hospital because she noticed that Chloe had not moved at all that day. A cardiotocograph (CTG) has shown reduced baseline variability with decelerations. At surgery, there is meconium-stained liquor. Chloe weighs 3.5 kg and has Apgar scores of 3[1] and 6[5]. She responds to bag and mask resuscitation but is admitted to the nursery because she is noticed to be pale and is grunting slightly. Her haemoglobin is 8 g/dl.

Q1. Is Chloe significantly anaemic? What is the expected haemoglobin for a baby of this age?

Q2. What are the most likely causes of the anaemia and how can this be investigated?

Q3. What is the appropriate management for Chloe and what is the prognosis?

Q1. Is Chloe significantly anaemic? What is the expected haemoglobin for a baby of this age?

The normal haemoglobin at birth is high compared to adult life at 15–23 g/dl, and any baby with a haemoglobin of less than 14 g/dl on a properly taken sample should be considered to have anaemia. Not all such babies will need a blood transfusion, but all such babies certainly deserve investigation into the cause. The haemoglobin level falls over the first few weeks of life in all babies, reaching a nadir of around 10 g/dl at about 2 months. Preterm babies have a more rapid and steeper fall.

Q2. What are the most likely causes of the anaemia and how can this be investigated?

There are three main groups of disorders that cause neonatal anaemia, and some babies have more than one problem at the same time. The groups are:
- Impaired red cell production
- Increased red cell destruction (haemolysis)

Maternal Kleihauer test

- Shows the presence of fetal red cells in the maternal circulation
- Important to diagnose fetomaternal haemorrhage as a cause of neonatal anaemia
- Often a history of reduced fetal movements and there can be CTG abnormalities
- Baby pale right from the start of life

Full blood count including reticulocyte count and film

- Low white cell count and platelet count combined with anaemia suggest a marrow problem
- Low reticulocyte count also suggests a primary failure of red cell production due to inherited disorder or congenital viral infection
- Elevated reticulocyte count suggests haemolysis
- Red cells may be seen to be an abnormal shape on blood film, e.g. spherocytosis

Blood group and Coombs' test

- Positive Coombs' test suggests alloimmune haemolytic anaemia due to blood group incompatibility between mother and fetus, e.g. ABO incompatibility, although the test is not always sufficiently sensitive
- Non-immune haemolysis is usually due to red cell membrane disorders, red cell enzyme deficiency or a haemoglobinopathy (e.g. thalassaemia)

Liver function tests

- Elevated unconjugated bilirubin level supports haemolysis
- Family history
- Some cases of congenital anaemia (e.g. Diamond–Blackfan anaemia in some families) are autosomal dominant
- Spherocytosis is also an inherited disorder with a history of intermittent aplastic crises in affected family members
- Ask about splenectomy in family members

- Blood loss.
  Investigations are described in Box 48.4.

Q3. What is the appropriate management for Chloe and what is the prognosis?

Consideration should be given to blood transfusion when a term baby is found to be significantly anaemic shortly after birth and in preterm babies who are ill with more modest anaemia. The appropriate blood product is leucocyte-depleted cytomegalovirus (CMV)-negative concentrated red cells, ideally from a cross-matched satellite pack. Irradiation is often used to ameliorate the risk of graft versus host disease, and is important for top-up or exchange transfusion in babies who received blood products in utero. Preterm babies need iron and folate supplementation. Erythropoietin can be used to treat the anaemia of prematurity, although the reduction in transfusion requirements has not been impressive.

Vitamin K deficiency bleeding

Newborn babies have low levels of vitamin K-dependent procoagulant factors, and continued vitamin K deficiency can lead to vitamin K deficiency bleeding (VKDB), sometimes termed haemorrhagic disease of the newborn. Vitamin K supplementation prevents most cases of VKDB. There is a very early form that occurs in mothers receiving medication that interferes with vitamin K metabolism, e.g. phenytoin, which requires maternal vitamin K administration in addition to neonatal supplementation. Originally, vitamin K was mainly given by intramuscular injection but since 1992 there has been controversy about the route of administration. The debate was generated by a study showing a link between intramuscular vitamin K and later childhood malignancy, and in spite of the fact that seven of nine further studies on the same topic have failed to confirm the link, the debate continues to rage. Oral vitamin K preparations are available and have not been shown to be linked to later malignancy, but there is concern about unpredictable absorption and parental compliance with the multiple oral doses that are thought to be required to prevent late-onset VKDB. With no vitamin K prophylaxis at all, the incidence of late-onset VKDB is about 7 in 100 000 births.

VKDB is much more common in breastfed babies because there are very low amounts of vitamin K in breast milk, and it has also been suggested that the gut bacterial flora of breastfed babies produces less vitamin K than that of formula-fed infants.

VKDB can be categorized as follows.

Early

- Presents within 24 hours of birth.
- Uncommon now with modern standards of obstetric care.
- Most likely to occur in babies born to mothers taking drugs such as anticonvulsants during pregnancy.
- Sites of bleeding and bruising involve areas related to birth trauma (e.g. cephalhaematoma)

- May present with melaena or intracranial haemorrhage.

Classic
- 40–50% of cases of VKDB.
- Presents between 1 and 7 days following birth.
- Primarily occurs in breastfed babies and those born to mothers taking procoagulant medications.
- Typically presents with bleeding from the cord stump.
- May also present with melaena, haematemesis or bleeding from the oral or nasal mucous membranes.
- Does not usually involve intracranial haemorrhage.

Late
- Mainly occurs in breastfed babies.
- May also occur as a complication in babies with conditions causing cholestasis, such as α_1-antitrypsin deficiency, and in babies with malabsorptive conditions such as cystic fibrosis.
- Infants who are treated with long-term broad-spectrum antibiotics may also be at risk because of reduction in bacteria that produce vitamin K.
- Classically presents with signs of sudden intracranial haemorrhage.

Diagnosis
The diagnosis is based on a prolongation of the pro-thrombin time. The platelet count is normal and so is the fibrinogen level; the baby does not have disseminated intravascular coagulation (DIC). In severe cases the partial thromboplastin time is also prolonged.

Management
Treatment is with vitamin K, either orally or intra-venously, depending on the severity of the situation. The prothrombin time rapidly corrects to normal once vitamin K is given. Fresh frozen plasma may also be required for babies with severe or continuing haemorrhage or intracranial haemorrhage.

Bleeding in the neonatal period is not always due to VKDB, and other causes to consider are:
- Trauma, including non-accidental
- DIC
- Inherited coagulation disorders, e.g. haemophilia
- Platelet problems (see below)
- Gastrointestinal pathology, e.g. necrotizing enterocolitis (NEC).

Haemolysis in the newborn

Haemolysis is a relatively common cause of neonatal anaemia. The diagnosis of haemolysis is suggested by anaemia, unconjugated hyperbilirubinaemia and a high reticulocyte count. The Coombs' test may be positive, suggesting a diagnosis of immune haemolytic disease. The main causes of haemolysis are:
- Haemolytic disease of the newborn (HDN), immune haemolytic anaemia
- Red cell membrane disorders
- Red cell enzymopathies
- Haemoglobinopathies.

The most common cause of Coombs'-positive haemolysis is HDN due to the transplacental passage of IgG antibodies against rhesus antigens or antigens of the Duffy (F^y) or Kell blood group systems. HDN can also be caused by antibodies to the ABO system, in which case it mainly occurs in babies born to mothers who are blood group O and whose babies are blood group A or B. Haemolysis due to anti-A is more common than that due to anti-B.

In modern obstetric practice mothers with rhesus antibodies are usually detected during pregnancy and carefully monitored. The timing of delivery is a matter for discussion and requires cooperation between obstetric and neonatal staff with input from specialists in transfusion medicine (in case fresh blood for an exchange transfusion is required). Fetal transfusion has revolutionized the management of severely rhesus-affected babies, so that hydrops is now rare. Further, the use of anti-D immunoglobulin given to rhesus-negative mothers in pregnancy and after the birth of a rhesus-positive baby (and at other times such as external cephalic version when fetomaternal haemorrhage could cause sensitization) has reduced the number of affected women substantially.

The treatment of severe haemolysis is with exchange transfusion, which corrects the anaemia and washes out the bilirubin. Babies with mild haemolysis can be managed with phototherapy initially and a 'top-up' transfusion, if required, later on. Folic acid must be given to all babies with haemolysis.

Glucose-6-phosphate dehydrogenase (G6PD) deficiency

This red cell enzyme disorder can present in the neonatal period, usually with marked jaundice but not with anaemia. G6PD deficiency is X-linked and hence is rare, but not unknown, in female babies. The disorder has a high prevalence in central Africa, the Middle East, tropical and subtropical areas of Asia and the Mediterranean. The geographical distribution mirrors, to some extent, that of malaria and G6PD deficiency is associated with a reduced susceptibility to malaria. Not all babies with G6PD develop marked hyperbilirubinaemia but many do and kernicterus can occur. Current thinking is that the combination of G6PD deficiency and Gilbert's syndrome is the explanation for the very severe hyperbilirubinaemia seen in some babies. Once the diagnosis is made, parents must be counselled about foods and medicines that can trigger acute haemolysis. Examples are antimalarial drugs, broad beans (fava beans) and sulphonamide antibiotics (e.g. Septrin). Most people with G6PD deficiency do not have chronic haemolysis and do not require folic acid.

Hydrops

Hydrops describes the condition that occurs when the fetus has excess body water, with massive subcutaneous oedema often accompanied by pleural and peritoneal effusions. Hydrops is not a diagnosis but is the end result of a number of disorders. The condition is serious, with a high mortality, and it is important to try to make a specific diagnosis in order to counsel parents about the likely outcome for future pregnancies.

Hydrops can be caused by fetal anaemia, in which case it does not usually develop in fetal life unless the fetal haemoglobin is less than 5 g/dl, and it is often around 3 g/dl. HDN due to rhesus immune disease can cause hydrops, and ABO incompatibility can be severe enough to cause hydrops in very rare cases. In the past, rhesus iso-immunization was the most common cause of hydrops, which is often classified into 'immune' and 'non-immune' categories as a result.

Other important causes of anaemia causing hydrops are erythrovirus 19 (parvovirus B19) infection. Alpha-thalassaemia major can also cause hydrops and predominantly affects families of South-East Asian origin. Both parents of a baby with α-thalassaemia major will be carriers of the gene (localized to chromosome 16) and will have hypochromic microcytic anaemia themselves.

The broad diagnostic categories of disorders that can cause hydrops are:
- Haemolytic disease of the newborn (rhesus iso-immunization)
- Cardiac disease causing raised central venous pressure
- Intrathoracic space-occupying lesions interfering with lymphatic drainage
- Liver and gut disorders
- Congenital infection
- Metabolic disorders
- Chromosomal disorders, e.g. trisomy 13, 18, 21
- Fetal anaemia
- Syndromes, e.g. Noonan's
- Placental abnormalities
- Maternal indometacin therapy.

The delivery of a baby with hydrops is an emergency, and intubation can be difficult because of oedema. An attempt should be made to resuscitate the baby and aspiration of pleural or peritoneal fluid may make resuscitation easier. Investigations should be set in train as soon as possible to investigate the cause because the baby may die early in spite of full intensive care.

Thrombocytopenia

The normal platelet count in the newborn is the same as that in adults: above $150 \times 10^9/l$. Thrombocytopenia is a common problem in the newborn period, particularly in sick preterm babies receiving intensive care when it is often an indicator of sepsis.

Many of the possible causes of thrombocytopenia are very rare, but for practical purposes there are only a few conditions that must be remembered and understood.

Early-onset (< 72 hours) thrombocytopenia

This is common in growth-restricted babies who have been subjected to placental insufficiency causing a degree of chronic intrauterine hypoxia. These babies have reduced numbers of progenitor cells, but the condition gradually resolves over a period of time. The thrombocytopenia is not usually very severe but on occasion platelet transfusions are required.

Babies who do not have intrauterine growth restriction (IUGR) but who are found to have early-onset thrombocytopenia may have the condition of neonatal alloimmune thrombocytopenia (NAITP). This is the platelet equivalent of HDN and occurs when a mother forms antibodies against her baby's platelets as a result of exposure during pregnancy (usually a platelet group HPA 1a-negative mother with a HPA 1a-positive baby). The condition can cause severe thrombocytopenia with platelet counts below $30 \times 10^9/l$, and the baby may present with petechiae, or intracranial haemorrhage in about 10% of untreated cases. Treatment is with compatible platelet transfusion if available or random platelet transfusion together with intravenous immunoglobulin.

Autoimmune thrombocytopenia

Caused by the placental transfer of platelet antibodies from a mother with idiopathic thrombocytopenic purpura (ITP) or conditions such as systemic lupus erythematosus, autoimmune thrombocytopenia may also occur in the neonate. The risk of intracranial haemorrhage is about 1%. In babies with platelet counts below $30 \times 10^9/l$, who are otherwise well, the current advised treatment is intravenous immunoglobulin.

Late-onset thrombocytopenia

This is often associated with systemic disease, either late-onset sepsis or NEC. Thrombocytopenia can also be a clue to congenital infection with CMV, *Toxoplasma* or rubella.

Platelet transfusions are indicated if the platelet count is below $30 \times 10^9/l$ in an asymptomatic baby, and below $50 \times 10^9/l$ in a baby who has a bleeding problem ($< 100 \times 10^9/l$ if there is major haemorrhage). The main risk of thrombocytopenia is intracranial haemorrhage.

Metabolism

Neonatal jaundice

Basic science of bilirubin metabolism

Bilirubin is produced as a breakdown product of haemoglobin. During the breakdown process the iron is reused and a molecule of carbon monoxide is excreted. Carbon monoxide can be measured in breath and the concentration is an index of bilirubin formation. Bilirubin is transported to the liver in the plasma, largely bound to albumin. This form of bilirubin is termed 'unconjugated' or 'indirect' bilirubin (the term indirect comes from the way the laboratory tests are used). There it is taken up by the hepatic conjugating system, forming 'conjugated' or 'direct' bilirubin. Conjugated bilirubin is water-soluble and is excreted into bile. Bile travels in the bile ducts to the small bowel and bilirubin undergoes further metabolism in the gastrointestinal tract. Some bilirubin in the small bowel is deconjugated again by an enzyme, β-glucuronidase, and it can be reabsorbed from the lumen of the small bowel. This adds to the load of unconjugated bilirubin. This 'enterohepatic recirculation' of bilirubin is a particular problem in babies who are not fully fed or whose bowel is not yet colonized by normal flora. In fetal life unconjugated bilirubin can easily cross the placenta for disposal by the maternal liver, and maternal liver disease can lead to high bilirubin levels at birth.

Jaundice (including biliary atresia)

Jaundice is extremely common in newborn babies and 60% of all white-skinned babies are visibly jaundiced in the first week of life. The key problems in neonatal jaundice are in determining when jaundice is a sign of more serious disease and in the prevention of kernicterus. Kernicterus occurs when unconjugated bilirubin crosses the blood–brain barrier. Once inside the brain bilirubin is toxic to the deep grey matter, the globus pallidus in particular. Children who survive acute bilirubin encephalopathy only to develop kernicterus are usually profoundly disabled by athetoid cerebral palsy and sensorineural deafness. Kernicterus can be prevented by avoiding high levels of unconjugated bilirubin, using phototherapy and exchange transfusion.

http://www.pickonline.org

Hyperbilirubinaemia. A US website for parents of children brain-damaged by bilirubin, including videos showing the long-term effects

Phototherapy works by providing photons of light energy in a wavelength likely to be absorbed by the bilirubin molecule, which enters an excited state. About 80% of the time the bilirubin molecule loses the excess energy and returns to normal, but about 20% of the time a photochemical reaction occurs; these reactions include configurational and structural isomerization, and photo-oxidation. The photoproducts (which include lumirubin) are thought to be more water-soluble than unconjugated bilirubin and hence more rapidly excreted in bile. The rate of bilirubin decline is proportional to the dose of phototherapy, and in babies with severe jaundice it is important to expose as much skin as possible to light of an appropriate spectrum and to use adequate irradiance (more bulbs, well maintained).

Haematological causes of neonatal jaundice are common and usually related to haemolysis (see above). They include:

- Immune haemolysis (HDN): rhesus, ABO, Duffy or Kell incompatibility with maternal antibodies
- Red cell membrane disorders, e.g. spherocytosis
- Red cell enzyme disorders, e.g. G6PD deficiency
- Haemoglobinopathy (rare)
- Infection causing haemolysis, e.g. CMV, toxoplasmosis, syphilis.

> **Problem-orientated topic:**
>
> ### late-onset jaundice
>
> Lucy is a 15-day-old baby who was born at 37 weeks' gestation and who required respiratory support for 3 days. She was slow to establish feeds but is now on full feeds of breast milk, partly through a nasogastric tube. She was first noted to be jaundiced at 7 days and the levels of bilirubin are slowly rising.
>
> Q1. What is the definition of late neonatal jaundice?
>
> Q2. What is the main differential diagnosis?
>
> Q3. How would you assess this child?

Q1. What is the definition of late neonatal jaundice?

Prolonged or late neonatal jaundice can be defined as visible jaundice — serum bilirubin > 85 μmol/l — persisting or occurring at 14 days of age in full-term babies and at 21 days in preterm infants.

Q2. What is the main differential diagnosis?

The most common cause of prolonged jaundice in full-term infants is benign and attributable to breastfeeding; up to 9% of breastfeeding infants are still jaundiced at 28 days of age. However, late-occurring jaundice can be an important sign of a number of relatively rare conditions, the long-term outcome of which may be favourably influenced by early diagnosis. These include congenital biliary atresia, congenital hypothyroidism and galactosaemia. Late jaundice can also be a sign of acute illness, such as urinary infection or septicaemia, or of persisting haemolysis.

In preterm infants the most common cause of conjugated hyperbilirubinaemia is parenteral nutrition.

Q3. How would you assess this child?

In assessing infants with late jaundice the following are important questions to address:
- Is the baby unwell?
- Is the urine dark and/or are the stools pale?
- Is the serum/plasma conjugated bilirubin concentration raised (> 15% of the total)?

A list of causes of prolonged/late jaundice is shown in Boxes 48.5 and 48.6.

BOX 48.5 Causes of late unconjugated hyperbilirubinaemia

- Breast milk jaundice
- Haemolysis:
  - Blood group incompatibilities (ABO and rhesus)
  - Spherocytosis
  - G6PD deficiency
- Increased enterohepatic circulation:
  - Pyloric stenosis
  - Bowel obstruction
- Endocrine/metabolic:
  - Hypothyroidism
  - Hypopituitarism
  - Hypoadrenalism
  - Galactosaemia
  - Sepsis:
    Systemic
    Urinary

The diagnosis can be suspected if there are reducing substances present in the urine, but this test is not sensitive or specific and must be confirmed by the analysis of erythrocyte galactose-1-phosphate uridyl transferase. Affected babies must be given a lactose-free diet, best achieved in infancy by using soy milk. Unfortunately the IQ is often permanently affected by the time a diagnosis is made and treatment begun, even though the liver disease recovers and the cataracts can be treated (or may regress somewhat). In the long term osteoporosis is a complication and dietary calcium supplementation is required. Young women with galactosaemia require hormone replacement therapy.

A screening test on the blood sample currently collected for phenylketonuria screening would be possible but is not considered cost-effective at present.

Galactosaemia

Galactosaemia is an extremely rare disease with a frequency of approximately 1:45 000 in the UK, and is a recessive genetic disorder. It is due to deficiency of the enzyme galactose-1-uridyl transferase, an enzyme involved in the conversion of galactose into glucose (galactose is derived from lactose, milk sugar, which is broken down to galactose and glucose). Classically, babies present towards the end of the first week with vomiting, diarrhoea, failure to thrive and jaundice. They may present with signs of VKDB due to the liver disease. There is an association with sepsis, most commonly an *Escherichia coli* urinary tract infection that can cause septicaemia. Cataracts often form very early on and, if not recognized and treated, lead to visual impairment from amblyopia.

Hypoglycaemia (see also p. 328)

Basic science of glucose metabolism

Healthy adults maintain serum glucose levels within a very tight range of 3.5–7 mmol/l during fasting or after meals, and they do this on a diet in which the main energy sources are fat- and sugar-based. Maintenance of serum glucose depends on a feedback loop involving the liver, the pancreas and the process of glycogenolysis (the breakdown of glycogen stores to make glucose) (Fig. 48.4). Gluconeogenesis is the process involved in the production of glucose from precursors such as amino acids, lactate, and glycerol derived from lipolysis. The fetus cannot make glucose from glycogen, and is wholly dependent on a supply of glucose via the placenta. The fetus does make glycogen, and the liver stores at term

BOX 48.6 Causes of conjugated hyperbilirubinaemia

Cholestasis

- Biliary atresia
- Choledochal cyst
- 'Inspissated bile' syndrome (following haemolysis)
- Congenital bile duct hypoplasia (Alagille's syndrome)
- Gallstones

Neonatal hepatitis syndrome

- Idiopathic neonatal hepatitis syndrome
- Intrauterine infections (e.g. 'TORCH' infections — *to*xoplasmosis, *r*ubella, *c*ytomegalovirus, *h*erpes simplex)
- Alpha$_1$-antitrypsin deficiency

Metabolic

- Total parenteral nutrition (TPN)
- Hypothyroidism
- Cystic fibrosis
- Abnormalities of carbohydrate metabolism, e.g. galactosaemia, fructosaemia
- Abnormalities of bile acid metabolism
- Abnormalities of lipid metabolism, e.g. Niemann–Pick type C
- Abnormalities of amino-acid metabolism, e.g. tyrosinaemia
- Congenital peroxisomal disorders, e.g. Zellweger's syndrome
- Hypopituitarism
- Sepsis
- Urinary tract infection

are sufficient for about 10–12 hours of fasting. At birth, the fetus is disconnected from the continuous supply of glucose and has to adapt quickly to the fast-feed cycle; glucose levels fall and there is a surge of glucagon and a fall in insulin levels. It takes more than a few hours for the newborn baby to switch on gluconeogenesis. During the inevitable fasting phase of the first few days of life (the volume of colostrum is very small, about 7 ml per feed) the baby's brain can use ketone bodies as an alternative fuel. There is a brisk ketogenic response in the normal baby, and the neonatal brain can extract and use ketones much more efficiently than the adult brain. There is a suggestion that formula feeding interferes with the ketogenic response, and this thinking is behind much of the current advice regarding initiation of breastfeeding.

Definition of hypoglycaemia

In recent years the tolerance for low blood sugar in newborn infants has increased so that it is now accepted that low blood sugar levels of < 2.6 mmol/l should be treated. Studies have suggested that blood sugar values below this are associated with poorer neurodevelopmental outcome and acute deterioration in neurological function measured by evoked potentials.

Causes of neonatal hypoglycaemia

See Box 48.7.

BOX 48.7 Causes of neonatal hypoglycaemia

Transient

- Developmental lags in gluconeogenesis and ketogenesis
- Transient hyperinsulinism; infants of diabetic mothers
- Reduced glycogen stores: IUGR, HIE

Persistent

- Hyperinsulinism:
  - Idiopathic hyperinsulinism
  - Potassium–adenosine triphosphate (ATP) channel
  - Beckwith–Wiedemann syndrome
- Counter-regulatory hormone deficiency:
  - Panhypopituitarism
  - Isolated growth hormone deficiency
  - Cortisol deficiency
- Glycogenolysis disorders:
  - Debrancher deficiency
- Gluconeogenesis disorders:
  - G6PD deficiency
  - Pyruvate carboxylase deficiency
- Fatty acid oxidation disorders

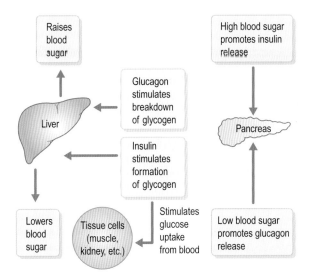

Fig. 48.4 Regulation of glucose

Hypocalcaemia, metabolic bone disease and vitamin D-deficient rickets

The serum ionized calcium level falls in the first 24 hours of life, as calcium continues to be taken up into newly forming bone, even though there is a cessation in the calcium supplied via the placenta and a postnatal surge in calcitonin. The failure to calcify newly forming bone adequately eventually causes rickets.

The definition of hypocalcaemia thus varies according to postnatal age, with a lower limit of normal during the first day. Total serum calcium should fall in the range 2.18–2.48 mmol/l (ionized 0.81–1.41) on the first day, and rise to 2.26–2.69 (ionized 1–1.5) by the end of the first week of life.

Signs of hypocalcaemia include:
- Irritability, twitching
- Seizures
- Lethargy
- Feed intolerance, vomiting.

Early hypocalcaemia is common in preterm babies, infants of diabetic mothers, babies whose mothers had poor vitamin D status during pregnancy (often immigrant mothers), and babies stressed by perinatal hypoxia.

Persistent hypocalcaemia suggests hypoparathyroidism, and a baby who is hypocalcaemic and who also has cardiac disease should be checked for Di George syndrome by examining the chromosomes for the characteristic 22q11 deletion. There are a number of other rare genetic causes of hypoparathyroidism such as HDR syndrome (*h*ypoparathyroidism, *d*eafness and *r*enal dysplasia).

The newborn baby has a store of vitamin D, which reflects the vitamin D status of the mother. Pre-term babies fed unsupplemented human milk may develop borderline vitamin D levels. Vitamin D supplementation improves calcium absorption and retention, although there is no evidence that massive doses (above 1000 IU per day) or administration of the active metabolite are of benefit. There is an argument for supplementation of all pregnant mothers and newborn babies in countries where sunlight is limited. In the British Isles, sunlight exposure is often not adequate for vitamin D manufacture, and in this situation dietary sources become essential. Rickets and vitamin D deficiency are a particular problem in immigrant families in the UK and northern Europe at the present time. Dietary sources of vitamin D in infancy have been shown to be marginal, and poor diet combined with indoor living, atmospheric pollution and increased use of sunscreen has been responsible for the resurgence of simple vitamin D deficiency rickets in recent years. The American Academy of Pediatrics has recently revised its vitamin supplementation policy to advise that all breastfed infants, and those on mixed feeding receiving less than 500 ml of formula daily, should be given 200 IU of vitamin D daily.

Rickets presents with the signs of hypocalcaemia and the bony changes are diagnostic. X-rays show cupping, fraying and splaying of the metaphysis of a long bone, and the changes are often best seen at the wrist. The skull bones are softened, termed craniotabes. Hypocalcaemia can present with seizures in the neonatal period. Rickets is most often due to simple dietary deficiency, but rarely can be due to a non-functioning vitamin D receptor (vitamin D-resistant rickets), renal disease or familial forms of hypophosphataemic rickets.

Preterm babies are at risk of developing metabolic bone disease, which can progress to rickets if left untreated, because the dietary supply of calcium and phosphate is insufficient to meet their needs. These babies usually have a low serum phosphate with a high alkaline phosphatase and their bones are demineralized on X-ray. Fractures can occur, particularly rib fractures.

The emergency treatment of symptomatic hypocalcaemia is with intravenous 10% calcium gluconate, given over 30–60 minutes. Babies can then be started on oral calcium and calciferol whilst confirmation of the diagnosis is sought with X-rays. Phosphate supplementation is not required, except for preterm babies. When a diagnosis of rickets is made in a baby who was born at term, of normal weight, evidence of osteomalacia should be sought in the mother, whose vitamin D status is likely to be marginal, and the other children in the family should be investigated for rickets.

Sepsis

Basic science

Babies are particularly vulnerable to infection for many reasons, including:
- There is reduced skin integrity.
- There is frequent damage to the respiratory epithelium from oxygen or ventilation.
- There is an immature response to organisms in the gastrointestinal tract.
- The neonatal neutrophil pool in the marrow is easily exhausted and the neutrophils are poor at migrating and ingesting opsonized pathogens.
- T and B cells are immature and are naïve with respect to foreign antigens and pathogens.

An understanding of the way in which the body reacts to pathogens is important and there has been an explosion of knowledge in the last 20 years. The inflammatory response includes a 'cytokine cascade'. Cells such as macrophages, when stimulated, release tumour

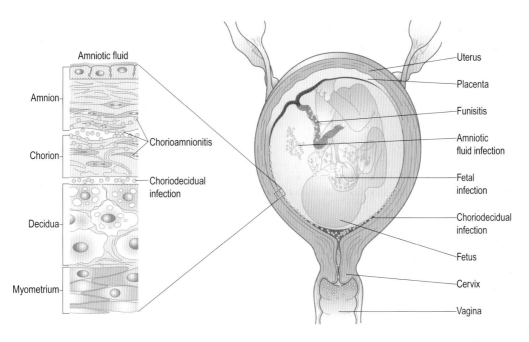

Fig. 48.5 Potential sites of bacterial infection within the uterus.
(From: Goldenberg RL et al 2000 New England Journal of Medicine 342:1500–1507)

necrosis factor and interleukin (IL)-1. These molecules trigger a cascade that includes other interleukins, platelet activating factor, prostaglandins and leukotrienes. There is upregulation of the adhesion molecules such as selectin and this helps leucocytes to roll along the endothelium directed by a chemotactic gradient, in order that they can reach the area of invasion.

Occasionally there is an over-zealous response, resulting in the 'systemic inflammatory response syndrome' (SIRS). This is responsible for the clinical features of septic shock: hypotension, thrombosis, pulmonary oedema with increased vascular permeability and multiple organ failure. SIRS is the reason why some babies with NEC and early-onset group B streptococcal (GBS) disease die very rapidly in spite of antibiotic therapy and full intensive care support.

There is increasing interest in the fetal inflammatory response syndrome too; infection is a common trigger for preterm delivery. Chorioamnionitis occurs when the maternal polymorphs gather under the chorionic plate, attracted there from the intervillous space (Fig. 48.5). Eventually they may invade it and cross to the amnion and the amniotic fluid. Chorionic vasculitis and funisitis are thought to be fetal inflammatory responses, and are associated with a 'cytokinaemia'; babies whose placenta showed funisitis have high levels of interleukins in cord blood, for example. There is a relationship between the fetal inflammatory response syndrome and later cerebral palsy, which is present for both chorioamnionitis and funisitis but is weaker for the former.

Problem-orientated topic:

early neonatal collapse

Harry is born by emergency caesarean section for failed induction, at term, weighing 2.5 kg. He is in good condition with a normal cord pH. The membranes were ruptured for 11.5 hours. Harry is noted to be grunting from the age of an hour; he is intubated because of rising oxygen requirements and given surfactant and antibiotics. Two hours later Harry has a cardiac arrest.

Q1. What are the most likely causes of the cardiac arrest?

Q2. How would you investigate this child?

Q3. Is any other management indicated?

Q1. What are the most likely causes of the cardiac arrest?

See Box 48.8.

Q2. How would you investigate this child?

See Box 48.9.

- Sepsis: particularly early-onset GBS disease
- Congenital heart disease, ductal-dependent, with closure of the ductus: e.g. hypoplastic aortic arch, coarctation of the aorta, hypoplastic left heart syndrome (p. 360)
- Arrhythmia: e.g. supraventricular tachycardia (SVT; usually babies cope well for many hours); ventricular tachycardia (VT; very rare in babies, suggests a myocarditis) (p. 360)
- Inborn error of metabolism (Ch. 34)
- Blood loss: e.g. massive subgaleal haematoma, ruptured liver, splenic rupture, intracranial haemorrhage with raised ICP
- Tension pneumothorax (p. 349): especially in an intubated and ventilated baby or a baby who required resuscitation or needling of the chest
- Cardiac tamponade: especially if there is a central venous line in place
- Gut perforation: think of this in a small preterm baby, particularly with NEC, but gastric and ileal perforation can occur due to ischaemic hypoperfusion; milk curd bezoars are rare causes of perforation but are reported

Q3. Is any other management indicated?

Babies with shock from any cause, particularly septic shock, have a high mortality and need full intensive care support and monitoring with aggressive treatment as soon as the condition is recognized. Assessment of acid–base and cardiovascular status is urgent, and ventilatory support is required whilst an attempt is made to elucidate the cause and offer specific treatment. Milk feeds should be stopped in case of inborn error of metabolism and because an ill baby will not absorb feeds, which may cause vomiting and aspiration.

Group B streptococcal (GBS) infection

GBS is a common vaginal commensal, which causes serious early-onset disease in about 1 per 2000 births. Risk factors for early-onset GBS disease include:
- Prematurity
- Heavy vaginal carriage
- Prolonged membrane rupture (more than 18 hours)
- Maternal pyrexia
- Previous affected baby (mother has no antibodies, usually against type III GBS).

- Electrocardiogram (ECG) monitoring, blood gas, blood pressure, saturation monitoring: to assess the need for inotropic support, volume replacement and cardiac rhythm
- Chest and abdominal X-ray: to exclude pneumothorax and to check the heart size and position; look for free air in the peritoneal cavity
- Blood culture, urine culture and surface swabs: to attempt to identify the organism in sepsis, not a rapid test
- Full blood count: a low white cell count or a very high one suggests infection. Babies do not mount a specific neutrophil response to bacterial sepsis. The platelet count often falls in sepsis or NEC
- C-reactive protein (CRP): the normal value varies between laboratories but is usually less than 1 mg/dl. Serial measurements are more valuable than a single estimate, and the CRP may take 48 hours to rise in response to sepsis. A normal value in the acute situation does not exclude sepsis
- IL-6: not yet available clinically, but more likely than CRP to be elevated early in the presence of infection
- Urea and electrolytes, lactate, ammonia: clues to inborn errors of metabolism
- Echocardiography: to detect congenital heart disease
- Cranial ultrasound scan: to detect intracranial bleeding but not a good technique for detection of subdural collections and will not diagnose subgaleal bleeding either. For this, careful clinical examination and serial head circumference measurements are helpful

Management

Intrapartum antibiotic prophylaxis is a proven effective treatment that can interrupt the vertical transmission of GBS infection from mother to baby. Intravenous penicillin 3 g should be given as soon as possible after the onset of labour and 1.5 g 4-hourly until delivery in women whose babies are at high risk of acquiring early-onset GBS disease. Women who are allergic to penicillin should receive clindamycin 900 mg intravenously 8-hourly. The current UK guidelines for intrapartum antibiotic prophylaxis adopt a risk factor-based approach; screening for GBS carriage at 35 weeks has been adopted in some countries but is not endorsed by the UK national screening committee.

http://www.gbss.org.uk

Group B Streptococcus support group; an excellent source of information, including leaflets for parents

http://www.nsc.nhs.uk

UK national screening committee

http://www.rcog.org.uk

The Royal College of Obstetricians comprehensive guideline on GBS, which is endorsed by the Royal College of Paediatrics and Child Health and the Royal College of Midwives in the UK

Most babies with early-onset GBS disease present soon after birth and virtually all present within 12 hours. Signs include raised respiratory rate, grunting, apnoea, poor feeding and mottling, and the disease can progress very rapidly to shock and death. The mortality is still around 10%.

Septicaemia

Apart from GBS, babies can acquire a bacteraemia from any one of hundreds of potential pathogens. Sepsis in the neonate is usually categorized as 'early-onset' and 'late-onset':

Early-onset:

- Presents by about 48 hours of age
- Is caused by organisms acquired from the birth canal or occasionally transplacentally, e.g. GBS, *E. coli*, *Listeria monocytogenes*

Late-onset:

- Presents after 48 hours of age
- Is usually caused by organisms acquired from the environment or nosocomially, e.g. coagulase negative staphylococci (CONS), *Staphylococcus aureus*, *E. coli*, *Klebsiella*, *Enterobacter*, *Serratia*, *Citrobacter*, *Acinetobacter*, *Pseudomonas*, *Candida* spp and other fungi, or viruses.

Exceptions to this pattern of acquisition and presentation include:

- Late-onset GBS
- Herpes simplex infection
- *Chlamydia* infection
- Congenital candidal and other fungal infections.

Infections caused by these organisms may be acquired at birth but present later. Anaerobic bacteria may also be a cause of sepsis, usually in association with bowel pathology.

It is important to remember viral infections including herpes virus, not least because aciclovir can be a life-saving treatment. Think of congenital candidiasis in preterm babies whose mothers have a history of chronic vaginal thrush and who had cervical cerclage, or who became pregnant with an intrauterine device fitted.

Babies with septicaemia usually present with non-specific signs such as poor feeding, mottling, lethargy, floppiness, apnoea and temperature instability. There may be tachypnoea and tachycardia. Quite often there is an ileus, with feed intolerance, dilated loops and abdominal distension, and these signs can be present even when the diagnosis is not NEC.

Treatment of septicaemia depends on accurate identification of the organism and appropriate use of antibiotics.

Meningitis

Think of meningitis in babies with signs of sepsis who are irritable. A full fontanelle and seizures are late signs, and meningitis should be diagnosed with LP before this stage is reached. LP is an essential tool in the diagnosis of meningitis, but it is known that in about 15% of cases the blood culture does not yield the organism.

The normal white cell count in neonatal CSF is higher than at other times of life, and in general counts of up to 30 per mm^3 are considered to be within the normal range. Differential white cell counts in CSF do not help to distinguish bacterial from viral meningitis in the newborn. If there is a high white cell count and no organisms are seen on Gram stain in CSF from a baby who has not received antibiotic treatment, think of viral meningitis and start aciclovir whilst awaiting PCR for herpes virus.

Meningitis carries a significant risk of brain damage and treatment must be carefully monitored. Brain imaging is important in order to detect ventriculomegaly and abscess (fortunately rare), and EEG can help in prognostication.

Eye infection

Sticky eyes are common in babies but serious eye infections are rare. The management depends on the organism, and an attempt should be made to identify *Chlamydia* because this may be 'masked' by treatment with topical chloramphenicol and requires systemic treatment with erythromycin (plus tetracycline eye drops) in order to treat any associated pneumonia. Staphylococcal infections are the most common.

Mild infections can be treated by cleaning with sterile saline, but if cultures are positive and discharge persists, topical antibiotics should be used. Chloramphenicol or neomycin eye drops are suitable. Gonococcal ophthalmia remains rare but, because the corneal damage can occur very quickly, it is important to consider this as a diagnosis, particularly when there is a profuse purulent discharge very early in life. The current recommended treatment is with intravenous ceftriaxone; the baby and mother must be isolated.

CHAPTER

49

Neonatology IV: Disorders requiring surgical intervention

LEARNING OUTCOMES

By the end of this chapter you should:

- Be able to understand the ways in which serious congenital anomalies may present
- Know how to manage babies suspected as having these conditions prior to and during transfer to a surgical centre
- Be aware of surgical complications that may occur in preterm babies
- Know when to refer babies with minor surgical conditions.

Introduction

Babies who require surgical referral in the neonatal period usually have one of the following three problems:

- A serious congenital anomaly
- An acquired surgical complication of prematurity
- A minor anomaly detected on routine examination.

Congenital anomalies are now often detected antenatally and delivery is planned at a regional surgical centre (e.g. gastroschisis, congenital diaphragmatic hernia). However, some conditions (e.g. most forms of congenital intestinal obstruction, oesophageal atresia) are rarely diagnosed antenatally and will be detected when symptoms develop postnatally. The correct early management of many of these conditions will influence morbidity and sometimes mortality.

Intestinal obstruction

Embryology

The intestine develops as a single tube from mouth to anus. At about 5 weeks of gestation the gut herniates through the umbilicus before returning to the abdominal cavity at about 10 weeks. As it returns

MODULE EIGHT

381

it rotates so that the stomach lies on the left, the duodenum starts on the right, looping round to the duodenojejunal (DJ) flexure on the left, the caecum is in the right iliac fossa and the colon extends from this point up the left side, across the upper abdomen and down the right side to the rectum. If this process fails to occur correctly, malrotation will exist.

The blood supply to the stomach and duodenum arises from the coeliac axis. The entire small bowel and right colon are supplied by the superior mesenteric artery and the remainder of the colon by the inferior mesenteric artery. Intestinal atresia occurs as a result of an antenatal ischaemic event. Innervation of the gut is thought to occur by migration of ganglion cells from neural crest tissue. Failure of this migration results in Hirschsprung's disease.

Problem-orientated topic:

intestinal obstruction

A well term male infant of 3.2 kg starts feeds on day 1 but develops bile-stained vomiting on day 2. The baby has not passed meconium. On examination the abdomen is distended but not tender.

Q1. What three specific clinical features are likely to be present?

Q2. How would you initially assess a baby with possible intestinal obstruction?

Q3. How should a baby with suspected intestinal obstruction be managed?

Q4. What are the possible causes of intestinal obstruction?

Q1. What three specific clinical features are likely to be present?

Intestinal obstruction is usually associated with three key features:
- Bile-stained vomiting
- Abdominal distension
- Failure to pass stool or flatus.

However, some of these features may be absent in specific causes of neonatal obstruction:
- Bile vomiting is absent in the one-third of babies with duodenal atresia in whom the atresia is proximal to the bile duct insertion.
- Distension may be absent in high intestinal obstruction (malrotation, duodenal atresia).

- Meconium may be passed by some babies with intestinal atresia if the atresia formed after the colon was filled with meconium.

Bilious vomiting

Bile is produced by the liver, is stored in the gallbladder and drains into the duodenum via the common bile duct (CBD). Bile is a golden-yellow/green colour but turns dark green on contact with gastric acid. Bile is not usually seen in gastric aspirate or vomit unless the intestine is obstructed beyond the point of entry of the CBD into the duodenum.

Mechanical obstruction to the lumen of the gut may be associated with impairment of the gut blood supply (e.g. volvulus, incarcerated hernia), which may progress to ischaemia, gut necrosis, peritonitis and death. Thus bile vomiting may be a warning sign of an impending catastrophe and should be assumed to be due to mechanical obstruction until proved otherwise.

Intestinal secretions

Considerable volumes of gastrointestinal secretions are produced each day. In the presence of obstruction fluid will accumulate within the gut lumen, which can affect fluid and electrolyte balance and cause intravascular volume depletion.

Passage of meconium

Around 98% of term babies pass meconium within 24 hours of delivery. Delay in passing meconium may occur with any of the causes of mechanical intestinal obstruction but may also be present if bowel function is altered, as may occur in many medical conditions (see below). Preterm babies, especially if very growth-retarded, may not pass meconium for 10 days or more, during which time they may develop significant abdominal distension.

Q2. How would you initially assess a baby with possible intestinal obstruction?

- Review maternal drug history.
- Assess the baby's general wellbeing; consider sepsis, metabolic causes and hypothyroidism.
- Assess the abdomen: most babies with a functional disorder will have a soft abdomen despite distension. Tenderness is a worrying sign and may require surgical review.
- Check hernial orifices.
- Check the anus is present.
- If mechanical obstruction is suspected, stimulate the rectum (e.g. glycerine suppository). If a plug passed or there is explosive decompression, discuss with surgeons.

- Nil by mouth
- Adequate-sized NGT (e.g. 8 Fr in term baby) on free drainage and hourly aspiration
- Establish i.v. access
- Assess hydration/perfusion
- Provide i.v. fluids:
  - Fluid resuscitation
  - Maintenance fluids
  - Nasogastric loss replacement ml for ml with normal saline + KCl

- If distension persists in the absence of a cause, discuss with surgeons.

Some babies have bilious vomiting that resolves and no cause is ever found.

Q3. How should a baby with suspected intestinal obstruction be managed?

Immediate management (Box 49.1) involves fluid resuscitation and strict attention to fluid and electrolyte balance. All enteral intake should be stopped and maintenance fluids given intravenously. A nasogastric tube (NGT) should be sited to prevent vomiting and aspiration. Gastric aspirates should be discarded but replaced by an equal volume of normal saline with potassium.

Q4. What are the possible causes of intestinal obstruction?

There are a number of causes of mechanical obstruction, some of which are described below. In some of these a precise diagnosis can be made by plain abdominal X-ray (AXR) or contrast radiology, but in many cases the precise diagnosis is not made until laparotomy.

Malrotation

This is the most dangerous cause of intestinal obstruction in the neonate because the position of the gut predisposes to midgut volvulus with subsequent ischaemia. The normally rotated gut is protected from volvulus because the base of the mesentery has a broad attachment from the DJ flexure to the caecum. In malrotation these two points lie side by side and the base of the mesentery is narrow and prone to twisting (volvulus; Fig. 49.1). If this occurs, the superior mesenteric artery may be occluded and the entire small intestine will become ischaemic; even if surgery takes place quickly, the whole of the gut may be lost.

Features of obstruction due to malrotation to note are:

- The abdomen is not usually distended.
- Bile vomiting may be intermittent.
- Blood may be passed rectally or found in the nasogastric aspirate.
- Although tenderness may be absent, volvulus may have already occurred, and by the time clinical features of an acute abdomen develop, the bowel may already be beyond salvage.
- Blood tests such as lactate and C-reactive protein (CRP) may initially be normal, even in the presence of gut ischaemia.
- The diagnosis is usually suggested by an abnormal AXR with a paucity of gas or an asymmetric gas pattern (Fig. 49.2).

If malrotation is suspected, the baby should:
- Be transferred immediately to a surgical centre

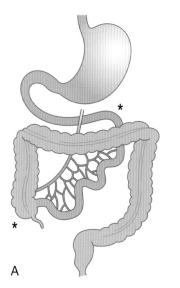
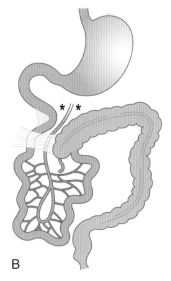

Fig 49.1 Malrotation
(A) Normal rotation; (B) typical malrotation. Note wide root of mesentery (indicated by *) in normal rotation compared to malrotation.

A   B

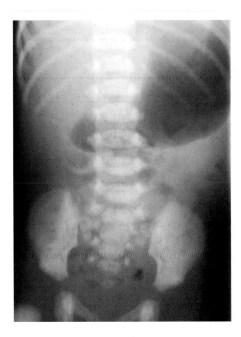

Fig. 49.2 Malrotation.
Note full stomach and duodenum but asymmetric gas pattern elsewhere.

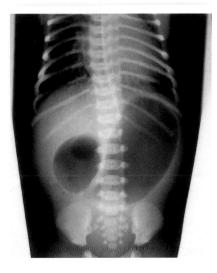

Fig. 49.3 Duodenal atresia 'double bubble'

- Have an immediate barium meal to identify the position of the DJ flexure
- Have immediate laparotomy if malrotation is confirmed.

Volvulus with ischaemia is fortunately quite rare and in most cases obstruction is due to a loose twist or bands and can be corrected easily. Surgery involves mobilizing the duodenum to correct any band obstruction and widening the base of the mesentery to reduce the risk of volvulus in the future.

Duodenal atresia/stenosis

In this condition there is obstruction in the second or third part of the duodenum.

Duodenal atresia:

- May be diagnosed antenatally
- Is associated with Down's syndrome in one-third of patients
- Is not usually associated with abdominal distension (although there may be epigastric fullness)
- Is associated with non-bilious vomiting in about 30% of patients because the atresia has occurred above the point of entry of the bile duct into the duodenum.

The diagnosis is made on AXR with a typical 'double bubble' appearance produced by air filling the stomach and the dilated proximal duodenum (Fig. 49.3). The presence of any air distal to the duodenum may indicate malrotation rather than atresia and urgent referral is indicated.

Corrective surgery is usually performed in the following 24–48 hours and involves an anastomosis to bypass the atresia (duodenoduodenostomy). Recovery of gut function postoperatively may be slow due to poor propulsion of feeds by the very dilated proximal duodenum. Long-term outcome is normal.

Small bowel atresia

Atresia is produced if a section of the intestine becomes ischaemic prenatally and this can occur at any stage, even in late pregnancy. Early atresia may be detected on prenatal scans. In late atresia the colon may have already filled with meconium and this may be passed postnatally, which may be confusing if a diagnosis of intestinal obstruction is being considered.

In babies with small bowel atresia:

- The abdomen becomes distended and dilated bowel loops may be visible. The more distal the atresia, the more distended the abdomen (Fig. 49.4).
- Contrast enema may be performed to try to distinguish obstruction caused by meconium ileus or meconium plugs (see below).
- Precise diagnosis may only be made at laparotomy.

Surgical correction usually involves primary anastomosis of the ends of the atresia. Subsequent recovery depends on how much, if any, intestine was lost at the time of the atresia formation. In most cases the amount lost is negligible. However, if a large amount of ileum has been lost, short bowel syndrome may occur and total parenteral nutrition (TPN) may be needed long-term.

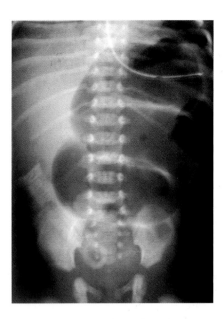

Fig. 49.4 Small bowel atresia (high).
Note only a few dilated loops with no gas beyond.

In the absence of short bowel syndrome long-term outlook is normal.

Meconium ileus

In this rare condition obstruction to the small intestine is caused by very sticky meconium. In almost all cases this is because the baby has cystic fibrosis. The diagnosis is usually only made by contrast enema or at laparotomy after transfer to a surgical centre.

Hirschsprung's disease (HD)

In this condition ganglion cells, which are responsible for the promotion of peristalsis along the length of the gut, are absent from the rectum upwards for a variable distance but usually extending to the sigmoid colon. This results in a functional obstruction to the colon.

In babies with HD:
- Abdominal distension is present.
- Obstruction is usually relieved by the passage of meconium and flatus on rectal examination.
- Continued decompression is usually possible by colonic washouts.
- Severe sepsis may occur due to Hirschsprung's enterocolitis.

If HD is suspected, the baby should be transferred to a surgical centre. Here decompression is usually achieved with colonic washouts, and a rectal suction biopsy is taken to confirm the diagnosis. Subsequent management is usually by continued washouts in the community until definitive surgery is performed in the first few months of life, although some surgeons opt for temporary colostomy formation, an intervention that will be required if washouts fail to decompress the bowel.

Although most babies with HD are clinically well, albeit obstructed, some present with or develop enterocolitis. This is characterized by:
- An ill baby with signs of severe sepsis
- Abdominal distension ± erythema or tenderness
- Bilious vomiting
- Offensive watery stool.

This serious complication of HD requires:
- Broad-spectrum intravenous antibiotics
- Regular decompression with colonic washouts
- NGT, nil by mouth.

Emergency laparotomy with colostomy may be required if these measures fail.

Anorectal malformation

The absence of an anal opening will obviously cause intestinal obstruction. It is therefore important to check the anus in any baby with obstruction. Even if the anus is present stenosis may occur and can cause obstruction. The anal size should be assessed by rectal examination in term infants, when the anal canal should permit the passage of a small fingertip. If doubt exists in the preterm baby, specialist referral is indicated. Stenosis can usually be treated by dilatation, although surgery is sometimes required.

Meconium plug

In some babies with clinical intestinal obstruction rectal examination or washout results in the passage of a meconium plug. This usually takes the form of a solid lump of meconium, sometimes with a white inspissated tip, followed by the passage of additional plugs or normal meconium. Most of these babies are normal but this may be the presenting feature of Hirschsprung's disease or meconium ileus. It is therefore essential that both conditions be excluded.

Obstructed inguinal hernia

See below.

Non-surgical causes of intestinal obstruction or delayed passage of meconium

- Normal transient delay (especially preterm babies)
- Sepsis

- Maternal diabetes, medications, narcotics
- Metabolic derangement: hypermagnesaemia, hypokalaemia, hypercalcaemia
- Hypothyroidism
- Congestive cardiac failure.

Diaphragmatic hernia

Problem-orientated topic:

respiratory distress at 1 hour of age

A term baby develops respiratory distress 1 hour after a normal vaginal delivery. On examination there is displacement of the trachea and cardiac apex beat to the right, there are reduced breath sounds on the left and the abdomen looks unusually flat.

Q1. What is the likely diagnosis?

Q2. What radiological investigations should be performed?

Q3. What immediate action should be undertaken?

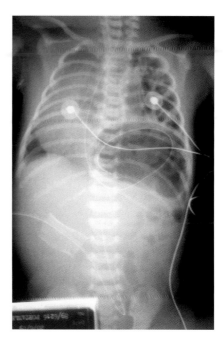

Fig. 49.5 **Left-sided congenital diaphragmatic hernia. Note stomach (with nasogastric tube) in chest, absence of bowel gas in abdomen and mediastinal shift to right.**

- Scaphoid abdomen (because the gut is in the chest)
- Bowel sounds heard in the chest.

Q1. What is the likely diagnosis?

A space-occupying lesion in the fetal chest (e.g. liver or bowel, as in congenital diaphragmatic hernia) will often prevent normal lung development and produce pulmonary hypoplasia, the severity of which will depend on the timing of herniation. Alveolar insufficiency and pulmonary vascular abnormality, both of which are features of pulmonary hypoplasia, commonly cause persistent pulmonary hypertension of the newborn (PPHN), which is the major cause of respiratory complications and determines outcome.

The above scenario will occur in a baby with a space-occupying lesion in the thorax. As well as diaphragmatic hernia, which is described below, it is important to exclude a tension pneumothorax. Cold light transillumination of the chest should be performed. Congenital cystic adenomatoid malformation of the lung (CCAM) may also cause this clinical picture but is rare.

In babies with congenital diaphragmatic hernia (CDH) there will be:

- Respiratory distress: varies from none (in those with normal lungs) to profound (in those with severe pulmonary hypoplasia)
- Mediastinal shift (trachea and cardiac apex beat), usually to the right, as 80% of hernias are on the left side

Q2. What radiological investigations should be performed?

- Diagnosis is made on chest and abdominal X-rays (Fig. 49.5).
- Loops of gut ± stomach are seen in the chest.
- There is mediastinal shift to the opposite side.
- There will be an abnormal intestinal gas pattern on AXR. It is essential to perform an AXR, as a cystic lung may look very like a CDH on CXR but will have a normal gas pattern below the diaphragm.

Q3. What immediate action should be undertaken?

Immediate management includes:
- Gastric decompression with large NGT (8 Fr)
- Avoidance of bag and mask ventilation, as this may expand the stomach and compromise lung expansion
- Appropriate respiratory support and intensive care: many babies will require immediate intubation and ventilation, umbilical arterial and venous access etc. but some will have minimal problems.
- Nil by mouth, i.v. access and fluids
- Transfer to a neonatal surgical centre.

Subsequent management includes:

- *Respiratory support.* In severe cases the lungs are too small to support life and the baby will die within hours. At the other extreme the lungs may be fully developed and there may be no respiratory problems. In most there is a degree of hypoplasia resulting in PPHN (p. 344).
- *Assessment of other congenital anomalies,* e.g. echocardiography. These are present in about 40% of cases.
- *Surgical repair of the diaphragm.* This is usually delayed for at least 24–48 hours, even in babies with minimal respiratory problems.

Timing of surgery

Survival and severity of clinical problems are determined by the degree of pulmonary hypoplasia and not by the presence of the gut in the chest. Surgery is performed when respiratory status allows. Some babies will never become this stable and will die without surgery. In others surgery may be delayed for several days.

Prognosis

The mortality from CDH is 30–40% and is due to lung hypoplasia or other congenital anomalies.

Abdominal wall defects

Problem-orientated topic:

abdominal wall defects

An emergency caesarean section is about to take place on a 36 weeks' gestation pregnancy with an antenatal diagnosis of an abdominal wall defect. The mother is on holiday in your area and does not know the name of the condition diagnosed in her baby but remembers being told that the intestine was on the outside.

Q1. What are the possible diagnoses?

Q2. What action will be needed at the delivery?

Q3. How will the baby need to be supported before and during transfer for surgery?

Q1. What are the possible diagnoses?

At about 5 weeks of gestation, probably as a response to rapid liver enlargement, the intestine herniates out of the abdominal cavity, returning at about 10 weeks of gestation, at which time the umbilicus closes. Failure of

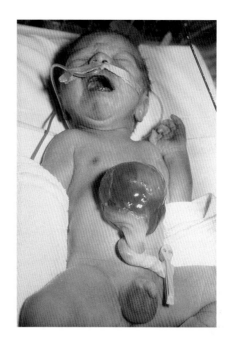

Fig. 49.6 Exomphalos.
Note sac covering gut.

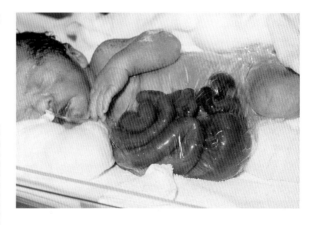

Fig. 49.7 Gastroschisis.
Note exposed gut without covering sac, Clingfilm wrap and towelling nappy under gut to support it in the midline.

development of lateral mesoderm is thought to result in exomphalos. In this condition the herniated viscera are contained within a semi-transparent sac, which may contain intestine alone or in combination with liver, depending on the size of the abdominal wall defect.

The embryology of gastroschisis is unclear but may be related to vascular changes at the umbilicus. The fetus initially has two vitelline veins; the left remains as the umbilical vein and the right obliterates. As the defect in gastroschisis is almost invariably to the right side of the umbilical ring, it has been suggested that abnormal obliteration of the right vitelline vein may result in the formation of gastroschisis.

The two primary conditions are exomphalos and gastroschisis (Figs 49.6 and 49.7). The features

Table 49.1 Comparison of exomphalos and gastroschisis

	Gastroschisis	Exomphalos
Anatomy	No sac	Sac
	Usually only gut out	Gut ± liver, spleen etc.
Abnormal karyotype	None	May be trisomy 18/13
Associated anomalies	Gut atresia only (5%)	Cardiac, renal, pulmonary hypoplasia, Beckwith syndrome etc.
Postnatal outcome	95% survival	50–80% live-born survive
		95% live-born survive if only abnormality

BOX 49.2 Principles of management in abdominal wall defects at delivery

- Pass NGT to decompress the stomach and prevent vomiting
- Prevent heat loss by wrapping the herniated viscera with Clingfilm
- Position herniated viscera in the midline to prevent vascular compromise
- Establish i.v. access and give an initial fluid bolus of 20 ml/kg, which may need to be repeated

of these conditions are shown in Table 49.1. The major differences are the presence of a sac and the associated anomalies in babies with exomphalos. It is the latter that contributes to the increased mortality in exomphalos. In both conditions, if isolated, the survival rate is 95%.

Q2. What action will be needed at the delivery?

See Box 49.2.

Q3. How will the baby need to be supported before and during transfer for surgery?

- Large-bore NGT left on free drainage with hourly aspiration
- Replacement of gastric aspirates with i.v. normal saline with added potassium
- Regular assessment of circulation, e.g. capillary refill time, with further bolus fluid replacement as required
- Regular assessment of colour of the herniated viscera with repositioning or rewrapping if required.

Immediate transfer to a surgical centre should be arranged. During transfer further fluid boluses will be

required and the viscera should be inspected regularly and repositioned as required to prevent venous engorgement or ischaemia.

In babies with exomphalos also be prepared for:

- *Lung hypoplasia*: some babies have severe respiratory problems.
- *Beckwith–Wiedemann syndrome*: macroglossia, gigantism, exomphalos. Associated with hyperinsulinism and thus hypoglycaemia — watch the blood sugar.
- *Trisomy 18, 13 or 21.*
- *Associated anomalies*: cardiac anomalies are the most relevant (20%).

Surgery is required for both conditions but is more urgent in gastroschisis as the exposed bowel will lose heat and fluid rapidly. Intravenous feeding is usually required for babies with gastroschisis as the bowel takes several weeks to function normally. Long-term outcome is normal in the absence of associated anomalies.

Oesophageal atresia

Problem-orientated topic:

oesophageal atresia

You are called to see a 12-hour-old term baby who has been noticed by the staff on the postnatal ward to have excessive oropharyngeal secretions. Staff on the neonatal unit have been unable to pass an NGT more than a few centimetres.

Q1. What are the possible causes of failure to pass the NGT?

Q2. How would you distinguish these?

Q3. How should a baby with oesophageal atresia be managed prior to transfer to a surgical centre?

Q1. What are the possible causes of failure to pass the NGT? (Box 49.3)

The foregut begins development as a single tube from which the oesophagus and trachea form in the early weeks of gestation. The exact process is not understood but it is thought that failure of full separation of these developing structures results in oesophageal atresia and tracheo-oesophageal fistula formation.

Choanal atresia

In this rare condition there is an obstruction at the back of the nose, at the level of the back of the hard

- Nasal obstruction:
  - Nasal oedema: common and resolves with time and/or decongestants
  - Choanal atresia
- Oesophageal atresia: with or without tracheo-oesophageal fistula

palate, about 3–4 cm from the opening of the nostril. It is more commonly unilateral, so if passing the tube fails on one side, try the other. There is a solid feeling to the obstruction as the NGT hits the atresia. Unilateral atresia does not require treatment in the neonatal period, with surgery being deferred until several years of age. Due to respiratory problems bilateral atresia will usually require surgery in the first few weeks of life.

Oesophageal atresia (OA) and tracheo-oesophageal fistula (TOF) (Box 49.4)

The usual anatomy is:

- Oesophagus ending blindly in the upper chest (OA)
- Lower oesophagus connected to the lower trachea (TOF) but other anatomical varieties exist.

BOX 49.4 Clinical problems in oesophageal atresia with tracheo-oesophageal fistula

- Problems caused by the atresia
- Failure to swallow saliva (mucousy baby)
- Cyanosis and choking with feeds as milk spills over to the lungs
- Problems caused by the fistula
- Lung irritation from acid reflux to trachea
- Gastric distension from air via trachea, especially if respiratory support is required
- Problems caused by associated malformations

Q2. How would you distinguish these?

To confirm the diagnosis of OA with TOF:

- Try to pass a large-bore (at least 8 Fr) naso- or orogastric tube. If successful, test aspirate with pH paper to confirm an acid reaction, as the tube could be coiled in the oesophagus.
- If the tube fails to pass, fix it as far as it will go and obtain CXR *and* AXR. This will show the tube in the upper chest, confirming atresia, and gas in the abdomen, confirming a fistula (Fig. 49.8). If the abdomen is gasless, there will be OA without TOF.

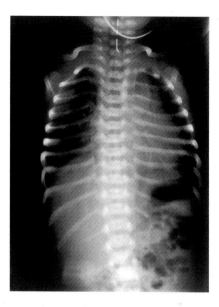

Fig. 49.8 Chest and abdomen in a baby with oesophageal atresia and tracheo-oesophageal fistula.
Note the tube arrested in the upper oesophagus and the air in the gut.

Q3. How should a baby with oesophageal atresia be managed prior to transfer to a surgical centre?

See Box 49.5.

BOX 49.5 Management of oesophageal atresia with tracheo-oesophageal fistula

- Remove the NGT and replace with a Replogle tube, if one is available. This is a 10 Fr sump suction catheter, which is connected to low-pressure continuous suction. Saline is flushed down the side-limb of the catheter every 15 minutes (or more often if necessary) to remove saliva from the oesophagus
- Nurse the baby head up to reduce flow of gastric acid into the trachea via the fistula. Prone position will further reduce the risk of reflux
- Establish i.v. access and commence maintenance fluids
- Notify regional surgical centre and arrange transfer, which should take place in the next few hours
- Continue above management during transfer

Respiratory management in OA with TOF

Most babies do not need respiratory support. Preterm babies, or those in who the diagnosis has been delayed until after aspiration pneumonitis has already occurred, may develop respiratory distress. Positive pressure ventilation will result in ventilator gases passing down the fistula and inflating the stomach. This can cause abdominal distension and worsen respiration. In severe cases gastric perforation and death may occur. If respiratory support is required, immediate transfer to a surgical centre should be arranged for emergency ligation of the fistula.

Management at surgical centre

Echocardiography is performed to exclude cardiac defects. Primary repair is performed in the first 24–48 hours. OA often occurs in association with other anomalies. Because of this, routine screening of other systems is performed (echocardiography, renal ultrasound).

Outcome

Long-term outcome is variable, with respiratory and gastrointestinal complications being commonplace.

Rectal bleeding

Problem-orientated topic:

rectal bleeding

Robbie, a 4-day-old breastfed term baby, is noted to have passed dark red blood into his nappy. He appears alert, active and well perfused.

Q1. What are the possible causes of rectal bleeding?

Q2. How would you assess this baby?

Q1. What are the possible causes of rectal bleeding?

The colour of blood passed rectally will usually give a clue to the anatomical site of bleeding. Bright red blood is usually coming from the rectum or anus, dark red blood from the colon or terminal ileum, and melaena from the oesophagus, stomach or duodenum. If there is massive bleeding then upper intestinal blood may emerge still red from the rectum, but the baby would show signs of acute hypovolaemia.

Causes of rectal bleeding are:

- Idiopathic: in many babies no cause is found
- Milk allergy: due to cow's milk protein in formula milk or ingested by the mother and secreted in breast milk
- Haemorrhagic disease of the newborn (HDN, p. 371)
- Anorectal trauma

- Necrotizing enterocolitis (NEC, p. 391)
- Intestinal ischaemia: e.g. volvulus
- Intestinal malformation: e.g. haemangioma, duplication cyst
- Swallowed maternal blood, from delivery or from a cracked nipple.

Q2. How would you assess this baby?

Assess the baby's general condition and abdomen. If the baby is haemodynamically unstable or if the abdomen is distended or tender:

- Establish i.v. access immediately
- Give a fluid bolus
- Cross-match blood
- Check clotting and vitamin K status
- Perform an AXR
- Inspect the anus for signs of trauma
- Check for an external haemangioma — this may be a marker for an internal one.

Management

- If the baby is systemically unwell or shocked, full resuscitation is required.
- If NEC is suspected on X-ray, stop enteral feeds and commence i.v. antibiotics.
- Treat vitamin K deficiency if HDN is proven.
- If the baby is well, wait. Most babies with milk allergy will stop bleeding either spontaneously or after change to milk devoid of cow's milk protein.

Scrotal swelling

Problem-orientated topic:

scrotal swelling

Andrew, a male infant born at 28 weeks' gestation and now 5 weeks old, is found on routine examination to have a non-tender swelling in the left scrotum, which is not reducible.

Q1. What are the possible causes of this swelling?

Q2. How can these be differentiated?

Q3. What action is required?

Q1. What are the possible causes of this swelling?

The processus vaginalis is an outpouching of the peritoneum, which extends through the inguinal canal. It develops in early gestation and is involved in the process of testicular descent. Passage of peritoneal fluid down the patent processus vaginalis (PPV) results in a hydrocele. In most cases the PPV is very narrow and the fluid cannot be reduced back into the peritoneum by manual pressure. If the PPV is wide enough, intestine can pass down it; this is an indirect inguinal hernia.

The testis develops from the gonadal ridge on the posterior abdominal wall and descends to the internal inguinal ring by mid-gestation. Between 28 weeks and term the testis emerges into the PPV and descends into the scrotum. In approximately 5% of boys at term the testis has not fully descended but by 6 months of age this figure has reduced to 1.5%. Undescended testis is more common in preterm and low-birth weight babies.

Inguinal hernia

- 1–2% of term babies will develop an inguinal hernia.
- In preterm babies under 1.5 kg the incidence rises to 20%.
- Boys are much more commonly affected than girls.

Hernias are usually reducible but may become irreducible, causing intestinal obstruction and ischaemia, a risk that seems to be greater in preterm babies than in older children. For this reason inguinal hernia repair is usually carried out before or soon after discharge from the neonatal unit.

In the case described the swelling is irreducible. If this is a hernia then:

- Signs of intestinal obstruction will develop.
- The swelling may become tender.
- It should not transilluminate (although this may be a difficult sign to elicit confidently).
- It should not be possible to get above the swelling — it should extend to the level of the inguinal canal.

Hydrocele

Hydroceles are common, affecting 10% of term babies. They are harmless and usually asymptomatic despite occasionally being very large. Hydroceles normally:

- Surround the testis
- Transilluminate
- Are usually confined to the scrotum.

Q2. How can these be differentiated?

The most common scrotal swelling is a hydrocele but it is important to exclude an inguinal hernia. Differentiation between the conditions can usually be made on clinical grounds:

- Check for signs of intestinal obstruction: vomiting, distension.
- Confirm that the swelling is not tender.
- Determine whether the swelling is discrete from the testis and that the testis is descended.
- Attempt transillumination of the swelling.

Table 49.2 Comparison of features of inguinal hernia and hydrocele

Clinical feature	Groin/scrotal swelling	
	Hernia	Hydrocele
Reducible	✓	✗ (usually)
Intestinal obstruction	May be present	✗
Tenderness	May be present	✗
Can get above it to feel spermatic cord	✗	✓
Transilluminates	✗	✓

Features of hernia and hydrocele are compared in Table 49.2.

Testicular torsion

Neonatal torsion usually occurs as a late prenatal event and the infant is typically found to have a hard discoloured non-tender hemiscrotum. The testis in such cases cannot be salvaged by surgery but surgical referral is essential, as many surgeons will opt to fix the contralateral testis. Acute postnatal torsion can also occur and any infant with a tender testis should be referred for emergency surgical assessment.

Q3. What action is required?

If a hernia is suspected, then urgent surgical opinion should be sought. Once diagnosed, there is no need for repeated reduction.

A hydrocele requires no treatment. Spontaneous resolution will occur in most cases over several weeks or months.

Pneumoperitoneum/ necrotizing enterocolitis

Problem-orientated topic:

pneumoperitoneum/necrotizing enterocolitis

Maya, a 25-week gestation baby now 8 days old, is noted to have abdominal distension with bilious aspirates. A pneumoperitoneum is noted on abdominal X-ray.

Q1. What are the causes of pneumoperitoneum?
Q2. How would you differentiate between them?
Q3. What are the management options?

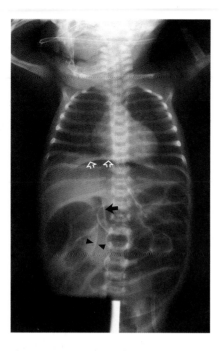

Fig. 49.9 Pneumoperitoneum.
Air is visible below the diaphragm (open arrows), on either side of the bowel wall (black triangles) and outlining the falciform ligament (black arrow).

Q1. What are the causes of pneumoperitoneum?

- Perforated NEC
- Spontaneous isolated intestinal perforation (SIP)
- In association with a pneumothorax.

The diagnosis of pneumoperitoneum is usually made easily on a supine AXR (Fig. 49.9), although sometimes a lateral decubitus X-ray of the abdomen is needed to show small air collections.

Q2. How would you differentiate between them?

Necrotizing enterocolitis (NEC)

Most babies do not require surgical referral but, in some, surgery will be life-saving. Surgical opinion should always be sought if there is a pneumoperitoneum or if clinical deterioration occurs despite maximal medical therapy.

The diagnosis of NEC is usually made on the basis of a combination of clinical and radiological features.

Clinical features are:
- Bile-stained aspirate
- Abdominal distension
- Blood in the stool
- Sepsis.

Radiological features are:
- Intramural gas
- Thickened bowel loops/free fluid
- Portal gas
- Pneumoperitoneum.

The diagnosis of pneumoperitoneum with pneumothorax should be obvious from the chest X-ray.

The diagnosis of SIP is by exclusion of NEC, but the diagnosis is usually not confirmed until laparotomy.

Q3. What are the management options?

When indicated, surgery involves a laparotomy with either resection and anastamosis or stoma formation. If there is a tense pneumoperitoneum compromising ventilation, insertion of a needle or peritoneal drain in the right iliac fossa prior to transfer may make transfer safer. Drain insertion should only be performed after discussion with a surgeon.

Spontaneous intestinal perforation

Perforation without NEC may occur and is most usually seen in very preterm babies in the first few days of life. Differentiation from perforated NEC may be difficult and the diagnosis is often not made until laparotomy. Occasional babies with isolated perforation can be managed by peritoneal drainage alone.

Pneumothorax and pneumoperitoneum

Air from a pneumothorax may track into the peritoneal cavity in the absence of intestinal perforation. Signs of abdominal sepsis will be absent.

Indications for surgery in NEC

- Intestinal perforation
- Failure of medical treatment:
  - Clinical deterioration: vital signs, abdominal mass, tenderness, erythema
  - Worsening laboratory results (platelets, electrolytes, acidosis, lactate)
- Stricture: usually presenting as obstruction some weeks after an episode of NEC and diagnosed by contrast radiology.

Bladder outflow obstruction

Problem-orientated topic:

bladder outflow obstruction

A male term infant is noted not to have passed urine at the age of 36 hours. On examination the abdomen is distended and a mass arising from the pelvis is palpable above the umbilicus.

Q1. What diagnoses should be considered?

Q2. What immediate investigations and intervention are required?

Q1. What diagnoses should be considered? (Box 49.6)

The failure to pass urine in the first day of life is not necessarily abnormal. Seven percent of healthy babies do not pass urine until the second day. However, the presence of an abdominal mass suggests an enlarged obstructed bladder, although other causes (e.g. abdominal teratoma) are possible.

Posterior urethral valves

Valves in the posterior urethra obstruct the flow of urine from the bladder. The degree of obstruction varies.

BOX 49.6 Causes of bladder outflow obstruction

Males
- Posterior urethral valves
- Prune belly syndrome (lax abdominal muscles, undescended testes, large bladder)
- Ureterocele

Females
- Ureterocele
- Cloacal anomaly (anorectal malformation, urogenital sinus)

Obstruction in fetal life may cause severe renal dysplasia, oligohydramnios and subsequent pulmonary hypoplasia (p. 34).

Clinical presentation in the neonate is very variable. At the worst end of the spectrum, babies may present with severe respiratory difficulty due to pulmonary hypoplasia and may die. Others with good lungs may present with failure to pass urine or have dribbling micturition, with abdominal distension due to an enlarged bladder and kidneys.

Q2. What immediate investigations and intervention are required?

- Prophylactic urinary antibiotics
- Urinary tract ultrasound
- Immediate referral to a paediatric urologist.

Key points
- Neonatal urea and electrolyte levels reflect maternal renal function in the first few hours of life and thus may be misleading.
- Bladder catheterization should not be performed without discussion with a paediatric urologist.
- Once the infant is catheterized, diuresis may be profound with rapid dehydration and hyponatraemia.

Surgical management

Endoscopic obliteration of the valves is usually performed, followed by long-term nephro-urology care. Some patients eventually develop end-stage renal failure.

Table 49.3 **Some of the common surgical conditions diagnosed at the postnatal check**

Condition	Refer to surgeon before discharge	Routine surgical outpatient appointment	Primary care services to refer if needed
Hypospadias		✓	
Undescended testis (uni- or bilateral)			✓
Impalpable testis (unilateral)			✓
Impalpable testes (bilateral)	✓		
Hydrocele			✓
Hernia: inguinal	✓		
Hernia: umbilical			✓
Accessory digit*		✓	
Pre-auricular skin tag*		✓	
Tongue tie with breastfeeding difficulty	Notify lactation nurse		
Request for religious circumcision			✓

* Refer to appropriate local surgeon. In some centres this may be plastic surgeon, ENT or paediatric surgeon.

Surgical conditions detected at postnatal check

Table 49.3 lists some of the common surgical conditions diagnosed at the postnatal check and states what action is required, if any.

Hypospadias

 This has three key features:

- *Abnormally sited urethral meatus*: anywhere from the underside of the glans to within the perineum
- *Chordee*: ventral curvature of the penis
- *Hooded foreskin*.

Surgery is not usually considered before 2 years of age. Routine outpatient surgical referral is required. However, if the testes are not both descended, more urgent referral is indicated, as this may constitute an intersex anomaly.

Undescended testis

Assessment of testicular descent forms part of the routine newborn check. An undescended testis will be found in 5% of term babies and in most the testis is palpable in the inguinal area. Routine surgical referral is not necessary, as testicular examination forms part of the routine Community Child Surveillance 6-week examination; referral will be made if necessary at that time or subsequently after the 8-month check.

Tongue tie

This affects about 3% of babies. It is debated whether this condition requires any treatment in the newborn period. There is some evidence that it may prevent effective breastfeeding. Local protocols for management usually exist.

Breda Hayes   Thomas G. Matthews

CHAPTER

50

Accidents, poisoning and apparent life-threatening events

LEARNING OUTCOMES

By the end of this chapter you should:

- Understand the contribution that accidents make to childhood death and disability
- Know which children with head injuries should be referred to hospital and what the indications are for brain imaging
- Understand the management of the common causes of poisoning in children
- Know and understand the risk factors of SUDI and how to minimize risk
- Know and understand the mechanisms by which a child may present with apparent life-threatening episodes (ALTEs)
- Know the appropriate advice to give to parents whose baby has had an ALTE.

MODULE EIGHT

Accidents (see also Ch. 17)

Injury is the principal cause of child death in all developed countries, accounting for almost 40% of deaths in the age group 1–15 years (Table 50.1). In the developed world, road traffic accidents account for approximately 41% of all injury-related deaths. Taken together, traffic accidents, intentional injuries, drownings, falls, fires, poisonings and other accidents kill more than 20 000 children every year in developed countries. In developing countries, an estimated 1 million children under 15 die each year from injuries.

For each death there is a very much larger number of non-fatal injuries, traumas and resulting disabilities. Annually about 10% of children suffer an accident necessitating contact with the health services. Accidents make up 29% of emergency department visits for children aged 0–5 years.

In general, accident causation varies from country to country and even within countries from region to region, as accidents depend on living conditions and the surrounding environment, both indoors and outdoors. However, in all countries the vast majority of all children's accidents involve falls, with a smaller number relating to motor vehicle accidents, fires, drownings, foreign body ingestion and poisoning. A child's risk for specific causes of injury is linked to developmental age, with studies showing differences in rates by 3-monthly intervals for children aged 0–3 years. Boys are 70% more likely to die by injury than girls.

Although it is true that child injury death rates have been falling for more than two decades, there is further

395

Table 50.1 Causes of death in children and young people

Top three causes of death	0–1 year	1–4 years	4–15 years	15–24 years
1	Developmental and genetic problems present at birth	Accidents	Accidents	Accidents
2	Sudden unexplained death in infancy (SUDI; sudden infant death syndrome, SIDS)	Developmental and genetic problems present at birth	Cancer	Homicide
3	Prematurity/low birth weight	Cancer	Homicide	Suicide

room for improvement. Sweden has had intensive child protection programmes running for over 35 years and has the lowest child injury death rate of any country.

The burden of accidental injury is disproportionately heavy on the most disadvantaged. Children from the poorest families are more likely to die from accidents, to be admitted to hospital and to be admitted with more severe injuries. The likelihood of a child being injured or killed is associated with single parenthood, low maternal education, low maternal age at birth, poor housing, large family size, and parental drug or alcohol abuse.

Accident prevention programmes need to be multi-faceted and to include poverty reduction programmes. Accident prevention is discussed in detail in Chapter 17.

Head injury

Minor closed head injury is one of the most frequent reasons for visits to a hospital. Only 1 in 800 results in any serious complications. The National Institute of Clinical Excellence (NICE) has described algorithms for referral to hospital and investigation of head injuries. The most recent recommendations for referral to hospital for further assessment include any of the following:

- Glasgow Coma Scale (GCS) < 15 (p. 308) at any time since the injury
- Any loss of consciousness as a result of the injury
- Any focal neurological deficit since the injury
- Amnesia for events before or after the injury in children > 5 years
- Persistent headache since accident
- Any vomiting since injury
- Any seizure since injury
- Any previous neurosurgical interventions
- High-energy head injuries (e.g. being struck by a car, fall from a height)
- Suspicion of non-accidental injury (Ch. 37)
- Finding of irritability or altered behaviour since the accident
- Any suspicion of skull fracture or penetrating head injury:

- Cerebrospinal fluid (CSF) from nose or ear
- Black eye with no associated trauma around eyes
- Bruising behind one or both ears
- Visible trauma to scalp or skull.

If the child is sent home, a reliable caregiver should be in charge at home and be given an instruction sheet for observation and for when to return the child to hospital.

Investigations

Skull radiography has no role in the evaluation and management of head injury. If neuroimaging is considered necessary, then computed tomography (CT) or magnetic resonance (MR) brain imaging is required. NICE recommends that urgent CT brain imaging should be undertaken if any of the following features is present:

- GCS < 13 at any time since the injury
- GCS 13 or 14 at 2 hours after the injury
- Focal neurological deficit
- Suspected open or depressed skull fracture
- Any signs of basal skull fracture
- Post-traumatic seizure
- > 1 vomiting episode.

 http://www.nice.org.uk

The GCS and the AVPU scales are described on page 308.

Head trauma may be due to child abuse or serious neglect by a parent or caregiver. In all cases a thorough history should be obtained of past injuries and of circumstances surrounding the present injury.

Road traffic accidents

While uncommon, motor vehicle accidents account for 40% of all fatal accidents in children. In the majority, the child is a pedestrian hit by oncoming traffic. In the remainder, the child is a passenger who is usually unrestrained or improperly restrained. Motor vehicle accidents are more common in underprivileged overcrowded areas with a lack of playground space. Adequate adult supervision is essential if children are outdoors, especially if there is access to passing traffic.

Child safety in cars needs to be addressed. All cars should be fitted with correct backseat child restraints, carefully selected according to the child's weight, height and length. Seat belts are designed for people 5 foot tall and over. Recommendations state that seat belts alone are inadequate until approximately 11 years of age.

Drowning

Drowning is ranked third overall as a cause of accidental death among children up to the age of 5. Incidence is closely related to climate, time of year and geographical zone. Toddlers account for the majority, with a second smaller peak incidence in adolescence. At all ages males are more at risk. Infantile drowning mainly occurs in the bath. Outdoor pools are the major sites of accidental drowning in toddlers. Children with epilepsy are up to four times as likely to suffer a drowning incident.

Immediate and effective cardiopulmonary resuscitation (CPR) is the largest determinant of outcome. Each minute that passes prior to implementation of CPR dramatically reduces survival and long-term outcome. Of near-drowning victims with cardiac arrest who received prehospital CPR, only 7–21% will be neurologically intact. Management is supportive, with attention to lung aspiration and hypothermia. Supervision of children around water is essential. Installation of pool fencing has been shown to be effective in preventing more than 50% of swimming pool drownings among young children.

Swallowed foreign body

Preschool children commonly swallow coins, toys and stones. The majority pass without complications. However, oesophageal hold-up requires urgent endoscopy. Sharp and long objects are the most likely to cause perforation. Abdominal pain and tenderness and failure of an object to progress radiologically in 24 hours are each independent indications for evaluation/endoscopy/surgical evaluation.

Poisoning

More than 50% of all poisonings occur in children 5 years or younger. Almost all are unintentional/accidental, with intentional poisoning becoming more common in the female adolescent. More than 85% of toxic exposures in children occur in the child's home, usually during the day and more commonly during school or public holidays. Most involve only a single substance. About 60% involve non-medicinal drug products, most commonly cosmetics, cleaning substances and hydrocarbons. Pharmaceutical products comprise the remainder, with analgesics, cough products, antibiotics and vitamins being the most common. More than 75% of paediatric poisoning exposures can be treated without direct medical intervention because either the product involved is not inherently toxic or the quantity involved is not sufficient to produce significant toxic effects. Death from acute poisoning in children less than 10 years has declined dramatically in the last decade. The two most important factors have been child-resistant containers and use of safer medicines.

Management

Detailed history, if possible documenting magnitude of exposure, timing of exposure, progression of symptoms and medical history, is vital to determine risk. Consultation with a poison control centre may assist in identifying active components within a product and likely side-effects. If further management is required, it is generally divided into two parts:

- *General management.* Supportive care is given, with management of airway, breathing and circulation and avoidance of hypoglycaemia.
- *Specific management.* The American Academy of Toxicology and the European Association of Poisons Centres and Clinical Toxicologists have released statements that the routine administration of ipecac syrup or other cathartics is not endorsed. Neither do they support gastric lavage or whole-body lavage, except in extreme circumstances.

Administration of activated charcoal should be considered as soon as possible after emergency department presentation, unless the agent and quantity are known to be non-toxic, the agent is known not to adsorb to activated charcoal, or the delay has been so long that absorption is probably complete.

Antidotes are available for only a limited number of poisons. Enhancing excretion is useful for only a few toxins. Few drugs or toxins are removed by dialysis in sufficient amounts to justify the difficulties and risks of dialysis in children. Blood levels are important in the management of poisoning with paracetamol, salicylates and iron. For other intoxicants quantifying levels may help in confirming the diagnosis but will not alter treatment.

Paracetamol

Paracetamol is the most widely used childhood analgesic and antipyretic. Unintentional paracetamol overdose in children rarely causes illness or death. This may be due in part to the immature cytochrome P450 (CYP) enzyme system in children. Fasting is a risk factor, possibly because of depletion of hepatic glutathione reserves. Concomitant use of other drugs that induce CYP enzymes, such as antiepileptics (including carbamazepine, phenytoin, barbiturates etc.), has also been reported as a risk factor. The acute toxic dose in children is considered to be 200 mg/kg.

Anorexia, nausea, vomiting and diaphoresis are common in the first 24 hours. If a toxic dose was absorbed, overt hepatic failure develops over 24–48 hours, peaking at around 72–96 hours. In massive overdoses, coma and metabolic acidosis may occur prior to hepatic failure.

Damage generally occurs in hepatocytes, as they metabolize the paracetamol. However, acute renal failure may also occur. This is usually caused by either hepatorenal syndrome or multisystem organ failure. Acute renal failure may also be the primary clinical manifestation of toxicity. In these cases, it is possible that the toxic metabolite is produced more in the kidneys than in the liver. A blood level 4 hours post ingestion is taken and plotted on a nomogram to determine whether antidotal treatment is indicated. Liver function tests and prothrombin time should be followed daily in those with potentially toxic levels. After large acute overdose activated charcoal should be considered. In cases of definite toxicity N-acetylcysteine should be started as soon as possible and has benefit up to 24–36 hours after ingestion.

Tricyclic antidepressants (TCAs)

TCAs are an extremely toxic source of poisoning in young children. The lowest toxic dose in the literature is 6.7 mg/kg. Overdoses of TCAs can cause coma, seizures, hypotension, cardiac arrhythmias and cardiac arrest. Central nervous system (CNS) symptoms occur in children more frequently than do cardiovascular effects. Treatment is directed at rapid assessment, monitoring and support of vital functions, halting drug absorption, and treating CNS and cardiac toxic effects. All children should be monitored for a minimum of 6 hours and many require admission to a critical care unit. The mainstay of therapy is alkalinization. Intravenous administration of sodium bicarbonate is the preferred treatment for hypotension, shock and arrhythmias. Hypotension is a poor prognostic sign. Blood pH should be monitored and should be maintained between 7.45 and 7.55. More specific drug therapy, cardioversion or artificial pacing may be required for refractory arrhythmias. Before the child is discharged from the hospital, strategies to reduce the risk of future poisonings should be discussed with the child's family.

Smoke inhalation

Referral for assessent after smoke inhalation is common after home fires. Physical examination, looking for signs such as singed hair, facial burns and carbonaceous sputum, aids in determination of extent of exposure. If there is hoarseness, stridor, increasing respiratory distress or difficulty handling secretions, the airway should be directly visualized by bronchoscopy or laryngoscopy. Signs of impeding airway obstruction due to mucosal oedema are an indication for elective intubation. Signs of carbon monoxide poisoning include headache, confusion, irritability and visual changes. Management includes blood carboxyhaemoglobin level (HbCO), haemoglobin level, arterial pH and urinalysis for myoglobin. Treatment includes close observation and oxygen until the HbCO level falls below 5%. Hyperbaric oxygen should be considered if there is a history of coma or seizures, or persistent metabolic acidosis in the case of a pregnant woman or neonate or for an HbCO level greater than 25%.

 http://omni.ac.uk/browse/mesh/
D011042.html

European Association of Poison Centres

Sudden unexplained death in infancy (SUDI; sudden infant death syndrome, SIDS)

It is proposed to discuss ALTEs after an introduction on SUDI, despite there being no proven link between the two conditions, primarily because both are unexpected unpredictable events predominantly affecting well/healthy infants in the first 6 months of life. Both remain largely unexplained and ALTEs cause considerable parental anxiety and distress because of the frightening nature of the episode and the worry of a future SUDI occurring.

SUDI is the term used for the sudden unexpected death of a well infant occurring during the first year of life (80% during the overnight sleep), which remains unexplained after a thorough case investigation, including a complete autopsy, examination of the death scene and review of the clinical history. In developed countries SUDI is the most common cause of death after the neonatal period in children less than 1 year, with the peak incidence between 2 and 4 months of age. SUDI is an unexplained death after investigation and is a diagnosis of exclusion. It is possible that, in about 50% of cases, incomplete case/postmortem investigations have been performed and a cause of the child's death has been missed.

Epidemiological studies have identified the prone sleeping position and maternal smoking during pregnancy as increasing the risk of SUDI, and 'reduce the risk of SUDI' campaigns in most developed countries have led to a dramatic decrease in the use of the prone sleeping position and an associated reduction in SUDI incidence over the last two decades from 2 to 0.6 per

1000 live births in Ireland. This fall in SUDI rates has resulted in the number of SUDI deaths falling from about 150 to 45 per year in Ireland, with no diagnostic transfer, and the overall infant mortality rate falling by the same amount. Maternal smoking rates have declined only slightly over the past few years, leaving smoking in pregnancy as the major current SUDI risk factor in Western countries, with a clear dose–response effect evident (this includes the number of cigarettes smoked by the mother and the number of smokers in the infant's environment).

Since the recent dramatic reduction in SUDI rates other epidemiological factors increasing the risk of SUDI have been sought. Risk factors include:
- Social deprivation.
- Infant–parent cosleeping. Sharing an adult bed for the entire night is a well-recognized risk factor and sharing a sofa is especially dangerous.
- Maternal smoking (risk of cosleeping being especially pronounced in infants of smoking mothers).
- Infant soother use has recently been shown to have some protective effect if used every night.

Despite much research the underlying aetiology of SUDI remains unknown. It is known that SUDI infants are lighter, with a smaller head (brain) size, than gestational age-matched controls at birth. SUDI infants also have demonstrable histological differences, probably an in utero growth restriction effect, in many different organs from lungs, diaphragm and kidneys to decreased brain myelination and increased brainstem gliosis, especially in areas crucial to autonomic/homeostatic control. Consequently it seems likely that SUDI infants are vulnerable in situations where the brain's controlling/protective systems (autonomic system) are heavily down-regulated (as in quiet/deep sleep, which is more prevalent in the prone sleeping position or after sleep disturbance/deprivation), often with an added stress from mild intercurrent illness or environmental stress such as overheating.

In the rare cases of recurrence of SUDI in a family (6/1000 families with a previous SUDI), other genetic disorders (e.g. central hypoventilation syndrome, metabolic disorders), as well as infanticide, should be excluded.

Apparent life-threatening episodes (ALTEs) (see also p. 317)

In 1986 a National Institutes of Health (USA) consensus conference on infantile apnoea and home monitoring defined an ALTE as:

an episode that is frightening to the observer and that is characterized by some combination of apnoea (central or occasionally obstructive), colour change (usually cyanotic or pallid but occasionally erythematous or plethoric), marked change in muscle tone (usually marked limpness), choking or gagging.

Essentially, such a broad definition can include any unexpected frightening episode in an infant. Most typically, ALTE episodes occur in the first few months of life and are mostly reported during the day, as caregivers are present and the events are witnessed. Infants are usually well or only slightly unwell before and after the event.

Some babies are described as being groggy, floppy or quiet and not themselves for a few hours after the episode. The level of resuscitation required dictates the level of worry regarding the possibility of SUDI occurring in a future episode, and although the literature in this regard is conflicting and confusing, there seems to be only a slight, if any, increased risk of future SUDI in these infants. The source of this confusion is clearly shown in the data from the Irish National SUDI Register on the relationship between a prior ALTE/apnoea/lifeless episode and SUDI. The data show that apnoea/lifeless episodes were significantly more frequent among SUDI cases than among controls (12/334 (3.6%) SUDI cases vs 6/1419 (0.4%) controls OR 2.81; CI: 1.65–4.76) on univariate analysis. However, on multivariate analysis the odds ratio of 2.56 for subsequent SUDI was not significant when adjusted for maternal age, education, smoking, alcohol consumption, urinary infection during pregnancy, social deprivation, tog value of bedding, problems in the last 48 hours, absence of usual soother use, cosleeping and being placed prone in the last sleep. The validity of continuing to add in the number of variables included in a multivariate analysis until the variable ALTE becomes not significant is highly debatable. Consequently, different authors have published that there is either a slightly increased (doubling) or no increased risk of SUDI in infants who have suffered a previous ALTE, depending on what has been included in the multivariate model.

An ALTE is a common reason for admission of infants to hospital and poses a problem for paediatricians as to what constitutes an adequate diagnostic workup and also as to how these infants and their worried parents should be managed. A careful history of the event, including a detailed description of the precipitating circumstances, the infant's appearance, the amount of resuscitation employed by the caregiver and its duration, will usually provide the pointers as to what may be appropriate investigations. Awake-onset episodes, whether associated with an obvious precipitating event such as crying, vomiting or gagging, fit most neatly into the spectrum of cyanotic/pallid breath-holding or reflex anoxic seizure type of events (Ch. 24), usually attributed to immature autonomic/brainstem control. These are mostly benign, sometimes with a positive family history, and are difficult to treat effectively. The presence of anoxic seizures should be obvious from the sequence of events in the history, as reflex-induced seizures in infants are extremely rare.

Sleep-related episodes logically fit most neatly within the realm of SUDI, with down-regulated protective reflexes (arousal responses to hypoxia or nasal occlusion are much slower during sleep and worse again during deep sleep) allowing otherwise normal infants to drift into slightly dangerous situations. The frequency of poor physiological responses to noxious situations in infants can be gauged from a study of healthy 6-week old infants, conducted many years ago, where 40% were unable to establish an oral airway within 25 seconds of the onset of nasal occlusion during sleep. Given the poor/immature background physiology, it is not surprising that some infants allow themselves to drift into slightly dangerous/frightening situations and present as an ALTE.

Causes

In children with ALTEs the factors described below are often considered as a possible cause.

Gastro-oesophageal reflux (GOR)

(see also p. 178)

A recent systematic review of the causes of ALTEs in the published literature revealed a remarkable heterogeneity in the quality of the published literature and diagnostic labels attached to ALTE cases (McGovern & Smith 2004). The fact that, of an initial 2912 papers, only 8 studies involving 643 infants could be included in the systematic review speaks volumes as to the poor quality of this literature. Even among the 8 papers used in the review, the definition of ALTE varied between the studies, as did study methodology, making it difficult to draw firm conclusions. Notwithstanding these limitations, this literature review found the most common 'diagnoses' reported as 'causing' ALTEs were GOR in 227, followed by a seizure (n-83), lower respiratory tract infection (n-58) and unknown (n-169). However, it is particularly important in this situation to distinguish between the chance temporal association of two events (an ALTE and another extremely common event in infants, such as GOR) and a causal relationship.

Most infants exhibit intermittent GOR in the first few months of life, due to immaturity of the gastro-oesophageal sphincter (p. 178). Recent studies have found no evidence for acid reflux either causing or exacerbating episodes of apnoea or oxygen desaturations or ALTE or SUDI, but there is an increased incidence of respiratory problems. In addition, treating GOR has not been shown to prevent recurrences of ALTEs or apnoea. Also given that most infants occasionally reflux acid stomach contents, an infant who has a massive over-reaction to a common event implies poor central control.

Consequently there is little support in the literature for GOR as the cause of either ALTEs or SUDI, making it difficult to justify the use of diagnostic tests (none of which is either sensitive or specific) aimed at establishing the presence of GOR. Also, the use of the varied treatments employed in treating this non-condition, which is mostly a variation of normal immature physiological development, is difficult to justify. However, clinically we do occasionally see infants with severe and/or recurrent ALTEs with the most severe GOR, both probably indicating poor central controlling mechanisms, where using a thickened feed may be justified.

Seizures

Seizures are the second most frequently diagnosed 'cause' of ALTEs in the published literature, yet it is rare that an ALTE is proven to be caused by a massive synchronous cerebral electrical discharge, i.e. epilepsy. The vast majority of ALTEs attributed to a seizure are either cyanotic breath-holding or pallid syncopal episodes. Breath-holding attacks are familiar to most doctors as non-epileptic episodes occurring in some infants and young children as a consequence of either a physical or a psychological hurt (Ch. 24). Diagnosis is usually not difficult when a detailed history of the sequence of events, with a clear triggering event, is available. The sequence of events involves either crying or breath-holding that raises intrathoracic pressure (a Valsalva manoeuvre) sufficiently to disrupt venous return and consequent cardiac output, resulting in cerebral ischaemia, loss of consciousness and sometimes a brief hypoxic seizure. Epilepsy in the first 6 months of life is rare and occurs in the presence of major underlying brain problems, as seen in severe birth asphyxia or infantile spasms with hypsarrhythmia. The stark normality of ALTE infants, once recovered from the event, excludes such a possibility.

Pallid syncopal episodes, by contrast, are due to periods of asystole induced by a mildly unpleasant experience such as being placed in a bath. Such infants have been shown to develop periods of asystole of up to 32 seconds (normal is < 2 seconds) following vagal stimulation by eyeball compression. Pallid syncopal attacks tend to feature extreme pallor, total limpness, the appearance of death and perhaps a cold sweat with a rapid return to normality, presumably once the heart restarts and a circulation is restored. Again, a brief tonic–clonic seizure, secondary to cerebral ischaemia and not underlying epilepsy, is not unusual. Diagnosis of these conditions is largely by history, management is by parental reassurance as to the benign nature of the episodes, and treatment (with atropine) highly specialized and not to be undertaken by the enthusiastic amateur.

Respiratory infections

Respiratory tract infections are the third most common 'cause' of ALTEs in the published literature. The literature clearly supports the concept of infants having 'funny' episodes while incubating an infectious disease such as whooping cough or bronchiolitis, often before other overt signs of infection. Consequently the presence of an evolving infection must always be considered. Infants who are incubating an infection have been demonstrated to be physiologically different, not showing the normal sleep-induced fall in core body temperature, for example, for several days before overtly becoming infected.

However, a major problem with this literature is the tendency to diagnose a respiratory infection based on the presence of snuffles, mucousy noisy breathing or a wheeze, all of which are extremely common in the healthy infant population and are usually not due to an infection. Unfortunately there are no case control studies showing infections (respiratory or otherwise) to be more common in ALTE infants than in carefully matched controls; consequently we have to rely on an anecdotal literature of case reports.

Other causes

Rarer causes of ALTEs, mostly single case reports, include metabolic or developmental problems, cardiac conduction defects or upper airway obstruction during sleep. Again a careful history of the event, a detailed family history and a history of the infant's preceding health and development will usually give clues to an underlying problem requiring investigation. In recurring ALTEs (10% of the total) inflicted or fabricated episodes pose a diagnostic and management dilemma, often with parents demanding ever more extensive investigations for an infant in rude good health (Chs 21 and 37).

Management

Management of ALTEs is made difficult by the poor-quality conflicting literature and often by the huge parental anxiety engendered by the witnessing of the apparent near-death of their infant. Understandably, if a healthy infant nearly dies, with no apparent cause, then parents feel their babies are at a greater risk of SUDI than if this episode had not happened. However, the literature would say that the subsequent risk of SUDI is at most 2–3 times higher than the baseline SUDI risk. It is important to translate this into an actual risk for parents; in non-smoking Caucasian non-socially deprived families the baseline SUDI risk is about 1/8000, so doubling or trebling this is still a very low risk situation. Obviously for smoking parents the baseline SUDI risk ranges from 1/980 (smoker) to 1/400 (most socially disadvantaged and a smoker).

Parents should be reassured that these events are mostly the result of poor/immature physiology, with infants maturing out of the danger of recurrence in a matter of months. As a rough guide, 50% of ALTE infants will have a second episode, with 10% having recurring episodes. Also the fact that very few SUDI cases have a prior warning event (3.6%) and that the actual risk of SUDI is still very low should help parents cope. Emphasizing the known risk reduction measures for SUDI also helps, as does the fact that the baby has essentially survived the first episode and is inherently likely to survive a second, should one occur. Unfortunately the literature on physiological testing/sleep studies in ALTE infants generally supports the concept of immature underlying (especially sleep) physiology, without suggesting any way of influencing this or predicting recurrent episodes.

Paediatricians generally take a pragmatic approach to the use of cardiorespiratory monitors at home in ALTE infants, despite there being evidence that their use does not prevent the rare subsequent occurrence of SUDI. Monitors used in the home tend to give frequent false alarms and generate considerable parental anxiety and stress. However, if parents are already very distressed by the ALTE — for example, if they are taking turns to stay awake at night to watch the baby — then the use of a monitor can help them to cope better. Easy access to the unit issuing the monitor is essential if there are any issues or worries, and this is a service parents value and rarely overuse. All parents should be taught basic resuscitation, whilst being reminded that whatever they did the first time worked and would probably do so again. Medication use for documented apnoea, including caffeine or aminophylline, has no evidence base and generally medicalizes and complicates the management without any proven benefit; it is best avoided. The use of 'sleep studies' is properly an area for research investigation and generally adds little to the diagnosis or management of the infant.

Reference

McGovern MC, Smith MBH 2004 Causes of apparent life-threatening events in infants: a systematic review. Archives of Disease in Childhood 89:1043–1048

Further reading

Carpenter RG, Irgens LM, Blair PS et al. 2004 Sudden unexplained infant death in twenty regions in Europe: case control study. Lancet 363:185–191

Committee on Injury, American Academic of Pediatrics 2005 Poison treatment in the home. Pediatrics 112:1182–1185

Matthews T 1992 The autonomic nervous system — a role in sudden infant death syndrome. Archives of Disease in Childhood 67:654–656

National Institutes of Health 1987 Consensus development conference on infantile apnoea and home monitoring. Pediatrics 79:292–299

James C. Nicholson   Matthew Murray

Oncology and palliative care

LEARNING OUTCOMES

By the end of this chapter you should:

● Have an understanding of the aetiology and epidemiology of childhood cancer
● Have the knowledge to assess a patient presenting with a malignancy
● Be able to select appropriate investigations for such a patient
● Be able to recognize and institute initial management of common complications of cancer patients
● Understand the principles of different modalities used to treat cancer
● Be aware of the short- and long-term side-effects of chemotherapy and radiotherapy
● Be aware of the indications for stem cell or bone marrow transplantation
● Appreciate the issues involved in the care of a child with a life-limiting illness, including symptom control
● Understand the concept of the paediatric oncology multidisciplinary team.

You should also take this opportunity to ensure that:

● Your history from, and examination of, the patient enable you to make an accurate assessment/differential diagnosis
● You can interpret the results of a full blood count and peripheral film
● You can interpret electrolyte disturbances secondary to tumour lysis syndrome.

Aetiology and epidemiology of childhood cancer

Childhood cancer is rare and accounts for only 0.5% of all cancers. The overall risk of developing cancer in childhood is 1 in 600 and there are 1500 new cases of childhood cancer in the UK each year, with a slight preponderance of males.

Malignancy is the most common cause of death in children in the 5–14-year age group and is second only to trauma and accidents between 15 and 19 years (Table 51.1).

Very little is known about the aetiology of most childhood cancers. Inherited predisposition accounts for less than 5% of cases and environmental factors play a minor role compared with adults. Examples

Table 51.1 **Most common causes of death by age** (England and Wales 2002)

Age (years)	Cause of death
< 1	Congenital abnormalities
	Sudden unexplained death in infancy (SUDI; sudden infant death syndrome, SIDS)
	Infection
1–4	Congenital
	Trauma/accidents
	Cancer
5–14	Cancer
	Trauma/accidents
	Congenital
15–19	Trauma/accidents
	Cancer
	Congenital

of inherited syndromes with a predisposition for cancer include familial Wilms' tumour, Beckwith–Wiedemann (10% develop tumours, of which Wilms' is most common) and neurofibromatosis-1 (NF-1, 40-fold greater risk of brain and spinal cord tumours than the general population).

Inherited predisposition to childhood cancer

Retinoblastoma is the most common example and provides a suitable model for understanding the principles of inherited predisposition, having been linked to a single gene locus. Familial retinoblastoma accounts for approximately 40% of cases and presentation is usually early (first year of life) and bilateral. Sporadic cases present later, are unilateral and are not associated with a positive family history. Survivors of familial retinoblastoma have a very high risk of developing second primary tumours, of which osteosarcoma is the most common.

These features of retinoblastoma were noted by Knudson and led him to propose the 'two-hit' mutational hypothesis in 1971. This states that two mutations are necessary in a cell for a tumour to develop. In hereditary cases the first mutation is germline, while the second is somatic. In sporadic cases two somatic mutations are required in the same cell for a tumour to develop.

Knudson's hypothesis was confirmed in the 1980s with the identification of the retinoblastoma tumour suppressor gene (*RB1*) on chromosome 13. Retinoblastoma results as a consequence of two mutations in the *RB1* gene within the somatic cells of the retina.

In comparison to retinoblastoma, familial clusters of other embryonal tumours are rare. For example, in Wilms' tumour, inherited cases are thought to represent only 1% of all cases. Beckwith–Wiedemann is the most common syndrome associated with Wilms'. Organomegaly, macroglossia, hemihypertophy, neonatal hypoglycaemia and exomphalos are all features of

this fetal overgrowth syndrome. Around 10% of cases develop tumours, of which Wilms' is the most common, and imprinting has been implicated as a causative mechanism. Patients with some forms of syndromes involving aniridia, genital abnormalities, nephritis and pseudohermaphroditism have up to a 50% risk of developing Wilms' tumour due to gene alterations.

NF-1 is inherited as an autosomal dominant condition, although many cases are new mutations. NF-1 is associated with a risk of brain and spinal cord tumours 40-fold greater than the general population and accounts for about 0.5% of all childhood cancers. Low-grade optic nerve gliomas are the most common brain tumours seen, with a 1000-fold increased risk.

Molecular mechanisms for the development of malignancies

Molecular mechanisms for the development of malignancies all relate to the alteration in structure or activity of genes that perform important regulatory functions of growth or differentiation of cells in the normal state. These may include:

- Mutation or deletion of a tumour suppressor gene. These genes code for proteins that have negative regulatory roles in the cell cycle. Complete loss of protein function is required to initiate the tumorigenic process and hence requires loss of both genomic copies.
- Activation of a 'proto-oncogene', which then becomes an oncogene, i.e. a tumour-promoting gene. This may occur through mutation or amplification.
- Translocation of a gene to a different locus may result in over-expression, as a result of juxtaposition with a 'promoter' region, or fusion with another gene that creates an oncogenic 'fusion product'.

Subsequent tumorigenesis is a multistep process involving the development of immortalization of cells, growth factor autonomy, inhibition of cell death pathways/apoptosis (programmed cell death), angiogenesis and the ability to invade local tissues/metastasize.

Tumour-specific acquired chromosomal abnormalities are seen in a wide range of solid and haematological malignancies. Whilst some of these appear to be random, others conform to recognized patterns with diagnostic or prognostic significance. The translocation t(9;22), resulting in the Philadelphia chromosome, was the first consistent cytogenetic abnormality to be described, occurring in chronic myeloid leukaemia (CML) and in some high-risk cases of acute lymphoblastic leukaemia (ALL).

Types of malignancy

The most common childhood malignancy is leukaemia, accounting for one-third of cases, followed by brain

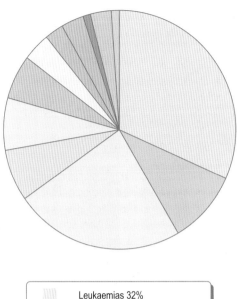

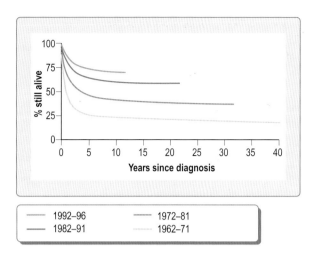

Fig. 51.2 **Survival of childhood cancer patients diagnosed in the UK from 1962 to 1996**
(Cancer Research UK 2004)

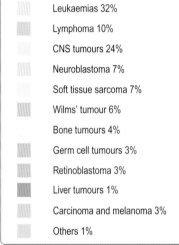

Leukaemias 32%

Lymphoma 10%

CNS tumours 24%

Neuroblastoma 7%

Soft tissue sarcoma 7%

Wilms' tumour 6%

Bone tumours 4%

Germ cell tumours 3%

Retinoblastoma 3%

Liver tumours 1%

Carcinoma and melanoma 3%

Others 1%

Fig. 51.1 **Percentage of cases by diagnostic group, ages 0–14 years, Great Britain 1989–98**
(Cancer Research UK 2004)

and spinal tumours, which constitute one-quarter of cases (Fig. 51.1). All the other solid tumours account for 45% of cases, of which lymphoma, neuroblastoma, rhabdomyosarcoma and Wilms' tumour are the most common extracranial solid tumours.

Principles of cancer therapy

Entry into trials and centralized treatment has been shown to be of direct benefit to patients. In the UK, most children are now treated on national or international studies, coordinated by the Children's Cancer and Leukaemia Group (CCLG) which was previously known as the UKCCSG and has close links with the International Society of Paediatric Oncology (SIOP).

 http://www.siop.nl

International Society of Paediatric Oncology

 http://www.ukccsg.org

Association for Children with Life-Threatening or Terminal Conditions (ACT)

Therapeutic strategies for childhood malignancies include chemotherapy, radiotherapy and surgery, alone or in combination. Chemotherapy forms the core of treatment for the majority and care is therefore usually coordinated by paediatric oncologists, working in designated centres. Geographical considerations dictate the provision of some treatment, including much of the supportive care, in local hospitals, and this 'shared care' is highly developed in parts of the UK.

A multidisciplinary team approach is central to management and should include paediatric oncologists, haematologists, surgeons, neurosurgeons, radiation oncologists, specialist nurses for inpatient and outpatient care, outreach nurses, dieticians, play therapists, social workers, teachers and psychologists.

Prognosis

Overall cure rates for childhood cancer now exceed 70% in the developed world (Fig. 51.2). There is a wide variation between different tumour types. For example, localized Hodgkin's disease is cured in well over 90% of cases, compared with around 20% in disseminated neuroblastoma. The current challenge facing oncologists is to develop and employ treatment strategies that minimize long-term side-effects of treatment without compromising cure.

Chemotherapy

Chemotherapy is the mainstay of treatment for most types of paediatric malignancy. Many cancers present as localized tumour masses, but previous experience has shown that local treatment with surgery and/or

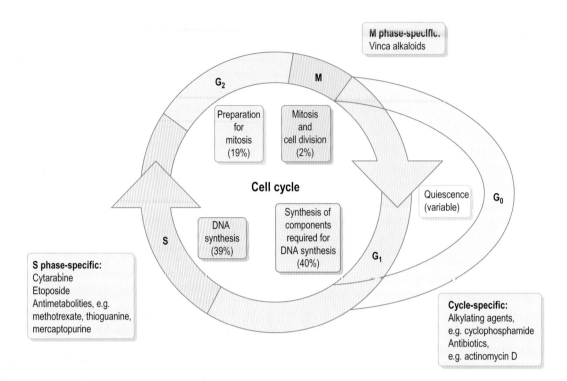

Fig. 51.3 Schematic representation of the normal cell cycle and action of chemotherapeutic agents

radiotherapy alone is insufficient for cure and may result in later recurrences at distant sites. For this reason, most patients receive systemic treatment with chemotherapy as well as local therapy. This has resulted in a dramatic improvement in overall cure rates in the last 20–30 years.

Chemotherapy may be given as adjuvant treatment (following surgery), neoadjuvant treatment (before surgery) or both. Combination therapy is usually employed to increase efficacy, reduce development of resistance and limit single-organ toxicity. In order to act as effective chemotherapeutic agents, drugs must either block cell replication or induce cell death.

The cell cycle itself is divided into four active phases — G_1, S, G_2 and M — and a resting phase, G_0 (Fig. 51.3). After cell division, cells enter G_1 or 'gap' phase and then synthesize DNA (S phase) before a second gap phase, G_2. Cells subsequently enter M phase, where mitosis occurs, resulting in cell division.

In aggressive tumours, many cells are actively undergoing mitosis, giving rise to a high 'mitotic index' when sections of these tumours are examined under the microscope. These tumours are more likely to respond to chemotherapy than slow-growing, indolent tumours with a low mitotic index in which a large proportion of cells are in the G_0 resting phase.

Almost all current agents employed interfere with cell division indirectly by:
- Damaging DNA
- Blocking DNA synthesis

- Interfering with DNA processing
- Disrupting mitosis.

The selectivity of cytotoxic drugs is dependent upon the fact that in malignancy a higher proportion of cells are undergoing division than in normal tissues. However, the difference between an effective treatment dose and a toxic one (the therapeutic index) is often quite small. Agents may be phase-specific (work at a particular phase of the cell cycle) or work through all phases (cycle-specific) (Fig. 51.3).

Most common short-term side-effects include vomiting, myelosuppression, alopecia and mucositis. Long-term effects on organ function (kidneys, gonads, hearing and heart) are variable (Box 51.1). Side-effects differ depending on the agents employed; examples of these are given below.

Administration of chemotherapy

Chemotherapy should only be given by fully trained individuals, aware of potential risks and complications, and working in centres fully equipped and accredited to support chemotherapy administration. Dosage is usually calculated according to surface area. Most chemotherapy is administered intravenously; central venous access is preferred. The risk of extravasation from peripheral veins is greatest with vinca alkaloids and anthracyclines. A number of agents are given orally as liquids or tablets, such as steroids, methotrexate and mercaptopurine in the 'maintenance' phase of leukaemia

Short-term

- Nausea and vomiting
- Alopecia
- Myelosuppression
- Mucositis, diarrhoea
- Hepatitis
- Haemorrhagic cystitis
- Nephrotoxicity/renal tubular leak
- Encephalopathy
- Radiation recall

Long-term

- Cardiotoxicity
- Pulmonary fibrosis
- Nephrotoxicity/renal tubular leak
- Infertility
- Hearing loss
- Secondary malignancy

treatment. Certain drugs (e.g. ifosfamide, cisplatin and methotrexate) are given with concomitant intravenous fluids to minimize potential toxicity. Mesna is given with cyclophosphamide and ifosfamide to protect the bladder from haemorrhagic cystitis, and folinic acid 'rescue' is given with high-dose methotrexate; folinic acid is selectively taken up by normal cells and helps to minimize mucositis and other side-effects. The benefit of cardioprotective agents (given with anthracyclines) remains unproven.

Intrathecal chemotherapy

Intrathecal methotrexate (i.t. MTX) is used for treatment or prophylaxis of central nervous system (CNS) disease in leukaemia and non-Hodgkin's lymphoma (NHL). Safety of arrangements for administration of intrathecal chemotherapy is paramount because of the catastrophic consequence of intrathecal administration of vincristine, which results in coma and death. Department of Health guidelines now state that administration of i.t. methotrexate and i.v. vincristine must take place in separate clinical areas and at different times. Doctors must be trained, be on the intrathecal register and be of registrar level or above. Some pharmacies will not dispense vincristine unless they witness a signed drug chart demonstrating that methotrexate has been given, and vice versa. *Vincristine should never be given intrathecally.*

Monitoring for toxicity depends on the agents used and may include the following during or between courses:

- Full blood count (FBC)
- Electrolytes and liver function
- Glomerular filtration rate (GFR) measurement
- Hearing tests
- Echocardiogram.

High-dose (HD) therapy and stem cell transplant

This involves 'conditioning', which is the delivery of myelo-ablative doses of chemotherapy and/or total body irradiation to the patient. This is followed by rescue with haemopoietic stem cells, which may be autologous, derived from the patient him- or herself, or allogeneic, for which the donor may be a sibling, matched unrelated donor or occasionally haplo-identical from a parent.

Conventional bone marrow transplant (BMT), in which stem cells are harvested directly from the bone marrow, is usually used for allografts. Peripheral blood stem cell transplants (PBSCT) are favoured for autografts. Stem cells are harvested by leucopheresis from peripheral blood using granulocyte colony stimulating factor (G-CSF) to mobilize them from the bone marrow after priming with chemotherapy. After high-dose chemotherapy, these pluripotential stem cells from BMT or PBSCT are reinfused intravenously and subsequently repopulate the marrow. Advantages of PBSCT include less risk of tumour contamination from marrow affected by disease, more rapid engraftment (usually 2–4 weeks), less severe infections and avoidance of anaesthetic for harvesting.

Indications for use in childhood malignancy include selected high-risk and relapsed leukaemias (allograft), high-risk solid tumours, including metastatic neuroblastoma, high-risk Ewing's sarcoma and relapsed tumours (autologous). The patient should be in remission prior to the procedure for it to be effective.

Causes of morbidity and mortality from stem cell transplant include graft failure, infection secondary to profound immune suppression, mucositis and veno-occlusive disease of the liver. Allografts carry greater risk, with approximately 10% procedure-related mortality. Graft versus host disease (GvHD) is a particular risk; it may affect any organ system but commonly skin and gastrointestinal system are involved. Ciclosporin A is given as prophylaxis and steroids may also be employed in treatment.

Radiotherapy

Radiotherapy is the clinical use of ionizing radiation to kill cancer cells. Dose and fractionation (number of treatments to deliver a total dose) vary according to the nature of the tumour and tolerance of the surrounding tissues. The target volume is determined by size and type of tumour and includes a safety margin. The aim is to deliver effective treatment to the target volume whilst sparing surrounding tissues.

Indications

Radiotherapy is indicated in selected cases of Hodgkin's disease, neuroblastoma, Wilms' tumour, soft tissue and Ewing's sarcomas and most subgroups of CNS tumours.

Studies have shown only limited benefit in osteosarcoma, extracranial germ cell tumours and NHL. In leukaemia, radiotherapy is limited to treatment of the CNS, to testicular disease and to conditioning for BMT (total body irradiation, TBI). Radiotherapy is also used for symptom control in palliative care, e.g. bony metastases, spinal cord compression.

Preparation for radiotherapy includes:

- Planning, by combination of computed tomography (CT) and magnetic resonance imaging (MRI)
- Immobilization using masks/shells, tattoos as markers, sedation or general anaesthesia for youngest children
- Protection of surrounding tissues (e.g. gonads) using lead shields
- Involvement of play therapists, who have a central role in this process.

Side-effects

Toxicity of radiotherapy is potentiated by certain chemotherapy agents, e.g. actinomycin D or anthracyclines. This may give rise to the phenomenon of 'radiation recall' when these drugs are used after radiotherapy, causing further damage to the organ/tissues. Side-effects can be classified as acute or late and depend on the dose and site to which radiotherapy is given, as well as the age of the patient at the time of radiotherapy (Box 51.2). Late effects of chemotherapy may occur months or even years after treatment, and are usually progressive and irreversible.

Surgery

Surgical interventions for solid tumours

- *Biopsy only*. Chemotherapy and/or radiotherapy may be curative without further surgery, e.g. Hodgkin's disease, NHL, rhabdomyosarcoma, germ cell tumours.
- *Resection, primary or following chemotherapy*. Completeness of excision influences subsequent need for adjunctive treatment (radiotherapy or chemotherapy), e.g. bone tumours, Wilms' tumour, hepatoblastoma and most CNS tumours.

BOX 51.2 Common side-effects of radiotherapy

Acute
- Nausea and vomiting
- Cutaneous erythema/desquamation
- Diarrhoea
- Myelosuppression
- Pneumonitis
- Hepatitis

Late
- Cardiotoxicity
- Lung dysfunction
- Renal dysfunction
- Musculoskeletal hypoplasia/asymmetry
- Hypothyroidism
- Spinal growth
- Hypopituitarism
- Neuropsychological sequelae
- Cataracts
- Infertility
- Second primary tumours (~5%)

Supportive and emergency care

- Management of the acute abdomen in neutropenic patients (patients may develop neutropenic colitis, also known as typhlitis).
- Raised intracranial pressure (ICP) and spinal cord compression (urgent referral to neurosurgical centre).
- Most children receiving chemotherapy will require a tunnelled central venous line: either a 'Hickman' line or a 'Portacath'.

Problem-orientated topic:

neck mass

Jodie, an 11-year-old girl, presents with a painless lump in the right side of her neck which was noticed 4 months ago. She has had two courses of antibiotics with no benefit. The lump was approximately the size of a broad bean when first noticed but has enlarged steadily, and a similar lump has appeared over the last 2 weeks on the left side. Jodie has lost a little weight over the last few weeks but has had no other constitutional symptoms. Examination reveals a firm, non-tender mass measuring 4 cm by 3 cm in the right anterior cervical triangle and a 2 cm lump in a similar position on the left side. Although she appears thin, there are no other positive findings on general examination.

Q1. What are the features pointing to a diagnosis of malignancy?

Q2. What other information from the history and examination would help in the differential diagnosis?

Q3. What is the differential diagnosis?

Q4. How should Jodie be managed?

Q1. What are the features pointing to a diagnosis of malignancy?

Enlarged cervical nodes in children are very common; the differential diagnosis is wide and malignancies account for only a very small fraction of cases. However, delay in diagnosis may have serious adverse consequences, in terms of extent of disease, intensity of treatment required and ultimate prognosis, so it is important to investigate cases thoroughly if there are features suggesting the possibility of malignancy.

Suspicious features in this case are:
- Absence of symptoms or signs of infection to account for lymphadenopathy
- Weight loss
- Size and characteristics of nodes. Nodes > 2 cm in diameter are a cause for concern and warrant consideration for biopsy. This patient has nodes that are significantly bigger than this and are progressively enlarging. Although they are not described as fixed or rubbery, terms particularly associated with malignancy, they are firm and non-tender, both features consistent with a diagnosis of malignancy.

Q2. What other information from the history and examination would help in the differential diagnosis?

Age
Of the malignant causes, Hodgkin's disease is more likely in older children, rarely occurring before the age of 5, whereas NHL and ALL are more likely to be seen in younger children. Disseminated neuroblastoma is unusual in children over 5 years old.

Systemic symptoms
These may help point towards the cause, whether infective or malignant. In particular, weight loss is a common finding in children with cancer and, when combined with fever and night sweats, is particularly associated with Hodgkin's disease (B symptoms).

Rate of progression
A timescale of days to weeks is more suggestive of NHL or ALL, whilst Hodgkin's disease tends to progress more slowly and the history may span many months.

Characteristics of nodes
In addition to size and presence or absence of tenderness, texture (firm, hard, craggy, rubbery, soft, fluctuant) and mobility (fixed, tethered, mobile) may be helpful.

Systemic examination
This may reveal evidence of a primary tumour or of pallor, bruising and/or petechiae, suggestive of pancytopenia. A child with advanced disease may look pale and non-specifically unwell. Presence of other palpable lymph nodes at all other stations and hepatosplenomegaly should be commented on. Supraclavicular or axillary lymphadenopathy is more likely to reflect an underlying malignant process.

Q3. What is the differential diagnosis?

Hodgkin's disease and NHL may both present with cervical lymphadenopathy, as may ALL. Distant spread from other solid malignancies is less common but neuroblastoma should be considered and rhabdomyosarcoma and nasopharyngeal carcinoma are also recognized causes in childhood. Hodgkin's disease is the most likely, given the age of the patient, the relatively slow progression and the lack of systemic disturbance that would be seen commonly with ALL or NHL.

Other possibilities to consider include bacterial infection, viral infection including cat scratch fever, toxoplasmosis, and rarely connective tissue disorders or Kawasaki disease. Atypical mycobacteria may produce large nodes in an otherwise well child that may be difficult to differentiate and will need (complete) excision biopsy (both to treat effectively and to exclude malignancy).

Q4. How should Jodie be managed?

Initial investigations
These should look for evidence of mediastinal and intra-abdominal pathology, and exclude other causes of lymphadenopathy:
- Chest X-ray (CXR)
- Abdominal ultrasound
- Full blood count and film: not very discriminating diagnostically, but if pancytopenia is present, this points to bone marrow involvement as part of a malignant process
- Viral serology.

Biopsy

This should be arranged without waiting for all the results of other investigations in this patient, because of the size of the nodes. It should be an excision biopsy to maximize the yield of diagnostic material and minimize the need for second-look surgery in the case of atypical mycobacterial infection. If the history were of lymph nodes that were more borderline in size (e.g. 1.5–2 cm) and the above investigations did not suggest malignancy, it would be reasonable to observe for 4–6 weeks and then proceed to biopsy if there had been no reduction.

Staging investigations

Further management, if malignancy is confirmed or considered highly likely, may include the following staging investigations:

- Bone marrow examination (aspirate and trephine)
- Lumbar puncture (if ALL or NHL)
- CT or MRI scan of chest and abdomen (not needed if ALL confirmed)
- Isotope scans (technetium or mIBG, meta-iodobenzylguanidine imaging), according to primary diagnosis
- Baseline fluorodeoxyglucose positron emission tomography (FDG-PET) scans may become routine, particularly for Hodgkin's disease.

Baseline investigations and procedures

Baseline investigations and procedures prior to starting treatment, related to recognized toxicities of chemotherapy, varying according to diagnosis and regimen employed. They may include:

- Echocardiogram
- Lung function tests
- GFR or creatinine clearance
- Audiometry
- Sperm cryopreservation.

Problem-orientated topic:

respiratory compromise

Naseem, a 9-year-old boy, has experienced episodes of wheezing for 3 weeks, steadily increasing in frequency and severity. He is now unable to sleep lying horizontally. He has been previously well with no hospital admissions, no history of asthma and no family history of atopy. His GP has given him a trial of inhaled bronchodilators but these seem to have made little difference. On examination, he is a little pale with obvious dyspnoea, recession, marked expiratory wheeze throughout the chest and some small 'shotty' cervical lymph nodes, none more than 0.5 cm in diameter.

Q1. Why should this not be treated as asthma without further investigation?

Q2. What is the differential diagnosis?

Q3. What investigations should be performed?

Q4. What is your initial management of Naseem?

Q1. Why should this not be treated as asthma without further investigation?

Any child presenting for the first time with wheeze, severe enough to need more than simple bronchodilators, warrants further investigation with a CXR, before being treated as asthmatic. Similarly, any marked change in pattern of wheeze in a known asthmatic should be investigated. Children with a mediastinal mass presenting with wheeze may have clinical signs that are atypical for asthma but this is not always so. These include evidence of compression of the superior vena cava (p. 415), protuberance of the chest wall secondary to the tumour mass, unilateral wheeze, effusion, pallor and petechiae. A trial of steroids for a presumptive diagnosis of asthma could be catastrophic in the event of malignancy, particularly lymphoblastic lymphoma or leukaemia (NHL or ALL), as life-threatening tumour lysis could be precipitated. Partial treatment of these conditions can also delay or prevent accurate diagnosis, and may impart a worse prognosis.

In this case, the history alone should raise suspicions. This boy has experienced rapid progression of his airway obstruction with poor response to bronchodilators, without a previous history of asthma. The presence of small lymph nodes (< 0.5 cm) is not in itself particularly helpful as they are extremely common in children and rarely significant.

Q2. What is the differential diagnosis?

Causes of mediastinal masses in children are shown in Table 51.2. In this case, the most likely cause is T cell NHL or ALL, based on the short history. Given this history, non-malignant causes are unlikely. Foreign body inhalation could present in this way, although the history would generally be much shorter — minutes or hours rather than days or weeks. Structural abnormalities are likely to have presented in infancy rather than this late in childhood. Heart failure may present in this way, after a viral illness causing a cardiomyopathy, but would be extremely rare.

Table 51.2 Differential diagnosis of mediastinal mass in childhood

	Anterior mediastinal	Posterior mediastinal
Malignant	T-cell NHL* ALL* Hodgkin's disease* Malignant germ cell tumour Rhabdomyosarcoma Ewing's sarcoma	Neuroblastoma* Ganglioneuroblastoma Sarcoma Phaeochromocytoma
Benign	Teratoma Cystic hygroma Haemangioma Thymic cyst	Ganglioneuroma Schwann cell tumour Neurofibroma Bronchogenic cyst

* Most common malignant causes of mediastinal mass. (NHL = non-Hodgkin's lymphoma; ALL = acute lymphoblastic leukaemia)

Q3. What investigations should be performed?

- CXR (preferably posterior–anterior and lateral) will be enough to demonstrate the presence of a mass causing these symptoms, together with any associated effusion.
- CT scan of chest and abdomen for staging may also provide useful additional information regarding compression of the airway if a general anaesthetic is being considered for subsequent procedures.
- Definitive 'tissue' diagnosis from one of the following:
  - FBC and film (may be sufficient if T cell ALL with high white cell count)
  - Bone marrow aspirate
  - Lumbar puncture (rarely positive but should be performed if possible)
  - Pleural tap
  - Biopsy of lymph node mass: via thoracotomy or mediastinoscopy if there are no significant peripheral lymph nodes
  - Serum tumour marker: α-fetoprotein (AFP) and human chorionic gonadotrophin (hCG) may be elevated in germ cell tumours, which arise in the midline and may rarely occur in the mediastinum.

If one of the above investigations provides the definitive diagnosis, then there will be no need to perform all of the others, the aim being to avoid the most invasive investigations.

Q4. What is your initial management of Naseem?

The child should be nursed on a high-dependency unit. He may well need elective intubation and mechanical ventilation to protect the airway, with transfer to an intensive care unit. Good intravenous access should be secured, ideally centrally, such as via a femoral line.

The order of further investigations and management will be dictated by the condition of the child, who may be at risk of severe acute respiratory failure. Caution should be exercised in laying any such child flat in a scanner without full anaesthetic support present. Avoid any sedation for scans in such children, as this may result in loss of airway tone and subsequent respiratory arrest.

The aim should be to obtain definitive diagnostic material and proceed swiftly to definitive treatment. However, in the event that open procedures or general anaesthetic are considered too hazardous, treatment with chemotherapy may have to commence without tissue diagnosis.

Commencing chemotherapy

If ALL or NHL is confirmed, then treatment with oral steroids (prednisolone or dexamethasone), with or without vincristine, may be sufficient as initial treatment in the sickest cases. Hyperhydration should accompany treatment, together with allopurinol or urate oxidase to minimize the risk of severe tumour lysis syndrome (p. 414).

Monitoring

The response to chemotherapy may be dramatic in T-cell lymphoblastic disease and the attendant risk of tumour lysis high. Renal function and electrolytes should be monitored 4–6-hourly initially, and monitoring should include assessment of calcium, phosphate and uric acid. Alkalinization of urine to help clear urate should not be necessary with the availability of urate oxidase and may exacerbate hyperphosphataemia.

Problem-orientated topic:

abdominal mass

A 2-year-old boy, John, attends the GP's surgery with his mother after she notices whilst bathing him that his abdomen appears distended. On reflection she admits that it may have been distended for 2 weeks but has become more obvious in the last 3 days. There is no other history of note.

Examination reveals a large firm mass in the right side of the abdomen. Blood pressure is 145/85 mmHg. Urinalysis reveals moderate protein only.

Q1. What are the two most likely diagnoses?

Continued overleaf

Q2. What else should you look for in your clinical evaluation?

Q3. What further investigations are warranted and why?

Q1. What are the two most likely diagnoses?

The two most likely diagnoses are right-sided Wilms' tumour (nephroblastoma) and neuroblastoma. These tumours account for 6% and 7% of total paediatric malignancies respectively. The incidental finding of an abdominal mass without other symptoms makes a Wilms' tumour the most likely diagnosis. The presence of significant hypertension can occur in both Wilms' tumour and neuroblastoma but is very rare in any other abdominal tumour.

The tumour may be difficult to differentiate from hepatomegaly or a liver mass such as hepatoblastoma, although it should be possible on examination to palpate above a Wilms' tumour or neuroblastoma. In addition primary liver tumours in paediatrics are very rare. Other rare causes of a malignant abdominal mass include B cell lymphoma and rhabdomyosarcoma, although the latter usually arises from within the pelvis.

Q2. What else should you look for in your clinical evaluation?

Wilms' tumour is associated with a number of syndromes. The presence or absence of clinical signs of these syndromes should be documented: for example, hemihypertrophy, Beckwith–Wiedemann (macroglossia, umbilical defects, horizontal earlobe crease), WAGR (aniridia, Wilms', microcephaly, cryptorchidism).

In addition, evidence of metastatic disease should be sought. Most Wilms' tumours present as localized disease. The most common site for metastases in Wilms' is the lungs but this is usually asymptomatic. However, most children with neuroblastoma present with advanced disease, and symptoms and signs often come from sites of metastasis, e.g. 'panda' eyes due to periorbital infiltration, or from constitutional symptoms associated with advanced disease such as cachexia and generalized wasting.

Q3. What further investigations are warranted and why?

- *Urine catecholamines* (homovanillic acid, HVA, and vanillylmandelic acid, VMA): elevated in neuroblastoma. A single spot sample is sufficient, as levels are expressed as ratios with creatinine.
- *Ultrasound* of the abdomen: to confirm renal or adrenal mass. Calcification is strongly suggestive of neuroblastoma.
- *CXR*: staging for Wilms'.
- *CT chest and abdomen*: further staging may demonstrate intra-abdominal lymphadenopathy more clearly than ultrasound.
- *ECG/echocardiogram*: patient is hypertensive and therefore evidence of heart strain should be sought. It is important to perform baseline investigations, as chemotherapy may include cardiotoxic agents.
- *Blood tests*, including FBC, clotting, urea and electrolytes, liver function tests, ferritin, lactate dehydrogenase (LDH) and neuron-specific enolase (NSE): NSE and ferritin are tumour markers for neuroblastoma.
- *Biopsy* to establish definitive diagnosis: ultrasound/CT-guided needle biopsy or open procedure.
- *Further staging*: may be required, depending on the results of other investigations, e.g. bone scan and bone marrow aspirates/trephines in neuroblastoma.

Problem-orientated topic:

limb swelling

Anna, a 14-year-old girl, has a 4-month history of pain in her right lower leg. The pain can wake her at night. Over the last month she has noticed a swelling over her right shin. She is a keen gymnast and her parents have attributed her symptoms to 'growing pains', although they note she had a fall from parallel bars 6 months previously.

On examination, she appears well. There is a tender smooth 12 × 8 cm swelling over the medial aspect of the upper third of the right tibia. The rest of the examination is unremarkable.

Q1. What is the most likely diagnosis? What benign condition may this be confused with?

Q2. What would you expect to see on plain X-ray?

Q3. What other investigations would you perform?

Q1. What is the most likely diagnosis? What benign condition may this be confused with?

Osteosarcoma is most likely. Bone tumours account for 4% of all paediatric malignancies, of which osteosarcoma and Ewing's sarcoma account for more than 90%. Both have a peak incidence at 12–14 years of age, classically presenting with pain and subsequent swelling over the affected area. Over 90% of osteosarcomas are located in the metaphysis (growth plate) of bone. Around 80% occur in the bones around the knee (i.e. distal femur, proximal tibia or fibula). In contrast, most Ewing's sarcomas occur in the diaphysis (mid-shaft) of the bone and only about one-third occur in the femur, tibia and fibula collectively. Ewing's is more often associated with fever, soft tissue masses and nerve root pain. It may be difficult to distinguish Ewing's from chronic osteomyelitis on the basis of history, clinical examination and radiological findings.

The benign condition which this may be confused with is Osgood–Schlatter's syndrome. This is apophysitis of the tibial tuberosity, occurring in children aged 10–14 years. It is usually bilateral. Pain is felt over the tibial tuberosity, just below the knee, and is worse with strenuous exercise. The tibial tuberosity is prominent and tender to palpation. Plain X-rays should be performed to exclude other pathology and demonstrate simple enlargement of the tibial tuberosity only. The condition is self-limiting and responds to rest and simple analgesics.

Significant diagnostic delay often occurs in such cases, as symptoms are attributed to 'growing pains'. The nature of the pain, being both unilateral and causing waking at night, is not consistent with this. It is also important not to be put off by a history of trauma; patients and families are frequently able to recall episodes of trauma in an attempt to explain symptoms that turn out to be presentations of malignancies.

Q2. What would you expect to see on plain X-ray?

Osteosarcomas have a classical appearance on X-ray of chaotic new bone formation, destruction of the cortex and cortical elevation. This is known as 'Codman's triad'.

In Ewing's sarcoma bone destruction gives rise to a 'moth-eaten' appearance. Cortical thickening also usually occurs. However, new bone formation is rare, unlike in osteosarcoma, and in addition, the soft tissue component of Ewing's may be visualized on plain X-ray.

Q3. What other investigations would you perform?

- *MRI of the primary lesion*: to allow accurate planning for biopsy as well as a baseline to assess response to chemotherapy prior to definitive surgery

- *CXR and CT chest*: to look for evidence of pulmonary metastases (10% in osteosarcoma, 25% in Ewing's)
- *Technetium-labelled bone scan*: if suggestive of metastatic lesions then these should be confirmed with MRI
- *Bone marrow aspirates and trephines*: in Ewing's up to 10% of patients have bone marrow involvement at diagnosis.

Problem-orientated topic:

headache (see also p. 13)

A 6-year-old girl, Lauren, presents to the accident and emergency department with a 3-week history of morning headaches and intermittent vomiting, having previously been well. Her parents have noted that she appears more clumsy than usual and that she has been falling over. As a result, her parents report that her attendance at school recently has been poor.

On examination she is apyrexial. Blood pressure is 90/55 mmHg. Ataxia and past-pointing are demonstrated. On fundoscopy bilateral papilloedema is seen to be present.

Q1. What is the most likely cause for this presentation?
Q2. What other conditions should be considered?
Q3. What investigations should be arranged?
Q4. What are the initial aims of management?
Q5. After establishing the diagnosis, what general management options can be pursued?

Q1. What is the most likely cause for this presentation?

Headaches and vomiting are the classical symptoms of raised ICP. This is associated with cerebellar symptoms such as ataxia, nystagmus and past-pointing. It should be noted that the absence of papilloedema does not exclude raised ICP. The most likely diagnosis is a posterior fossa tumour. The most common tumours at this site are medulloblastoma or low-grade astrocytoma, but ependymoma is also seen. A long history points more to an astrocytoma than a medulloblastoma. However, an astrocytoma may have been present asymptomatically for some time before acutely presenting with a short history of raised ICP when the tumour reaches a critical size. Thus a short history per se cannot reliably distinguish between the two.

Q2. What other conditions should be considered?

Ataxia can occur following varicella infection but this would rarely present with headaches and papilloedema. Benign intracranial hypertension presents with headache, raised ICP and papilloedema but cerebellar symptoms would be uncommon. A cerebral abscess would be unlikely in a previously well child.

Q3. What investigations should be arranged?

- *CT head with contrast*: if MRI is not readily available. This will identify the tumour and the presence of any hydrocephalus and will dictate the urgency of referral to a neurosurgical centre.
- *MRI head and spine*: MRI head more clearly delineates the tumour than a CT head and allows for planning of surgery. As a medulloblastoma is the most likely diagnosis, given the history, we also need to image the spine to look for evidence of spinal metastases.
- *Lumbar puncture*: to look for evidence of microscopic tumour cells in CSF. This is usually performed 2–3 weeks post-operatively to allow any cellular debris from surgery to resolve. Even presence of microscopic disease, which is not visible on neuroimaging, imparts a poorer prognosis and is therefore important staging information to ascertain.

Q4. What are the initial aims of management?

- *Control raised ICP*. Raised ICP is caused by direct infiltration of the tumour itself or the compression of other brain structures. A rapidly growing tumour often has significant surrounding oedema and this may contribute to raised ICP. Steroids such as dexamethasone are used to reduce oedema and provide an improvement in symptoms. However, raised ICP may also be secondary to obstruction of CSF by the tumour. Urgent neurosurgery may be required for a CSF diversion procedure, e.g. extraventricular drain (EVD) or third ventriculostomy if raised ICP persists despite administration of steroids.

- *Control pain, seizures or electrolyte disturbances*. Seizures and electrolyte disturbances are more common with tumours of the cerebral hemispheres and suprasellar regions respectively.
- *Establish a tissue diagnosis*. In most cases attempt at complete excision is appropriate and associated with better outcome. Neurosurgery should be performed promptly but allowing for appropriate preoperative investigation and stabilization.

Q5. After establishing the diagnosis, what general management options can be pursued?

The subsequent management depends on histology and may range from surveillance imaging alone in completely resected astrocytomas, to further surgery if there is interval growth or symptoms from the tumour, and use of radiotherapy and/or chemotherapy. Radiotherapy-based strategies are avoided in young children, wherever possible, particularly in those less than 3 years of age, because of the impact on the developing brain. Chemotherapy regimens have a place alongside radiotherapy, particularly in medulloblastoma, and may be used in young children to spare toxicity of radiotherapy, by allowing dose or field reductions, or by delaying or avoiding it altogether.

Presentation of malignancy

The list shown in Table 51.3 is not exhaustive. A child presenting several times with the same problem and without a firm diagnosis should be investigated appropriately.

Paediatric oncology emergencies

Tumour lysis syndrome

This syndrome (Box 51.3) is caused by the rapid lysis of malignant cells on initiating chemotherapy, with subsequent release of intracellular contents, exceeding renal excretory capacity and physiological buffering mechanisms, and leading to risk of acute renal failure. It is mainly seen in 'bulky' disease such as high-count ALL and NHL (especially B cell); it may occur spontaneously or be precipitated by a single dose of steroids.

Prevention and close monitoring are the keys to management:
- Hyperhydration before and during initiation of therapy (e.g. 2.5% dextrose 0.45% saline) with no added potassium.

Table 51.3 **Presentation of malignancy**

Presenting complaint	Suspicious features and comments
Pancytopenia	• Pallor/lethargy due to low haemoglobin • Recurrent fever/infection due to low white count • Bruising and/or petechiae due to low platelets Occurs due to displacement of marrow by leukaemia or disseminated malignancy. Note that not all cell lines may be equally affected
Lymphadenopathy/unexplained mass	• Diameter greater than 2 cm • Progressive enlargement • Non-tender, rubbery, hard or fixed character • Supraclavicular or axillary location • Associated with other features, e.g. pallor or lethargy • Hepatosplenomegaly
Respiratory symptoms	• New episode or change in pattern of wheeze Suggestive of intrathoracic mass
Bone and joint pain and swelling	• Persistent back pain — rarely innocent in children May reflect bone marrow infiltration with leukaemia, metastases or a spinal tumour
Abdominal mass	• Progressive enlargement • Association with general malaise, e.g. neuroblastoma N.B. May be painless and isolated finding, e.g. Wilms' tumour
Raised intracranial pressure	• Early morning headache • Vomiting • Ataxia • Papilloedema • III and VI cranial nerve palsies (false localizing signs)
Neurological signs	• Cranial nerve deficits • Cerebellar signs, including head tilt • Visual disturbances or abnormal eye movements • Abnormal gait • Motor or sensory signs • Behavioural disturbance • Deteriorating school performance or milestones • Increasing head circumference in infants
Endocrine or systemic disturbances	• Poor feeding or failure to thrive (diencephalic syndrome) • Diabetes insipidus • Growth hormone deficiency • Precocious puberty

BOX 51.3 Biochemical features of tumour lysis syndrome

- Hyperkalaemia
- Hyperuricaemia
- Hyperphosphataemia
- Hypocalcaemia
- Metabolic acidosis, if severe

- Ensure good renal output, with furosemide if necessary.
- Urate precipitation: reduced with allopurinol, or urate oxidase in high-risk cases.
- Hyperphosphataemia/hypocalcaemia: increase fluids, use haemofiltration in extreme cases.
- Hyperkalaemia: salbutamol, calcium resonium, dextrose/insulin, haemofiltration.

Hyperviscosity syndrome

This is associated with high-count leukaemias (presenting peripheral white blood count > $200 \times 10^9/l$), leading to sludging of venous blood in cerebral vessels. To treat/prevent, commence prompt leukaemia treatment: hydration, urate oxidase and chemotherapy. Transfuse slowly and only if essential for symptomatic anaemia, as this may exacerbate hyperviscosity. In severe cases, leucopheresis may relieve symptoms.

Superior vena cava (SVC) obstruction

This is caused by mediastinal masses (Table 51.2); airway obstruction may also occur. It may present with dyspnoea, chest discomfort, hoarseness or cough, and findings include plethora, facial swelling, engorgement of veins of the chest wall and venous dilatation of optic fundi. Sedation or anaesthesia for diagnostic purposes is hazardous and empirical treatment may therefore be based on imaging alone.

Acute abdomen

The most common cause in a child with an underlying malignancy is neutropenic enterocolitis or typhlitis, particularly associated with leukaemia, where bacterial invasion of bowel wall leads to inflammation, full-thickness infarction, perforation, sepsis and coagulopathy with high mortality. Symptoms may be masked by steroid use in ALL induction. Management includes prompt institution of antibiotics, resting of the bowel and close monitoring with surgical review. Most cases resolve with conservative management.

Raised intracranial pressure

Raised ICP is a neurosurgical emergency (p. 313). High-dose dexamethasone should be commenced immediately to reduce associated oedema.

Spinal cord compression

This presents with back pain, abnormal gait, sensory loss, and bladder and bowel disturbance. Causes include neuroblastoma, sarcoma, lymphoma and CNS tumours (also infection, osteomyelitis and abscess). Multidisciplinary input is vital; urgent MRI and surgical decompression and biopsy must precede steroids to avoid tumour lysis under anaesthetic. Perform other essential diagnostic procedures (e.g. lumbar puncture, bone marrow examination) under the same anaesthetic if possible. Treatment depends on cause but may include subsequent steroids, radiotherapy and supportive bladder and bowel management.

Supportive care

All paediatric oncology treatment centres should have clear local guidelines for supportive management, which should be referred to for details. This section should not be regarded as a substitute for such guidelines.

Infection

Fever should be treated as an emergency, as immuno-compromised children may succumb to overwhelming sepsis within hours. Greatest risks are associated with count nadirs, usually 10 days into a course of chemotherapy. Central venous catheter (CVC) infection should be considered regardless of count, particularly with symptoms such as rigors, associated with line flushing.

Febrile neutropenia

Febrile neutropenia is fever > 38°C and a neutrophil count < 1.0×10^9/l, resulting in increased risk of bacterial infection.

Causes of neutropenia
- Chemotherapy
- Spinal radiotherapy
- Bone marrow disease.

Organisms
- Skin or gut flora
- Greatest risk from Gram-negative organisms, including *Pseudomonas*
- Gram-positive organisms may be from a CVC.

Examination
Include inspection of the skin, mouth, intravenous line sites, surgical sites and perianal area.

Investigations
- FBC and differential, CRP
- Culture of blood, urine, stool
- Swabs of throat, nose, suspicious skin lesions or central line exit sites
- Plain CXR or abdominal X-ray if indicated by symptoms or signs.

Management
Broad-spectrum antibiotics should be commenced without delay as infection with Gram-negative bacilli may be fatal within hours. Choice of antibiotics will vary by institution and local resistance patterns but must include adequate cover for both Gram-negative (including *Pseudomonas*) and Gram-positive organisms, and for anaerobes in the presence of abdominal pain, diarrhoea or mucositis.

Viral infections in immunocompromised patients

If there has been varicella zoster (VZV) contact and the patient is non-immune, give prophylactic aciclovir or zoster immune globulin. Active chickenpox or shingles should be treated aggressively with intravenous aciclovir. Herpes simplex (HSV) may cause painful oral ulceration; treat early with aciclovir. Cytomegalovirus (CMV), adenovirus, respiratory syncytial virus (RSV) and adenovirus may all cause pneumonitis, associated with high morbidity and mortality, especially in BMT patients. Other antiviral therapy may be employed in these cases.

Fungal infections

Consider in prolonged febrile neutropenia and treat promptly. Clinical spectrum includes pulmonary aspergillosis, hepatic candidiasis and abscess formation. Risk is highest during intensive chemotherapy, such as reinduction for relapsed leukaemia and following BMT. Mortality remains high, although it is reduced by newer agents, e.g. liposomal amphotericin. Prophylaxis is used in high-risk treatment regimens.

Pneumocystis carinii (jirovecii) pneumonia (PCP)

Interstitial pneumonitis, associated with prolonged immunosuppression, presents with tachypnoea, dry cough and oxygen requirement. Co-trimoxazole prophylaxis is usual for patients on chemotherapy lasting over 6 months. Treatment involves high-dose co-trimoxazole and steroids in severe cases.

Haematological support

The usual threshold for blood transfusion is 8 g/dl but teenagers are often symptomatic at higher levels. Caution should be used if there is high-count leukaemia, long-standing anaemia or heart failure. Platelets should be maintained above $10 \times 10^9/l$ if the patient is well or $20 \times 10^9/l$ if febrile or for minor procedures (e.g. lumbar puncture), but higher for brain tumours, after significant bleeds or for major surgery. Thresholds may vary between institutions and should be overridden in the event of bruising or bleeding. Blood products should be leucodepleted to reduce viral transmission and incidence of reactions, which may be treated with antihistamine and/or steroid. Irradiated products are required in certain circumstances, such as following BMT and in patients with Hodgkin's disease.

Renal toxicity

Glomerular or tubular toxicity may result from chemotherapy, antibiotics and antifungals, particularly in combination. Close attention should be paid to electrolytes, including magnesium and phosphate levels. Hypercalcaemia rarely complicates disseminated paediatric malignancies.

Nausea and vomiting

Chemotherapy varies in its emetogenicity, from oral antimetabolites and vincristine requiring no prophylaxis, to cisplatin and ifosfamide requiring multiple agents. Aim to prevent rather than treat severe symptoms:

- First line: domperidone or metoclopramide
- Second line: add in ondansetron (5-hydroxytryptamine (5-HT) antagonist)
- Dexamethasone: a useful adjunct
- Cyclizine: may be particularly useful for children with CNS tumours
- Nabilone or chlorpromazine in severe cases.

Nutrition and mucositis

Good nutritional status is essential for recovery from chemotherapy, surgery and radiotherapy, but is compromised by the presence of malignancy, direct effects of treatment on appetite and taste, mucositis and infection. Mucositis may be caused by chemotherapy or radiotherapy and may cause significant pain and diarrhoea. Treatment includes analgesia, often with opiates, good oral hygiene and antiseptic mouthwashes to reduce infection. Nasogastric or gastrostomy feeding should be employed early; total parenteral nutrition (TPN) is used only when the enteral route is inadequate.

Table 51.4 summarizes management of common symptoms.

Palliative care

Palliative care is the active total care of patients whose disease is no longer curable and whose prognosis is limited. It needs to embrace physical, emotional, social and spiritual needs of children and their families.

Children with cancer constitute the largest paediatric group requiring palliative care and over one-quarter will die, mostly from progressive disease. Recognition of the appropriate time to stop active 'curative' treatment is always difficult and is compounded by differing views of family members and professionals. Palliative treatment may still involve chemotherapy, radiotherapy or surgery, as these may be effective for symptom control. Many families are willing to explore experimental treatments, as part of phase I or II studies, at a time when conventional treatment has no more to offer. Death from complications of treatment is more likely to be rapid, with limited opportunity for preparation.

In discussions with families, an honest and open approach is essential and careful consideration should be given to the needs and wishes of the child. It is important to emphasize that the focus of treatment is changing to quality of life and symptom control. Families should be discouraged from keeping the truth from older children through their desire to protect them, as this is likely to create problems of trust when the truth can no longer be hidden.

Table 51.4 Other common symptoms and examples of treatment

Symptoms	Treatment options
Nausea, vomiting	Domperidone, cyclizine (particularly for raised ICP), levomepromazine, haloperidol
Constipation	Laxatives when starting opioids Use less constipating opiates where possible
Bowel obstruction	Antispasmodics, stool softeners, octreotide reduces secretions and vomiting
Convulsions, cerebral irritation, terminal restlessness	Diazepam, midazolam
Spinal cord compression	Dexamethasone, radiotherapy, bladder and bowel management
Dyspnoea	Non-pharmacological measures (position, relaxation, play therapy, fan), opioids, benzodiazepines, oxygen, steroids
Excess secretions	Hyoscine, glycopyrronium
Anxioty, doproooion	Diazepam, levomepromazine or amitriptylline
Pruritus	Cimetidine if due to disease Antihistamine if opioid-induced
Haematological	Anaemia, haemorrhage, bruising; transfuse only for symptomatic improvement and quality of life Topical tranexamic acid or adrenaline (epinephrine) for troublesome mucosal bleeding

Organization of care

Few children will have their palliative care coordinated by a paediatrician specializing in palliative care. The role of the multidisciplinary team is vital and may include specialist nurses, social workers, psychologists and play therapists, with the medical lead taken by either a general or a specialist paediatrician supported by the GP. Most children die at home, through family preference, but some prefer to be in a hospice and a minority in a hospital ward setting.

 http://www.act.org.uk

Association for Children with Life-threatening or Terminal Conditions (ACT)

Symptom control

Symptoms will vary according to diagnosis and should be anticipated as far as possible, with the aim of correcting underlying causes, such as constipation and infection. Good communication and consideration of psychosocial and spiritual factors will contribute to good control, which may include pharmacological and non-pharmacological measures. See Table 51.4 for common symptoms.

Pain

- Stepwise progression is from paracetamol and non-steroidal drugs to opioids of increasing strength.
- Oral route is preferred; transdermal route employed for some agents.
- Subcutaneous infusion is used for the terminal phase, often in combination with antiemetics, sedatives or anticonvulsants.

- Combining different agents is more effective than escalating dose of single one.
- Adjuvants are additional drugs used in pain management. They include gabapentin for neuropathic pain, antispasmodics (hyoscine, glycopyrronium), muscle relaxants (diazepam) and steroids.

Specific malignancies

Leukaemia

Leukaemia is the most common malignancy of childhood. Approximately 80% of cases are acute lymphoblastic leukaemia and 20% acute myeloid leukaemia, other types being rare. The risk of developing leukaemia in Down's syndrome is increased 30-fold compared with the general population.

Acute lymphoblastic leukaemia (ALL)

ALL has an annual incidence of about 1 in 25 000 children, with a peak age of 2–5 years. It results from malignant proliferation of 'pre-B' or T-cell lymphoid precursors. Mature B-cell ALL is a separate entity that is treated with more intensive chemotherapy, similar to B-cell NHL. The cause of ALL is unknown, but genetic predisposition and patterns of childhood infection may account for some cases. Most present between 2 and 6 years of age.

Clinical features

Presentation is of short history (days/weeks) of symptoms reflecting pancytopenia, pain (bone marrow expansion) and lymphadenopathy (Table 51.3). Clinical examination should include testes in boys.

Investigations

These include bone marrow examination and CSF for Cytospin (CNS involvement is rare). A CXR will exclude a concomitant mediastinal mass.

Management

Treatment involves remission induction, consolidation/CNS-directed therapy and then prolonged maintenance with one or two intensive blocks during the first year.

Induction lasts for 4 weeks as an inpatient and the aim is to have a morphological remission (< 5% blasts) when the bone marrow is reassessed at day 28. The consolidation phase provides CNS prophylaxis and includes weekly doses of intrathecal methotrexate. Maintenance phase involves continuation treatment to a total of 2 or 3 years for girls or boys respectively. Oral chemotherapy includes daily 6-mercaptopurine (6-MP) and weekly methotrexate; doses are adjusted according to blood count, aiming for mild marrow suppression without prolonged neutropenia. Patients attend for monthly intravenous vincristine with a 5-day pulse of oral dexamethasone and 3-monthly intrathecal methotrexate. Intensive blocks of chemotherapy interrupt the first year of maintenance, with combinations of oral, intravenous and intrathecal chemotherapy.

Prognosis

Prognosis is improving steadily and overall survival is ~80% for standard-risk patients with current treatment. Adverse prognostic indicators are listed in Box 51.4.

Molecular techniques are currently being developed to evaluate minimal residual disease (MRD), which allows the detection of low levels of disease, undetectable by conventional morphology. This may lead to stratification of treatment according to risk.

Relapsed ALL may be confined to bone marrow or involve extramedullary sites (mainly CNS, testes). Treatment involves intensive reinduction and consolidation for all, with a further 2 years of maintenance for low-risk and BMT for higher-risk cases. Cure rates are variable but highest in isolated extramedullary relapse more than 2 years off treatment.

Acute myeloid leukaemia (AML)

AML results from the malignant proliferation of myeloid or non-lymphoid precursors. It is subclassified by morphology, according to the 'FAB' (French, American, British) classification, M1 to M7, each with different behaviour and cytogenetics. Favourable prognosis is associated with translocations t(15;17), t(8;21) and inv(16), and poor prognosis with monosomy 7 or complex abnormalities.

Clinical features

This is similar to ALL. Lymphadenopathy is less prominent and intrathoracic and extramedullary disease are also less common than in ALL.

Management

Treatment differs fundamentally from that of ALL. Four or five courses of intensive myelosuppressive chemotherapy are given, with no prolonged maintenance therapy. High-risk cases, including those slow to respond, are transplanted in the first remission.

Prognosis

Prognosis has improved dramatically due to intensive treatment and supportive care, with overall survival more than 60%. Relapses may be salvaged with BMT.

Lymphoma

Lymphomas are malignant proliferations of lymphoid precursor cells at various stages of differentiation. However, non-Hodgkin's lymphoma (NHL) and Hodgkin's disease are distinct disease entities and differ in terms of natural history, presentation and management. Both are more common in males than females.

Non-Hodgkin's lymphoma

Clinical features

Presentation varies according to site, including palpable lymphadenopathy, pain, obstruction or ascites from abdominal mass, respiratory symptoms or SVC obstruction from mediastinal mass, and pancytopenia (Table 51.3).

Investigations

Investigation includes bone marrow examination, lumbar puncture, imaging according to site, biopsy for histology with immunophenotyping and cytogenetics.

BOX 51.4 Adverse prognostic indicators in childhood leukaemia

- Male gender
- Age < 2 or > 10 years
- High white cell count (> 50×10^9/l) at diagnosis
- Unfavourable cytogenetics:
  - Philadelphia chromosome: t(9;22)
  - MLL gene rearrangements: e.g. t(4;11) in infants
  - AML1 amplification
- Poor response to induction treatment
- High levels of minimal residual disease at end of induction*

* See text.

The majority in childhood are high-grade tumours, divided according to histology, immunophenotype and cytogenetics:

- *Lymphoblastic* (90% T-cell, 10% pre-B): 30% of NHL cases. Most present with an anterior mediastinal mass. If there are > 25% blasts in bone marrow, then disease is regarded as ALL.
- *Mature B cell* (Burkitt's or atypical Burkitt's): 50% of cases occur in the abdomen, head and neck, bone marrow and CNS, and may grow very rapidly. Endemic or African Burkitt's is associated with early Epstein–Barr virus (EBV) infection and frequently affects the jaw, a site rarely involved in sporadic disease.
- *Anaplastic large cell lymphoma* (ALCL): < 20%.

Management

Lymphoblastic (T cell, pre B cell) lymphoma is treated similarly to its ALL counterparts, treatment lasting up to 2 years.

Mature B cell disease and ALCL are treated with short series of dose-intensive chemotherapy, including significant doses of alkylating agents. The risk of tumour lysis is high.

Prognosis

More than 70% of children with NHL survive overall and over 90% of cases with localized disease survive with limited treatment. Relapse tends to occur early. Although the cure rate for primary NHL is high, salvage options are limited and few relapsed patients survive.

Hodgkin's disease

Hodgkin's disease is characterized by the presence of neoplastic Reed–Sternberg cells in a reactive lymph node infiltrate. It is much slower-growing than NHL and rare under 5 years, incidence rising with age. Some cases show evidence of previous EBV infection. Hodgkin's disease is classified as classical or lymphocyte-predominant; the latter usually involves localized disease and has a better prognosis.

Clinical features

There is progressive painless lymph node enlargement, cervical in around 80%, mediastinal (often asymptomatic) in 60%. Dissemination to other organs occurs late. Fever, night sweats and weight loss constitute 'B' symptoms, which are more common in advanced stages.

Ann Arbor staging

Stage I   Single site
Stage II   > 1 site of disease, on one side of the diaphragm
Stage III   > 1 site of disease, on both sides of the diaphragm
Stage IV   Disseminated disease.

Investigations

These are as for NHL, without lumbar puncture but including EBV serology.

Management

Stage I disease may be cured with either involved field radiotherapy or a short course of chemotherapy. All other stages require chemotherapy, which usually includes significant doses of anthracyclines and/or alkylating agents. The additional use of radiotherapy is subject to national and institutional variation, but is usually employed in bulky mediastinal and disseminated disease, as well as in resistant or relapsed cases, when further intensive chemotherapy is also indicated.

Prognosis

Overall survival at 5 years exceeds 90%, ranging from 70% for stage IV to 97% for stage I.

Late effects remain a significant concern, as both radiotherapy and the chemotherapy regimens carry risks (p. 407). The role of functional imaging with PET scans shows promise in Hodgkin's disease and may help to identify good-risk disease requiring less toxic treatment.

CNS tumours

Brain tumours are the most common solid tumours, as they constitute 25% of childhood malignancies, but they represent a wide spectrum of histological subtypes with widely different features, management and outcome:

- Infratentorial tumours predominate (> 50%), usually associated with raised ICP, headaches, vomiting and cerebellar ataxia.
- Supratentorial tumours present with raised ICP and/or focal signs according to site, hypothalamic/pituitary dysfunction or visual impairment.
- Primary spinal tumours are very rare and are managed similarly to their intracranial counterparts; they may present with cord compression (p. 416).
- CNS metastases of extracranial tumours are rare in children.

Delay in diagnosis is common, as few cases present classically. For every childhood brain tumour there are around 5000 children with migraine.

Involvement of the multidisciplinary team is central to management and should involve neurosurgeons, paediatric oncologists, radiotherapists and endocrinologists.

Initial management

- Diagnostic imaging: CT provides essential information for emergency management of hydrocephalus. MRI provides better tumour definition combined with spinal imaging for staging.
- Raised ICP requires prompt management, particularly if onset is rapid: prompt referral and transfer to a paediatric neurosurgical unit, using dexamethasone to control oedema, and intensive care unit (ICU)/ventilation in severe cases.
- Initial surgery may involve CSF diversion only (third ventriculostomy or external ventricular drain to relieve hydrocephalus), or biopsy or complete resection, depending on location and likely diagnosis.
- Other investigations may include CSF cytology and tumour markers.
- Postoperative scan within 48 hours of surgery avoids confounding artefact from post-surgical change (haematoma/oedema).

Low-grade glioma (~45%)

Most have histological characteristics of pilocytic astrocytoma (grade I) and behave in an indolent fashion, with variable responses to treatment. Outcome depends on site, with cerebellar tumours usually cured by surgery alone. Unresectable cases that progress or are symptomatic, such as optic pathway or hypothalamic gliomas with diencephalic syndrome or threat to vision, are treated with chemotherapy. Radiotherapy may be employed in older children, except in NF-1-associated cases (~50%), in which the risks of second primary tumours and cerebrovascular complications are increased.

High-grade glioma (~10%)

These may be World Health Organization grade III or IV. They occur predominantly in older children and teenagers, and supratentorial sites predominate. They are usually incompletely resectable and cure is rarely achieved. Radiotherapy is the treatment of choice but responses are rarely sustained and chemotherapy is of limited benefit.

Brainstem glioma (< 5%)

Intrinsic pontine gliomas are usually diagnosed on characteristic MRI appearances alone. They are high-grade and inoperable, and their response to radiotherapy is variable and short-lived. Chemotherapy has failed to improve median survival of < 1 year. Tumours growing outwards from the brainstem (exophytic) may be low-grade and amenable to biopsy with less morbidity, and have a better outcome.

Primitive neuroectodermal tumours (PNETs) (~25%)

This is the most common group of malignant brain tumours of childhood, with peak incidence at 5 years. The majority occur in the cerebellum (where they are called medulloblastoma), and present with raised ICP and ataxia. Supratentorial PNETs, including pineoblastomas, have a worse prognosis. CSF-borne metastases occur in 10–15% of cases. Excision and craniospinal radiotherapy form the basis of treatment, but chemotherapy provides further benefit. About 70% of localized cases are cured but long-term morbidity from radiotherapy is significant, particularly in young patients.

Ependymoma (~10%)

Ependymomas usually arise in and around the ventricles, with presenting features according to site of origin but usually including obstructive hydrocephalus. Complete surgical excision confers the best outcome (> 70% survival, compared with < 50% for those in whom complete surgical excision is not possible) and involved field radiotherapy is then given. Chemotherapy may delay or occasionally remove the need for radiotherapy in younger patients.

Craniopharyngioma (5–10%)

Craniopharyngioma is a slow-growing midline benign epithelial tumour that arises in the suprasellar area from remnants of Rathke's pouch. Treatment involves complete resection in 80% and partial resection with focal radiotherapy in the remainder. Management of complications of the disease and its treatment — including damage to the hypothalamus, vision and behaviour — remains the greatest challenge, particularly as most become long-term survivors.

CNS germ cell tumours (5%)

These are described on the MasterCourse website.

Neuroblastoma

Neuroblastoma is a malignant embryonal tumour derived from the neural crest and represents 7% of childhood malignancies. It has a median age of onset of 2 years with the majority of cases arising in the adrenal glands, abdomen or thorax, usually related to the sympathetic chain. Small numbers occur in the pelvis, neck and elsewhere. Disease is often advanced at diagnosis with metastases to bone, bone marrow, liver, and occasionally CNS and lungs. There is a wide spectrum of behaviour according to age of patient and disease stage.

Clinical features
Presentation is often non-specific, depending on site, spread and metabolic effects:
- Lymphadenopathy or palpable masses
- Compression of structures, including nerves (e.g. Horner's, spinal cord), airway, veins, bowel
- Pancytopenia
- Bone pain, limp
- Sweating, pallor, watery diarrhoea and hypertension.

Investigations
Specific diagnostic tests include:
- Imaging of affected area for staging purposes (CT or MRI)
- Urine VMA/HVA creatinine ratios (urine catecholamines); raised in > 80% cases and may be used for monitoring of disease progress
- ^{131}I-mIBG uptake by primary tumour and metastases, in the majority; if negative for primary, ^{99}Tc bone scan is required
- Bilateral bone marrow aspirates/trephines (disease infiltration may be patchy)
- Biopsy of lesion
- Cytogenetic analysis of biopsy, bone marrow and blood.

Management
Treatment ranges from surgery only for resectable localized (stage 1) neuroblastoma to induction chemotherapy, surgery, high-dose chemotherapy with autologous stem cell rescue and radiotherapy in stage 4 (disseminated) and *MYCN*-positive stage 3 disease.

Infant neuroblastoma characteristically presents with disseminated disease restricted to bone marrow, liver and skin (stage 4S), which usually resolves spontaneously; chemotherapy is only required for life-threatening symptoms.

Prognosis
Disseminated neuroblastoma is only cured in 20–30%, despite intensive treatment. Survival in low-stage cases in infants is more than 90%. Adverse prognostic indicators are listed in Box 51.5.

Wilms' tumour

Wilms' tumour, or nephroblastoma, is an embryonal tumour of the kidney accounting for 6% of childhood malignancies. Around 75% of cases occur in patients less than 4 years.

Clinical features
Presentation is most commonly as a visible or palpable mass, often painless, in a well child. Haematuria and

---

> **BOX 51.5 Adverse prognostic indicators in neuroblastoma**
>
> - Age > 1 year
> - Stages 3 and 4
> - Raised tumour markers: ferritin, lactate dehydrogenase (LDH), neuron-specific enolase (NSE)
> - Unfavourable histology
> - Cytogenetic abnormalities: *MYCN* amplification, 17q gain, 1p loss

hypertension are found in one-third. Most tumours are localized at diagnosis but lung metastases may occur. Bilateral (stage 5) disease accounts for 10% of cases and is more likely to be associated with an inherited predisposition (p. 404).

Investigations
These include:
- Abdominal ultrasound
- CT scan of abdomen
- CXR or CT chest
- Urine catecholamines to exclude neuroblastoma (prior to anaesthetic)
- Full blood count and coagulation studies (a transient acquired von Willebrand-like syndrome is recognized in 1% of cases)
- Biopsy.

Management
Definitive surgery usually follows a short course of chemotherapy. Subsequent treatment depends on stage and histology, ranging from a short course of vincristine to 6 months of three- or four-drug anthracycline-based chemotherapy. Radiotherapy is required for incompletely resected disease and most cases with lung metastases. In bilateral disease (stage V), the aim is to maximize response to chemotherapy prior to performing nephron-sparing surgery to avoid the need for dialysis.

Prognosis
Overall survival ranges from ~70% for stage IV disease to > 95% in stage I. Follow-up should include regular CXR as well as abdominal ultrasound, as pulmonary relapse is more common than local recurrence.

Other renal tumours are rare in childhood. Mesoblastic nephroma occurs in infants and most cases can be cured with surgery alone. Clear cell sarcoma requires more intensive treatment than Wilms' tumour, and malignant rhabdoid tumour carries a very poor prognosis.

Osteosarcoma and Ewing's sarcoma

Bone tumours are rare in childhood, accounting for 4% of all paediatric malignancies.

Incidence increases with age, peaking in teenage years and early adulthood. The majority of cases are osteosarcoma or Ewing's sarcoma, histologically distinct and with differing patterns of disease and response to treatment but with many common features. All cases should be referred to a specialist bone tumour centre for surgical management.

Clinical features

This is with pain, swelling, pathological fracture, and rarely overlying erythema. Osteosarcoma occurs mostly in long bones and around the knee in 80%. In Ewing's the axial (central) skeleton is involved more often and the pelvis is the most common site. Delay in diagnosis is a common feature. Metastases are more common at diagnosis in Ewing's (25%) than osteosarcoma (10%), and in lungs more commonly than bone, with bone marrow metastases in Ewing's only.

Investigations

Diagnostic investigations include:
- Plain X-rays of bony lesion
- MRI of primary site to define extent of tumour and aid surgical planning
- Definitive diagnosis requires biopsy, which should be carried out at a specialist centre where definitive surgery will be performed
- CT chest
- Isotope bone scan
- Bone marrow aspirates and trephines (bilateral): Ewing's only.

Management

Surgery, with the aim of limb preservation, is preceded and followed by chemotherapy in all cases. Prostheses are designed to allow lengthening as the patient grows. Radiotherapy is an effective adjunct and alternative to surgery, particularly in axial Ewing's, but its role in osteosarcoma is restricted mainly to palliation.

Prognosis

Overall survival for both groups is around 60%, but adverse outlook is associated with large primaries, axial sites, poor response to preoperative chemotherapy and metastatic disease.

Rhabdomyosarcoma

Rhabdomyosarcoma (RMS) is the most common soft tissue sarcoma in childhood and represents 6% of childhood malignancies. Most cases occur before the age of 10 years and are sporadic.

Clinical features

This depends on site, mostly bladder, pelvis, nasopharynx, parameningeal or paratestis, and may include palpable mass, pain or bladder outflow obstruction. Metastases are uncommon.

Investigations

Diagnosis and staging involve:
- Imaging of primary: ultrasound, followed by staging CT or MRI
- Biopsy: for histology and molecular cytogenetic analysis. Alveolar RMS is associated with adverse prognosis and is characterized by the presence of t(2;13) or t(1;13), which produce fusion products of *PAX* and *FKHR* genes
- Bone marrow examination
- Bone scan
- Lumbar puncture for parameningeal disease.

Management

Treatment involves 6–9 courses of combination chemotherapy. Some cases achieve complete remission with chemotherapy alone. Surgery for accessible sites (paratesticular, peripheral) occurs after three or six courses of chemotherapy. Radiotherapy is also required in cases with residual disease and for alveolar histology.

Prognosis

This depends on risk factors and ranges from around 10% for bony metastatic disease to over 70% for completely excised paratesticular tumours with favourable histology. The outcome for metastatic relapse and local recurrence within a previous radiotherapy field is extremely poor.

Rare tumours

Many other forms of cancer occur in children but all are very rare. They include:

Germ cell tumours	3% of childhood cancers
Retinoblastoma	3% of childhood cancers
Liver tumours	1% of childhood cancers
Histiocytosis	1:200 000 children
Chronic myeloid leukaemia	Very rare in childhood
Juvenile myelomonocytic leukaemia	Very rare in childhood

 Some of these are described in more detail on the MasterCourse website.

Index

DVD Player access instructions

- Place the DVD in the DVD player and press play. Use the Up, Down, Left and Right arrows on your remote control to navigate the menus. Press **Enter** or **Play** to make a selection.

DVD-ROM access instructions

Windows

- Locate the DVD icon in **My Computer** or select **"Start"**, **"Programs"** and the name of the DVD software
- Click the DVD icon or the name of the DVD software and the **Main Menu** will appear.

Mac

- The DVD will auto-start unless **auto-start** has been disabled in **System Preferences**.

System requirements

This is a Region 0 enabled DVD so is compatible with any DVD player.
A NTSC-compatible television/monitor is required to display the content correctly.

Windows PC

PC Based Pentium 450 MHZ
Windows 2000 or higher
256 MB RAM or higher
32 MB or higher Graphics Card
4X DVD-ROM drive
Display Resolution of 800 × 600 or greater
Sound Card and Speakers
Software which supports DVD-Video playback

Mac

Power PC G4 300MHZ, I-Mac, I-Book
Macintosh OS 9.2 or higher
256 MB RAM or higher
32 MB or higher Graphics Card
4X DVD-ROM drive
Display Resolution of 800 × 600 or greater
Sound Card and Speakers
Software which supports DVD-Video playback

Technical support

Technical support for this product is available between 7.30 a.m. and 7.00 p.m. CST, Monday through Friday.
Before calling, be sure that your computer meets the minimum system requirements to run this software.
Inside the United States and Canada, call 1-800-692-9010.
Inside the United Kingdom, call 0-0800-6929-0100.
Rest of World, call +1-314-872-8370.
You may also fax your questions to +1-314-523-4932,
or contact Technical Support through e-mail: technical.support@elsevier.com.

Elsevier DVD-Video licence agreement